DISEASES OF THE LIVER AND BILIARY SYSTEM

Gabriel Duarte

ALLIED
HEALTH
PRESS

Diseases of the Liver and Biliary System

Author: **Gabriel Duarte**

Allied Health Press
4164 Lakeshore Road
Burlington ON L7L 1A4
Canada
www.alliedhealthpress.com
Email: orders@arclereducation.com

ISBN: 978-1-77956-803-8

ABOUT THE AUTHOR

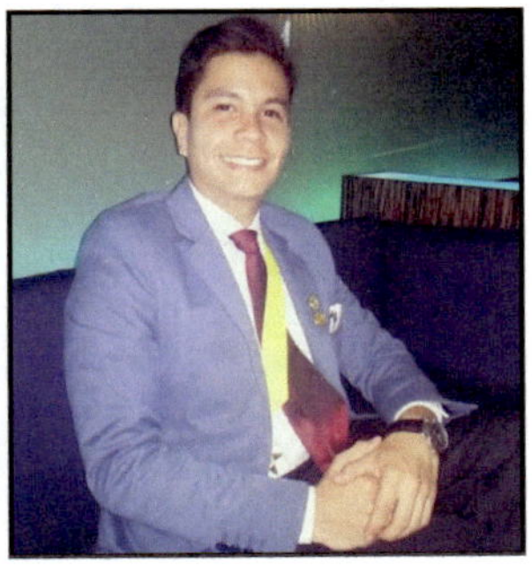

Gabriel is a doctor, passionate about radiology and diagnostic imaging with a solid clinical background. He completed his medical studies at the Universidad de Los Andes, Venezuela; and later he dedicated himself to the approach in anatomy, ultrasound, diagnosis and tomography studies. Besides, he has special training in teaching for undergraduate studies, human anatomy chairs and educational consulting. His passion for writing, editing and scientific research has led him to create experience as an author of many publications. Gabriel is a highly trained professional committed with teaching and high-quality professional medical practice.

Brief Table of Contents

Detailed Table of Contents

CHAPTER 5

Non-Alcoholic Fatty Liver Disease (NAFLD) 139

CHAPTER 6

Alcoholic Liver Disease 177

CHAPTER 7

Metabolic and Genetic Liver Disorders 211

CHAPTER 10

Biliary Tract Diseases 309

CHAPTER 11

Biliary Atresia and Pediatric Liver Diseases 345

CHAPTER 12

Primary Biliary Cholangitis (PBC) and Primary Sclerosing Cholangitis (PSC) 375

CHAPTER 15

LIST OF FIGURES

PREFACE

The liver and biliary system are a marvel of physiological engineering, harmonizing a variety of crucial functions to sustain human life. From its central location in nutrient metabolism to its involvement in detoxification and immunoprotection, the organ system ensures that material ingested is metabolized, toxic substances are detoxified, and essential biomolecules are synthesized. The gallbladder and bile ducts augment liver function by providing storage and regulated discharge of bile, a requirement for the digestion and absorption of lipids. Disturbances in these tightly controlled processes can lead to a range of disorders, each with its own clinical challenges and management concerns for the patient.

During the last three decades, advances in diagnostic imaging, molecular biology, and therapy have transformed our understanding of liver and biliary disease. Sophisticated techniques allow clinicians to detect subtle early warnings of disease, characterize genetic and metabolic determinants, and develop treatments with unprecedented precision. Concurrently, the global burden of liver disease—from viral hepatitis to metabolic disease—is increasing, reaffirming the need for widespread resources that span foundation science and current clinical practice.

Diseases of the Liver and Biliary System aims to bridge the gap between basic physiology and the evolving role of hepatology. It presents readers with a rationale, clinically organized overview of hepatic and biliary disease, integrating evidence-based advice with lessons derived from new research. With clear explanations and well-planned chapters, the book attempts to equip healthcare professionals with the knowledge required to diagnose, manage, and eventually improve outcomes in patients afflicted with these complex diseases.

Chapter 1 provides liver and biliary anatomy and physiology as a basis for understanding subsequent disease states. The chapter defines hepatic lobular organization, parenchymal cellular elements, bile formation and bile transport, and key aspects of nutrient metabolism and detoxification pathways. Vivid accounts of principles of basic hepatocyte function, sinusoidal blood flow, and enterohepatic circulation are given to prepare the reader for clinical correlation.

Chapter 2 covers hepatitis, acute and chronic, and covers viral etiologies—A, B, C, D, E, and non-viral etiologies including autoimmune and drug-induced injury. Diagnostic criteria are compared, serological markers are covered, and staging systems are compared, while therapeutic choices, including antiviral therapy and newer immunomodulatory therapy, are examined.

Chapter 3 discusses cirrhosis and complications. Mechanisms of fibrogenesis and portal hypertension are explored, then an introduction to complications such as ascites, variceal hemorrhage, hepatic encephalopathy (HE), and hepatorenal syndrome (HRS) is given. Treatment algorithms for decompensated and compensated cirrhosis are displayed, as well as updates from recent guidelines.

Chapter 4 discusses liver failure, distinguishing between the acute liver failure (ALF) syndromes and the insidious deterioration of chronic hepatic insufficiency. The prognostic scoring models, criteria for referral to transplantation, and supportive care strategies, including artificial liver support technologies, are discussed extensively.

Chapter 5 provides an overview of non-alcoholic fatty liver disease (NAFLD), charting its epidemiological rise along with obesity and metabolic syndrome. Pathophysiological correlations between insulin resistance (IR), adipokine dysregulation, and hepatic steatosis are discussed. Clinical staging, risk of progression to steatohepatitis and cirrhosis, and lifestyle and pharmacologic interventions are covered.

Chapter 6 covers alcoholic liver disease (ALD), such as consumption patterns, ethanol's metabolism, and the spectrum from steatosis to steatohepatitis and cirrhosis. Screening, counseling, and medical management strategies with a focus on nutrition and anti-inflammatory agents are discussed.

Chapter 7 discusses metabolic and genetic liver disorders, specifically Wilson's disease, hemochromatosis, alpha-1 antitrypsin deficiency, and glycogen storage diseases (GSDs). The genetic testing technologies, pathophysiology, and linked therapies, including chelation and gene therapy possibilities, are discussed.

Chapter 8 addresses benign and malignant liver tumors. Focal nodular hyperplasia (FNH), hemangiomas, and adenomas are distinguished from hepatocellular carcinoma (HCC) and metastatic lesions in the chapter. Features for diagnostic imaging, biopsy problems, staging systems, and treatment strategies—surgical, ablative, and systemic—are covered.

Chapter 9 covers vascular liver diseases, including Budd–Chiari syndrome, portal vein thrombosis (PVT), and sinusoidal obstruction syndrome (SOS). The etiologic background, Doppler ultrasound, cross-sectional imaging diagnosis, and radiologic intervention for recanalization and shunt creation are explained.

Chapter 10 discusses biliary tract diseases such as cholelithiasis, cholangitis, and cholestatic syndromes. Diagnostic methods, including endoscopic retrograde cholangiopancreatography (ERCP) and magnetic resonance cholangiopancreatography (MRCP), and therapeutic procedures such as endoscopic stone clearance and stenting are covered.

Chapter 11 discusses biliary atresia and pediatric liver disease. Neonatal screening protocols, surgical alternatives such as the Kasai procedure, and the care in the long term, including issues of transplantation, are highlighted as well as metabolic and infectious disorders unique to the pediatric population.

Chapter 12 addresses primary biliary cholangitis (PBC) and primary sclerosing cholangitis (PSC), contrasting their autoimmune etiopathogenesis, clinical syndromes, serologic assays, and cholangiograms. Modern and investigational treatment, including ursodeoxycholic acid (UDCA), obeticholic acid, and immunosuppressive drugs are discussed.

Chapter 13 covers parasitic and infectious liver disease, excluding viral hepatitis, such as parasites such as *Entamoeba histolytica*, *Schistosoma* species, and *Leishmania*. Life cycles, modes of transmission, diagnostic serologies, imaging characteristics, and anti-parasitic therapy are covered.

Chapter 14 covers drug-induced liver injury (DILI). The mechanisms of hepatotoxicity—metabolic idiosyncrasy, dose-dependent toxicity, and immune-mediated injury—are discussed. Diagnostic algorithms, causality assessment tools, and treatment approaches, including withdrawal regimens and rechallenge considerations, are covered.

Chapter 15 then looks to the future of progress in hepatology and the potential. New biomarkers for the early detection of disease, new antivirals and biologics, regenerative medicine, and the potential of personalized therapy through genomic and proteomic profiling are covered.

This volume is directed towards the diverse audience: medical students seeking an in-depth foundation, residents and fellows desiring refinement in their clinical practice, hepatologists and gastroenterologists requiring ready reference, and allied health care professionals complementing multidisciplinary liver care teams. Researchers and public health workers will be similarly served with the incorporation of current evidence and the delineation of gaps ripe for further investigation.

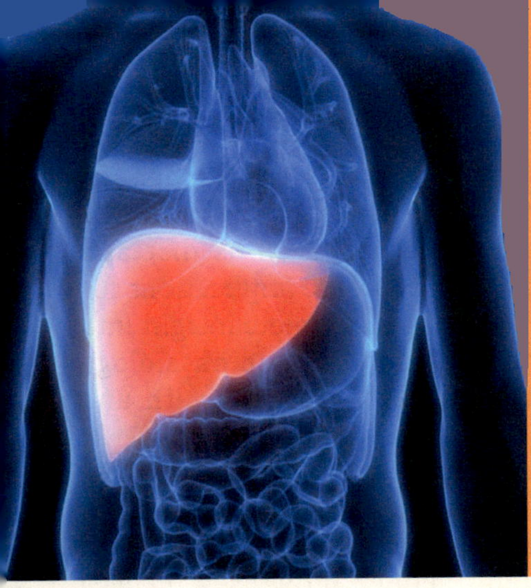

Chapter 1

INTRODUCTION TO LIVER AND BILIARY ANATOMY AND PHYSIOLOGY

Contents

Introduction

Not only is the liver the biggest internal organ, but it also has a critical role in many of the physiological functions essential to homeostasis maintenance within the human body. Detoxification, protein synthesis, and the production of biochemicals needed for digestion are just a few of its multifaceted functions. The liver also takes part in carbohydrate, fat, and protein metabolism, which testifies to its central position in energy balance and nutrient utilization. Understanding of the liver's complex composition and physiology is crucial in describing how it is coordinated with the biliary system. The interconnection between them is responsible for bile formation and secretion, helping in emulsification, absorption, and digestion of ingested lipids, validating the liver's importance to the digestive system and having an influence on overall well-being and health. The biliary system, such as the gallbladder and bile ducts, operates in concert with the liver to aid digestive processes. Bile, produced by hepatocytes of the liver, is stored in the gallbladder until food intake stimulates release. The regulation of relaxation of sphincters and gallbladder contraction ensures the timely transfer of bile into the duodenum, where dietary fats are digested. The biliary system's responses are highly sensitive to the body's physiological requirements, which may be controlled by a number of factors such as diet and endocrine regulation. Also, alterations in biliary performance can have considerable implications for liver function and digestive efficiency, emphasizing the importance of having a complete insight into both liver and biliary anatomy and physiology. Learning liver and biliary anatomy and physiology is not merely an academic endeavor, since it has broad application to both public health and clinical practice. Such pathological processes as hepatitis, cirrhosis, and biliary obstruction serve to emphasize the necessity of learning these systems in informing diagnosis and treatment regimens. Furthermore, technological progress, such as that of transjugular intrahepatic portosystemic shunt (TIPS) use, illustrates the necessity for an adequate understanding of the pertinent anatomy to optimize patient outcome (Lee *et al.*, 2023). Knowledge of sex and gender influences in liver disease and sensitivity to treatment can optimize therapeutic approaches further towards a less obtrusive method of patient care (F-Jarvis *et al.*, 2020). Finally, a complete understanding of liver and biliary physiology and anatomy provides the foundation for improving the quality of care and health outcomes for patients with liver disease.

Overview of the Liver's Role in the Body

The liver, which is the biggest organ inside the body, is vital for keeping the body's functions steady and supporting many important processes. In the upper right part of the abdomen, it is involved in breaking down macronutrients, removing harmful substances, and producing needed proteins. The liver takes up carbohydrates during digestion, changes them into glucose, and stores the glucose as glycogen, which can be used later to keep blood sugar levels steady. In addition, it breaks down fats and proteins to make the metabolites needed for energy and tissue repair. So, the liver's role in metabolism is very important for good health, since any issues can result in metabolic disorders and liver diseases. The liver is especially suited to filter and handle blood coming from the digestive tract before it goes to other parts of the body. The liver manages the levels of substances such as toxins, hormones, and nutrients because of the special way the hepatic artery and portal vein work together in hepatic circulation.

The organ breaks down harmful drugs and metabolites using enzymes and other biochemical processes, then sends them out of the body through bile or urine. Interestingly, recent research has shown that the liver's vascular system is intricately organized, providing insights into liver function and its pathologies, such as cirrhosis and hepatic encephalopathy (HE) (Casteleyn *et al.*, 2014). With this, the liver is shown to be important in metabolism and in defending the body against harmful substances. In addition, the liver helps make important proteins, including clotting factors and albumin, which support normal blood pressure and coagulation. Because it is the most common protein in blood plasma, albumin helps carry hormones, vitamins, and enzymes, which affect many body processes. The liver can regenerate, which helps it heal after injury and continue its functions. However, prolonged damage from CLD can hinder this regenerative ability, leading to fibrotic changes and loss of hepatic functionality (Viil *et al.*, 2016). Understanding the liver's multifaceted roles highlights its importance in both health and disease, informing therapeutic approaches to liver-related ailments and the role of transplantation for end-stage liver diseases (Figure 1.1).

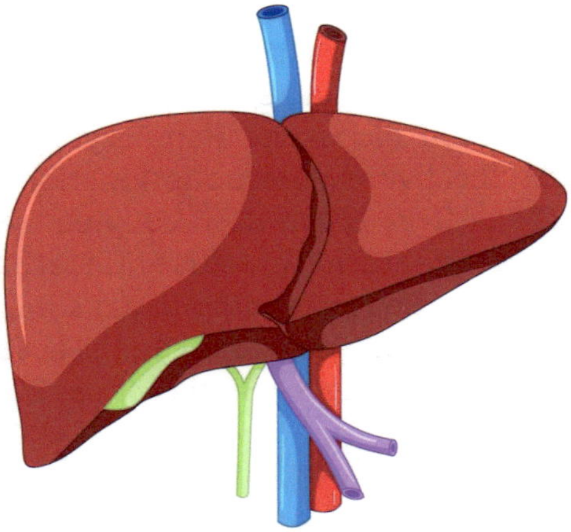

Figure 1.1. Liver.

Source: https://img.freepik.com/vector-gratis/anatomia-higado-cuerpo-humano_1308-81771.jpg?semt=ais_hybrid&w=740&q=80

Importance of the Biliary System in Digestion

The biliary apparatus plays an important role in the emulsification of fats and the control of bile within the body as a whole. Within the liver and extending through a chain of ducts, the apparatus is responsible for the generation, storage, and transport of bile to emulsify fats ingested in food. Fat emulsification enlarges the surface area of the fat, making it easier for lipases—fat-degrading enzymes—to function. Without a functional biliary system, digestion and absorption of lipids would be severely compromised, causing malnutrition and gastrointestinal disease. The coordinated high functioning of the biliary system shows how imperative it is in allowing efficient breakdown of complicated lipids, and this highlights its function in the digestion process and utilization of nutrients. Apart from facilitating the digestion of fats, the biliary system also plays a critical role in the excretory pathway of toxic and waste products. Bilirubin, a breakdown product of red blood cells, is excreted into the bile by the liver, and this is then transmitted by the bile ducts to the intestine. This not only plays the role of excreting potentially toxic chemicals but also determines the colour of feces, a commentary on its functional status. In addition, the biliary system maintains the physiological pH balance of the intestines via the alkaline character of the bile, neutralizing gastric acid when chyme enters the duodenum.

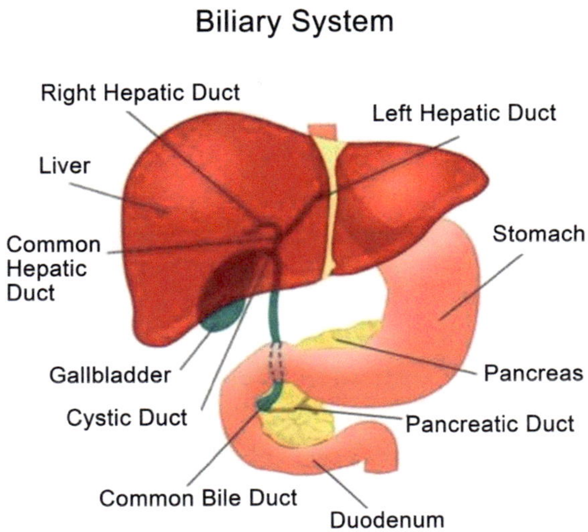

Figure 1.2. Biliary system.

Source: https://healthiack.com/wp-content/uploads/Pictures-of-Biliary-System-1193.jpg.

Through both the digestion and detoxification roles, the biliary system thus further illustrates its integral contribution towards the sustenance of homeostasis and support for essential physiological functions in the digestive tract. Recent studies have illustrated the intricate interactions between the biliary apparatus and other cellular constituents of the liver, highlighting its structural and functional importance. Hepatocytes and bile duct cells come into close interaction with each other, forming a dynamic microenvironment to sustain liver tissue regeneration and function. At the time of injury, such as in the case of biliary colic, the ductal cells can act as progenitors and regenerate the lost epithelium because they have been discovered to become activated and proliferate according to physiological demand (Espinoza *et al.*, 2019). Moreover, management of biliary ailments, including evaluation of therapies such as Apamarga paniya kshara for Udarashula, underscores the clinical importance of the study of the role of the biliary system in ensuring gut well-being (Krushnadev *et al.*, 2015). By and large, the biliary system is no less crucial to digestion, as it is a cornerstone component in liver health and regeneration (Figure 1.2).

1.1. Anatomy of the Liver

The liver, which is the largest organ inside the human body, is arranged in a very organized way. Lobules are the functional units in the liver, and hepatocytes found in each lobule mainly do metabolic work, detoxify substances, and create proteins. Around each lobule are portal triads made up of the hepatic artery, portal vein, and bile duct, which organize the movement of blood and bile. Because the liver gets highly oxygenated blood from the hepatic artery and nutrient-rich blood from the portal vein, it is able to handle many different functions and process items absorbed by the gastrointestinal tract. Additionally, the liver houses specialized cells, such as Kupffer cells and hepatic stellate cells (HSCs), that are integral to the organ's immune response and tissue maintenance, emphasizing the liver's role as a central hub of metabolic and immunologic activity. As well as its main role in metabolism and detoxification, the liver is important for maintaining homeostasis by using its unique vascular system to regulate blood flow. The liver can handle up to a quarter of the blood pumped by the heart, which gives it a large capacity to filter out toxins, so it is a main target for chemicals. The liver's sinusoids, which are lined with liver sinusoidal endothelial cells, allow blood to move directly from the portal and hepatic artery into the central vein. The way the liver is built helps nutrients, waste products, and pathogens move easily between blood and hepatocytes, which supports the liver's metabolic functions. The dynamics of liver blood flow, coupled with its extensive detoxification processes, underline the importance of understanding hepatic anatomy in the context of liver-related diseases and toxicological responses (Hinton *et al.*, 2017).

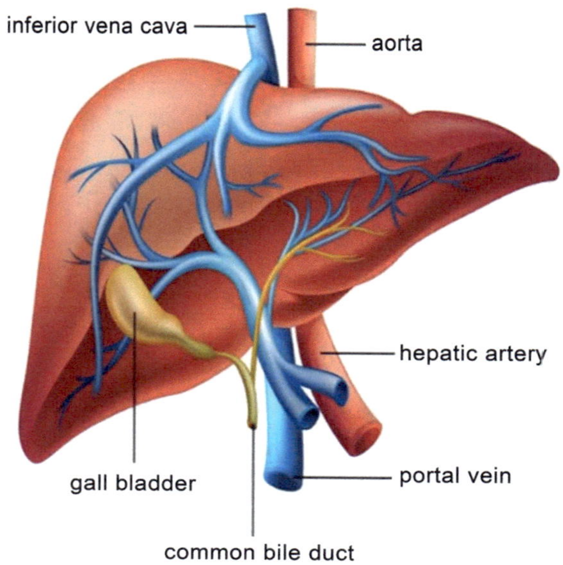

Figure 1.3. Human liver anatomy.

Source: https://swheal.com/wp-content/uploads/2024/03/Screenshot-2024-03-30-at-12.53.11%E2%80%AFPM.png.

The liver is very important for making and removing bile, which is needed for digesting and absorbing fats. Bile production occurs primarily in hepatocytes, where bile acids (BAs) are synthesized and then secreted into bile canaliculi, small ducts that collect bile from multiple hepatocytes. After the bile is produced, it goes through a number of bile ducts and is stored in the gallbladder until needed for digesting fats in the intestine. It is very important for digestion and also for getting rid of waste products from metabolism. Also, any problems with the biliary system such as those in cholangiocytes, can impact the liver and the body's overall balance. As oxidative stress plays a critical role in the pathogenesis of various liver diseases, including inflammation and fibrosis, insights into liver and biliary anatomy are essential for developing effective therapeutic strategies (Banerjee *et al.*, 2023) (Figure 1.3).

1.1.1. Location and Size of the Liver

The liver, the body's second most extensive organ, is located in the upper right corner of the abdominal cavity beneath the diaphragm and partly protected by the rib cage. This positioning not only gives the liver physical protection from outside trauma but also allows for efficient access to the hepatic circulation so critical to the organs' metabolic functions. The adult liver weighs approximately 1.5 kilograms and measures approximately 15 centimeters in length, with its highly vascular and complex morphology. It consists of a number of lobes separated by fissures, wherein the organ's shape is distinctive to facilitate its multi-tasking role in digestion, detoxification, and metabolism. Awareness of the location and size of the liver is the foundation for health care professionals because it informs diagnostic imaging, surgery, and assessment of hepatic pathologies that can be caused by anatomical defects or trauma. Location and size of the liver are inherent to its essential physiological functions, particularly in the circulatory system. Anatomically, the liver is supplied with blood by both the hepatic artery, which provides oxygen-carrying blood, and the portal vein, which provides blood from the gastrointestinal tract rich in nutrients. The fact that the liver has a dual blood supply points to its significant role in processing nutrients and expelling toxic substances. The precise nature of the hepatic vasculature's structure is of extreme importance as it allows for the circulation of blood within the organ to be conducted smoothly. New technological advances in techniques such as vascular corrosion casting and micro-CT scanning have vastly enhanced the understanding of the vascular anatomy of the liver. These techniques allow for accurate morphological analysis, which has generated an awareness of the complexity of the hepatic microcirculation and offered insight into how anatomical variation can affect liver function and illness (Casteleyn *et al.*, 2014).

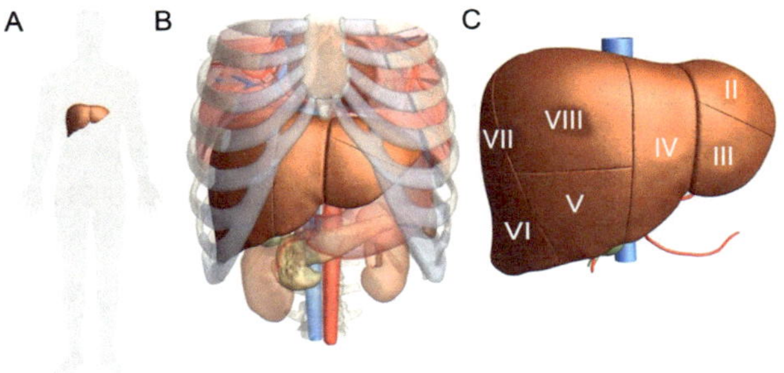

Figure 1.4. (A) Orientation image showing the approximate position of the liver in an adult. (B) The liver is positioned within the ribcage adjacent to organs such as the lungs, heart, and stomach. C The liver is divided into eight segments as shown by their roman numerals. Segment I is between segments VIII and IV. Segments II and III constitute the left liver lobe and the remaining segments constitute the right liver lobe.

Source: https://www.researchgate.net/profile/Mikael-Forsgren/publication/325441551/figure/fig1/AS:631879027920897@1527663108981/A-Orientation-image-showing-the-approximate-position-of-the-liver-in-an-adult-B-The.png.

Apart from its position and dimensions, the anatomical connection of the livers to adjacent structures also contributes to its functional dynamics. Situated alongside the gallbladder, pancreas, and segments of the small intestine, the liver is a central part of the biliary system, which helps in the digestion of bile. Recognition of these anatomical neighbours is crucial in understanding biliary tract disorders and surgical implications. Its position is also what exposes it to some illness, and hence the need for contextual anatomical knowledge in the clinical environment. For instance, cirrhosis or liver tumors can alter its size and its relations around it, which must be carefully assessed and treated. The incorporation of anatomical information into clinical practice illustrates the need to study human anatomy, not as a conceptual analysis, but as a usable application at the core of many medical disciplines (Mejino *et al.*, 2007) (Figure 1.4).

1.1.2. Lobular Structure and Blood Supply

Hepatocytes, the main working cells in the liver, are arranged in a very organized way in the liver lobules. The shape of a liver lobule is roughly hexagonal, and it has a central vein with plates of hepatocytes radiating from it. The structure of the liver allows it to deal with blood and substances in the most efficient way. Because of the structure, hepatocytes and blood are always interacting, which is necessary for functions like detoxification, protein production, and bile creation. Because of the way cells are arranged, bile is able to move through canaliculi to the bile ducts, which highlights the role of lobular architecture in the liver's many functions. The liver lobules are functional because of vascularization, which ensures the proper supply and drainage of blood for metabolic balance. The liver gets its blood from the hepatic artery, which brings oxygen-rich blood, and the portal vein, which delivers blood full of nutrients. Blood from the gastrointestinal tract and spleen is carried by the portal vein to the liver, which allows the liver to process the absorbed nutrients well. This is very important because hepatocytes depend on both oxygen and metabolites, which show the liver's dual role in metabolism. When blood flows through the hepatic sinusoids, it comes into close contact with the hepatocytes, helping to absorb nutrients and secrete different substances, which is why a good blood supply is important for the liver. Also, the way blood vessels are arranged around the liver lobules facilitates the efficient movement of blood and the exchange of nutrients. The peribiliary plexus, which is found around bile ducts, is important for controlling bile flow and drainage. In this way, bile secretion and blood flow in the liver are well synchronized, which is important for its metabolic activities. Also, the veins in the lobular structure either connect to the central vein or drain straight into the lobular vein, which demonstrates the liver's and blood system's close working relationship. Such intricate vascular dynamics are essential not only for liver physiology but also for understanding hepatic pathology when these systems become compromised, as often observed in liver diseases (Figure 1.5).

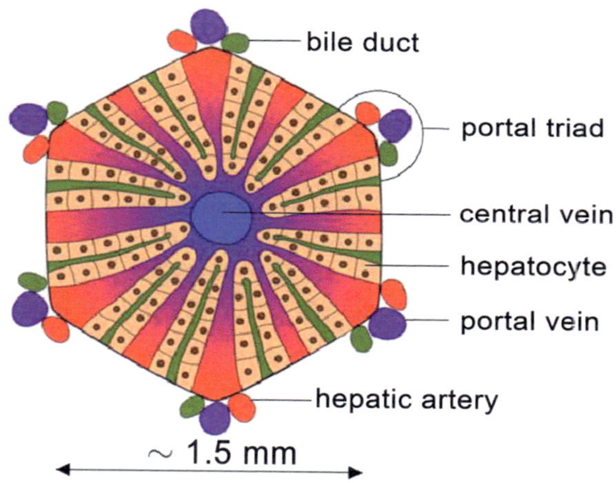

Figure 1.5. Structure of a liver lobule.

Source: https://www.researchgate.net/profile/Tim-Ricken/publication/265863835/figure/fig2/AS:392351789928449@1470555364190/Structure-of-one-liver-lobules.png.

1.1.3. Major Ligaments and Surrounding Structures

The liver, a vital organ in human anatomy, is supported by a series of crucial ligaments that play a key role in stabilizing the liver's position in the abdominal cavity. The falciform ligament, a typical one, originates from the anterior wall of the abdomen and separates the liver's right and left lobes. This ligament also forms the vital route for the round ligament of the liver, the remains of the obliterated umbilical vein. The coronary ligament is another vital structure that suspends the liver to the diaphragm and secures it in its anatomical position. Triangular ligaments also surround the liver and provide further fixation. The position of these ligaments is to provide integrity and function to the liver by allowing it to perform its life-sustaining functions, such as metabolism and detoxification, without unnecessary movement. In addition to the ligaments, the liver also comes into direct contact with other surrounding organs whose combined function and integrity contribute to that of the liver. The liver is closely associated with the gallbladder, a pear-shaped organ used for storing bile secreted by the liver. This anatomic relationship is important, because synchronized release of bile into the small intestine allows for fat digestion and absorption. Oxygenated blood is supplied to the liver by the hepatic artery, and nutrient-supplied blood from the gastrointestinal tract is supplied by the portal vein. These blood vessels are vital to liver function, and their proximity indicates the dependency of the liver on its related anatomic structures. Moreover, the inter-relationship of these structures underscores the complexity of the role of the liver in the digestive system, which is used to further highlight the need for integrative knowledge in the clinical environment. The clinical implication of such knowledge of the ligaments of the liver and adjacent structures cannot be stressed enough, particularly in surgery. Technological advancements in medical sciences, including applications of 3D printing, have enhanced pre-surgery planning for biliary and liver surgery. As highlighted, this technology is applied to generate patient-specific models of anatomy, enabling surgeons to rehearse complex procedures and improve outcomes of surgery (Meyer-Szary *et al.*, 2022). Further, data from these structures can be employed to inform approaches to liver diseases, such as cirrhosis and tumors. Understanding the key ligaments and supporting structures not only aids surgical technique but also targeted therapies that address specific pathological processes that affect liver physiology. With advancing science, the relevance of these anatomical specifics remains paramount in enhancing both surgical practice and therapeutic management.

1.2. Functions of the Liver

The liver is important for the body because it carries out many functions that help maintain balance. A major part of its function is to regulate metabolism by breaking down nutrients taken in by the digestive system. Hepatocytes, which are the main cells in the liver, take part in making glucose, storing glucose as glycogen, and processing carbohydrates, fats, and proteins. Additionally, the liver helps make albumin and clotting factors, which are important proteins. Because it controls blood sugar and reacts to hormones, the liver is essential for maintaining energy balance and storing nutrients, which affects metabolic health. This part of the liver helps the body by providing energy and supporting its proper functioning, which is why it is so important to the liver and the whole body. As well as metabolism, the liver is important for detoxifying and biotransforming substances to keep the body safe from harmful substances. It takes toxins, drugs, and metabolic waste out of the blood from the gastrointestinal tract. These harmful substances are made harmless by hepatic cells through enzymatic reactions, mainly with the help of the cytochrome P450 enzyme family. Detoxification is necessary to prevent the spread of toxins and to keep the body balanced. The liver is also important for immunity because Kupffer cells, which live in the hepatic sinusoids, help remove pathogens. The liver filters substances and also plays a key role in the immune system, which highlights its many roles in health. Bile, which is needed for digesting and absorbing fats, is produced and secreted by the liver. Hepatocytes make bile, which is kept in the gallbladder until digestion begins. It has bile salts, bilirubin, cholesterol, and other factors that help emulsify fats in the intestine, which makes it easier for them to be broken down and absorbed. This shows how the liver and digestive organs are connected, so that liver health influences both nutrition and digestion. Disturbances in bile production or secretion can lead to a range of clinical conditions, emphasizing the liver's essential role in maintaining digestive health and overall metabolic homeostasis within the body (Figure 1.6).

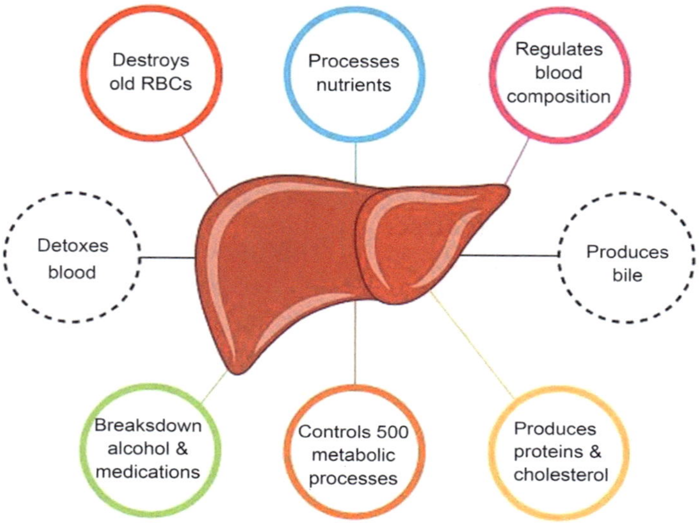

Figure 1.6. Essential liver functions.

Source: https://qph.cf2.quoracdn.net/main-qimg-8c2c9200a1c9564ef2cd5d054a960bec-lq.

1.2.1. Metabolism of Carbohydrates, Proteins, and Fats

The liver is a primary organ for carbohydrate, protein, and fat metabolism, regulating complex biochemical processes necessary for homeostasis. Metabolism of carbohydrates consists primarily of gluconeogenesis and glycolysis, which are critical pathways that maintain blood glucose levels. During times of sufficient glucose availability, the liver stores it as glycogen to satisfy immediate energy needs during fasting. Besides, any excess glucose can be converted into fatty acids through lipogenesis, indicating the interconnectedness of carbohydrate and lipid metabolism. Such adaptability in metabolism is significant as it allows the liver to adapt to variations in sources of diet and energy demands of the body, thus playing a critical role in overall metabolic well-being as well as in preventing such disorders as insulin resistance (IR). Proteins are metabolized in a complex manner in the liver, underpinning the organ's central role in amino acid homeostasis and nitrogen status. The liver bears the responsibility for the process of deamination, where amino groups are removed from amino acids, enabling them to be utilized as glucose or fats and thus be involved in energy production and storage. Additionally, the liver secretes plasma proteins like albumin and clotting factors employed in maintaining osmotic pressure preservation and enabling normal blood coagulation. All this variation in protein metabolism consequently mirrors the integration of the function of the liver into nutrient assimilation, detoxification, and synthesis, all contributing collectively to maintain significant physiological processes toward life. Protein metabolism and intake are regulated most importantly in catabolic conditions, when the muscle protein is utilized by the body as energy to regulate the liver. The liver metabolism of fat includes a series of mechanisms that yield energy and produce necessary biomolecules. The liver synthesizes, oxidizes, and stores fatty acids and is involved in cholesterol metabolism. During fasting or endurance exercise, the liver breaks down stored triglycerides into free fatty acids to be metabolized as a secondary fuel source. The complexities of lipid metabolism are further highlighted by the phenomenon of liver zonation, in which various parts of the liver specialize in different metabolic roles, making lipid synthesis and degradation more efficient. It is significant to comprehend these pathways of metabolism, especially with the rising prevalence of metabolic diseases such as non-alcoholic fatty liver disease (NAFLD) that compromises the regular function of the liver and makes one susceptible to systemic disease (Cunningham *et al.*, 2021). Comprehension of these interactions provides hints on the probable therapeutic approaches against liver diseases and general metabolic health (Vinarov *et al.*, 2021) (Figure 1.7).

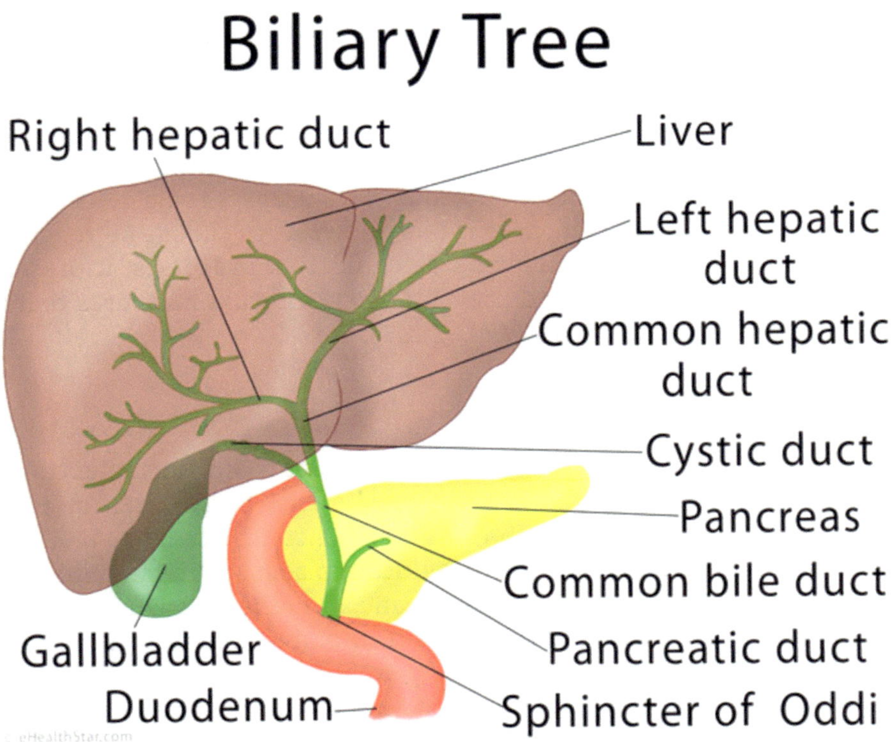

Figure 1.7. Major metabolic functions of the liver.

Source: https://www.researchgate.net/profile/John-Chiang-4/publication/271910276/figure/fig3/AS:667598400262156@1536179270549/Major-metabolic-functions-of-the-liver-During-the-fed-state-glucose-is-stored-in-the.png.

1.2.2. Detoxification and Drug Metabolism

The liver is responsible for clearing toxins and breaking down drugs in the body, which is key to keeping homeostasis. As a chemical factory, the liver takes care of many substances, changing toxic substances into safer forms. Drug metabolism happens through several enzymes, mainly those belonging to the cytochrome P450 family, which are necessary for getting rid of drugs. Enzymes in the liver make it possible for lipophilic drugs to become hydrophilic, which helps the kidneys remove them from the body. Furthermore, advancements in systems biology have elucidated the intricate relationship between liver function and systemic metabolic processes, underscoring the liver's contribution not only to detoxification but also to the pathogenesis of liver diseases, including metabolic dysfunction-associated steatotic liver disease (MASLD) (Liao *et al.*, 2025). The liver's ability to detoxify is also affected by circadian rhythms, which manage when drugs enter, move through, are processed, and removed from the body. Studies done recently point out that these rhythmic processes in the body play a big role in how the liver handles different drugs, highlighting how enzyme and transporter functions change throughout the day. For instance, transporters from the ATP-binding cassette (ABC) and solute carrier (SLC) families play pivotal roles in both the absorption of drugs and their subsequent detoxification within the liver. The rhythmic nature of these functions suggests that timing can impact drug efficacy and toxicity, prompting the exploration of chronotherapy—tailoring medication administration to align with the body's circadian rhythms to optimize therapeutic outcomes (Okyar *et al.*, 2024). Also, the process of drug metabolism is not only chemical; it is also affected by sex differences and what a person eats. It appears that the way males and females metabolize drugs can be affected by the different enzymes and their activities, which are regulated by circadian control. Also, fructose and other dietary components can have a significant effect on how the liver works, which may explain some metabolic disorders. Understanding the various ways drugs interact with each other helps us understand how individuals react to medications and allows us to choose better treatment options. As our knowledge deepens regarding the liver's detoxification processes, it presents avenues for innovation in therapeutic interventions and preventative healthcare measures that account for the dynamic nature of drug metabolism (Liao *et al.*, 2025).

1.2.3. Synthesis of Essential Proteins and Hormones

Liver plays a pivotal function in the biosynthesis of vital proteins and hormones involved in various physiological processes vital to maintaining homeostasis. One organ vital for the synthesis of a variety of proteins like albumin, clotting factors, and enzymes that catalyze metabolic reactions is the liver. The biosynthesis of albumin, the most significant plasma protein, is vital in that it helps to maintain osmotic pressure and transport other substances via the bloodstream. Moreover, the liver also synthesizes clotting factors such as fibrinogen, prothrombin, and factors V, VII, IX, and X, which are major contributors to coagulation and preventing excessive bleeding. Hence, the liver's ability to synthesize these proteins complements its pivotal role in cardiovascular function and overall body function. Apart from protein synthesis, the liver has an important function of generating hormones that regulate essential metabolic pathways. Above all, the liver secretes insulin-like growth factor-1 (IGF-1), a critical growth and metabolism factor that affects cellular function throughout the body. The liver also secreted hormones such as angiotensinogen and hepcidin, which control blood pressure and iron homeostasis, respectively. Synthesis of these hormones is closely linked to the metabolic function of the liver, with secretion of these hormones being controlled by changes in nutrient status, hormone levels, and general health. Understanding the synthesis and action of these hormones provides a basis for understanding the liver's broader physiological roles and its impact on overall health and disease. The relationship between liver function and cholesterol metabolism acts to emphasize the organ's role within hormone synthesis that governs many biological processes. Not only does the liver produce cholesterol, a precursor molecule for steroid hormones, but it also regulates their quantity in response to nutritional intake and hormonal signals. Cholesin, for instance, is a recently discovered hormone tightly linked with dietary absorption of cholesterol, illustrating the regulatory role of the liver on lipid metabolism and homeostasis. As observed in its interaction with receptors like G protein-coupled receptor 146 (GPR146), the synthesis and regulation of cholesin underscore the liver's central role in cholesterol synthesis regulation and its effect on metabolic well-being (Gilliam-Vigh *et al.*, 2025; Huang *et al.*, 2024). Therefore, liver synthesis of proteins, including hormone proteins, is a complex and vital function of human physiology, especially highlighting its relative importance in maintaining health and preventing disease (Figure 1.8).

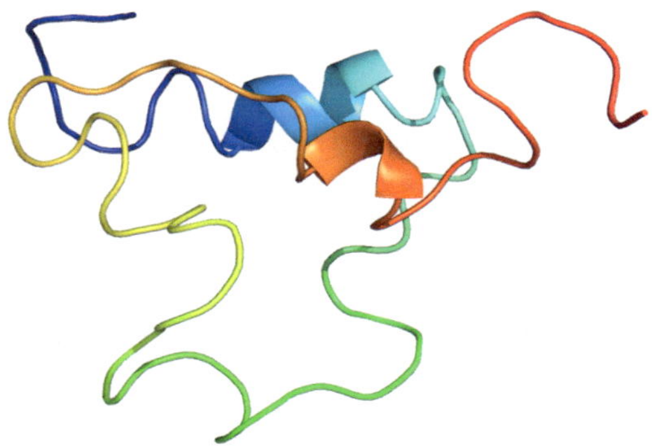

Figure 1.8. Structure of the IGF1 protein.

Source: https://upload.wikimedia.org/wikipedia/commons/e/e3/Protein_IGF1_PDB_1bqt.png.

1.3. Anatomy of the Biliary System

A network of structures in the biliary system produces, moves, and stores bile, which is a key digestive fluid made by the liver. The liver, gallbladder, and some ducts are included in the anatomy of this system, which helps bile move through the body. The liver is separated into areas by its biliary ducts, which unite to make the right and left hepatic ducts. All these ducts come together to make the common hepatic duct, which carries bile to the cystic duct, going to the gallbladder. The gallbladder holds bile and sends it to the duodenum through the common bile duct when digesting fat is needed. Knowing the anatomy of this system is very important for diagnosing and treating biliary problems, so it is a primary focus in the study of liver and biliary anatomy and physiology. The role of the biliary system goes beyond bile storage; it is crucial for balancing the hepatic portal system. Bile, which contains bile salts, cholesterol, and bilirubin, helps the small intestine absorb lipids. The enterohepatic circulation also helps bile salts be reused, which makes them even more effective for digestion. If there is biliary obstruction or cholestasis, the digestive process can be greatly affected, which can lead to digestive issues and problems with liver function. Research emphasizing human biliary tree stem/progenitor cells (hBTSCs) reflects a growing interest in alternative therapies for hepatic diseases, highlighting the clinical relevance of understanding biliary anatomy. The successful manipulation of these cells could revolutionize treatments for liver pathologies, indicating the need for ongoing exploration in this specialized field (Aliberti *et al.*, 2017). Moreover, examining the biliary system's anatomy in clinical studies points out the importance of using exact surgical methods while performing a cholecystectomy. After reviewing the cases, it was found that age, previous surgeries, and demographic factors had little effect on the conversion rate, but acute cholecystitis and stones in the common bile duct were very important. Because of these findings, it is crucial to use good pre-operative imaging to check the biliary anatomy, as problems from variations can result in more difficulties and a higher chance of surgery being converted. Understanding the intricate details of biliary pathways not only informs surgical practice but also guides clinical decision-making in gastroenterology, thus reinforcing the significance of the biliary system within the broader context of liver anatomy and physiology (Osman *et al.*, 2011).

1.3.1. Components of the Biliary Tree

The biliary tree, which plays a crucial role in bile transportation and liver function, is comprised of varying components that work together for digestion. The process begins with bile formation, primarily done via hepatocytes within the liver. The bile then flows out of the hepatocytes into small canaliculi, then pools into bigger bile ductules known as interlobular bile ducts. These ducts merge to form the larger intrahepatic bile ducts. The intrahepatic bile ducts have a lining of cholangiocytes, specialized epithelial cells that play the most critical roles in the modification of bile composition and in controlling bile flow. As the bile ducts go outward, they unite to form the common bile duct, which is the conduit for bile to flow into the duodenum and assist in fat digestion. From the liver, the common bile duct unites with the pancreatic duct to form the ampulla of Vater before discharging into the duodenum. Regulation of bile flow into the duodenum is crucial since it is controlled by the hormone cholecystokinin (CCK), which acts to cause gallbladder contraction to secrete preformed bile. The gallbladder, a pear-shaped, elongated organ situated below the liver, is a temporary reservoir for bile. It is dehydrated by extracting water and electrolytes, making bile more efficient for the emulsification of lipids during digestion. It also has a protective function in that it stores bile in a less toxic state until the digestive system is ready for its release. Therefore, the cooperative function of the components of the biliary tree maximizes the digestion and absorption of dietary fats without causing bile acid toxicity. The anatomy of the biliary trees is very integrated with the overall function of the liver, affecting many metabolic processes and defining hepatic well-being. For instance, changes within the biliary tree, such as strictures or cholestasis, may lead to serious hepatic complications, such as inflammation of the liver and fibrosis. Moreover, conditions like cholangiopathy, or structural diseases of the biliary tree, may be caused by portal hypertension or bile duct obstruction. It is the recognition of these potential stressors that becomes critical, and indeed, can progress underlying liver diseases and lead to progressive conditions of the liver like cirrhosis and hepatocellular carcinoma (HCC). The connection between the structure of the biliary trees, bile production, and liver function highlights the importance of this system in maintaining the overall hepatic well-being and the fact that pathologies in it can have a considerable impact on liver physiology (Banerjee *et al.*, 2023; Premkumar *et al.*, 2021) (Figure 1.9).

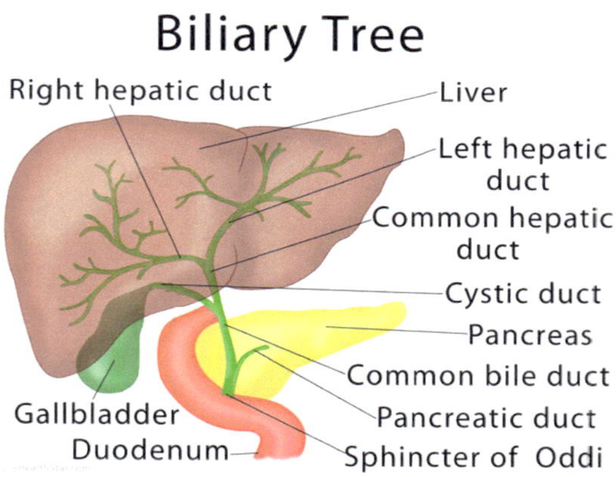

Figure 1.9. Biliary tree.

Source: https://www.ehealthstar.com/wp-content/uploads/2016/03/Biliary-tree.jpg.

1.3.2. Gallbladder Structure and Function

The gallbladder is very important in the digestive system because it stores and concentrates bile, a fluid from the liver. The gallbladder, which is below the liver, is a small pear-shaped organ that stores about 30 to 50 milliliters of bile. The emulsification and digestion of fats in the small intestine are greatly helped by bile. Eating fatty foods causes CCK to be released, which makes the gallbladder contract and allows stored bile to move into the biliary tract. It highlights the gallbladder's key role in digestion and nutrient absorption, which fits within the larger picture of liver and biliary physiology. The structure of the gallbladders tells us about their multiple functions. There are several layers in the organ, among them the mucosal layer, the muscular layer, and the serosa. Specialized cells in the mucosal layer take water and electrolytes from bile, which makes the bile salts and pigments more concentrated. Concentrating the bile helps it work better during the digestion process. Also, the muscular layer helps the gallbladder to contract well during digestion, which is very important for controlling bile release. Any changes in the gallbladder, including swelling or the formation of stones, can disrupt the process and may result in cholecystitis or other gallbladder problems, highlighting the organ's delicacy. Although treatments have improved, gallbladder removal or cholecystectomy is still a common surgery for gallstone disease. While laparoscopic cholecystectomy has become the gold standard due to its minimally invasive nature and rapid recovery, some patients continue to experience post-operative symptoms suggestive of residual gallstone disease, with studies indicating that 6% to 39% of patients are affected (Daud *et al.*, 2001). They reveal that gallbladder function is not simple, and its surgical removal may influence digestive health. The increasing interest in nonsurgical options reflects a need for further research into alternative treatments, evaluating the balance of efficacy and safety in managing gallstone disease while addressing the fundamental need for proper gallbladder function in maintaining digestive harmony (Weinberg *et al.*, 2011) (Figure 1.10).

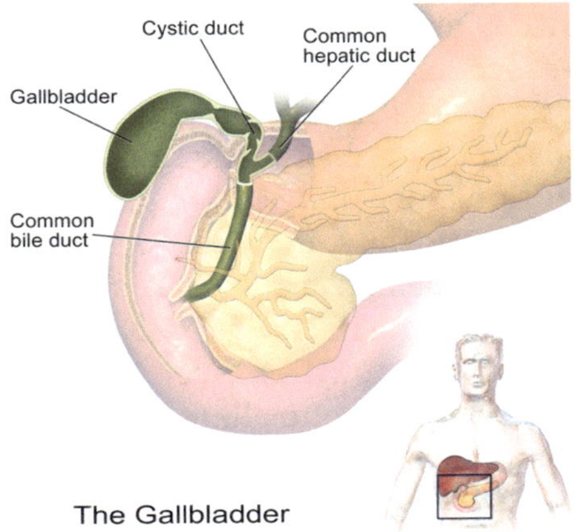

Figure 1.10. Gallbladder.

Source: https://upload.wikimedia.org/wikipedia/commons/thumb/e/ed/Gallbladder_%28organ%29.png/800px-Gallbladder_%28organ%29.png.

1.3.3. Relationship Between Liver and Biliary System

The liver and biliary system share a close relationship, with both playing key functions in digestion and metabolism. The liver is the largest organ of the body and synthesizes bile, an essential product in emulsifying and absorbing fats in food. Bile is continuously secreted by hepatocytes and is stored in the gallbladder to be released into the small intestine, where it facilitates lipid digestion. This interactive process focuses attention on the liver's function, not just in metabolic activity but in mechanical digestion of nutrients as well. Additionally, bile carriage from the liver to the intestine needs a complex ductal system within the biliary system, reflecting how closely these systems cooperate in maintaining physiological homeostasis. Further yet, the anatomical relationship of the liver with the biliary system is essential in understanding many clinical conditions. For instance, anatomical differences can significantly influence the treatment of liver transplant patients. In such cases, knowledge of the routine procedures for the anastomosis of the vascular and biliary structures is essential for the procedure's success. Awareness of these associations facilitates the radiologists and surgeons in their diagnostic and therapeutic interventions. By mapping blood and bile inflow and outflow in these environments, clinicians can maximize outcomes and minimize complications from biliary disease, emphasizing the critical harmony of liver function and biliary anatomy in controlling chronic disease and postoperative management (Al-Ogaili *et al.*, 2024). The connection between the biliary system and the liver also equates to disease pathology and interactions with the microbiome. Recent studies have indicated a rising incidence of biliary system disorders, which may indicate a complex interaction between microbial health and liver function. The biliary system is a conduit between the liver and the intestine with an important role in the body's metabolic processes. Disruption in the system has secondary implications for liver health, with conditions like gallstones and biliary tract cancer (BTC) exhibiting heterogeneity in microbial communities. This interaction is important because knowledge of it not only aids in the diagnosis and treatment of biliary disease but also in refocusing attention on the integrative physiological function that is essential to much health status (Wang *et al.*, 2024).

1.4. Physiology of Bile Production

The way bile is produced by the liver is essential for digestion and metabolism. Bile, which is greenish-yellow and produced by hepatocytes, has bile salts, bilirubin, cholesterol, and other components important for breaking down fats in food. Hepatocytes produce primary BAs by using cholesterol, which are then joined with glycine or taurine to become bile salts. Because of these bile salts, lipids in the small intestine are broken down into micelles, which makes them easier for the body to use and absorb. Bile is produced all the time by the liver, which secretes between 500 and 700 milliliters of bile daily. Because it constantly moves, it is necessary for breaking down fats in food and for removing waste, which is important for maintaining a healthy metabolism. When production is complete, bile travels into the bile canaliculi, which are small spaces between neighbouring hepatocytes. After leaving the canaliculi, bile goes through larger and larger bile ducts, ending up in the common bile duct, which can send the bile to the duodenum or store it in the gallbladder. The gallbladder helps by focusing bile, which makes the digestion of fatty foods more effective. The hormone CCK, which is released when fats enter the duodenum, mainly controls the release of bile into the intestine. So, the liver, gallbladder, and intestinal mucosa work together to highlight how bile production and secretion are complex and very important for digestion and nutrient absorption. Bile production depends on the health of the liver, because stressors can influence the function of liver cells and their ability to produce bile. Oxidative stress (OS) induced by factors such as viral infections, alcohol, and high-fat diets can lead to impaired bile acid transport, which contributes to hepatocellular toxicity and inflammation. Impaired secretion of BAs in the liver can cause the BAs to build up, which can lead to hepatocyte death and make liver diseases worse, resulting in cholestasis and non-alcoholic fatty liver disease. So, studying the body's processes for making bile and secreting it is necessary for treating liver diseases and designing effective treatments. This represents a significant area of research, especially in the context of the increasing prevalence of liver-related disorders in contemporary society, highlighting the interconnectedness of bile physiology with broader metabolic and immune responses in the body (Banerjee *et al.*, 2023; Rychik *et al.*, 2019).

1.4.1. Composition and Role of Bile

Bile is a complex fluid excreted by the liver and plays a crucial role in digestion, particularly emulsification and absorption of lipid nutrients. Its main components are bile salts, cholesterol, bilirubin, electrolytes, and water. The chief BAs, which are cholesterol-derived, are conjugated with glycine or taurine and form bile salts, which are accountable for lipid digestion by breaking down globules of fat into minute-sized micelles. Also, the bilirubin, a byproduct of hemoglobin breakdown, is responsible for giving bile its yellow pigment and plays a part in the removal of toxic waste products. The sensitive balance of these components is paramount as a shift would lead to gallstones or cholestasis, underlining the role of bile in gastrointestinal well-being and the overall homeostasis of the body. The liver hepatocytes produce and secrete bile, thus exemplifying the interrelationship between the health of the liver and bile. Not only do the hepatocytes produce bile, but they also transport the bile to allow passage into the gallbladder for concentration and storage. The hepatocytes also possess a sophisticated membrane trafficking system, enabling them to secrete proteins and also bile independently through distinct cellular domains. This dual function is instrumental to the maintenance of regular metabolic processes, whereby bile aids digestion and lipid absorption and helps in the detoxification of toxic material and metabolic waste. In addition to being part of the body's detoxification processes, bile functions as a multi-purpose substance that is vital in ensuring the function of the liver as a whole and, consequently, the function of the entire gastrointestinal tract (Schulze *et al.*, 2019). Bile metabolism also has important pharmacokinetic consequences, particularly with regard to drug absorption and efficacy. Variation in bile composition may significantly change the solubility and absorptive function of orally administered drugs and is therefore an essential consideration in therapeutic design. Gastric emptying time and pH of the gastrointestinal tract also regulate drug absorption, with cholestatic illness potentially exaggerating these effects. This difference highlights the important interaction between bile content and drug bioavailability within the body. Current research shows that understanding these dynamics not only improves oral drug design but also contributes to the relief of variability of therapeutic effects (Vinarov *et al.*, 2021). Thus, an appreciation of the form and function of bile is important for both gastrointestinal health and the effective delivery of drugs and hence it takes on importance within the general scheme of liver and biliary anatomy and physiology (Figure 1.11).

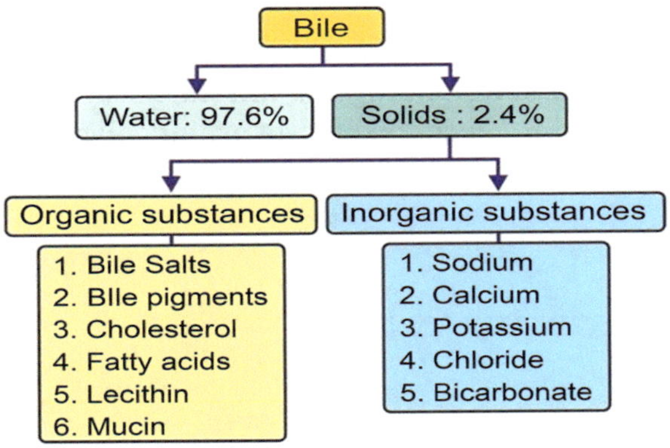

Figure 1.11. Composition of bile.

Source: https://d45jl3w9libvn.cloudfront.net/jaypee/static/books/9789385999468/Chapters/images/195-1.jpg.

1.4.2. Mechanisms of Bile Secretion

Many cellular processes work together to help bile be produced and move from the liver through the gallbladder and into the intestines. One of the primary components of this process is the action of specific membrane proteins known as aquaporins (AQPs). They are needed for the movement of water and solutes across the membranes in the hepatobiliary system. In the liver, AQP8 and AQP9 help move water, which is necessary for keeping the right level of bile. AQPs such as AQP1 and AQP4 also help to reabsorb and secrete water in the biliary tract, which affects the composition and concentration of bile. The dysfunction or dysregulation of AQPs has been linked to various hepatobiliary disorders, underscoring their importance in the physiological and pathophysiological contexts of bile secretion (Khalil *et al.*, 2024). Apart from AQPs, BAs are also very important in setting up the mechanisms for bile secretion. The liver makes bile acids by using complex biochemical reactions, mainly using cholesterol. Amino acids are then joined to these BAs, which makes them easier to dissolve and facilitate their release into the bile. Ursodeoxycholic acid (UDCA) exemplifies a bile acid with therapeutic properties, particularly in the context of cholestatic liver diseases. It appears that UDCA acts in several ways to help: it protects cholangiocytes from harmful hydrophobic BAs and also promotes their excretion from the liver. UDCA also seems to stop apoptosis in liver cells that results from bile acid retention, which is a common problem in cholestasis. The modulation of bile acid synthesis and secretion is thus crucial for maintaining hepatic health, making understanding these mechanisms essential for effective treatment strategies in liver diseases (Cifuentes-Silva *et al.*, 2023). Another important way bile is secreted depends on the action of transport proteins that move bile acids across the cell membrane. These transporters, which include the bile salt export pump (BSEP) and the sodium-taurocholate cotransporting polypeptide (NTCP), are responsible for the uptake of BAs into hepatocytes and their subsequent secretion into the bile canaliculus. Any problems with these transport proteins can prevent bile acids from being secreted properly, which may result in cholestasis and NAFLD. Also, hormones and different foods affect the way these proteins function, so bile secretion is not just automatic, but is well-controlled by the liver. As such, understanding the intricate workings of bile acid transporters is essential for elucidating the broader mechanisms governing bile secretion and their implications in health and disease (Figure 1.12).

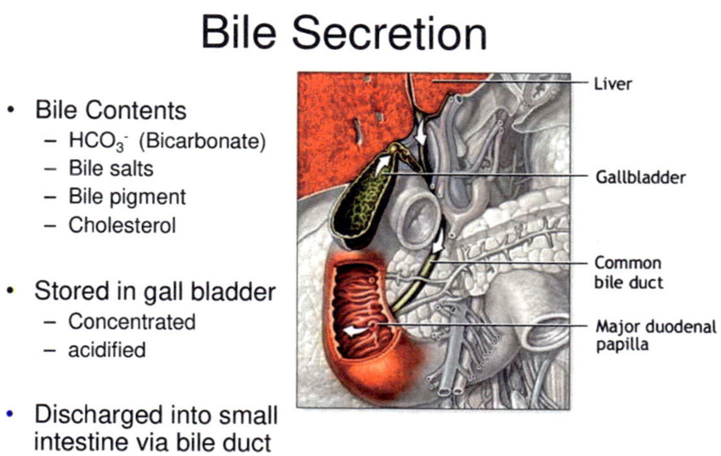

Figure 1.12. Bile secretion.

Source: https://slideplayer.com/slide/16931651/97/images/21/Bile+Secretion+Bile+Contents+Stored+in+gall+bladder.jpg.

1.4.3. Regulation of Bile Production

Regulation of bile secretion is a complex physiological process that is at the core of digestion and lipid metabolism. The liver, the primary organ for the synthesis of bile, relies on hepatocytes for the generation of bile acids, which are stimulated by multiple physiological stimuli and hormonal inputs. Leading among them is cholecystokinin (CCK), a hormone released from the intestine after food intake. CCK not only contracts the gallbladder to release stored bile but also stimulates liver production of bile. Additionally, enterohepatic circulation of the BAs, where the BAs are absorbed from the intestines and transported back to the liver, is a feedback process that regulates bile acid synthesis, ensuring that it is produced in quantities proportional to the body's digestive needs. Along with that, regulation of bile is a multifaceted process involving various types of cells in the liver, the most prominent being the Kupffer cells, which play a crucial role in the homeostasis of the liver. In conditions such as intrahepatic cholangiolithiasis (IBDS), the balance of bile flow and composition may be disrupted with severe complications. Present studies have revealed that inflammation and Kupffer cell polarization to an M2 type can affect bile duct obstruction and alter the secretion of pro-inflammatory cytokines like interleukin-6 (IL-6) from the cells. Elevated levels of IL-6 can then affect the proliferation of hepatic bile duct epithelial cells, as seen in IBDS cases. This points towards the importance of immune cell regulation in the overall process of bile production, illustrating a complex interaction between metabolic and inflammatory pathways in liver physiology (Li *et al.*, 2024). Further, understanding biochemical pathways regulating bile production is important to developing insights into liver disease. Hormonal cues, particularly from the enterohepatic apparatus, modulate bile acid biosynthesis by enzymes like cholesterol 7α-hydroxylase, the rate-limiting enzyme in bile acid biosynthesis. Regulation of dietary fat modifies the formation and regulation of bile salts and thus integrates nutrition with liver function. Understanding the molecular mechanisms of bile acid regulation and synthesis is of particular significance, particularly in the context of the therapeutic implications of liver diseases. By knowing how obesity and metabolic syndrome cause inflammation of the liver and affect bile regulation, we can create personalized interventions that improve the production of bile and the health of the liver, revealing the intricate interplay between diet, metabolism, and hepatic function (Al-ibrahimi *et al.*, 2025).

1.5. Pathophysiology of Liver Diseases

Liver diseases include many different health problems that cause hepatic function to change, which has major effects on the whole body. Many different things can cause liver disease, and prevalent causes are viral infections, drinking alcohol, and metabolic disorders. For instance, chronic hepatitis B (CHB) and C (CHC) viruses can instigate inflammatory responses that progressively damage hepatocytes, eventually culminating in fibrosis and cirrhosis. NAFLD is now one of the main reasons for liver problems, and it is often linked to obesity and metabolic syndrome. As a result of these pathologies, the liver affects the whole body and increases the risk of heart disease, which shows how important the liver is for maintaining general health and the need for complete care. A major part of liver disease pathology is changes in the liver's circulation. Since the liver gets blood from the hepatic artery and the portal vein, its blood vessels must be thoroughly understood. New studies using advanced imaging have exposed the detailed structure of the liver blood vessels, which greatly influences how blood flows when disease develops. Cirrhosis may result in portal hypertension, which changes the usual blood flow, and this can lead to varices and ascites.

These vascular changes need to be understood because they make liver disease worse and add challenges to surgical and medical treatments. Recognition of these changes informs clinical practice and guides both diagnostic and therapeutic modalities for liver diseases (Casteleyn *et al.*, 2014). Targeting the main causes of liver diseases is important to prevent further harm and improve how patients feel. For example, antiviral treatments have made it possible to cure hepatitis C for many patients, which can also repair some liver damage. Also, both lifestyle changes and medicines are important for managing NAFLD, mainly by focusing on weight loss and controlling metabolic problems. Also, using teams made up of different specialists can help patients with liver diseases receive the care they require. Working together, specialists in hepatology, nutrition, and mental health can help patients receive more effective treatment, and a better quality of life. As our understanding of liver pathophysiology advances, so too does the potential for novel therapeutic avenues, highlighting the importance of ongoing research in this vital organ system (Chaviano *et al.*, 2017) (Figure 1.13).

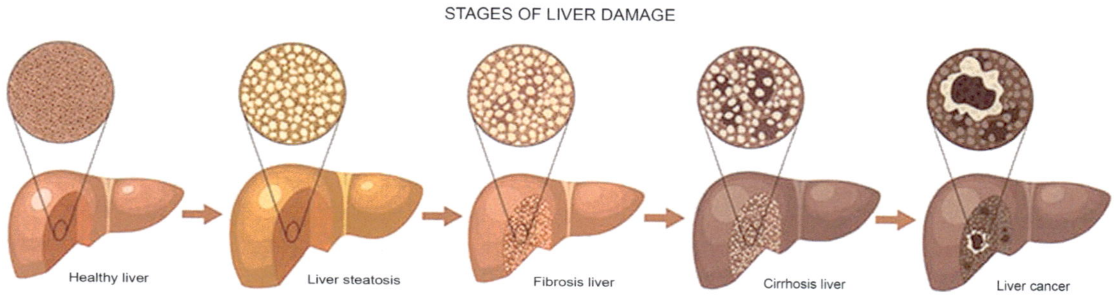

Figure 1.13. Stages of liver damage.

Source: https://kauveryhospital.com/blog/wp-content/uploads/2021/05/stages-liver-damage-after-cancer.jpg.

1.5.1. Common Liver Diseases (Hepatitis, Cirrhosis)

The liver is an essential organ that carries out different physiological functions, and its status defines the overall health. Hepatitis and cirrhosis are the most prevalent diseases of the liver and completely disable its function. Hepatitis, or inflammation of the liver, can be caused by viral infections, alcohol consumption, or an autoimmune process. It can be in acute and chronic form, and viral hepatitis types A, B, and C are major causes globally. Prevalent among the majority of populations, viral hepatitis can lead to serious complications, including liver failure and the risk of developing hepatocarcinoma. Elucidation of the pathogenetic processes of hepatitis is essential for guiding treatment modalities and improving patient survival, as novel developments in antiviral therapies are constantly being developed, allowing better control of the disease. Cirrhosis represents the late development of chronic liver damage, most often the result of prolonged insults such as hepatitis, alcoholism, or NAFLD. Cirrhosis involves progressive replacement of normal liver tissue with fibrotic scar tissue, leading to impaired liver function and complications such as portal hypertension and hepatic encephalopathy. Recent research opposes the old paradigm of cirrhosis as an irreversible lesion, with it now being unveiled that reversal of disease can occur with the help of certain therapies and lifestyle modifications after the removal of etiologic factors. As reported, "new concepts create new responsibilities and opportunities for the pathologist to contribute to the understanding of liver pathology" (Quaglia *et al.*, 2016). This emerging awareness underlines the importance of early detection and intervention in cirrhosis care, affecting treatment outcomes and improving the quality of life for patients. Treatment of liver disorders is also extended to advanced techniques such as liver transplantation, offering a lifeline for individuals with end-stage liver failure due to cirrhosis or fulminant hepatitis. Multidisciplinary strategy for transplantation incorporates candidate evaluation, nutrition support, and control of recurrent disease post-transplant. Recommendations by expert panels are crucial in optimizing results for transplantation candidates with regard to early referral and direct-acting antiviral (DAA) drugs in patients with hepatitis (Burra *et al.*, 2018). With ongoing research and expert advice guiding clinical practice, the future for the treatment of liver disease is rosy, with new therapies being married to growing understanding of disease mechanisms. Lastly, integration of liver anatomy, physiology, and pathophysiology is essential for innovation in prevention, diagnosis, and treatment strategies for commonly encountered liver diseases.

1.5.2. Impact of Liver Disease on Biliary Function

Liver disease and its impact on biliary function are important to study when looking at the wider effects of hepatic diseases. Illnesses of the liver, such as cholestasis, block the movement of bile, which causes a large buildup of BAs in the liver. In cholangiopathies and fatty liver diseases, the biliary tree is damaged, which blocks the normal flow of bile and causes disruption. Problems with biliary function may cause jaundice, which is usually due to a rise in plasma bilirubin. The correlations between liver function tests (LFTs) and biliary obstruction are particularly revealing; for instance, plasma bilirubin serves as a key discriminator in diagnosing conditions like common bile duct stones versus malignant strictures, underscoring the liver's pivotal role in maintaining biliary health (Karvonen *et al.*, 2009). Also, liver disease can influence the gallbladder and cause serious changes in its function. Because it is part of the biliary system, the gallbladder can show signs of trouble as liver function declines. Chronic cholestasis may result in damage to the gallbladder, which can cause inflammation, gallstone formation, and sometimes perforations. The relationship points out that the biliary tree and the gallbladder, which are lined with similar epithelial cells, are both at risk of liver diseases. As such, understanding the interconnectedness of these organs is crucial for appropriate therapeutic strategies that address both liver and biliary disorders comprehensively (Alpini *et al.*, 2023).

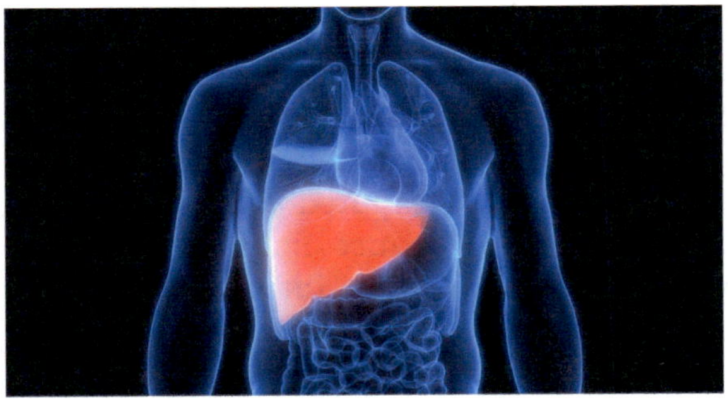

Figure 1.14. Biliary Function

Source: https://www.medstarhealth.org/-/media/project/mho/medstar/blogs/blogmedstar2021/thomas-liver-disease-desktop.jpg.

In addition, treating liver disease often means looking after both the liver and the biliary system. ERCP and similar clinical treatments can both remove bile duct blockages and reduce the risk of ongoing liver problems. Since many cholestatic diseases can cause serious health problems and complications, it is very important for doctors to understand how liver and bile function are related. It is clear from long-term results that treating the bile ducts in conjunction with addressing the underlying liver disease is very important. By fostering such comprehensive approaches, healthcare providers can enhance diagnostic accuracy and therapeutic efficacy in managing the multifaceted impacts of liver disease on biliary function (Karvonen *et al.*, 2009) (Figure 1.14).

1.5.3. Diagnostic Methods for Liver Diseases

The liver is a vital organ that carries out numerous functions, including metabolism, detoxification, and bile production. Thus, diagnosis of liver disease involves various sophisticated diagnostic methods that enable effective evaluation and planning for treatment. Blood tests such as LFTs are routinely the initial investigation. These tests define the enzymes, proteins, and constituents, such as bilirubin levels, to enable clinicians to diagnose cholestasis or hepatocellular injury. In addition to the above, imaging techniques, including ultrasonography, computed tomography (CT), and magnetic resonance imaging (MRI), are beneficial in providing information on the morphology and function of the liver. Using these modalities, doctors can identify conditions such as gallstones, tumors, or inflammatory diseases and limit their differential diagnosis and guide further investigations (Korenevskiy *et al.*, 2025). In more complex cases, especially when initial tests are inconclusive, liver biopsy (LBx) may be needed. This invasive procedure makes it possible to directly analyze liver tissue for histopathologic examination and to exclude or confirm the presence of certain diseases such as cirrhosis or hepatitis. In addition, integration of molecular diagnostics such as next-generation sequencing (NGS) is revolutionizing the field of hepatology. Such technologies make it possible to detect genetic predispositions and rare disorders, widening the universe of diagnostically available conditions for practitioners. It is important to understand these various modalities because, besides enhancing diagnostic accuracy, they also enable tailored treatment approaches that take into account the pathophysiology of liver disease (Liu *et al.*, 2024). There has also been a recent development in enhancing the efficacy of diagnostic procedures for liver disease. For instance, non-invasive assessment of fibrosis techniques such as transient elastography and magnetic resonance elastography are gaining widespread use. The new imaging modalities help determine liver stiffness, which is equivalent to the extent of fibrosis, thereby making biopsy unnecessary. In addition, the use of artificial intelligence (AI) in diagnostics can potentially improve accuracy and predictive capabilities. With professionals now beginning to use these technologies, their faith in diagnosing liver disease rises. With diagnostic methods constantly improving, clinicians are increasingly capable of providing enhanced care, ultimately leading to better patient outcomes as they fight the complexities of biliary and liver anatomy and physiology (Korenevskiy *et al.*, 2025) (Figure 1.15).

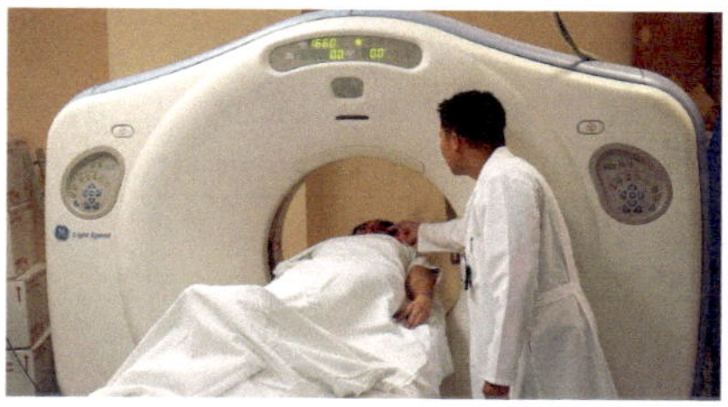

Figure 1.15. Diagnosing liver disease.

Source: https://liverfoundation.org/wp-content/uploads/2022/07/Liver-Cancer-Screening-1280x720-1.jpg.

1.6. Clinical Significance of Liver and Biliary Anatomy

Because of their role in metabolic regulation, detoxification and bile production, liver and biliary structures are very important in clinical medicine. The liver is essential for maintaining metabolic balance by affecting how carbohydrates, proteins, and fats are processed. Because it receives blood from both the hepatic artery and the portal vein, the liver can process the blood from the digestive tract, which is important for breaking down nutrients and drugs. Also, if the liver has abnormalities or diseases such as tumors or cirrhosis, it can result in important clinical problems. Being familiar with the lobes, segments, and blood vessels of the liver is necessary for hepatologists and surgeons because it helps them decide on the best surgical and diagnostic approaches for different diseases of the liver and bile ducts. Problems in liver and bile duct anatomy, for example, situs inversus, reveal the strong link between the structure of organs and health outcomes. Sometimes, when someone has situs inversus, other gastrointestinal problems can develop and remain unnoticed until they cause serious health problems. In a number of cases, those with situs inversus do not have symptoms, and the disorder is only found after death during an autopsy. It emphasizes that a good knowledge of liver anatomy is needed to catch any complications during surgery. Surgical teams must remain vigilant in identifying anatomical variations that may not conform to textbook descriptions, as these variations can significantly affect surgical access and outcomes during procedures, thereby underscoring the need for detailed anatomical knowledge in clinical practice (William *et al.*, 2019). Better imaging technology has made it easier to understand the liver and biliary system, which has helped improve both diagnosis and treatment in hospitals. The implementation of computer-assisted combined indocyanine green (ICG) molecular fluorescence imaging has revolutionized the preoperative planning and intraoperative detection of liver tumors. Because it shows anatomical structures in three dimensions, this technology helps surgeons figure out the tumor's edges and decide on the best way to operate. It makes it possible to find small lesions that can be missed by regular imaging techniques. The seamless integration of ICG fluorescence imaging into surgical practice not only enhances the accuracy of tumor resections but also minimizes the risk of complications such as biliary leakage following surgery, thereby improving patient care outcomes significantly (Medical Association of Chinese Medical Association Digital, 2019).

1.6.1. Surgical Interventions (Liver Transplant, Cholecystectomy)

Surgical intervention is a key component of managing liver and biliary system disorders, particularly when non-surgical management is insufficient. Among these procedures, liver transplantation has become a life-saving intervention for individuals with end-stage liver disease or acute liver failure (ALF). Liver transplantation not only eliminates the signs of liver failure but also corrects the underlying physiological abnormalities responsible for systemic health deterioration. The complexity of such procedures requires precise anatomical knowledge, especially concerning the vascular and biliary complex to be saved or recreated. The physicians would also need to weigh potential complications, including rejection and infection, that can affect postoperative outcomes significantly, thus demanding an interdisciplinary approach with hepatologists, transplant surgeons, and critical care physicians. Cholecystectomy, or surgery for the removal of the gallbladder, is another standard procedure for biliary pathology, particularly for gallstones or cholecystitis. Laparoscopic cholecystectomy, now the norm due to its brief recovery and fewer complications compared to open cholecystectomy, is performed for it. The gallbladder and the surrounding structures, including the cystic duct, the hepatic ducts, and the liver, are essential in anatomy for surgeons to navigate through in surgery. Advances in laparoscopic and robotic procedures further cemented these interventions. As revealed in recent publications, the interventions have been determined to have comparable oncologic outcomes, decreased intraoperative blood loss, and shorter hospital stays, thus proving their efficacy and enhancing recovery of the patient (Shimizu *et al.*, 2022). Therefore, an appreciation of liver and biliary anatomy is essential in order to optimize surgical planning. Further, as surgical technique improves, so too does the scope of conditions that can potentially be curatively treated, including malignant and benign biliary and hepatic tumors. Improvements in technology, for instance robotics, have seen vast improvements with regard to precision and minimality. Studies have established that robot-assisted hepatic procedures are associated with less intraoperative blood loss and shorter lengths of hospital stay compared to open standard surgery, maintenance of significant oncological results, and even augmented rates of R0 resections (Shimizu *et al.*, 2022). In addition, knowledge of the liver microvascular architecture is imperative while considering interventions that can impact organ function. For instance, alterations in vascular segments therapeutically guide surgical methods and postoperative care. In this respect, therefore, synergy between new surgical methods and good anatomical principles continues to play a central role in determining effective treatment paradigms in biliary and liver surgery (Figure 1.16).

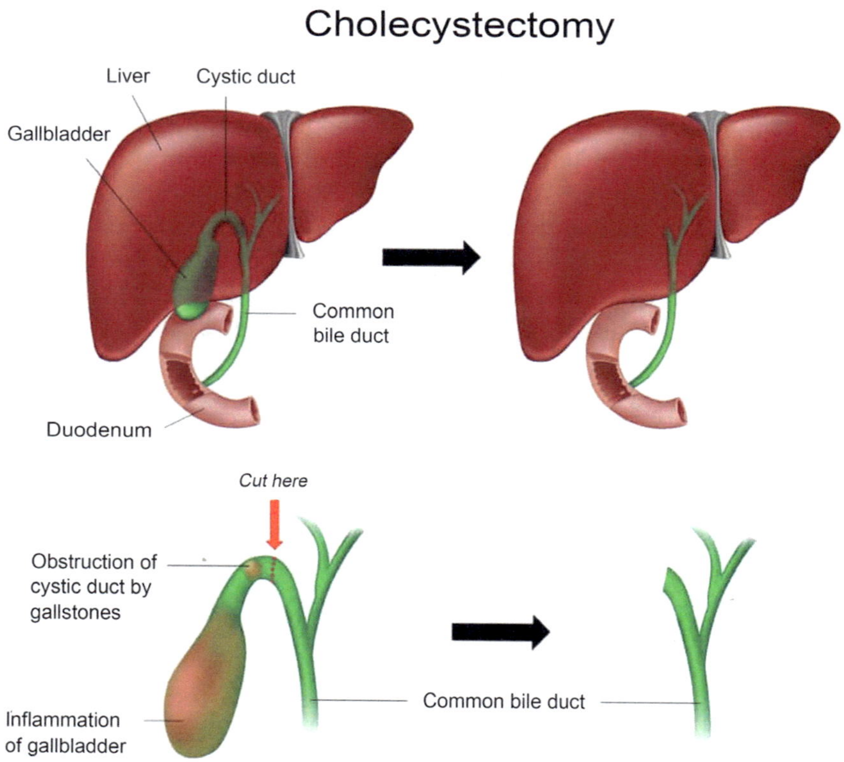

Figure 1.16. Cholecystectomy.

Source: https://uppergisurgery.com.au/wp-content/uploads/cholecystectomy.jpg.

1.6.2. Implications for Pharmacology and Drug Delivery

How drugs are processed and removed from the body is greatly affected by the liver and bile ducts, which are key to the liver's metabolism. The liver, which is responsible for most drug metabolism, has a special sinusoidal structure that facilitates the uptake of substances. The design of the intestine affects the way drugs are taken up and also how they are processed before being released into the bloodstream. Also, knowing how liver function varies from person to person is important for giving the right medicine. Advances in predictive modeling, such as physiologically based pharmacokinetic (PBPK) models, allow for the consideration of population heterogeneity in drug absorption, distribution, metabolism, and excretion (ADME) processes, thereby enhancing drug delivery strategies to target liver-related conditions effectively (Bois *et al.*, 2010). Also, problems with the liver can change how drugs work and their effectiveness in treating diseases. Liver fibrosis causes the liver to not work properly, which makes it hard for doctors to decide on the right drug dosage. Chronic liver injury, characterized by the activation of hepatic stellate cells (HSCs) and subsequent extracellular matrix accumulation, complicates pharmacological interventions due to altered drug clearance rates. As highlighted by recent studies, exploring the roles of molecular pathways, such as those influenced by transforming growth factor beta 1 (TGFβ1), provides insight into how drugs can be tailored to mitigate the adverse effects of liver disease (Elnagdy *et al.*, 2021). Knowing how these changes happen is very important for making effective drugs to treat liver problems and other diseases. Also, new ways to deliver drugs, especially targeted therapies, are expected to help improve the outcomes of liver diseases. Applying nanotechnology and controlled release can help drugs target their intended sites better, work more effectively, and cause fewer general side effects. They are designed to use the special features of the liver, such as a lot of blood and special types of cells, to help drugs get absorbed where they are needed most. Using knowledge of liver and biliary functions, researchers can create better treatments when combining these advanced delivery methods. Working together, pharmacologists, hepatologists, and bioengineers can develop new treatments that address the liver's complex structure, which will help manage liver diseases and improve drug delivery.

1.6.3. Importance in Nutrition and Metabolic Disorders

The liver is at the hub of nutrition and metabolic health, serving as an important hub for the disassembly and distribution of nutrients. It metabolizes carbohydrates, protein, and fat, ensuring these macromolecules are properly converted to energy or stored for future use. In cases of metabolic disease, such as obesity and diabetes, the liver's function can be interrupted, with calamitous effects on health. For example, IR, which is prevalent among overweight individuals, can disrupt glucose metabolism and incline individuals towards fatty liver disease. Hence, understanding the liver's role in nutrient metabolism is pivotal while establishing effective interventions in addressing such metabolic disorders (Burra *et al.*, 2018). With proper knowledge of liver physiology, healthcare practitioners will be able to personalize nutritional strategies to avoid such health risks. Nutrition directly affects the function of the liver and thus shapes the profile of various metabolic disorders. In patients with diseases such as NAFLD, nutrition treatment gains crucial relevance in managing the disease course. Nutrient deficiencies can exacerbate metabolic abnormalities, while properly balanced diets with optimal nutrients can enhance hepatic function and aid in recovery. The operation of the micronutrients, such as vitamins and minerals, is particularly important, as they assist in enzymatic reactions in liver metabolism. Furthermore, as quoted by the Italian Association for the Study of the Liver, malnutrition is also a problem with patients waiting for liver transplantation. Successful management of these nutritional deficiencies is required to maximize outcomes for patients and illustrate the interrelatedness of liver function, nutrition, and metabolic well-being (Burra *et al.*, 2018). In contemporary health terminology, the increasing obesity rates present an emergent public health crisis that cannot be underestimated. The World Health Organization's designation of obesity as an international epidemic illustrates the necessity for a prompt response. Obesity greatly impacts the liver's health, resulting in steatosis and fibrosis, among other diseases, that heighten the risk of other liver diseases. Strategies for managing obesity must incorporate nutrition education as a central component. Physical fitness activities and healthy food habits fueled by societies can be used to reverse the increasing trend of obesity. Although the evidence is mounting for the role of diet in metabolic disorders, it is increasingly clear that there is a need for an integrated approach to manage these disease conditions at the individual and community levels (Kyrou *et al.*, 2010).

SUMMARY

The intricate anatomy and physiology of the liver and biliary apparatus underscore their critical roles in ensuring health and homeostasis in general. The liver not only serves as a metabolic center but also plays a significant role in detoxification, protein synthesis, and the storage of vital nutrients. Diseases of this complex system, such as LC and HCC, highlight the need for continuous research and development in diagnostic and therapy strategies. The promise of osteopontin, as detailed, highlights its potential as both a biomarker and a therapeutic target for treating liver, pancreas, and bile disease, and thus highlights the need for continuous studies on its multifaceted functions (Liu *et al.*, 2024). The significance of liver transplantation also needs to be considered, especially since demand exceeds the number of suitable donors. Some conditions, like alcohol-induced LC and viral hepatitis, rank among the causes of the increased patient populations applying for transplant services. Understanding the epidemiological profile of transplant recipients provides insight into the broader health issue of liver disease, as revealed by the observational study that showed population trends among the patients (Souza Lopo *et al.*, 2024). This information serves to inform public health actions and healthcare resource allocation so that treatment is directed at those who are most at risk. Last, the interconnected nature of liver and biliary anatomy and associated illnesses necessitates an integrated understanding of health care and inquiry. The recognition of the critical roles of the liver and the complexity of its disease—especially through biomarkers like osteopontin—is spurring the development of diagnostic and therapeutic strategies. This pooled information has the potential to improve outcomes and quality of life in patients with liver disease, providing access to novel treatments and enhanced management strategies for the practice of hepatology. Future research to elucidate the genetic and molecular underpinnings of liver disorders will undoubtedly inform directed interventions and further understanding of these life-sustaining mechanisms.

Biliary and hepatic systems play a critical role in achieving physiological homeostasis through their complex anatomy and interdependent functions. The liver is central to the system since it is the focal point where bile acid synthesis, metabolism, and storage occur. Cholesterol-derived BAs are involved in lipid absorption and digestion in the intestines. Their bioassembly is well-regulated, with the central regulating protein Fibroblast growth factor 19 (FGF19) playing a central regulating role in the negative feedback regulation of bile acid synthesis in the bile acids. An increase in bile acids induces the release of FGF19 from the terminal ileum, which informs the liver to reduce bile acid synthesis, thereby maintaining homeostasis (Johansson *et al.*, 2020). The subtle balance of these elements underscores the liver's vital function in lipid metabolism and digestive function. Also, the biliary tree, as a ductal system that directs the liver to the gallbladder, provides for the prompt delivery of bile into the intestine. This anatomical design is vital for maintaining the bile flow required for lipid emulsification and nutrient absorption. However, biliary tree disorders such as bile duct obstruction or dilatation lead to profound health impacts. Dilatation of bile ducts must be diagnosed in order to find conditions such as stones or tumors, which have wide-ranging implications for liver function and overall health. Recent studies have developed computer-assisted image processing for the early diagnosis of abnormalities of the biliary tree, which supplements clinical evaluation and patient treatment (AL-Munaizel *et al.*, 2021). This overlap of anatomy and technological advancement is what helps to affirm the necessity of early detection and treatment in hepatic and biliary disease. Last but not least, the liver's capacity for regeneration, along with its regulatory functions, places it uniquely within the overall context of human anatomy. A model of the interaction of BAs, FGF19, and hepatocyte function guides the liver's response to varying metabolic demands and pathology. In cholestatic disease, for instance, where bile flow is impeded, FGF19 levels may rise, reflecting bile acid dynamics and hepatic adaptation. Notably, such regulatory action is not unique to the liver; the bidirectional interaction between FGF19 and BAs is an indicator of an autocrine signaling pathway that may affect the production of bile acids in human hepatocytes. As future research continues to unravel these complex pathways, the potential for new innovative therapeutic interventions towards the management of liver and biliary diseases increases (Johansson *et al.*, 2020). These advances have significant implications for achieving the maximum liver health and optimizing the results of treatment in patients with biliary disease.

CLOSER LOOK

TRANSJUGULAR INTRAHEPATIC PORTOSYSTEMIC SHUNT (TIPS)

A Transjugular Intrahepatic Portosystemic Shunt (TIPS) is a procedure that creates a connection between two blood vessels in the liver, the portal vein and the hepatic vein, to reduce portal hypertension. This is done to alleviate complications like variceal bleeding and ascites, which can arise from high pressure in the portal vein (Figure 1.17).

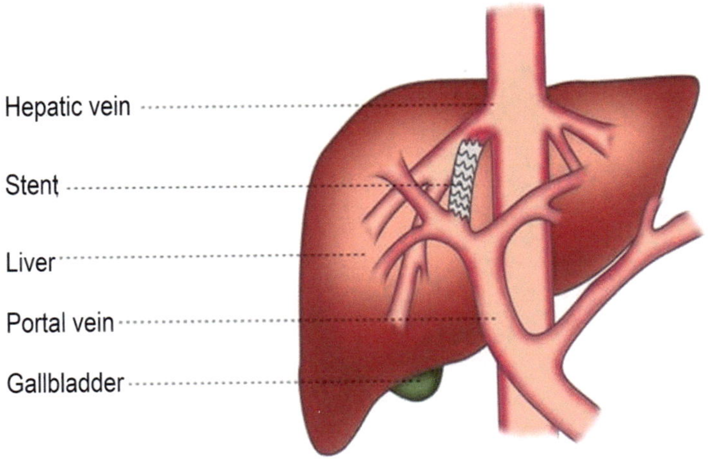

Figure 1.17.

Source: https://www.cirse.org/wp-content/uploads/2018/08/TIPS600x420-1-600x420.jpg.

Purpose

TIPS aims to relieve high pressure in the portal vein, which can cause complications like esophageal variceal bleeding (bleeding from enlarged veins in the esophagus) and ascites (fluid buildup in the abdomen).

Procedure

A thin tube, called a stent, is placed between the portal vein and the hepatic vein, creating a direct path for blood flow, bypassing the damaged liver tissue.

Benefits

TIPS can reduce the risk of variceal bleeding, decrease ascites, and improve overall quality of life for patients with portal hypertension.

Risks

Potential complications include infection, bleeding at the insertion site, or damage to blood vessels. There's also a risk of HE, a brain disorder that can result from the buildup of toxins in the blood.

Alternatives

In some cases, TIPS can be an alternative to surgery or liver transplantation for managing portal hypertension.

Revisions and Occlusion

If the TIPS becomes narrowed or blocked, it can be revised or reopened with a procedure called angioplasty. In certain situations, the TIPS might be intentionally closed (occluded).

References

1. Aliberti, C., Alvaro, D., Bastianelli, C., Berloco, P., *et al.* (2017). Cryopreservation protocol for human biliary tree stem/progenitors, hepatic and pancreatic precursors. https://core.ac.uk/download/98348621.pdf (accessed on 24 May 2025).
2. Al-Ibrahimi, L. A., & Hussein, Z. M. (2025). Study of liver development in laboratory mice embryos *Mus musculus. International Journal of Current Science Research and Review.* https://www.semanticscholar.org/paper/1865d4e73b45b99288b216d96f81476026fed80a (accessed on 24 May 2025).
3. AL-Munaizel, T., AL-Oudat, M., Alomari, S., Azzeh, M., *et al.* (2021). An interactive automation for human biliary tree diagnosis using computer vision. https://core.ac.uk/download/478789430.pdf (accessed on 24 May 2025).
4. Al-Ogaili, M., Baldawi, J., Wallace, A., Alzubaidi, S., Oklu, R., Knuttinen, G., Naidu, S., *et al.* (2024). Post-liver transplantation vascular and biliary anatomy: A pictorial review. *Digestive Disease Interventions.* https://www.semanticscholar.org/paper/0472aac6a23f5bef2187ca849ee94a299e602f80 (accessed on 24 May 2025).
5. Alpini, G., Baiocchi, L., Ceci, L., Francis, H., Gaudio, E., Han, Y., Kennedy, L., *et al.* (2023). Gallstone and gallbladder disease: Biliary tract and cholangiopathies. https://core.ac.uk/download/599513205.pdf (accessed on 24 May 2025).
6. Alsaab HO, Alharbi FD, Alhibs AS, Alanazi NB, Alshehri BY, Saleh MA, Alshehri FS, Algarni MA, Almugaiteeb T, Uddin MN, Alzhrani RM. (2022) PLGA-Based Nanomedicine: History of Advancement and Development in Clinical Applications of Multiple Diseases. Pharmaceutics. 6;14(12):2728. doi: 10.3390/pharmaceutics14122728.
7. Banerjee, P., Gaddam, N., Chandler, V., & Chakraborty, S. (2023). Oxidative stress–induced liver damage and remodeling of the liver vasculature. *American Journal of Pathology, 193,* 1400–1414. https://doi.org/10.1016/j.ajpath.2023.06.002.
8. Bois, F. Y., Clewell, H. J., & Jamei, M. (2010). PBPK modelling of inter-individual variability in the pharmacokinetics of environmental chemicals. https://core.ac.uk/download/52669006.pdf (accessed on 24 May 2025).
9. Burra, P., Caraceni, P., Ferri, F., Giannini, E., *et al.* (2018). Specific issues concerning the management of patients on the waiting list and after liver transplantation. https://core.ac.uk/download/159268374.pdf (accessed on 24 May 2025).
10. Casteleyn, C., Cornillie, P., Debbaut, C., Dierick, M., *et al.* (2014). Analyzing the human liver vascular architecture by combining vascular corrosion casting and micro-CT scanning: A feasibility study. https://core.ac.uk/download/55806749.pdf (accessed on 24 May 2025).
11. Chaviano, F., Orazi, A., Pizzi, M., Rugge, M., *et al.* (2017). A lucky mistake: The splenic glands of Marcello Malpighi. https://core.ac.uk/download/154325705.pdf (accessed on 24 May 2025).
12. Cifuentes-Silva, E., & Cabello-Verrugio, C. (2023). Bile acids as signaling molecules: Role of ursodeoxycholic acid in cholestatic liver disease. *Current Protein & Peptide Science.* https://www.semanticscholar.org/paper/97f19c202ef733b91435cc0ac7f843376bd1354b (accessed on 24 May 2025).

13. Cordero Espinoza, L. (2019). The mesenchymal regulation of ductal-driven liver regeneration. https://core.ac.uk/download/227519049.pdf (accessed on 24 May 2025).
14. Cunningham, R. P., & Porat-Shliom, N. (2021). Liver zonation–revisiting old questions with new technologies. *Frontiers in Physiology, 12*. https://doi.org/10.3389/fphys.2021.732929.
15. Daud, M., & Ashraf, M. (2001). Post cholecystectomy syndrome: After two years and beyond 127 successful laparoscopic cholecystectomies in the Hospital University Sains Malaysia. https://core.ac.uk/download/89468917.pdf (accessed on 24 May 2025).
16. Elnagdy, M. (2021). PDE4 inhibition: A novel therapeutic strategy in liver fibrosis. https://core.ac.uk/download/482116877.pdf (accessed on 24 May 2025).
17. Gilliam-Vigh, H., Suppli, M., Heimbürger, S. M. N., Lund, A., Knop, F. K., & Ellegaard, A. M. (2025). Cholesin mRNA expression in human intestinal, liver, and adipose tissues. *Nutrients, 17*. https://www.semanticscholar.org/paper/32780f37e4e9393261f610250986d052f11cdfc3 (accessed on 24 May 2025).
18. Goyal, W. S. (2019). Embryological and clinical significance of situs inversus totalis: Rare case presenting with cholelithiasis and choledocholithiasis. *Indian Journal of Clinical Anatomy and Physiology*.https://www.semanticscholar.org/paper/d02b876837e40a3bd3345f5cc084b4d1fe153e64 (accessed on 24 May 2025).
19. Hinton, D. E., Segner, H., & Braunbeck, T. (2017). Toxic responses of the liver. In C. D. Klaassen (Ed.), *Casarett and Doull's Toxicology: The Basic Science of Poisons* (8th ed., pp. 305–344). CRC Press. https://doi.org/10.1201/9781315109244-4.
20. Huang, R., Pang, Q., Zheng, L., Lin, J., Li, H., Wan, L., & Wang, T. (2024). Cholesterol metabolism: Physiological versus pathological aspects in intracerebral hemorrhage. *Neural Regeneration Research, 20*(6), 1015–1030. https://www.semanticscholar.org/paper/ede9b582b7e45031b81f16122d84eb9e30d6d638 (accessed on 24 May 2025).
21. Johansson, H. (2020). *The Role of Fibroblast Growth Factor 19 In Human Liver*. https://core.ac.uk/download/322854617.pdf (accessed on 24 May 2025).
22. Karvonen, J. (2009). *Bile Duct Stones, Strictures and Iatrogenic Lesions: Studies on Early Diagnosis and Treatment*. https://core.ac.uk/download/197988914.pdf (accessed on 24 May 2025).
23. Khalil, M., Gena, P., Di Ciaula, A., Portincasa, P., & Calamita, G. (2024). Aquaporins in biliary function: Pathophysiological implications and therapeutic targeting. *International Journal of Molecular Sciences, 25*. https://www.semanticscholar.org/paper/792efb5c8ff13fe0d882aad4c16bb478f1b41bd0 (accessed on 24 May 2025).
24. Korenevskiy, N., Al-kasasbeh, R., Shaqadan, A., Al-Habahbeh, O. M., Telfah, A., Mousa, M. S., Rodionova, S., *et al.* (2025). Computerized decision support system and fuzzy logic rules for early diagnosis of pesticide-induced diseases. *Critical Reviews in Biomedical Engineering, 53*(1), 1–22. https://www.semanticscholar.org/paper/5ac274771a4f1de44b354568e3ddd710833f7469 (accessed on 24 May 2025).
25. Kyrou, I., & Weickert, M. O. (2010). Clinical problems caused by obesity. https://core.ac.uk/download/46324.pdf (accessed on 24 May 2025).
26. Lee, E., Eghtesad, B., García-Tsao, G., Haskal, Z. J., Hernández-Gea, V., Jalaeian, H., Kalva, S. P., *et al.* (2023). AASLD practice guidance on the use of TIPS, variceal embolization, and

retrograde transvenous obliteration in the management of variceal hemorrhage. *Hepatology, 79*, 224–250. https://doi.org/10.1097/hep.0000000000000530.

27. Li, L., Peng, H., Li, Z., Zhou, F., & Yu, Q. (2024). FTO-mediated regulation of Kupffer cell polarization and interleukin-6 secretion promotes biliary epithelial cell proliferation in intrahepatic bile duct stones. *CytoJournal, 21*. https://www.semanticscholar.org/paper/5fb1df5ec3b1c4aac576df824ba0d026cd1cec17 (accessed on 24 May 2025).
28. Liao, Y., Davies, N. A., & Bogle, I. D. L. (2025). Computational modelling in liver system and liver disease. *Physical Sciences Reviews*. https://www.semanticscholar.org/paper/8b9f6017367d342088cf31409941739c94a2cbc1 (accessed on 24 May 2025).
29. Liu, L., Niu, K., Yang, Z., Song, J., Wei, D., Zhang, R., & Tao, K. (2024). Osteopontin: An indispensable component in common liver, pancreatic, and biliary related disease. *Journal of Cancer Research and Clinical Oncology, 150*. https://www.semanticscholar.org/paper/78d1568aa6eca827aa00be75a3feb1e3259d80a6 (accessed on 24 May 2025).
30. *et al.*Jarvis, F., Bairey Merz, C. N., Barnes, P. J., Díaz Brinton, R., Carrero, J. J., DeMeo, D. L., De Vries, G. J., *et al.* (2020). Sex and gender: Modifiers of health, disease, and medicine. *The Lancet, 396*, 565–582. https://doi.org/10.1016/s0140-6736(20)31561-0.
31. Medical Association of Chinese Medical Association Digital, *et al.* (2019). Guidelines for application of computer-assisted indocyanine green molecular fluorescence imaging in diagnosis and surgical navigation of liver tumors (2019). *Journal of Southern Medical University, 39*(10), 1127–1140. https://www.semanticscholar.org/paper/c296821c685874c7952aaa9ea7051f38bb070ac4 (accessed on 24 May 2025).
32. Mejino, J. L. V., & Rosse, C. (2007). *The Foundational Model of Anatomy Ontology*. https://core.ac.uk/download/pdf/9412334.pdf (accessed on 24 May 2025).
33. Meyer-Szary, J., Luis, M. S., Mikulski, S., Patel, A., Schulz, F., Tretiakow, D., Fercho, J., *et al.* (2022). The role of 3D printing in planning complex medical procedures and training of medical professionals—Cross-sectional multispecialty review. *International Journal of Environmental Research and Public Health, 19*, 3331. https://doi.org/10.3390/ijerph19063331.
34. Okyar, A., Ozturk Civelek, D., Akyel, Y., Surme, S., Pala Kara, Z., & Kavakli, I. (2024). The role of the circadian timing system on drug metabolism and detoxification: An update. *Expert Opinion on Drug Metabolism & Toxicology, 20*, 503–517. https://www.semanticscholar.org/paper/be9b49474587303438b79920bf0281e0889eb64e (accessed on 24 May 2025).
35. Osman, M. F. (2011). Laparoscopic cholecystectomy conversion rate and associated factors. https://core.ac.uk/download/141499427.pdf (accessed on 24 May 2025).
36. Premkumar, M., & Dhiman, R. K. (2021). Portal cavernoma cholangiopathy: Indian perspective. *Clinical Liver Disease, 18*, 127–137. https://doi.org/10.1002/cld.1130.
37. Qamar, A. ., Khan, H. G., Khan, M. M., Kiani, M. R. B., Kundi, H., & Mushtaq, F. (2024). Statin Induced Changes in Rat Pancreatic Tissue: A Histological and Biochemical Perspective. Journal of Rawalpindi Medical College, 28(1). https://doi.org/10.37939/jrmc.v28i1.2367
38. Quaglia, A., Dhillon, A. P., Balabaud, C., Snover, D. C., van Leeuwen, D. J., Crawford, J. M., Ferrell, L., *et al.* (2016). Role of etiology in the progression, regression, and parenchymal remodeling of liver disease: Implications for liver biopsy interpretation. https://core.ac.uk/download/79506237.pdf (accessed on 24 May 2025).

39. Rychik, J., Atz, A. M., Celermajer, D. S., Deal, B. J., Gatzoulis, M. A., Gewillig, M., Hsia, T. Y., *et al.* (2019). Evaluation and management of the child and adult with Fontan circulation: A scientific statement from the American Heart Association. *Circulation, 140*. https://doi.org/10.1161/cir.0000000000000696.

40. S. Aharinejad, A. Lametschwandtner, P. Franz, W. Firbas. (1991) The vascularization of the digestive tract studied by scanning with special emphasis on the teeth, esophagus, stomach, small and large intestine, pancreas, and liver. Scanning Microscopy. Vol 5, num 3. (Pages 811-849). https://core.ac.uk/download/427316097.pdf.

41. Schulze, R. J., Schott, M. B., Casey, C. A., Tuma, P. L., & McNiven, M. A. (2019). The cell biology of the hepatocyte: A membrane trafficking machine. *The Journal of Cell Biology, 218*(7), 2096–2112. https://doi.org/10.1083/jcb.201903090.

42. Shiralkar M, Shiralkar D, Krushnadev S, Wagh R. (2015). To evaluate the effect of Apamarga Paniya Khara in the management of Udara Shula with special reference to biliary colic. Ayushdhara. Vol 2. Nro 3. https://core.ac.uk/download/333809501.pdf

43. Shevchenko KV, Yeroshenko GA, Yakushko OS, Kazakova KS, Kramarenko DR. Morphometric description of the exchange segment of microvasculature of rats' salivary glands in normal conditions and chronic ethanol intoxication. (2019). Wiad Lek. ;72(3):323-326. PMID: 31050975.

44. Shimizu, A., Ito, M., & Lefor, A. K. (2022). Laparoscopic and robot-assisted hepatic surgery: An historical review. *Journal of Clinical Medicine, 11*, 3254. https://doi.org/10.3390/jcm11123254.

45. Souza Lopo, L. H. C., da Paixão, L. S., Reina, F. N., dos Santos Lima, I., & de Freitas, L. A. R. (2024). Clinical and epidemiological profile analysis of patients submitted to hepatic transplantation in a reference pathological anatomy laboratory in Salvador-BA. *International Journal of Complementary and Alternative Medicine*. https://www.semanticscholar.org/paper/ed3130c02eec183f29b328b08679d3c8c2092089 (accessed on 24 May 2025).

46. Viil, J. (2016). *Terve Ja Kahjustatud Maksa Regeneratsioonis Ning Dupuytren'i Kontraktuuri Progressioonis Osalevate Rakuliste Ja Molekulaarsete Mehhanismide Uurimine* [Doctoral dissertation]. https://core.ac.uk/download/79114844.pdf (accessed on 24 May 2025).

47. Vinarov, Z., Abdallah, M., Agúndez, J. A. G., Allegaert, K., Basit, A. W., Braeckmans, M., Ceulemans, J., *et al.* (2021). Impact of gastrointestinal tract variability on oral drug absorption and pharmacokinetics: An UNGAP review. *European Journal of Pharmaceutical Sciences, 162*, 105812. https://doi.org/10.1016/j.ejps.2021.105812.

48. Wang, H., Gong, J., Chen, J., Zhang, W., Sun, Y., & Sun, D. (2024). Intestinal microbiota and biliary system diseases. *Frontiers in Cellular and Infection Microbiology, 14*. https://www.semanticscholar.org/paper/e235f3b50969656bc56765429d53cb111392f03c (accessed on 24 May 2025).

49. Weinberg, D. (2011). *Is the Gallbladder Really Unnecessary? An Evaluation of Gallstone Treatment* [Master's thesis]. https://core.ac.uk/download/217329338.pdf (accessed on 24 May 2025).

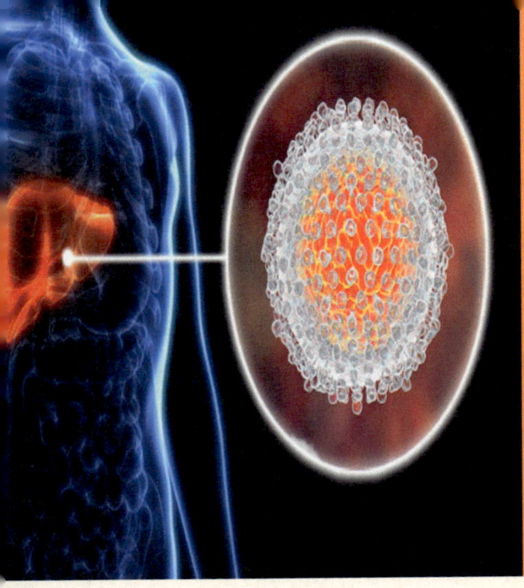

Chapter 2

HEPATITIS (ACUTE AND CHRONIC)

Contents

Introduction

The subject of hepatitis encompasses a wide range of liver injury and inflammation, classified primarily as acute and chronic forms, both having different characteristics and implications for public health. Acute hepatitis is usually described with the sudden onset of manifestations, including fatigue, jaundice, and abdominal pain, typically due to viral infections, toxins, or autoimmune reactions. On the other hand, chronic hepatitis is characterized by persistent liver inflammation for over six months, increasingly associated with long-term health consequences such as cirrhosis and hepatocellular carcinoma (HCC). The prevailing prevalence of liver disease necessitates a better understanding of etiology and disease evolution because the liver's multifunctional role in metabolism, detoxification, and immunity exposes it to multiple insults. Also, the multifaceted pathology of hepatitis highlights key factors that could exacerbate or modulate liver damage. For instance, the relationship between systemic inflammation and liver function is complex; since liver disease often develops in the context of significant immunological alterations, understanding these relationships is crucial for effective treatment and management of the disease. Liver functionality alterations, such as decreased biotransformation capacity and impaired immune response, could make the clinical syndrome more complicated, particularly in the elderly. Metabolic and immune alterations developing over time can predispose patients to hepatitis complications, supporting the need for targeted therapeutic interventions. The need for timely identification of such alterations requires healthcare professionals to shift away from a reductionist strategy in both acute and CLD management. The applicability of addressing hepatitis is not only limited to the individual health domain but also extends to affect broader public paradigms for health. Most importantly, the advent of novel biomarker research has catalyzed diagnostic potential and risk stratifications, paving the way for improved prognostic models. Berezin *et al.* (2024) demonstrate how serum and urine biomarkers could be used to forecast the advancement from acute kidney injury (AKI) to chronic kidney disease (CKD), outlining the dire need for early detection and intervention. In the same vein, appreciation of systemic consequences of hepatic inflammation, especially in the setting of acute-on-chronic liver failure (ACLF), is critical. Alzamili *et al.* (2024) unveil how changes in immunological functions and organ reserve propel the pathophysiology of liver diseases, with a call for early diagnosis and full care to optimize patient outcomes. Such observations call for ongoing research and education on hepatitis, with the goal of minimizing the disease burden on individuals and health systems.

Definition of Hepatitis

Hepatitis is a condition where the liver, which is responsible for metabolism, detoxification, and making proteins, is inflamed. The main factors leading to liver disease are viruses, too much alcohol, immune system problems, and injuries caused by drugs. Hepatitis is most often caused by viruses, and these are known as the hepatitis A, B, C, D, and E viruses. All these variants are spread differently and have different effects on the body, which leads to the variety seen in affected individuals. Since hepatitis is a major public health issue, it can cause both quick and long-term health problems, and chronic forms of the disease may result in cirrhosis or HCC. To understand hepatitis, we must look at its causes, signs, and the effects it has on health. Part of defining hepatitis is looking at the criteria used to diagnose it, which are very important for its management. Usually, doctors use clinical exams, blood tests for liver enzymes, and imaging to find out how much the liver has been damaged. Looking for viral markers is important for determining the type and stage of hepatitis a person has. Notably, drug-induced liver injury (DILI) is an area of growing concern, particularly concerning medications used in conditions such as tuberculosis. New guidelines stress that doctors should be aware of risk factors, biochemical markers, and histological findings in diagnosing DILI, which means they must be careful when prescribing anti-tuberculosis drugs and other hepatotoxic agents. Thus, fostering an in-depth awareness of various forms and diagnostic methods for hepatitis is vital for optimizing patient outcomes and treatment pathways (Abdyazdani *et al.*, 2024). Also, hepatitis should be defined in a way that includes its effect on society and the economy, mainly because chronic types of the disease impact some populations more than others. Recent studies indicate that metabolic disorders associated with obesity and Type 2 diabetes can significantly exacerbate liver conditions, often complicating the clinical picture in patients with chronic hepatitis B (CHB). Asian Americans are becoming more affected by both metabolic syndrome and liver disease, which has led to greater attention being given to their relationship. This link between metabolic problems and liver disease stresses why it is important to find and treat these problems early. Addressing the challenges of managing hepatitis in populations at risk can not only alleviate the personal health burden but also reduce the broader societal impacts associated with chronic liver conditions (Dong *et al.*, 2024). Thus, the multi-faceted definition of hepatitis extends beyond its clinical manifestations to encompass the underlying risk factors that contribute to its progression and management (Figure 2.1).

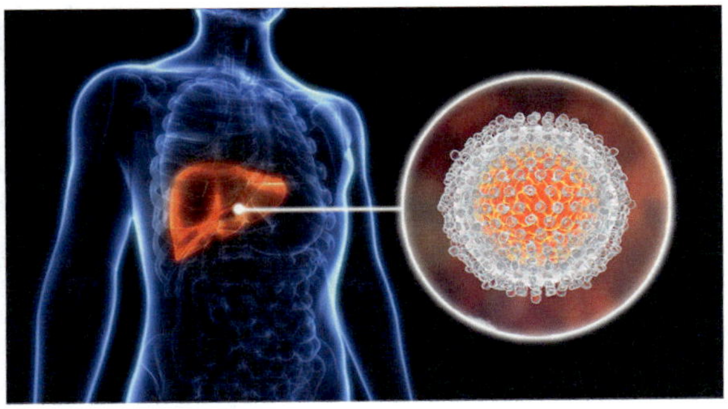

Figure 2.1. Hepatitis

Source: https://www.cdc.gov/hepatitis-c/media/images/2024/04/what-is-hepatitis-c-thumbnail.jpg.

Importance of Understanding Hepatitis

In treating the health crisis induced by hepatitis, it is necessary to understand the intricacies of its two variants, acute and chronic hepatitis. Understanding the pathogenesis of hepatitis allows practitioners to formulate successful treatment methods and prevention mechanisms. The special mechanisms of entry into host cells, replication, and induction of immune responses by the different hepatitis viruses are the focus of these therapeutic approaches. For instance, knowledge of viral replication cycles can be applied in the development of antiviral treatments that inhibit such processes, with a direct positive effect on patients. Additionally, the identification of each type of hepatitis serologic marker aids in the accurate diagnosis of infection. Such extensive knowledge inspires a better-informed response to preventive measures, such as vaccination and screening, required to curb the spread of hepatitis among various populations (Ronald *et al.*, 2023). The epidemiological context of hepatitis also underscores the importance of understanding its mode of transmission, particularly in high-prevalence areas. For instance, recent research done in Spiti Valley, India, has demonstrated that the hepatitis B virus (HBV) genotypes are endemic and revealed that specific strains dominate in specific areas. Molecular characterization is significant in understanding how different HBV genotypes are transmitted and the resultant public health implications involved. By identifying HBV genotypes circulating, public health professionals can tailor vaccination and therapeutic interventions to combat the specific strain infecting the population in a specific area. Additionally, having such epidemiological factors facilitates a more accurate assessment of risk likelihoods of transmission, particularly through vertical transmission upon delivery or through improper injection techniques (Pacholi *et al.*, 2022). Localized research and targeted intervention are therefore essential for limiting outbreaks of hepatitis. An understanding of the significance of knowing hepatitis does not only transcend individual health consequences; it is also about broader public health goals and global health justice. Stigma around hepatitis tends to discourage people from accessing appropriate medical care, worsening the disease burden in communities. Educational programs and stigma-reduction campaigns, based on the most up-to-date research and thorough knowledge of the disease, can decrease stigma. By establishing a culture in which individuals feel comfortable coming for treatment, communities can guarantee greater early diagnosis and therapy initiation, thereby decreasing the frequency of complications due to chronic hepatitis. Furthermore, safe sex education, vaccination, and harm reduction can be an effective tool to empower high-risk groups to make well-informed choices, eventually as a part of overall global hepatitis elimination. Through continued research and advocacy, we can narrow the gap between knowledge and action in the battle against hepatitis (Ronald *et al.*, 2023).

Overview of Acute and Chronic Hepatitis

A study of hepatitis, whether it is acute or chronic, shows that viruses, the immune system, and liver changes are closely related. A viral infection, for example, hepatitis A, B, or E, is usually the cause of acute hepatitis, which results in sudden liver inflammation. The symptoms of this condition may be mild, such as tiredness and yellow skin, or may be very severe, such as ALF. The symptoms a patient has often depend on what is causing them, and their overall health. For instance, acute-onset liver failure (ACLF) signifies a rapid deterioration in liver function and represents a critical health threat, often requiring immediate medical intervention. As identified in the literature, the prevalence of liver disease in the American population, with over 30 million afflicted, underscores the urgent need for a comprehensive understanding and prompt management of acute hepatitis to prevent further complications and deaths (Alzamili *et al.*, 2024). In this case, chronic hepatitis is caused by ongoing liver inflammation, which is often the result of a long-lasting infection such as hepatitis B or C. When inflammation lasts a long time, it can cause fibrosis, cirrhosis, and HCC after many years or decades. Most people affected by chronic hepatitis show few symptoms until the liver is seriously damaged, which makes it hard to diagnose and treat the disease on time. In addition, seniors are at greater risk because changes in liver function with age can intensify chronic liver problems. Because of decreased organ function and immune changes, clinical symptoms and treatment reactions may be quite different in these patients. Consequently, understanding the chronic phase's nuances is crucial in developing effective treatment strategies and optimizing patient outcomes (Alzamili *et al.*, 2024). New studies are pointing out that hepatitis E can cause problems outside the liver, which is not always well known. Between 2014 and 2022, a study found that 19% of patients with acute hepatitis E showed symptoms outside the liver, such as low platelet counts and kidney problems. This points out that diagnosing hepatitis can be difficult when the symptoms are not just related to the liver. If a person has other medical issues or infections, their hepatitis diagnosis may come later, which shows why a better approach is needed. Noticing these extrahepatic symptoms matters a lot, as they can change the course of the disease and the effectiveness of treatments. So, having a detailed approach for diagnosing hepatitis helps improve patient care and health for people in different groups.

2.1. Types of Hepatitis

It is imperative to understand the forms of hepatitis in order to realize the spectrum of liver diseases encompassed by this condition. Hepatitis A and E are commonly recognized as viral infections leading to acute hepatitis and are mostly transmitted via the fecal-oral route, often being associated with inadequate sanitary practices. Hepatitis A and E types tend to recover spontaneously without causing chronic liver disease (CLD). On the other hand, Hepatitis B, C, and D have the potential to cause chronic infection, a significant liver disease burden worldwide. Chronic infections can progress to severe health conditions like cirrhosis and hepatocellular carcinoma (HCC) and require awareness, prevention strategies, and timely treatment among high-risk populations. The realization of such distinctions assists medical practitioners in customizing their prevention, immunization, and treatment for different populations infected with these viruses. Chronic Hepatitis due to Hepatitis B and C viruses poses a great public health problem worldwide. Hepatitis B is a DNA virus that can produce chronic infection with characteristics of ongoing inflammation and possible progression to CLD and cancer. It is transmitted through blood, sex, and mother to child at birth. In contrast, Hepatitis C, which is an RNA virus, is primarily spread through blood-to-blood contact in the form of needle sharing between intravenous drug abusers. Importantly, chronic hepatitis C can be symptom-free for decades before significant liver damage, and thus early diagnosis and treatment are hard. Recent advances in antiviral therapy of Hepatitis C, especially direct-acting antivirals (DAA), have revolutionized the treatment to the extent that cure is now possible in the majority of patients, thereby alleviating the load of chronic complications that were otherwise thought to be inevitable in such patients. The pathogenesis of hepatitis infections varies remarkably based on the virus type, thereby influencing clinical management directly. For instance, while acute-on-chronic liver failure (ACLF) features severe clinical features and mortality, the contribution of immune dysfunctions to the disease pathogenesis remains a critical area to investigate. In ACLF, studies have highlighted the importance of B cells and their subsets in influencing immune responses and how this disordered immune milieu may lead to amplified liver failure (Wang *et al.*, 2025). Secondly, knowledge of the virological differences in replication and persistence mechanisms between Hepatitis B and C is helpful in designing targeted prophylaxis and therapies. Clinical and epidemiological research into such virological differences and their immunological implications is crucial for not only successful treatment options but also for formulating public health policy to prevent the incidence and prevalence of both acute and chronic hepatitis disorders (Martin *et al.*, 2024) (Figure 2.2).

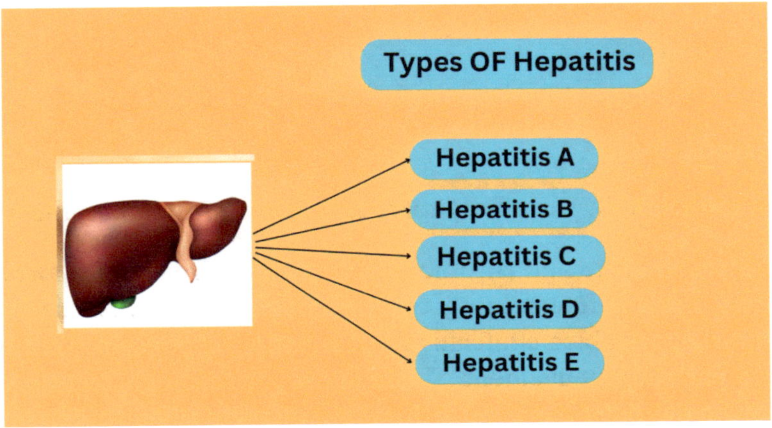

Figure 2.2. Types of hepatitis.

Source: https://drchetankalal.com/wp-content/uploads/2023/07/Hepatitis-Virus-Treatment-in-Mumbai.png.

2.1.1. Viral Hepatitis (A, B, C, D, E)

Because of their special ways of spreading, the symptoms they cause, and the risk of becoming a chronic infection, viral hepatitis A, B, C, D, and E are a major public health concern. Hepatitis A virus (HAV) and hepatitis E virus (HEV) are predominantly acquired through the fecal-oral route, often resulting in self-limiting acute infections. In contrast, hepatitis B virus (HBV) and hepatitis C virus (HCV), transmitted through blood and other bodily fluids, can lead to CLD, including cirrhosis and HCC. Hepatitis D virus (HDV) requires the presence of HBV for its replication, complicating the clinical picture. Knowing how diseases are transmitted is necessary to prevent them. In regions like Bangladesh, where sporadic outbreaks occur frequently, targeted public health interventions are paramount to mitigate the risks associated with these viral infections (Ronald *et al.*, 2023). The presence of certain serologic markers is very important for both diagnosing and treating viral hepatitis. For example, the detection of hepatitis B surface antigen (HBsAg) indicates an active HBV infection, while anti-HCV antibodies signify exposure to HCV. In the case of HAV and HEV, the presence of specific IgM antibodies can confirm acute infection (Figure 2.3).

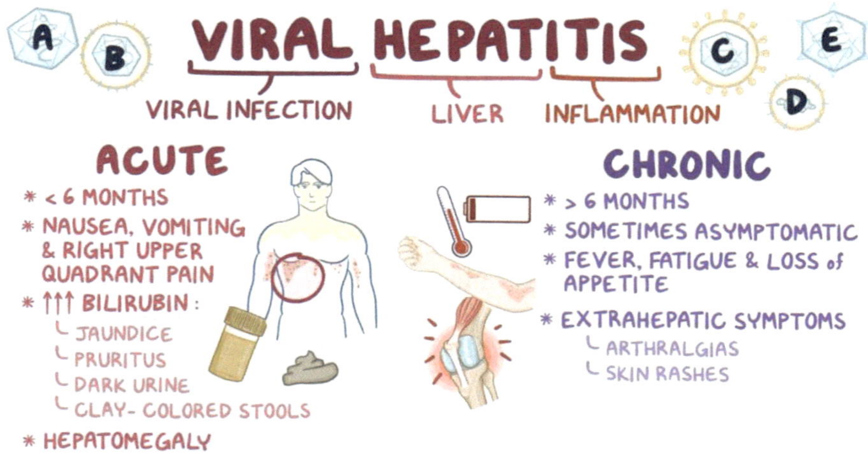

Figure 2.3. Viral hepatitis.

Source: https://enabilityot.com/wp-content/uploads/2023/07/unnamed-file.jpeg.

The distinction between acute and chronic infections is of greatest importance in determining regimens of treatment and in determining the prognosis of the disease. Furthermore, serial monitoring of these markers enables clinicians to determine response to treatment and recognize the need for continued patient management. Through proper serologic testing, clinicians can safely steer patients through their disease process, thereby enhancing health outcomes and potentially curbing transmission of these viruses in vulnerable populations (Ronald *et al.*, 2023). Prevention of viral hepatitis is done through a broad array of strategies depending on the virus. Prevention of hepatitis A and B can be done through vaccination, which drastically reduces the incidence of infection with these viruses.

Public health programs, including safe injection and screening of blood and organ donors, contribute importantly to curtailing transmission of HAV, HBV, and HCV. Inducement of safe sex also prevents HBV and HCV transmission. Prevention of HEV, which takes place mainly in areas of poor sanitation, requires the enhancement of access to clean water and sanitation education. Prevention of HBV through vaccination is the main prevention strategy for hepatitis D, a reflection of the interdependence of the viruses. A multi-faceted approach, involving vaccination, education, and screening, is necessary in effectively tackling the burden of viral hepatitis in the world (Kayesh *et al.*, 2022).

2.1.2. Non-Viral Hepatitis (Alcoholic, Autoimmune, Drug-Induced)

The realm of non-viral hepatitis encompasses a variety of conditions, including alcoholic hepatitis, autoimmune hepatitis (AIH), and drug-induced liver injury (DILI), each presenting distinct pathophysiological mechanisms and clinical implications. Too much alcohol causes alcoholic hepatitis, which leads to inflammation and the death of liver cells. If the liver is damaged, it may develop fibrosis and cirrhosis in people who have risk factors such as genetics, malnutrition, and other liver diseases. It is essential to diagnose and treat liver disease early to stop acute-on-chronic liver failure from happening. It is also often challenging for doctors to tell alcoholic hepatitis apart from other liver diseases, which calls for thorough checks of a patient's medical history and how their liver is functioning. AIH is a kind of non-viral hepatitis, where the immune system attacks the liver cells by mistake. Some patients can be asymptomatic for a long time, but then suddenly develop jaundice and other signs of liver problems, which is described in several clinical reports. The identification of specific autoantibodies, such as antinuclear antibodies (ANA) and anti-smooth muscle antibodies (SMA), is vital in establishing a diagnosis. Delayed treatment can precipitate life-threatening complications, including cirrhosis and acute liver failure (ALF), underscoring the importance of early recognition and the initiation of corticosteroid therapy to mitigate inflammatory damage. As the diagnosis relies significantly on the exclusion of other CLD etiologies, thorough clinical assessments remain paramount in managing AIH effectively (Hernández *et al.*, 2024). Patients on anti-tuberculosis medications, especially in DILI, are at a major risk during their therapy. The occurrence of DILI shows that healthcare staff must be attentive, knowing the signs and risk factors for drug-related liver problems. Recommendations from recent guidelines underscore the necessity for precise baseline testing, periodic liver function monitoring, and the avoidance of re-exposure to identified hepatotoxic agents (Abdyazdani *et al.*, 2024). Because of these practices, any DILI symptoms are identified early, which can help prevent serious liver problems or failure. Given the complexity of diagnosing DILI amid polypharmacy, a careful and systematic approach is essential to improve patient outcomes in those at risk (Figure 2.4).

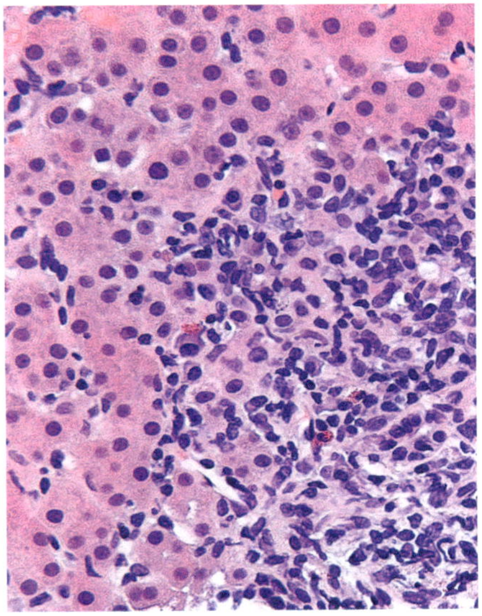

Figure 2.4. Very high magnification micrograph of autoimmune hepatitis.

Source: https://upload.wikimedia.org/wikipedia/commons/thumb/0/0c/Autoimmune_hepatitis_-_cropped_-_very_high_mag.jpg/800px-Autoimmune_hepatitis_-_cropped_-_very_high_mag.jpg.

2.1.3. Comparison of Acute vs. Chronic Hepatitis

The comparison between acute and chronic hepatitis is crucial to an appreciation of how liver disease progresses. Acute hepatitis, caused most frequently by viral infection such as hepatitis A or B, arrives abruptly with jaundice, fatigue, and nausea, normally resolving within six months. The body's immune response effectively eliminates the virus in most instances, re-establishing liver health and function. Conversely, chronic hepatitis is more than six months in duration and could lead to serious complications, including cirrhosis and HCC. Chronic viral hepatitis, especially hepatitis B and C, could be asymptomatic for years while causing irreversible liver damage, and therefore, early detection and treatment become challenging. This critical distinction helps direct treatment planning, since treatment for acute hepatitis is very different from that required for chronic infection, where ongoing follow-up and therapy are required to minimize complications and maintain liver function. Chronic hepatitis constitutes a significant public health concern due to its long-term impact and higher morbidity rates compared to acute infection. Pathologic mechanisms of chronic hepatitis involve a repeated cycle of liver cell injury and regeneration, leading to fibrosis and ultimately liver failure. Unlike acute hepatitis, where recovery is often achievable, chronic hepatitis can lead to irreversible damage, necessitating strict observation in patient management and treatment. Modern medical practice relies significantly on regular screening and early intervention methods for high-risk populations, particularly in the presence of an underlying illness such as alcohol liver disease or co-infection with other viral infections. This is supported by the aggressive approach advocated by the American Association for the Study of Liver Diseases, which adheres to total care paradigms for not only treating the virus but also comorbidities associated with the virus and patient education regarding lifestyle modifications to improve outcomes (Northup *et al.*, 2020). In treating acute and chronic hepatitis, there is a distinct difference in treatment approaches. Acute hepatitis is largely reliant on supportive care and symptom management because the majority of patients recover spontaneously through the body's immune mechanisms. Chronic hepatitis is more complex in treatment protocols, normally with antiviral medications to inhibit viral replication and prevent further liver damage. This may be in the long term with DAA in Hepatitis C or nucleoside analogues in Hepatitis B, showing the trend in the current treatment in this field. Besides, patients with chronic hepatitis must be regularly assessed to monitor liver function and for screening of HCC, given the increased risk owing to chronic infection. This wide management program underlines the heterogeneity in the course of the disease and the requirement for individualized strategies in the continuum of care for hepatitis (Crabb *et al.*, 2019) (Table 2.1).

Table 2.1. Acute vs. Chronic Hepatitis

	Acute	Chronic
Duration	< 6 months	> 6 months
Outcome of immune activities	Clearance	Not able to clear
Age at highest predisposition	Infection at adulthood	Infection in childhood
Presentation	More dramatic	Less dramatic – unless complicated

Source: https://i.ytimg.com/vi/lHw2cwkDeMw/maxresdefault.jpg?sqp=-oaymwEmCIAKENAF8quKqQMa8AEB-AHUBoAC4AOKAgwIABABGDsgTih_MA8=&rs=AOn4CLCywMj_Me1l9idIAzsDPweG_OlX-Q.

2.2. Causes and Risk Factors

There are many factors that can lead to hepatitis, acute or chronic, and these are not the same for every type of viral hepatitis. The main source of acute hepatitis is usually Hepatitis A and E viruses, which are spread by contaminated food and water. Unlike Hepatitis B and C, which are mainly spread by blood or bodily fluids, Hepatitis A is usually acquired through contaminated food or water. Some demographic traits, for example, age and social class, can increase a person's risk. For example, living in areas with poor sanitation increases the chance of getting hepatitis A and E, and intravenous drug use or unsafe sex can cause Hepatitis B and C. Public health efforts to stop outbreaks and reduce transmission rely on knowing these causes. Certain risk factors can increase the seriousness of hepatitis infections, which are caused by individual factors. Among all these factors, drinking alcohol is a major cause of liver disease worsening. In patients with Hepatitis B, studies have shown that alcoholic behaviour correlates with the likelihood of developing acute-on-chronic liver failure, a condition with high morbidity and mortality rates (Zhang *et al.*, 2022). Also, diabetes, obesity, and fatty liver disease can make the condition more difficult to manage. They raise the chance of infection and also make it harder to treat and recover from the infection. For this reason, spotting high-risk groups and teaching them about possible risks can be very important for controlling the disease and improving health outcomes. Besides, because the population is aging, there are now new difficulties in handling hepatitis. As the population ages, the prevalence of comorbidities such as obesity and CLD is likely to rise, which can leave individuals more susceptible to severe forms of hepatitis E and its complications (Fang *et al.*, 2022). Aging and existing liver problems often cause people to be hospitalized more often and to stay sick for a longer time. So, by identifying these high-risk groups, healthcare providers can plan customized screening and intervention plans. Managing both acute and chronic hepatitis requires dealing with the causes and risk factors to improve prevention and health results for people affected by the disease.

2.2.1. Transmission Methods for Viral Hepatitis

Understanding the various modes of transmission of viral hepatitis is crucial in planning effective public health interventions. Hepatitis A (HAV) and hepatitis E (HEV) are primarily spread by the fecal-oral route from contaminated food and drinking water supplies. These viruses pose a high risk in areas without adequate sanitation and hygiene measures, particularly among the poor. There has been a significant link established between unsanitary conditions and HAV and HEV outbreaks, which highlights the need to enhance hygiene levels within communities to reduce the risk of transmission. Furthermore, HEV is also transmitted via blood transfusion, particularly in immunocompromised patients, emphasizing a double challenge associated with its transmission, for instance, in prevalence studies that require screening of blood donors for HEV RNA to safeguard blood supplies (Niederhauser *et al.*, 2024). Hepatitis B (HBV) and hepatitis C (HCV) are primarily disseminated via parenteral transmission and sexual activity. These types of hepatitis are usually related to chronic infection that may lead to severe liver diseases, e.g., cirrhosis and HCC. Behavioural risk factors like unsafe sex and intravenous needle sharing between drug abusers are also important in spreading these viruses. The seroprevalence surveys of specific groups have shown that elderly individuals and men are disproportionately infected with HCV and HBV, typically because of higher rates of exposure among these age groups. Solutions to these patterns of transmission call for targeted interventions, such as harm reduction programs and education, to reduce levels of high-risk behaviours for transmission of viral hepatitis (Schaer *et al.*, 2022). Prevention of transmission of viral hepatitis requires a multifaceted process with particular emphasis on vaccination against preventable forms and behaviour change among those at risk of exposure to risk factors for HBV and HCV. The production of hepatitis A and B vaccines has played a crucial role in reducing incidence rates, particularly among vulnerable groups. Furthermore, ensuring safe practices in healthcare facilities and among susceptible groups has the potential to stem the tide of parenterally transmitted hepatitis virus strains. Concurrently, the screening and treatment availability for infected individuals, particularly in light of the chronic nature of HBV and HCV, needs to be improved. Through public health sector collaboration as well as collaboration between public health sectors and community organizations, it is possible to introduce total strategies to decrease infection rates and eventually relieve the public health burden of viral hepatitis (Niederhauser *et al.*, 2024; Schaer *et al.*, 2022) (Figure 2.5).

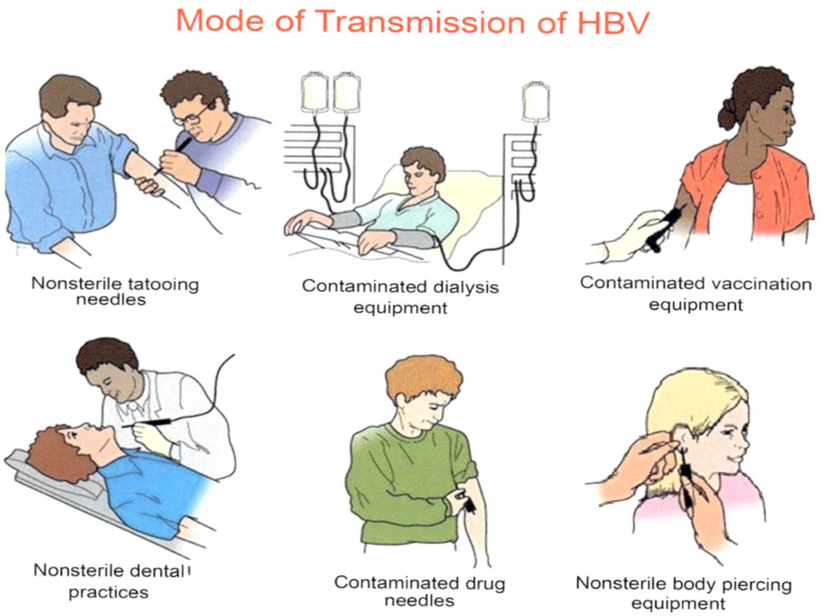

Figure 2.5. Modes of transmission of hepatitis B.

Source: https://medicoinfo.org/wp-content/uploads/2018/12/Medicoinfo.in-Hepatitis-B-3-virus.jpg.

2.2.2. Lifestyle Factors Contributing to Non-Viral Hepatitis

Non-viral hepatitis, which often occurs due to lifestyle choices, shows that what we do can influence our liver health. Alcohol consumption stands out as a primary contributor to alcoholic liver disease (ALD), which presents a spectrum from simple fatty liver to severe liver cirrhosis (LC). Drinking a lot over a long period causes liver inflammation and damage, which can lead to alcoholic hepatitis and might result in cirrhosis if not treated. It shows that knowing how alcohol impacts the liver and using preventive methods to reduce alcohol intake is very important. Intervening in drinking behaviours not only helps mitigate liver-related health issues but also emphasizes broader public health issues surrounding alcohol usage and its societal implications, as highlighted in recent guidelines that recommend comprehensive screening for alcohol use (Bourgonje *et al.*, 2020). Liver health is strongly affected by what you eat, and a poor diet can result in non-viral hepatitis. High-calorie diets, particularly those rich in sugar and unhealthy fats, are associated with non-alcoholic fatty liver disease (NAFLD), which can progress to non-alcoholic steatohepatitis (NASH). Such conditions may cause severe scarring and liver problems as time goes on. Besides controlling calorie intake, the balance of carbohydrates, fats, and proteins in one's diet has been linked to liver health. For example, a diet high in fructose can cause more fat to build up in the liver, which shows how what you eat can affect liver disease. As the prevalence of obesity rises, addressing dietary habits becomes imperative for reducing the incidence of non-viral hepatitis and ensuring better clinical outcomes (Bourgonje *et al.*, 2020). Also, not being physically active and having metabolic syndrome can greatly increase the risk of getting non-viral hepatitis. A lack of physical activity encourages obesity, IR, and inflammation of the liver. Metabolic syndrome, which involves central obesity, problems with blood lipids, high blood pressure, and high blood sugar, is now known to be a major risk factor for NAFLD and NASH. How much you exercise affects your liver; regular exercise helps you lose weight and keep your metabolism in check, which decreases fat in your liver. With more evidence showing the advantages of staying active, encouraging people to exercise can be very important for preventing and managing liver disease in those at risk. Consequently, addressing these lifestyle factors through comprehensive health strategies is essential for mitigating the global burden of non-viral hepatitis (Crabb *et al.*, 2019).

2.2.3. Genetic Predispositions and Environmental Influences

The synergy between genetic susceptibility and environment is central to the aetiology of hepatitis, acute or chronic. Genes determine an individual's susceptibility to viral infections, such as hepatitis B and C, which are major causes of chronic hepatitis. Specific alleles can enhance or reduce the immune response to the infections, determining the severity and outcome of the disease. Furthermore, some genetic variants are associated with individuals who have different reactions to viral antigens, which affect the probability of developing CLD. Therefore, knowledge of these genetic factors helps us understand why some people are likely to experience worse manifestations of hepatitis, while others are asymptomatic. Apart from genetic predispositions, environmental influences play a strong role in hepatitis outcomes. Socioeconomic status, hygiene conditions, and access to healthcare are critical factors in exposure to the virus as well as the availability of treatment. For example, communities living in areas with inferior sanitation conditions are likely to face hepatitis A infection as a result of contaminated water sources, while those living under inferior healthcare access conditions are likely to experience late detection of chronic hepatitis, worsening their condition. In addition, behaviours in life such as drinking and illicit drug use can interrupt genetic vulnerabilities, so that one is more susceptible to developing advanced liver disease. Therefore, both the environment and genetics need to be considered in order to understand the epidemiology of hepatitis. Research indicates that increasing rates of disease are frequently the result of external factors rather than purely heritable traits. As an example, the rising prevalence of atopic disorders in industrialized nations demonstrates how environmental components, including diet alteration and urbanization, lead to augmented expression of disease. Consistent with this is the appreciation that hepatitis-related disorders may also result through interactions between environmental elements and inherited tendencies. The explosive rise in the incidence of hepatitis over the last decades can in part be explained by changes in lifestyle and access to healthcare, underlining the necessity for employing a multidisciplinary approach in the prevention and control of disease. From both genetic predispositions and environment, healthcare workers can devise holistic approaches geared toward reducing the number of cases and improving the management of hepatitis cases effectively (Figure 2.6).

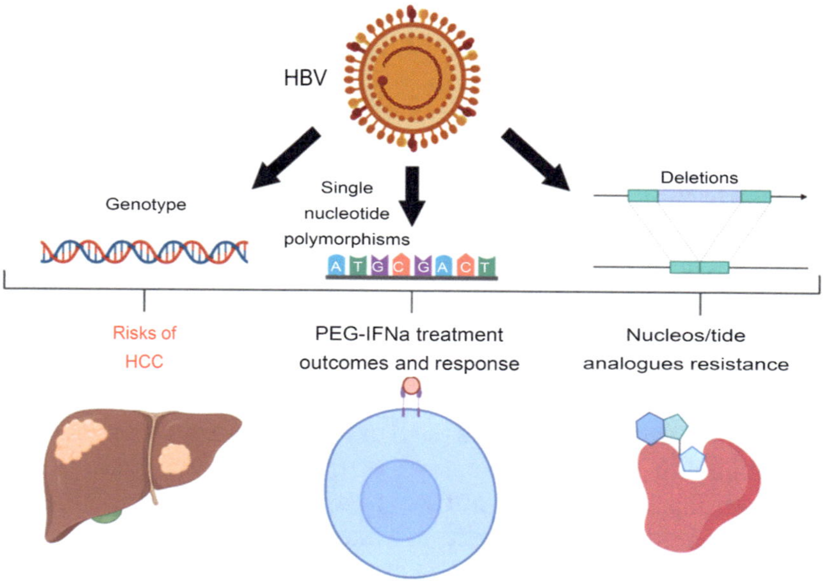

Figure 2.6. Impacts of hepatitis B virus (HBV) genetic variants including genotype, single nucleotide polymorphisms, and deletions of genetic regions.

Source: https://www.researchgate.net/publication/344613073/figure/fig2/AS:11431281387855893@1745141375186/Impacts-of-Hepatitis-B-Virus-HBV-genetic-variants-including-genotype-single-nucleotide.tif.

2.3. Symptoms and Diagnosis

Identifying hepatitis symptoms early is very important for proper diagnosis and care of acute or chronic cases. Patients with acute hepatitis B usually have jaundice, decreased appetite, abdominal pain, nausea, and vomiting. Most of these symptoms are caused by the liver's inflammation, which happens as the body responds to HBV infection. Severe cases may cause ALF, which is a condition where the liver quickly fails, and the chances of survival are very low if not treated promptly. Healthcare providers must remain vigilant in identifying these signs, as the mortality rate for patients with ALF due to hepatitis B can reach alarming levels within just weeks of hospitalization, emphasizing the urgency of early, accurate diagnosis and management strategies, as indicated by the salient symptoms (Antari *et al.*, 2025). Chronic hepatitis usually does not cause serious symptoms until years have passed, and these symptoms are often not noticed. In AIH and PBC, the first symptoms are usually fatigue, weight loss, and a general feeling of not being well, which makes it hard to detect the diseases early. Due to the similar symptoms, it is sometimes hard to tell these diseases apart, so a thorough examination, including tests for specific antibodies and LFTs, is needed. The overlap syndrome (OS) predominantly features elevated serum transaminases and detectable autoantibodies, complicating the clinical picture. It underscores the importance of considering differential diagnoses when evaluating patients with suspected liver disease to facilitate early intervention and improve prognostic outcomes (Barbosa *et al.*, 2024). To make a definite diagnosis of hepatitis, imaging studies and liver biopsies are critical. Imaging modalities, including ultrasonography and computed tomography (CT), can reveal important structural changes in the liver, such as cirrhosis or biliary obstruction. Additionally, a liver biopsy (LBx) remains a gold standard for assessing the degree of liver damage and differentiating between various liver diseases, including hepatitis types and conditions like OS. If a patient has high transaminase levels and typical symptoms, an LBx may show important changes in the liver and help decide on the treatment. With advancements in diagnostic techniques and a greater understanding of the pathophysiology of liver diseases, healthcare providers are poised to make informed decisions that enhance patient outcomes and decrease morbidity associated with both acute and chronic hepatitis (Antari *et al.*, 2025; Barbosa *et al.*, 2024).

2.3.1. Common Symptoms of Acute Hepatitis

Acute hepatitis is characterized by a collection of symptoms that occur as a result of liver inflammation. They typically begin with malaise and fatigue, which may be felt in the form of general ill health that significantly impacts daily functioning. These typically begin at various times in various patients, with some having an acute onset of discomfort while others develop insidious onset over several days. Jaundice, where the skin and eyes turn yellow, also occurs due to decreased liver function, which permits the accumulation of bilirubin in the blood. Jaundice is a critical indicator that the liver is stressed, and its onset often convinces individuals to visit doctors. Recognition of these symptoms is important to aid in early diagnosis and treatment since they can be associated with a range of conditions that are characterized by acute hepatitis. Acute hepatitis patients also often present with symptoms that affect the gut, such as loss of appetite, nausea, and vomiting. These contribute to the development of malnutrition, thereby complicating the patient's condition. Particularly, the anorexia can be troublesome since it will exacerbate malaise and fatigue, setting a vicious circle that will not allow recovery. Also, abdominal pain and discomfort can be related to these gastrointestinal symptoms, typically in the right upper quadrant where the liver lies. Such discomfort may be of variable intensity and could mimic other intra-abdominal diseases, so diagnosis is rendered more difficult. It is of great significance that healthcare providers can differentiate these presentations from those of other gastrointestinal diseases in a way that ensures proper management and suitable treatment measures are taken. With the recognition of these signs, physicians can better treat the multifaceted nature of acute hepatitis. In certain cases, acute hepatitis can result in more severe complications, such as ALF, which presents unexpectedly and requires immediate medical intervention. Confusion, disorientation, and reduced level of consciousness are symptoms that have the potential to point towards declining liver function and the potential for hepatic encephalopathy (HE). The neuropsychiatric symptoms are observed as the toxins in the blood build up due to the failure of the liver to remove them efficiently. Abnormalities in coagulation with the risk of bleeding and bruising can also be felt by the patients. Identification of the transition from mild to severe complications is very important because, with timely intervention, the outcome might dramatically change. The complex interaction of symptoms of acute hepatitis emphasizes the importance of extensive evaluation and management strategies in clinical practice. Hence, a proper understanding of these symptoms in a careful manner is necessary for health care workers as well as patients for proper management of the disease course (Figure 2.7).

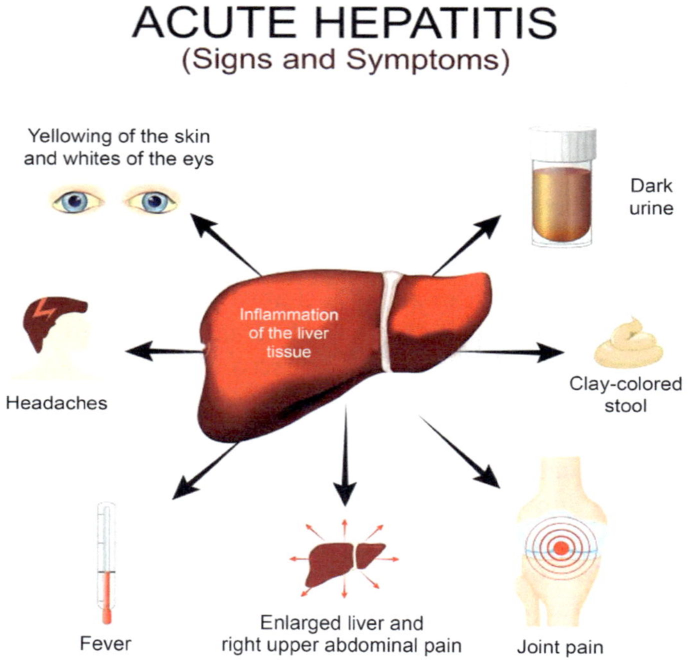

Figure 2.7. Acute hepatitis signs and symptoms.

Source: https://www.shutterstock.com/image-vector/acute-hepatitis-signs-symptoms-viral-260nw-2406270231.jpg.

2.3.2. Symptoms of Chronic Hepatitis and Their Progression

Symptoms of chronic hepatitis usually develop slowly which makes it hard to diagnose early. Patients might first feel tired, unwell and have a vague pain in the abdomen which could be mistaken for other common, harmless conditions. When the disease gets worse, jaundice, dark urine and pale stools can appear which point to problems with the liver. Additionally, patients may present with itching (pruritus) due to the accumulation of bile salts in the bloodstream. Although some people do not show symptoms for a long time, untreated chronic hepatitis can eventually cause cirrhosis and liver failure. Being careful to notice these milder early symptoms plays a key role in helping healthcare providers intervene early which could change the course of the disease. How chronic hepatitis develops depends a lot on the cause and viral hepatitis B and C are often involved. Infection that lasts for a long time usually causes inflammation and scarring in the liver which may result in cirrhosis. In patients suffering from chronic hepatitis, significant liver deterioration can result in acute exacerbations that manifest as severe acute exacerbation (SAE). Independent risk factors such as LC and low levels of alanine aminotransferase (ALT) have been identified as primary contributors to this deterioration, indicating a need for tailored monitoring and management strategies (Yuan *et al.*, 2019) (Figure 2.8).

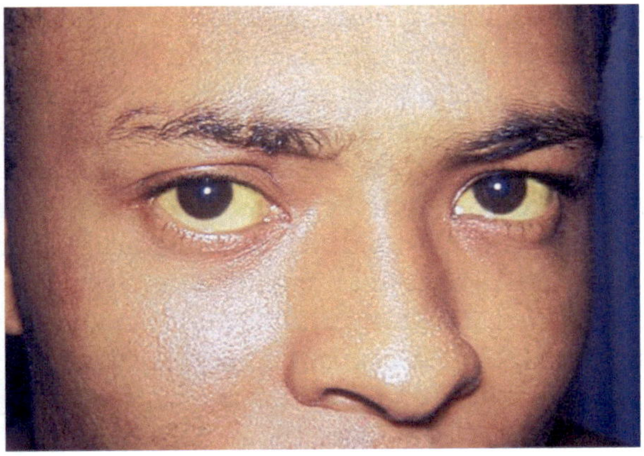

Figure 2.8. Jaundiced eyes.

Source: https://upload.wikimedia.org/wikipedia/commons/d/de/Jaundice_eye.jpg.

With deteriorating liver function, the patients become prone to developing acute-on-chronic liver failure, a significant reason for heightened morbidity and mortality. Thus, awareness about risk factors responsible for disease progression becomes essential for better patient outcomes. In the clinic, the management of chronic hepatitis calls for ongoing surveillance and a flexible therapeutic strategy, especially with alterations in symptoms. Patients presenting signs of liver decompensation require immediate therapeutic intervention to prevent further damage and acute deterioration. The evidence shows that a significant percentage of patients do not receive appropriate care, which denies them the necessary treatment (Ylli *et al.*, 2023). Identifying patients at risk of disease progression using clinical assessment and laboratory investigations becomes crucial to provide maximal care. There is a need for continuous investigation into the symptomatology and progression of chronic hepatitis, as this will help develop better clinical guidelines. This greater insight will ultimately help healthcare providers deliver effective and proactive treatment for individuals grappling with the challenges posed by chronic hepatitis (Figure 2.9).

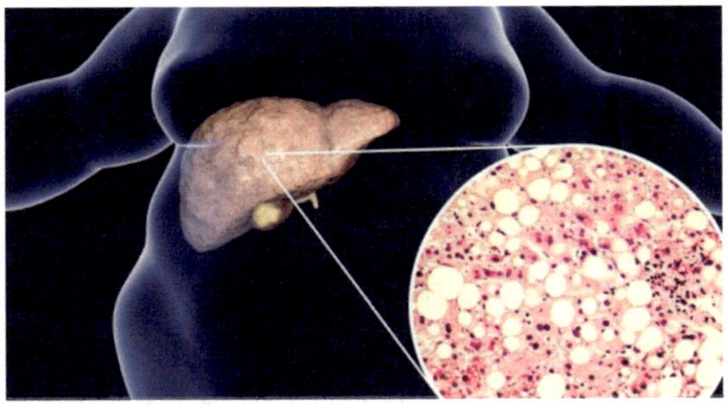

Figure 2.9. Chronic hepatitis

Source: https://media.post.rvohealth.io/wp-content/uploads/sites/3/2020/01/327062_2200-1200x628.jpg.

2.3.3. Diagnostic Tests and Procedures

Correct diagnosis of acute and chronic hepatitis is highly dependent on various diagnostic tests and procedures that yield essential information regarding the condition's etiology, course, and possible complications. The first stage usually includes serological testing to identify particular antibodies and antigens associated with the hepatitis viruses (A, B, C, D, and E). For instance, the presence of antibodies to HBsAg is proof of active infection, whereas the presence of antibodies to the hepatitis C virus (anti-HCV) could signify either current or past infection. Serological markers are monitored by clinicians to ascertain the cause of the hepatitis and to dictate future management strategies, illustrating the importance of early diagnosis in preventing the spread of the disease and enabling early intervention (Ancarani *et al.*, 2006). Following serological testing, molecular diagnostic tests such as polymerase chain reaction (PCR) are employed to quantify viral load and assess active viral particle replication. This is particularly important in hepatitis C since the degree of HCV RNA determines the risk of chronic infection and the potential for guiding therapy. Because the natural course of hepatitis infections is so unpredictable from person to person, it is important to obtain these quantitative estimates. In acute hepatitis C, research indicates that many patients may observe spontaneous clearance within three months. Thus, serial HCV RNA monitoring over this duration can advise clinicians whether or not emergency antiviral therapy is necessary or whether a conservative approach is best (Ancarani *et al.*, 2006). Other than serological and molecular tests, imaging examinations such as ultrasound may also be utilized in order to evaluate the structural integrity of the liver and scan for complications like cirrhosis or HCC. In children, where presentation of liver ailments is typically nondescript, imaging is even more important in order to provide an appropriate diagnosis. Advances in imaging technology have enhanced the detection of hepatic pathology, facilitating earlier diagnosis and better management outcomes for hepatitis-related disorders. Interplay between diagnostics from laboratory tests and imaging technology culminates in an efficient holistic strategy in treating liver disease, underscoring the complexity of hepatitis as a public health problem (Figure 2.10).

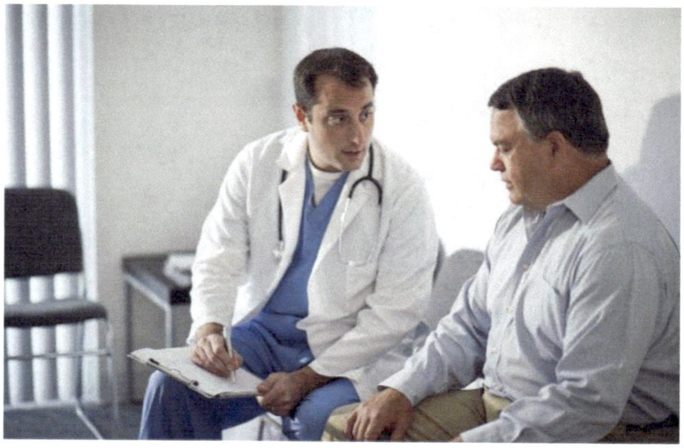

Figure 2.10. Diagnostic Tests and Procedures

Source: https://www.verywellhealth.com/thmb/XKk3YsotZz9uqKrVG4qf4-quSDo=/1500x0/filters:no_upscale():max_bytes(150000):strip_icc()/109439697-56a6114b3df78cf7728b2ebc.jpg.

2.4. Treatment Options

It is essential to distinguish between acute and chronic hepatitis when planning how to treat the disease. For acute hepatitis, which can happen after Hepatitis A or B, most of the time, the immune system handles the infection, and care is mainly supportive. Treatment options may be rest, drinking water, and controlling symptoms like nausea and abdominal pain. In some severe cases, patients need to be hospitalized and closely monitored to handle complications. Chronic cases of hepatitis, mainly Hepatitis B and C, call for more treatment, including antiviral drugs to handle the infection and help protect the liver. It is very important to know how long these treatments work and how effective they are to avoid serious complications such as cirrhosis or liver failure. CHB causes many public health issues for people around the world, with almost 296 million affected. CHB does not have a cure now, but antiviral medicines have been shown to help control the virus. Long-term management typically involves the use of nucleos(t)ide analogues (NAs), which require lifelong, consistent adherence to prevent disease progression. Even though NAs do not often lead to HBsAg loss, some patients might be able to stop treatment if their HBsAg and HBV RNA levels are low. Even so, this way of treating addiction is not without controversy, and more research is required to develop clear rules for stopping treatment and managing possible relapses. This clarity is crucial, as emerging studies signal a variable response to relapse and treatment outcomes depending on the specific agent used in NA therapies, highlighting the need for individualized treatment plans (Korkmaz *et al.*, 2024). Moreover, the therapeutic landscape for chronic hepatitis is complicated by the risk factors contributing to LC, which often stem from various etiological factors like alcohol consumption, autoimmune diseases, and viral infections (Cioarca-Nedelcu *et al.*, 2024). Treatment should target the reason for liver damage and also look after the problems that come with advanced fibrosis or cirrhosis. It might require making lifestyle changes, using medicines, and, for severe cases, thinking about a liver transplant. It is essential to do detailed assessments and differentiate between conditions, especially when patients have portal hypertension, HE, or ascites. Handling these challenging factors can greatly affect how a patient feels and improve their chances of recovery, which highlights why a full treatment strategy is necessary in chronic hepatitis.

2.4.1. Antiviral Medications for Viral Hepatitis

The treatment setting for viral hepatitis has profoundly altered in the past two decades, with new antiviral drug developments being the prime mover. For hepatitis B, nucleos(t)ide analogues have become the first-line treatment for chronic infection. Entecavir and tenofovir are some of the antiviral drugs that are effective in reducing viral load and ultimately suppressing the course of liver disease. Periodic follow-up is also critical to evaluate the effectiveness of these treatments, as well as the formation of possible drug resistance. Based on recent studies, sustained viral suppression by these medications not only improves liver function but also slows down the formation of end-stage complications such as cirrhosis and liver carcinoma. The action of these medications highlights the importance of further research and development for hepatitis treatment. And yet another significant advance in the treatment of viral hepatitis has been the introduction of interferon therapies, including pegylated interferon alpha, that stimulate the immune system against the hepatitis virus. While this can be an effective intervention, it is typically also accompanied by a range of side effects and thus not ideal for all patients. However, pegylated interferon can produce a sustained virological response in a subset of patients, particularly those with hepatitis C. The choice between DAA drugs, which target specific stages in the virus's life cycle, and interferon-based therapy relies on many variables, including patient profile and viral genotype. The discovery of DAAs has revolutionized the therapy of hepatitis C to achieve high cure rates with fewer side effects, thus redefining hepatitis C patient clinical treatment (Alexander *et al.*, 2020). In addition to the standard antiviral therapies, the care of viral hepatitis is now shifting towards a more personalized approach. The age of patients, liver condition, and comorbidities are considered for formulating a treatment plan. New treatments are being studied, with a focus on maximizing cure rates and minimizing side effects. Those regulatory agencies have been active in approving new antiviral drugs, thus increasing the number of choices for care providers. With further research expanding the field, the pairing of new treatments with established treatment regimens could enhance patient outcomes and further decrease the global burden of viral hepatitis. Availability of such drugs is central to effective control, requiring persistent efforts towards improvement in screening and treatment among risk populations (Alexander *et al.*, 2020) (Figure 2.11).

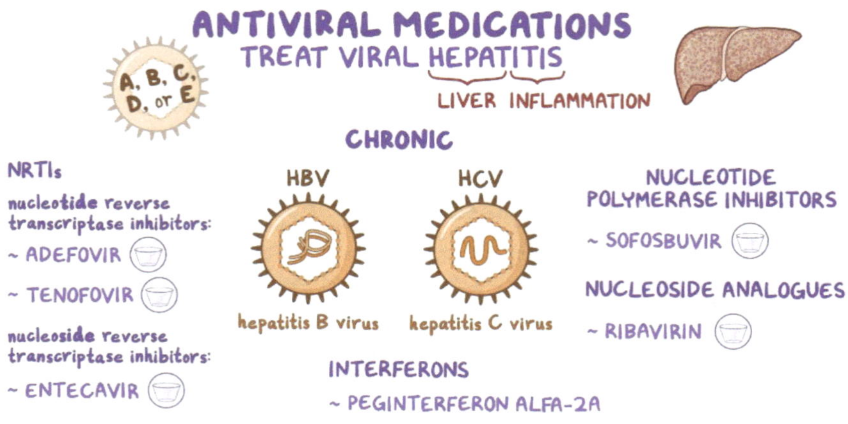

Figure 2.11. Antiviral medications.

Source: https://www.osmosis.org/_next/image?url=https%3A%2F%2Fd16qt3wv6xm098.cloudfront.net%2FVSgNPZVERKOzLWPMOitFYyKoTZajyYZI%2F_.jpg&w=3840&q=75.

2.4.2. Lifestyle Changes and Supportive Care for Non-Viral Hepatitis

People with non-viral hepatitis should change their lifestyle to protect their liver and manage the disease well. A key change is to eat a healthy diet full of nutrients that help your liver. Eating fruits and vegetables that contain antioxidants and drinking plenty of fluids can reduce inflammation in the liver and help you recover. It is also necessary to reduce alcohol and processed foods, since they can make liver damage worse and reduce how well treatment works. Staying active regularly can help circulation, support the immune system, and help control weight, which can prevent more liver problems. Making these changes together is very important for non-viral hepatitis patients to live healthily and protect their liver. Supportive care is just as important for non-viral hepatitis, since it supports a complete approach to treatment and recovery. Health professionals may suggest joining support groups and seeing a counselor, which can help a lot with the emotional side of chronic illness. Most patients feel anxiety, depression, or become isolated from others, so emotional support is very important for successful treatment. Monitoring and check-ups with healthcare providers help to notice any changes in the liver, symptoms, or general health. In addition, educational resources help patients learn more about what is happening with their health and the options for treatment. Being part of support groups can boost motivation and help people who have the same difficulties feel connected. All of these elements work together to give better support and lead to better long-term health. The use of new therapies, for example, stem cell treatment, is being introduced and developed in the management of hepatitis. Stem cell therapy shows great promise because it can repair damaged tissue and alter immune responses, which is very important for people with CLD. Even though studies are mostly about viral hepatitis, the positive outcomes in animals suggest that it might be useful for other forms of the disease too. At the same time as researchers try out various approaches, such as using autologous bone marrow-derived stem cells, it is important to strengthen positive lifestyle changes and care to make the treatment more effective. Paying attention to lifestyle and mental health will increase the chances of success with new treatments and will help manage non-viral hepatitis and improve the health of patients in many ways.

2.4.3. Emerging Therapies and Research Directions

Novel treatments and research directions for hepatitis, acute and chronic, continue to become more promising, with significant advances in understanding the inherent mechanisms of the disease. One of the primary areas of research is in pattern recognition receptors (PRRs), which are essential to the innate immune system. PRRs recognize pathogens and are central to inducing immune responses. The ongoing quest for mechanisms by which PRRs recognize viral components linked with hepatitis will eventually lead to novel therapies that enhance the host's innate defense against infection. Clarification of the structural features and signaling networks of various PRRs, as described in recent literature, has established new prospects for the targeting of immune-mediated pathways in hepatitis. Such promising findings highlight the prospects for leveraging natural immunity to optimize patient outcomes and effectively combat acute and chronic hepatitis (Li *et al.*, 2021).

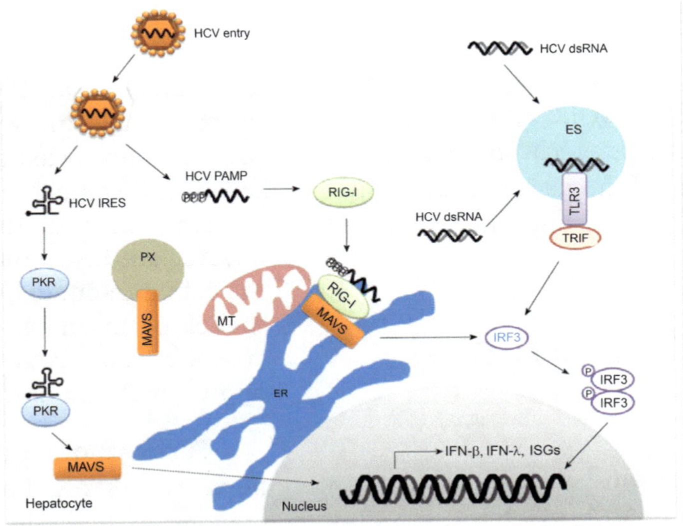

Figure 2.12. Immune sensing of hepatitis C virus by pattern recognition receptors.

Source: https://www.researchgate.net/profile/Darong-Yang/publication/274728054/figure/fig1/AS:567417999773696@1512294401716/mmune-sensing-of-hepatitis-C-virus-by-pattern-recognition-receptors-During-hepatitis-C.png.

The use of DAAs has transformed the therapy for hepatitis C, delivering outstanding cure rates with lower risks of side effects when compared to traditional drugs. Ongoing studies aim to expand the availability and efficacy of DAAs for the therapy of hepatitis B, a significant global health problem. Researchers are also exploring combination therapy with DAAs and immune-modulators to enhance the antiviral effect and eradicate chronic infection. The identification of new classes of antiviral compounds, together with the development of personalized medicine, promises to provide tailored therapy according to the unique patient's profile. This step towards precision therapy not only aligns with patient-centered care but also with the bigger trend in hepatitis research towards the discovery of the genetic and immunological determinants that govern response to therapy, paving the way for improved therapeutic strategies (Li *et al.*, 2021). Aside from pharmacological progress, recent studies indicate that prevention by vaccines could also unlock the potential for vaccine development to prevent not just acute but chronic hepatitis infections. New technologies, including mRNA technology, which are becoming frontline players during the COVID-19 pandemic, promise new avenues to find solutions for developing effective vaccines against hepatitis viruses. Research targets identifying antigenic targets that can elicit strong immunity, thereby facilitating early and long-term immunity in susceptible populations. Additionally, ongoing global surveillance of hepatitis virus mutations informs vaccine development and facilitates flexibility in an ever-changing viral landscape. This focus on vaccine manufacturing not only emphasizes prevention as imperative, but it is also synchronized with public health targets to reduce the occurrence of hepatitis infections worldwide. Through these synchronized research efforts, the future of hepatitis therapeutic interventions is brighter and more vibrant (Figure 2.12).

2.5. Complications of Hepatitis

The liver complications of hepatitis are a significant public health problem because long-term infections with chronic hepatitis can lead to severe liver injury. The most severe complication is the development of HCC, which is a major liver cancer that can occur in CHB or CHC-infected patients. Studies have established that individuals with elevated HBsAg levels have a significantly increased risk of tumor development. This correlation suggests the necessity for vigilant monitoring and intervention strategies for such patients to lower the risk of having HCC. The development of prognostic instruments, including nomograms to quantify recurrence risk in HCC patients, reflects the importance of ascertaining the impact of hepatitis in clinical practice. Thus, identification and response to the complications of hepatitis can improve patient outcomes and provide a foundation for more effective management.

Apart from assisting in liver cancer development, hepatitis may also result in cirrhosis, which is a complication involving permanent scarring of the liver. Cirrhosis is a consequence of chronic inflammation and damage to liver tissue caused by longstanding hepatitis infection. Complications such as portal hypertension, HE, and ascites are common among patients with cirrhosis. Such complications are of serious quality-of-life impact and may require other medical treatment, including potential liver transplantation. The impact of chronic hepatitis has also been exacerbated by concomitant overlapping health emergencies, for instance, the pandemic of COVID-19, which intervened in standard follow-up care and treatment protocols for a vast majority of patients. Under the circumstances of the stress on healthcare systems, the patients were at increased risk of adverse outcomes, and it was critical to maintain the commitment to hepatitis care. It is important that clinicians understand the pathways to these complications from hepatitis so that they can apply timely interventions.

Furthermore, the comorbidities caused by hepatitis extend beyond hepatic health and may have systemic effects. Chronic hepatitis infection patients can form comorbidities, including cardiovascular disease and metabolic syndrome, that bring a higher mortality risk. Pathophysiologic correlates of CLD with systemic complications validate the hypothesis that untreated hepatitis exerts complex effects on well-being. For instance, the chronic inflammation produced by hepatitis may contribute to elevating the risk of cardiovascular complications, and hence it is important to have integrated approaches to patient care. Ongoing screening and monitoring of liver status as well as other potential complications are vital to improving patient outcomes. Emphasis on the interconnected nature of these health issues will be a key feature of public health strategies to combat the impact of hepatitis on individual patients and society as a whole.

2.5.1. Chronic Hepatitis and Liver Damage

Chronic hepatitis is a major health problem worldwide because it can lead to serious damage to the liver. The disease usually starts without symptoms, and patients often do not realize they have it until their liver is seriously damaged. Severe liver infections with hepatitis B and C viruses can result in scarring of the liver (fibrosis), cirrhosis, and, in some cases, HCC. Because of constant inflammation and the death of liver cells, normal recovery processes are stopped, which makes liver damage worse over time. Early diagnosis and appropriate management strategies are crucial; without intervention, the likelihood of developing severe liver-related events increases, stressing the importance of continual monitoring for at-risk populations (Figure 2.13).

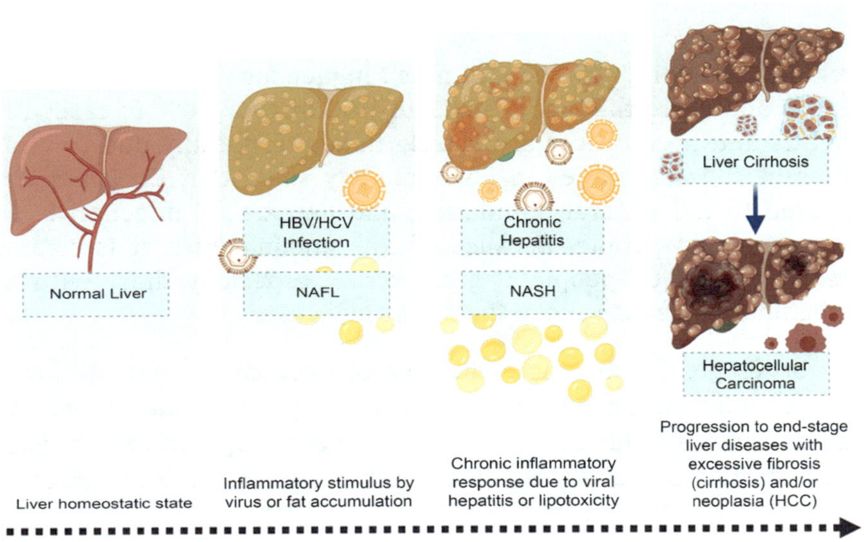

Figure 2.13. Clinicopathological stages of chronic liver diseases. The liver in its homeostatic state performs its normal physiological functions, which can be altered by viral infections with HBV or HCV and by the accumulation of fat (NAFL) due to systemic dysfunctions associated with different conditions such as diabetes and obesity. Non-resolution of viral infection leads to chronic hepatitis, and the continuous accumulation of fat in the liver increases the chances of developing NASH via lipotoxicity events.

Source: https://www.researchgate.net/publication/359020862/figure/fig1/AS:11431281177704124@1690569153861/Clinicopathological-stages-of-chronic-liver-diseases-The-liver-in-its-homeostatic-state.png.

New studies underscore the pivotal relationship between specific virological indicators and the evolution of liver disease in individuals with chronic hepatitis. For instance, in chronic HDV infection, indicators such as the extent of LC and patient age have been found to be significant predictors of liver pathology. The research indicates that patients with advanced cirrhosis possessed significantly low quantitative anti-HBc levels, thereby illustrating how certain immunological markers are able to reflect worsening liver function. With meticulous monitoring of such markers, clinicians can more accurately predict which patients are at greater risk of developing severe complications and hence apply timely interventions that could prevent the widespread liver damage from chronic hepatitis.

Complicated by co-infections and vulnerable patient populations, the treatment of chronic hepatitis is more difficult, particularly in vulnerable populations such as children and pregnant women. Hepatitis C, for example, can lead to extensive liver pathology and sequelae among these populations, but treatment guidelines are frequently limited and complex. The demand for careful monitoring and individually tailored treatment strategies is underscored by the risk of mother-to-infant transmission during pregnancy that may complicate both maternal and neonatal health outcomes. The evolving dynamic of hepatitis management must answer to the specific needs of such individuals, fostering systemic reform that extends accessibility and encourages early diagnosis and best management in an effort to avoid long-term effects of chronic liver damage.

2.5.2. Risk of Liver Cancer

The danger of liver cancer, mainly HCC, is still much higher for those who have chronic hepatitis infections. Hepatitis B and C are the main causes of HCC in over 90% of cases related to chronic liver disease. Hepatitis and liver cancer are closely linked, especially due to viral infections and cirrhosis from different causes. Studies in epidemiology show that CHB infection increases the risk by 15% compared to the general population, and hepatitis C infection is 18% higher than the 12% risk in non-infected people. Because of this unequal rate, it is clear that prevention and intervention should focus on people at greater risk, especially those with limited access to healthcare and screening, which can make liver cancer worse.

Alcohol use disorder greatly increases the risk of liver cancer, mainly for those who have chronic hepatitis infections. Among people in the LGBTQ community, there is a much higher rate of alcohol use disorder—about 25%, while the general population only has 16%. Hepatitis infections, together with the increased risk, increase the chances of liver cancer. Besides lifestyle, metabolic syndrome plays a role, and it affects 22% of LGBTQ individuals. Because of these many connected causes, it is necessary to use thorough screening tools and public health efforts that target all these risks. Strategies aimed at enhancing healthcare access and equity for underserved populations can play a pivotal role in mitigating liver cancer risks associated with hepatitis-related conditions (Figure 2.14).

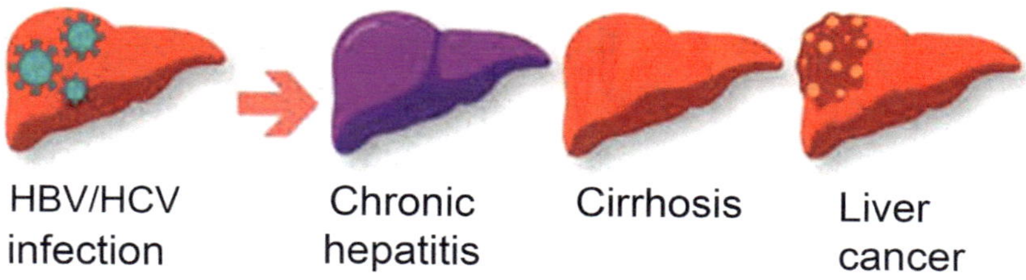

Figure 2.14. Hepatitis and liver cancer.

Source: https://encrypted-tbn0.gstatic.com/images?q=tbn:ANd9GcQDyV0udTAHiuYXM71V5yODoZHgQJ2Bag1oDg&s.

In addition to addressing the individual risk factors, systemic healthcare programs play a vital role in eradicating liver cancer disparities due to hepatitis. Current screening rates for liver cancer have been determined to be too low, particularly in underprivileged populations, at around 40% compared to the population rate of 60%. Stigma and discrimination act as barriers to early detection and treatment, highlighting the need for culturally sensitive healthcare practices. Targeted interventions such as the implementation of hepatitis B vaccination regimens and increased access to the treatment of hepatitis C are key interventions in primary and secondary prevention. Furthermore, awareness and education of risky populations about hepatitis-liver cancer associations can empower the individual to seek medical attention, ultimately aligning with the overall purpose of reducing liver cancer burdens attributed to hepatitis infections.

2.5.3. Impact on Overall Health

The impact of hepatitis on general health transcends the short-term aftermath of the virus, having a significant impact on the long-term health of infected persons. Chronic hepatitis infection can lead to serious complications, including cirrhosis and HCC, which severely cut life span and quality of life. In addition, most patients with hepatitis also have other ailments, including liver-related symptoms and systemic manifestations such as fatigue, depression, and anxiety. These comorbid illness issues are to blame for a poorer quality of life and increased healthcare costs. By means of research, integrating health care in the form of supportive health interventions like lifestyle modification and psychological therapy can fortify individuals against some of these adverse effects and improve their overall health profile in the case of hepatitis-related issues. Thus, acknowledging and addressing the complicated impact of hepatitis on health is crucial in designing whole-person care strategies.

The psychological impact of hepatitis cannot be downplayed since the diagnosis can cause intense emotional disturbance and anxiety in patients. The chronic nature of hepatitis predisposes individuals to experience feelings of isolation, anxiety, stigma, and uncertainty about the outcome of health, worsening mental disorders. Research underscores the significance of psychological support as an integral part of the regimen for patients with hepatitis. Mental health service integration has the potential to improve treatment adherence, thus overall health outcomes. Furthermore, patients with fewer symptoms of psychological distress are linked with greater health-related quality of life. Accordingly, attempts to provide mental health services in addition to medical care for hepatitis should be prioritized because they are a key element in decreasing the overall burden of the disease. It highlights the need for end-to-end health care strategies that focus on the physical and mental health of hepatitis patients.

In understanding the social determinants of health for hepatitis, it is obvious that socioeconomic status has a role in dictating the health outcomes of those infected. The areas with less healthcare access have higher rates of untreated infection for hepatitis, which then correlates to higher health burdens overall. Inadequate insurance, low health literacy, and limited healthcare facilities are among the obstacles to early diagnosis and treatment. Public health interventions for improving access to screening and healthcare can bridge these gaps and reduce the incidence of advanced liver diseases to a large extent. Greater knowledge and awareness regarding hepatitis are also essential in promoting preventive methods and beginning early interventions. Engaging communities in activities that improve health can help individuals become health-oriented and reverse the effects of hepatitis on their overall well-being. These social determinants need to be addressed in order to create a healthier future for patients with hepatitis.

2.6. Prevention Strategies

Preventing hepatitis, whether acute or chronic, involves efforts from public health and changes in individual behaviour. Having a vaccination is one of the best methods to prevent hepatitis A and B, which can cause serious health problems if caught. A lot of these infections have become much less common in different populations because of universal vaccination. Also, public health initiatives that explain the need for vaccinations encourage more people to join the effort. By focusing efforts on educative measures, health authorities can encourage high-risk groups, such as travelers and healthcare workers (HCWs), to receive the hepatitis vaccines, thereby decreasing the overall disease burden. Apart from vaccination, using safe injection methods and having effective blood screening are key to stopping hepatitis B and C. Since blood and needles are common ways for these viruses to spread, making sure blood donation is well-regulated and harm reduction is promoted among people at risk is very important. Both needle exchange programs and supervised injection sites have helped lower the spread of hepatitis among intravenous drug users. These interventions not only provide immediate protection against infection but also serve as entry points for individuals to access treatment and addiction services, thus promoting overall health in vulnerable communities (Shahini *et al.*, 2024). It is also crucial to educate people about safe ways to have sex to reduce the risk of hepatitis. People can contract hepatitis B and C during sexual contact, which makes it necessary to teach sexual health education that highlights the use of protection and the risks related to having sex with several partners. When hepatitis prevention is taught with sexual health, it can support openness about safe behaviours and reduce the stigma associated with hepatitis. Moreover, regular testing for sexually transmitted infections (STIs) can facilitate early detection of hepatitis infections, allowing for timely intervention and management. By creating an informed populace, the spread of hepatitis can be curtailed, ultimately contributing to the alleviation of this global health issue (Shahini *et al.*, 2024).

2.6.1. Vaccination for Hepatitis A and B

Vaccination is very important for stopping hepatitis A and B, which are serious health problems worldwide. Most cases of HAV occur when water or food is contaminated by fecal matter, which is the main way HAV is spread. People who are at risk, such as travelers to areas where hepatitis A is common, those in contact with infected people, and those with CLD, should be vaccinated. Studies have proven that the hepatitis A vaccine works well, giving most people lasting immunity, which makes it very useful for public health. In places where hepatitis A is widespread, vaccination efforts can cut down on outbreaks and improve the health of the community, which can also reduce expenses for treating acute hepatitis A and its complications. Unlike HCV, HBV can cause CLD, including cirrhosis and liver cancer, which adds to the challenge. Because of the hepatitis B vaccine, the number of new infections has gone down significantly across the globe, mainly among infants and health care workers. Research indicates that vaccination has significantly decreased mortality rates associated with HBV-related liver diseases, which account for a substantial proportion of global deaths annually (Danpanichkul *et al.*, 2025). Vaccinating newborns, children, and those at high risk is very important for stopping the spread of HBV. If all governments use universal vaccination, they can fight the hidden hepatitis B epidemic and greatly reduce the number of cases of liver disease. It is also essential to keep checking and evaluating hepatitis B vaccines after they are given. Studies have shown that while many HCWs develop adequate immune responses post-vaccination, booster doses may be necessary to maintain protective antibody levels, especially in older individuals and those who received their vaccinations many years prior (Alkhaldi *et al.*, 2024). Also, it is important to ensure that HCWs are well vaccinated, not only for their safety but also to prevent patients from getting HBV in hospitals and clinics. As such, public health initiatives should emphasize the importance of vaccination coupled with robust educational strategies to inform at-risk populations about the necessity of timely vaccinations and potential booster shots to prevent both acute and chronic hepatitis infections effectively (Figure 2.15).

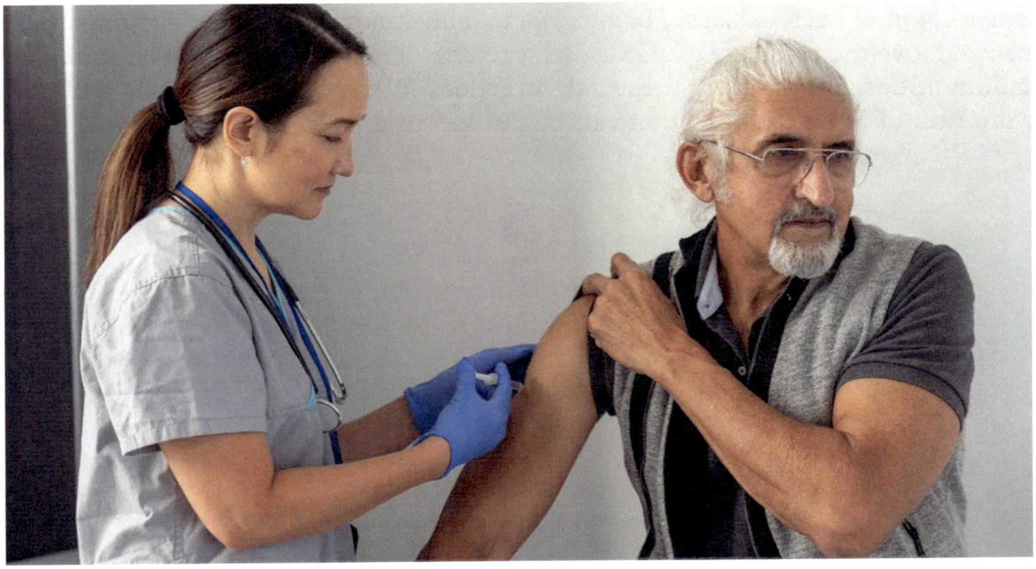

Figure 2.15. Hepatitis B vaccination.

Source: https://www.cdc.gov/hepatitis-b/media/images/2024/04/hepatitis-b-vaccination-thumbnail.jpg.

2.6.2. Safe Practices to Reduce Transmission

The transmission of Hepatitis viruses, particularly Hepatitis B and E, can be greatly avoided by adopting safe practices in various fields, including health care, food safety, and community mobilization. In the health care system, the use of gloves, sterilization of instruments, and proper disposal of syringes are the most crucial standard precautions. Health workers must be educated to recognize high-risk circumstances, especially in dealing with blood and body fluids. In addition, although Hepatitis B is easily preventable by vaccination, screening of blood for donation is most vital, particularly in endemic regions. Studies indicate that preventive strategies such as the universal screening of blood donations for HEV RNA are crucial to avoid transmission of Hepatitis E, especially to immunocompromised individuals who are more at risk of severe outcomes (Niederhauser *et al.*, 2024). Food safety also plays a vital role in preventing the transmission of Hepatitis viruses, particularly that of Hepatitis E, which has a tendency of being acquired through the consumption of contaminated food items, like raw pork. The efficacy of food safety interventions is experienced in agricultural practice and public policy on health, which must concentrate on the significance of proper cooking practices and hygiene in food preparation. Public campaigns can be employed to educate consumers on the risk posed by some sources of food and the need for proper cooking to safe temperatures. By following the application of knowledge in foodborne pathways, communities can come together to reduce the infection rate and protect vulnerable populations (Yulida *et al.*, 2024). Finally, awareness and education community-level interventions play a role in safe practice towards Hepatitis transmission reduction. Interventions should entail mass information dissemination on modes of transmission for Hepatitis B and E, vaccination mobilization, and screening of high-risk populations. Efforts to educate high-risk behaviours, such as the sharing of needles or unprotected sex, need to become a priority in an effort to address the social determinants of disease transmission of such viruses. Further, the establishment of support systems for vulnerable populations can move them closer to healthcare services, thus decreasing transmission and building healthier communities. By adopting these safe practices in day-to-day activities and public health measures, the rate of Hepatitis infection can be curbed to a large extent (Figure 2.16).

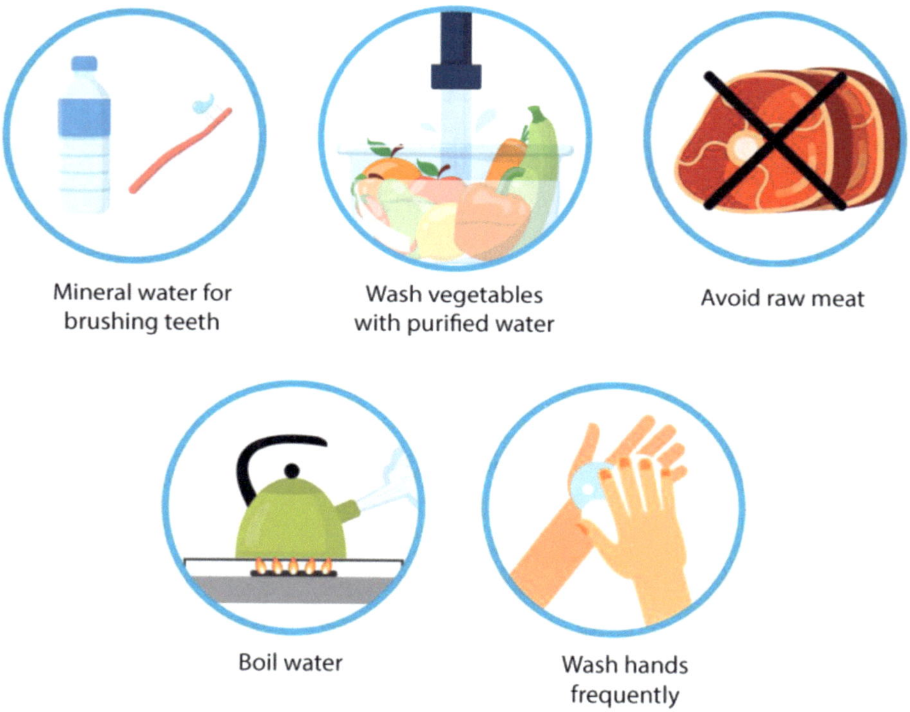
Mineral water for brushing teeth
Wash vegetables with purified water
Avoid raw meat
Boil water
Wash hands frequently

Figure 2.16. Hepatitis B prevention.

Source: https://askthenurseexpert.com/wp-content/uploads/2023/09/how-to-prevent-hepatitis.png.

2.6.3. Public Health Initiatives and Education

Educational programs designed by public health help to deal with the different aspects of hepatitis, whether it is acute or chronic. Good public health campaigns inform people about the ways hepatitis is transmitted, the factors that increase risk, and how to prevent it. Public health measures that educate intravenous drug users and people in correctional facilities help a lot in stopping the spread of the disease. For example, teaching people about strategies to reduce harm, such as proper needle disposal and the need for regular health check-ups, is very important in these efforts. Communities benefit not only from a decrease in infection rates but also from the elevation of overall public health literacy concerning hepatitis and its effects on society (Crespo *et al.*, 2017). In addition, working together with community organizations helps healthcare professionals improve public education about hepatitis. Nurses, social workers, and peers from marginalized communities working together help build a support system for people who are at risk of or have hepatitis. Education programs made for certain groups can help them overcome specific problems and stick to treatment. When education and social support are included, studies indicate that more marginalized people become involved in treatment. For example, the application of community outreach in settings like methadone programs or correctional facilities not only informs patients about their health but also encourages them to seek necessary medical interventions, which is essential for reducing the prevalence of HCV (Ford *et al.*, 2007). Public health programs should be flexible and checked regularly to address the problems of hepatitis in all communities. Because treatments for hepatitis are improving and becoming more available, education programs should also keep up with these changes. Using new ways to teach patients, such as digital tools and peer-based activities, can improve how much information they remember. It is crucial to make sure these educational frameworks support the national and global strategies for hepatitis management. Ultimately, promoting a culture of health literacy, preventive care, and support can empower individuals to take charge of their health, leading to a profound impact on public health outcomes related to hepatitis prevention and treatment (Crespo *et al.*, 2017) (Figure 2.17).

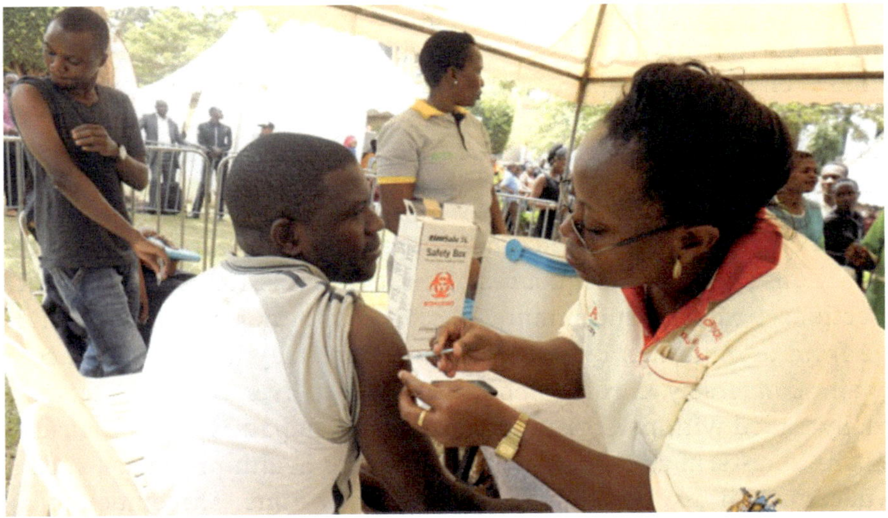

Figure 2.17. Vaccination

Source: https://www.publichealth.com.ng/wp-content/uploads/2019/08/Where-To-Get-Hepatitis-B-Vaccine-In-Nigeria-1.jpg.

SUMMARY

In balancing out the intricate dynamics of hepatitis, both acute and chronic, the conclusion addresses the utmost significance of effective understanding and practical handling. The distinction between acute and chronic hepatitis must be clearly conveyed to physicians and patients as well, since both entail different diagnostic challenges and treatment measures. Further, new evidence suggests the necessity for new diagnostic methods, such as antigen testing of urine for HEV, with the potential to markedly increase the accuracy of diagnosis, especially where there is high infection prevalence. Through emphasis on the improvement of testing modalities, the medical community can trigger interventions in a timely fashion and reduce morbidity associated with hepatic infection (Stahl *et al.*, 2023). The role of individual patient circumstances in the management of hepatitis cannot be overstated. For example, the case of an immunocompromised patient who had become chronically infected with HEV despite high antibody titers demonstrates the complexity of the immune response and the risk of chronicity in certain groups. The reliance solely on the antibody presence as a surrogate for immunity is misleading and brings home the importance of vigilant surveillance through techniques such as RT-PCR, which can identify active infection despite apparent immunity. This proves to be the difference while making decisions regarding therapy, particularly in specialized patient groups (Panning *et al.*, 2019). This ultimately supports the theory of no single approach to hepatitis care. Lastly, to combat the limitations of both acute and chronic hepatitis, ongoing research, enhanced diagnostic techniques, and targeted treatment protocols must be met. The integration of innovative approaches to infection diagnosis, as seen with advances in HEV antigen detection, holds promise for enhanced patient management. In addition, the recognition of the limitations of current antibody-based models, especially in high-risk groups, aids in the development of more effective therapies. The ongoing research into immune responses and their role in infection control holds promise for future advances in the management of hepatitis, which requires continued improvement in clinical practice and public health policy for viral hepatitis (Panning *et al.*, 2019; Stahl *et al.*, 2023).

In the evaluation of the key points concerning hepatitis, either acute or chronic, it is essential to value clinical distinctions and the consequences of these diseases. Acute hepatitis often occurs as the result of viral infections, toxins, or autoimmune diseases with the acute onset of liver inflammation, which may range from asymptomatic to severe. Symptoms may include jaundice, fatigue, nausea, and abdominal pain. Conversely, chronic hepatitis develops over the years from a previous acute attack and is usually linked with persistent infections with hepatitis C and B viruses. The effects of chronic hepatitis are long-term and can progress to severe health problems, such as cirrhosis and HCC, hence the necessity to diagnose and treat the two on time. The epidemiologic perspectives of hepatitis reflect the disproportionate prevalence and impact of the disease globally. Hepatitis A is typically associated with endemic epidemics and is to a large extent vaccine-preventable, while hepatitis B and C are persistent public health issues due to their potential for chronic infection and associated morbidity. According to recent findings, antimicrobial resistance control for viral hepatitis also requires combating it because the disease burden of drug-resistance infection complicates treatment (Murray *et al.*, 2022). Public health measures through vaccination, screening, and health education on risk factors for transmission are also important for preventing incidence and prevalence of hepatitis among populations, particularly in high-endemicity settings. Public health interventions for hepatitis need to extend beyond treatment protocols for individuals to encompass preventive interventions on a larger scale. This involves enhancing access to vaccination and screening services, particularly in high-risk groups, and the implementation of efficient education programs on safe procedures in infection prevention. With evolving research, novel treatment strategies are being developed, the most significant of which is in chronic hepatitis C, where DAA agents are showing promise in achieving SVR rates (Rini *et al.*, 2019). Still, this matter of health disparities and access is a significant concern, most significantly in low-resource settings where morbidity and mortality from hepatitis are disproportionately high. Effective management of hepatitis thus must be tackled with a multi-pronged approach of integrating medical therapy with holistic public health initiatives towards ultimately promoting better global health outcomes.

CLOSER LOOK

HEPATITIS B VIRUS (HBV)

HBV is a virus that causes hepatitis B, a potentially life-threatening liver infection. It can lead to both acute and chronic infections, with chronic infections potentially leading to severe complications like cirrhosis and liver cancer. HBV is transmitted through contact with infected blood or body fluids, and a vaccine is available to prevent infection (Figure 2.18).

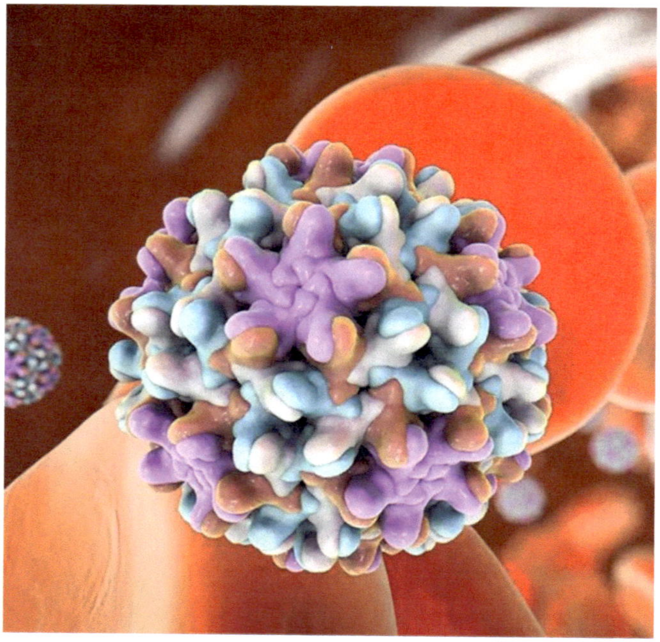

Figure 2.18.

Source: https://www.ganeshdiagnostic.com/admin/public/assets/images/product/1668162566-Hepatitis%20B%20Virus%20(HBV)%20Genotyping%20Test.webp.

Transmission

HBV spreads through contact with infected blood, semen, or other body fluids. Common transmission routes include sexual contact, sharing needles, and from mother to child during birth.

Infection

HBV infection can be acute (short-term) or chronic (long-term). Chronic infection can lead to long-term liver damage and an increased risk of cirrhosis and liver cancer.

Symptoms

Initial symptoms of HBV can be mild or absent. Some individuals may experience fatigue, nausea, vomiting, abdominal pain, and jaundice (yellowing of the skin and eyes).

Prevention

A safe and effective vaccine is available to prevent HBV infection. Vaccination is recommended for infants and at-risk individuals, says the WHO.

Treatment

Antiviral medications can help reduce the amount of virus in the body and slow liver damage. Treatment is typically recommended for individuals with CHB, especially those with liver disease.

References

1. Abdyazdani, N., Arabnezhad, A., Keyhanvar, N., Namdar, N., *et al.* (2024). Leveraging stem cells to combat hepatitis: A comprehensive review of recent studies. https://core.ac.uk/download/644527362.pdf (accessed on 24 May 2025).
2. Alexander, G. C., Stoller, K. B., Haffajee, R. L., & Saloner, B. (2020). An epidemic in the midst of a pandemic: Opioid use disorder and COVID-19. *Annals of Internal Medicine, 173*, 57–58. https://doi.org/10.7326/m20-1141.
3. Alkhaldi, S., Aldousari, H., Alfaresi, S., Alqabandi, S., Khafagi, W., Sheha, M., Sanhoury, M., *et al.* (2024). Measuring immunoglobulin titers among healthcare workers after hepatitis B vaccination: A cross-sectional study in Kuwait. *Cureus, 16*. https://www.semanticscholar.org/paper/6bdcad42d3fb625d15f5e1b6a3cde3d6e9a6eeb3 (accessed on 24 May 2025).
4. Alzamili, F. (2024). Acute-on-chronic liver failure in older patients: An overview. *Academic International Journal of Medical Sciences*. https://www.semanticscholar.org/paper/9e92d66701bc32b26f45db75e41a494623278a06 (accessed on 24 May 2025).
5. Ancarani, F., Antonucci, G., Babudieri, S., Cariti, G., *et al.* (2006). Risk factors and outcome among a large patient cohort with community-acquired acute hepatitis C in Italy. https://core.ac.uk/download/11686659.pdf (accessed on 24 May 2025).
6. Antari, N. K. R. J., & Pramarta, D. Y. (2025). Patients with acute liver failure due to Hepatitis B: A case report. *International Journal of Advances in Medicine*. https://www.semanticscholar.org/paper/dcfb950ea8f97d623f8b7bdb38cbece68c7f0668 (accessed on 24 May 2025).
7. Berezin, A., Berezina, T., Hoppe, U. C., Lichtenauer, M., & Berezin, A. (2024). An overview of circulating and urinary biomarkers capable of predicting the transition of acute kidney injury to chronic kidney disease. *Expert Review of Molecular Diagnostics*. https://www.semanticscholar.org/paper/1f606deb7dc1a01de59233caef7a671ff4fbb9ac (accessed on 24 May 2025).
8. Bourgonje, A. R., Abdulle, A. E., Timens, W., Hillebrands, J. L., Navis, G., Gordijn, S. J., Bolling, M. C., *et al.* (2020). Angiotensin-converting enzyme 2 (ACE2), SARS-CoV-2 and the pathophysiology of coronavirus disease 2019 (COVID-19). *The Journal of Pathology, 251*, 228–248. https://doi.org/10.1002/path.5471.
9. Chen, X., Gao, F., Pan, Q., Huang, C., Luo, R., Lu, X., Chen, X., Li, T., Huang, H., Wu, J., Yu, J., Li, L., & Cao, H. (2024). aCCI-HBV-ACLF: A Novel Predictive Model for Hepatitis B Virus-Related Acute-On-Chronic Liver Failure. Alimentary Pharmacology & Therapeutics, 61, 286 - 298.
10. Cioarca-Nedelcu, R., Atanasiu, V., Istratie, B. E., Nistor, D., Proks, M., Maghet, E., Preda, M., *et al.* (2024). Liver cirrhosis in a patient with alcohol dependence and autoimmune hepatitis. *European Review for Medical and Pharmacological Sciences, 28*(8), 3099–3103. https://www.semanticscholar.org/paper/a3485aede9410eb5ad157ce4b340fb341e094166 (accessed on 24 May 2025).
11. Corman, J. L., Iwatsuki, S., Peters, R. L., Porter, K., *et al.* (1979). Liver allograft: Its use in chronic active hepatitis with macronodular cirrhosis, hepatitis B surface antigen. https://core.ac.uk/download/12203751.pdf

12. Crabb, D. W., Im, G. Y., Szabó, G., Mellinger, J. L., & Lucey, M. R. (2019). Diagnosis and treatment of alcohol-associated liver diseases: 2019 practice guidance from the American Association for the Study of Liver Diseases. *Hepatology, 71*, 306–333. https://doi.org/10.1002/hep.30866.

13. Crespo, J., Llerena, S., Cobo, C., & Cabezas, J. (2017). Is HCV elimination possible in prison? *Revita Española de Sanidad Penitentiaries, 19*, 70–73. https://www.semanticscholar.org/paper/1be759a388a1d00192f530a648f945856386016a (accessed on 24 May 2025).

14. Dalamagka, M. (2024). Acute Pain and Analgesia in children. GSC Advanced Research and Reviews. https://www.semanticscholar.org/paper/Acute-Pain-and-Analgesia-in-children-Dalamagka/fd404f3fb72fa771059492652a76c68aa1bbb687

15. Danpanichkul, P., Duangsonk, K., Chen, V. L., Saokhieo, P., Dejvajara, D., Sukphutanan, B., Aboona, M. B., *et al.* (2025). Global burden of HBV-related liver disease: Primary liver cancer due to chronic HBV infection increased in over one-third of countries globally from 2000 to 2021. *Hepatology*. https://www.semanticscholar.org/paper/f494c37134e24701ca764d978b3ab39793a1a259 (accessed on 24 May 2025).

16. Della Corte C, Mosca A, Vania A, Alterio A, et al. (2015) Pediatric liver diseases: Current challenges and future perspectives. Expert Review of Gastroenterology & Hepatology, DOI: 10.1586/17474124.2016.1129274

17. Dong, L., Le, H., Gong, O., Lu, W., Ma, X., Pan, C., Ma, G. X., *et al.* (2024). Abstract A063: Exploring metabolic and liver steatosis comorbidities among Asian Americans with chronic Hepatitis B using All of Us research program datasets. *Cancer Epidemiology, Biomarkers & Prevention*. https://www.semanticscholar.org/paper/e4a2b2aed33e3e7620bd07bd1ef0d7086b81d814 (accessed on 24 May 2025).

18. Fang, L., Zhang, J., Chen, H., Lv, F., Yu, Y., & Du, X. (2022). Epidemiological characteristics and clinical manifestations of Hepatitis E in a tertiary hospital in China: A retrospective study. *Frontiers in Microbiology, 12*. https://www.semanticscholar.org/paper/9ce2fe5372aaa206e2d12a5ee58a91bff3887bed (accessed on 24 May 2025).

19. Ford, J., & Cheong-Lee, C. (2007). The role of hepatology nurse in the difficult-to-treat hepatitis C population. *Canadian Journal of Gastroenterology, 21*(6), 353–354. https://www.semanticscholar.org/paper/064085cb34f9b875826545869742df174f9f44c9 (accessed on 24 May 2025).

20. Martin Garcia , E. P., Dominguez-Perez, L., Galan, D., Davila, E., Vicent, L., Durante, A., Bruna, V., *et al.* (2024). Comparison between acute and chronic refractory cardiogenic shock: Is prognosis different? *European Heart Journal: Acute Cardiovascular Care*. https://www.semanticscholar.org/paper/c6c32864d5cd449155a7ce7e08e7a47f78359a58 (accessed on 24 May 2025).

21. M.D, R.P., & Mlt, R.C. (2023). Overview of Related Features of Viral Hepatitis: From Pathogenesis to Prevention, Treatment, and Complications. Formosa Journal of Multidisciplinary Research. DOI:10.55927/fjmr.v2i5.4321

22. Grierson, J., Pitts, M., & Koelmeyer, R. (2013). *HIV Futures Seven: The Health and Wellbeing of HIV Positive People in Australia*. https://core.ac.uk/download/pdf/30672666.pdf.

23. Guvenir M, Arikan A. Hepatitis B Virus: From Diagnosis to Treatment. Pol J Microbiol. 2020 Dec;69(4):391-399. doi: 10.33073/pjm-2020-044. Epub 2020 Dec 27. PMID: 33574867; PMCID: PMC7812357.

24. Hernández, Y. E. B., Molina Calderón, A. J., & Tamay, D. G. (2024). Acute-on-chronic liver failure in an adult secondary to autoimmune hepatitis: A case report. https://core.ac.uk/download/620836690.pdf (accessed on 24 May 2025).

25. Job, S.M., & Chacko, B. (2024). Outcomes of Critically ill Patients with Acute on Chronic Liver Failure in a Tertiary Intensive Care Unit: A Retrospective Cohort Study. Indian Journal of Critical Care Medicine : Peer-reviewed, Official Publication of Indian Society of Critical Care Medicine, 28, S493 - S495.

26. Kayesh, M. E. H., Kohara, M., & Tsukiyama-Kohara, K. (2022). Epidemiology and risk factors for acute viral hepatitis in Bangladesh: An overview. *Microorganisms, 10.* https://www.semanticscholar.org/paper/d54dd39ffbff80f68c55f04a6cff3d7401c5c8b4 (accessed on 24 May 2025).

27. Kim, J.H., Kim, K., Kwon, H., Kim, S., Jun, I., Song, J., & Hwang, G.-. (2024). Impact of Chronic Hepatitis C Virus on Acute Kidney Injury After Living Donor Liver Transplantation. Anesthesia and analgesia. https://www.semanticscholar.org/paper/Impact-of-Chronic-Hepatitis-C-Virus-on-Acute-Kidney-Kim-Kim/f993d714c8392b753c9b3976a05ff258ef966609

28. Korkmaz, P., & Demirtürk, N. (2024). Discontinuation of nucleos(t)ide analogues in HBeAg negative chronic Hepatitis B patients: Risks and benefits. *Infectious Diseases & Clinical Microbiology, 6*, 70–77. https://www.semanticscholar.org/paper/a484252e4990e5fd29ac99613e623516ef978639 (accessed on 24 May 2025).

29. Lee, W., Chaudhary, F., & Agrawal, D.K. (2024). Environmental Influences on Atopic Eczema. Journal of environmental science and public health, 8 2, 101-115 . https://www.semanticscholar.org/paper/Environmental-Influences-on-Atopic-Eczema.-Lee-Chaudhary/ffccf63a4aa9512d5e5d0a1028ed405072b52281

30. Li, D., & Wu, M. (2021). Pattern recognition receptors in health and diseases. *Signal Transduction and Targeted Therapy, 6.* https://doi.org/10.1038/s41392-021-00687-0.

31. Li, M., Wang, Y., Li, K., Lan, H., & Zhou, C. (2022). Characterization of highly expressed novel hub genes in Hepatitis E virus chronicity in rabbits: A bioinformatics and experimental analysis. *BMC Veterinary Research, 18.* https://www.semanticscholar.org/paper/990037ab5709a88d70405bcf71024e6ec0c13bee (accessed on 24 May 2025).

32. Li, Z., Luo, Q., Wang, P., Wang, L., Zheng, X., Zhang, Y., Xu, W., *et al.* (2024). Efficacy and safety of individual nutrition support in patients with hepatitis B virus-related acute-on-chronic liver failure at nutrition risk: A study protocol for a randomized controlled clinical trial. *BMJ Open, 14.* https://www.semanticscholar.org/paper/7e7f71febc625293b59c732cc07825e83216ed99 (accessed on 24 May 2025).

33. Molina Calderón, A.J., Tamay, D.G., & Hernández, Y.E. (2024). Acute-on-chronic liver failure in an adult secondary to autoimmune hepatitis: a case report. International Journal of Research in Medical Sciences. https://www.semanticscholar.org/paper/Acute-on-chronic-liver-failure-in-an-adult-to-a-Calder%C3%B3n-Tamay/63e8830a0e3b140dae685460f09c1a02bba1f942

34. Murray, C. J. L., Ikuta, K. S., Sharara, F., Swetschinski, L. R., Robles Aguilar, G., Gray, A. P., Han, C., *et al.* (2022). Global burden of bacterial antimicrobial resistance in 2019: A systematic analysis. *The Lancet, 399*, 629–655. https://doi.org/10.1016/s0140-6736(21)02724-0.

35. Niederhauser, C., Gowland, P., Widmer, N., El Dusouqui, S. A., Mattle-Greminger, M., Gottschalk, J., & Frey, B. (2024). Prevalence of acute hepatitis E virus infections in

Swiss blood donors 2018–2020. *Viruses, 16*. https://www.semanticscholar.org/paper/c282923ea86a851d06e102768d398fc76ef3d293 (accessed on 24 May 2025).

36. Northup, P. G., García–Pagán, J. C., García-Tsao, G., Intagliata, N. M., Superina, R., Roberts, L. N., Lisman, T., *et al.* (2020). Vascular liver disorders, portal vein thrombosis, and procedural bleeding in patients with liver disease: 2020 practice guidance by the American Association for the Study of Liver Diseases. *Hepatology, 73*, 366–413. https://doi.org/10.1002/hep.31646.

37. Pacholi, S., Bishwal, S. C., & Barde, P. (2022). Identification of hepatitis B virus genotypes detected in Lahaul & Spiti district of Himachal Pradesh, India. *The Indian Journal of Medical Research, 156*, 779–785. https://www.semanticscholar.org/paper/1f91ee7ea0198b4bf851c76afc97a23309b3a818 (accessed on 24 May 2025).

38. Panning, M., Basho, K., Fahrner, A., & Neumann-Haefelin, C. (2019). Chronic Hepatitis E after kidney transplantation with an antibody response suggestive of reinfection: A case report. *BMC Infectious Diseases, 19*. https://www.semanticscholar.org/paper/02e12e35ccea3e83c7468c2c8f23b0467ec7a470 (accessed on 24 May 2025).

39. Pishmisheva-Peleva, M., Kotsev, S., Golkocheva-Markova, E., & Argirova, R. (2024). Extrahepatic manifestations in patients with acute Hepatitis E–Pazardzhik, Bulgaria 2014–2022. *Problems of Infectious and Parasitic Diseases*. https://www.semanticscholar.org/paper/4d40409d2c8bc96709129cd390678e38a91e8626 (accessed on 24 May 2025).

40. Rini, B. I., Plimack, E. R., Stus, V. P., Gafanov, R., Hawkins, R. D., Nosov, D., Pouliot, F., *et al.* (2019). Pembrolizumab plus axitinib versus sunitinib for advanced renal-cell carcinoma. *New England Journal of Medicine, 380*, 1116–1127. https://doi.org/10.1056/nejmoa1816714.

41. Barbosa Rodrigues, B., Pereira, L., Campante, F., & Pona, A. P. (2024). Chronic liver disease, not everything is what it seems: Autoimmune hepatitis/primary biliary cholangitis overlap syndrome. *Cureus, 16*. https://www.semanticscholar.org/paper/029ffb9ed89759457c69285e5fc34258cdf92809 (accessed on 24 May 2025).

42. Sacleux, S., & Saliba, F. (2023). How to Optimize the Results of Liver Transplantation for Acute-on-Chronic Liver Failure. Life, 13. https://www.semanticscholar.org/paper/How-to-Optimize-the-Results-of-Liver-for-Liver-Sacleux-Saliba/b36fbf4b9b3db8a2a01fdc6dd0e776eb9c87e7b9

43. Schaer, R., Bastos, F., Simões, J., da Encarnação Silva, J., Trindade, S., Nascimento, R., Freire, S., *et al.* (2022). Seroprevalence of viral Hepatitis of enteric (A and E) and parenteral/sexual (B and C) transmission of individuals aged 30 to 70 residents in Salvador-Brazil. *Studies in Health Sciences*. https://www.semanticscholar.org/paper/5ce0b4d9b3908bff01497665c012c04951166141 (accessed on 24 May 2025).

44. Shahini, E., Argentiero, A., Andriano, A., Losito, F., Maida, M., Facciorusso, A., Cozzolongo, R., *et al.* (2024). Hepatitis E virus: What more do we need to know? *Medicina, 60*. https://www.semanticscholar.org/paper/4b95864ef73a45bf1f84e273479d031fc86b0fcb (accessed on 24 May 2025).

45. Stahl, Y., Kabar, I., Heinzow, H., Maasoumy, B., Bremer, B., Wedemeyer, H., Schmidt, H., *et al.* (2023). Enhanced monitoring and detection of recent genotype 3 hepatitis E virus infection through urine antigen testing. *Emerging Microbes & Infections, 12*. https://www.semanticscholar.org/paper/6e90412a3cbf7e8d5fd8775b8a1929bfd85074fd (accessed on 24 May 2025).

46. Varghese, N., Majeed, A., Nyalakonda, S., Boortalary, T., Halegoua-DeMarzio, D., & Hann, H. (2024). Review of Related Factors for Persistent Risk of Hepatitis B Virus-Associated Hepatocellular Carcinoma. Cancers, 16. https://www.semanticscholar.org/paper/Review-of-Related-Factors-for-Persistent-Risk-of-B-Varghese-Majeed/5261584eb5ce5c75d95d5c7adf0e0383b2950c16

47. Wang, H., Xu, C., Yao, R., Zhang, W., Wang, S., Qin, X., Liu, Q., *et al.* (2025). Single-cell transcriptome identifies a proinflammatory B-cell subset in Hepatitis B Virus associated acute-on-chronic liver failure. *Journal of Viral Hepatitis, 32*(3), e70012. https://www.semanticscholar.org/paper/9a8ec6d05c8aab721951f91635d9d627a7f605e1 (accessed on 24 May 2025).

48. Ylli, T., Stea, T., & University of Kristiansand. (2023). Quantifying missed opportunities in health sector for women and girls' victims of violence in Albania. *The European Journal of Public Health, 33.* https://www.semanticscholar.org/paper/d688cb75ffe7c955622c822973fc4e5ba1257af0 (accessed on 24 May 2025).

49. Yuan, L., Zeng, B., Liu, L. L., Ren, Y., Yang, Y., Chu, J., Li, Y., *et al.* (2019). Risk factors for progression to acute-on-chronic liver failure during severe acute exacerbation of chronic Hepatitis B virus infection. *World Journal of Gastroenterology, 25*, 2327–2337. https://www.semanticscholar.org/paper/1796e592e901f76a32ccc8353775f9bd81b223cf (accessed on 24 May 2025).

50. Yulida, Y., Wiranto, A. S., Faisal, F., Karim, M. A., & Soesanto, O. (2024). SACR epidemic model for the spread of hepatitis B disease by considering vertical transmission. *BAREKENG: Journal Ilma Mathematica dan Terrapin*. https://www.semanticscholar.org/paper/97a969125f42240db55c546791637dc99031438f (accessed on 24 May 2025).

51. Zhang, Q., Shi, B. L., & Wu, L. (2022). Characteristics and risk factors of infections in patients with HBV-related acute-on-chronic liver failure: A retrospective study. *PeerJ, 10*. https://www.semanticscholar.org/paper/56fe2c524eca47e2d1a87239f8f47568f28cfb4e (accessed on 24 May 2025).

52. Zhao, G., Shi, X., Zhang, L., & Liang, H. (2024). Comment on "Diabetic MAFLD is associated with increased risk of hepatocellular carcinoma and mortality in chronic viral hepatitis patients". International Journal of Cancer, 154.

53. Zubair AS, McAlpine LS, Gardin T, Farhadian S, Kuruvilla DE, Spudich S. Neuropathogenesis and Neurologic Manifestations of the Coronaviruses in the Age of Coronavirus Disease 2019: A Review. JAMA Neurol. 2020;77(8):1018–1027. doi:10.1001/jamaneurol.2020.2065

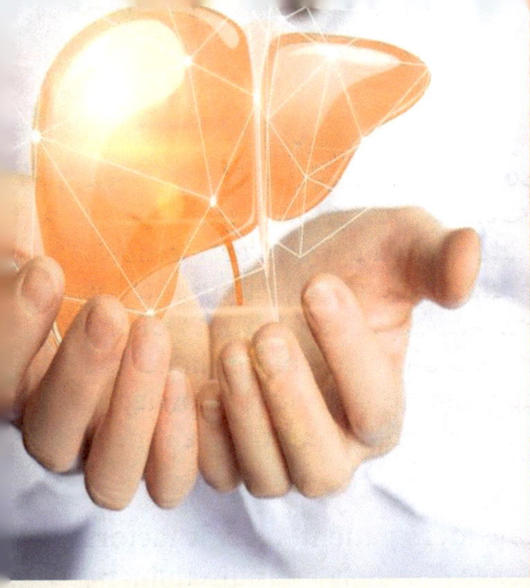

Chapter 3

CIRRHOSIS AND ITS COMPLICATIONS

Contents

Introduction

Cirrhosis is the result of chronic liver disease (CLD) with diffuse fibrosis and architectural reorganization of the liver tissue. It is a progressive illness produced by several etiologies, including alcohol abuse, viral illnesses like hepatitis, and metabolic disorders. The inevitability of cirrhosis, once a particular level of liver injury has occurred, generates a wide range of complications that can severely compromise the quality of life of patients and lead to premature death. One should note that cirrhosis itself is not a precise disease but rather a syndrome generated by a variety of underlying injuries to the liver. Consequently, strict control and prompt treatment are vital for the prevention of the progression of liver injury and the resultant complications of this fatal disease. The complications of cirrhosis are a multifaceted challenge for clinicians, as they represent both physical and psychological consequences. One of the most alarming ones is the occurrence of hepatocellular carcinoma (HCC), a major liver cancer that often arises in cirrhotic individuals. The relationship between cirrhosis and HCC is best understood through the complex interaction between liver disease and carcinogenesis. Cirrhotic patients are also at risk of venous thromboembolic conditions, such as portal vein thrombosis (PVT), as evident from studies that detail the prothrombotic state induced by liver cirrhosis (LC) and HCC. Also, advanced liver disease has a propensity to precipitate complications such as ascites, variceal bleeding, and hepatic encephalopathy (HE), which are key determinants of the morbidity of the disease (Burra *et al.*, 2018; Hu *et al.*, 2006). One should also comprehend the multifaceted pathophysiology of cirrhosis and its complications, demanding sufficient knowledge of the pathophysiological process involved as well as the diagnostic approach behind the treatment strategy.

The treatment of cirrhosis is a comprehensive evaluation that considers patient-specific factors and specific complications that arise in each. As treatment of liver disease is usually multidisciplinary, hepatologists, oncologists, and other specialists need to work together to optimize outcomes for the patient. Additionally, technical advancements and screening modalities for managing complications such as HCC and PVT continue to evolve, which gives hope in the form of improved management methods. Therefore, a better understanding of cirrhosis and its consequences is key to enhancing clinical practice and, ultimately, reducing the burden of CLD.

Definition of Cirrhosis

Cirrhosis causes healthy liver tissue to be replaced by scar tissue, which clogs both the blood and bile flow within the organ. Several things can lead to this condition, such as long-term alcohol abuse, viral hepatitis, or NAFLD. When the liver is very scarred, it has less ability to remove toxins, help in digestion, and make proteins. Because cirrhosis can get worse over time, it is very important to detect and control the disease early to reduce the risks. By learning how liver inflammation can develop into cirrhosis, one can find out how to prevent it and treat the causes. As well as the initial liver damage, cirrhosis can lead to many serious and disabling complications. A key problem is portal hypertension, which happens when blood pressure goes up in the portal vein system because the liver is blocked by scar tissue. As a result of this condition, blood vessels may become enlarged and could burst, which can be very dangerous. In some cases, fluid can build up in the abdominal cavity, known as ascites, which can be uncomfortable and raise the risk of infection. Cirrhosis increases the likelihood of HCC, which is a main liver cancer often found in people with severe liver disease. Management strategies must therefore focus on addressing these complications to improve patient outcomes, as suggested by recent expert recommendations in the field of transplant hepatology (Burra *et al.*, 2018). Treating cirrhosis well means handling its complications and also bringing together different specialists to find out the causes and support the liver. Both lifestyle changes, such as avoiding alcohol and eating well, and medical treatments which target viral hepatitis, may be part of the treatment plan. When less invasive treatments are not enough, liver resection has been useful in treating certain liver tumors, mainly HCC. Research into surgical techniques indicates that meticulous approaches like kellyclasia, coupled with careful management of hemostasis and biliostasis, yield favorable outcomes despite potential complications such as liver insufficiency (Grazi *et al.*, 2007). Therefore, the holistic treatment of cirrhosis not only focuses on the disease itself but also encompasses the need for careful, expert management throughout the patient's treatment journey (Figure 3.1).

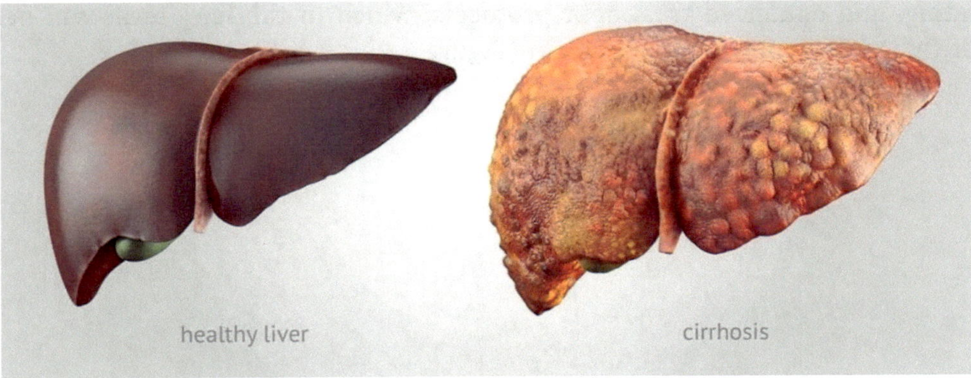

Figure 3.1. Healthy liver and cirrhosis.

Source: https://liverfoundation.org/wp-content/uploads/2022/06/Healthy-V-Cirrhosis.jpeg.

Importance of Understanding Cirrhosis

Cirrhosis is a long-term liver disease that is defined by the replacement of normal liver tissue with fibrosis or scar tissue, which makes the liver unable to work properly. An overall understanding of cirrhosis is very important for all stakeholders, including healthcare professionals, patients, and policymakers. Cirrhosis has been recognized as a major cause of morbidity and mortality globally, particularly in the United States, and awareness can contribute to earlier diagnosis and management. Awareness of the etiology and natural history of cirrhosis facilitates targeted intervention, enabling the health practitioner to implement supportive care and prevention early in the course of the disease. This emphasis on early diagnosis is not only advantageous for the individual patient's results but also for the overall public health priority of managing liver disease, which is an important cause of healthcare cost and resource use. Moreover, awareness of cirrhosis complications significantly enhances patient management and education. Patients with LC suffer from a tremendous range of complications such as HE, portal hypertension, and heightened vulnerability to infections, for example, Clostridium Difficile. Such infections are particularly a concern, as they are linked with high morbidity and mortality in cirrhotic patients due to complications like prolonged hospitalization and disease-driven immune dysfunction, as seen in the identification of cirrhosis-associated immune dysfunction (CAID).

By informing the patient and caregiver about such risks, practitioners are able to empower them with proactive self-care of their health, treatment compliance, and with detection of signs of complication, optimizing quality of life and survival. Understanding cirrhosis is relevant to the healthcare policy framework, where resource planning and funding decisions can be guided by a better understanding of the disease burden. Given the fact that cirrhosis is among the leading causes of death in the US, with chronic hepatitis and alcoholism being primary causes, investment in education and research is necessary (Dugas *et al.*, 1982). Furthermore, the understanding of cirrhosis and its complications, along with the role that liver transplantation plays – pioneered by institutions such as the University of Pittsburgh since 1967 – emphasizes the need for comprehensive approaches in managing advanced liver disease (Dugas *et al.*, 1982). By their contribution to an enlightened discussion on cirrhosis, stakeholders can advocate for early screening programs, better research funding, and enhanced treatment protocols, which in the long term will help to check the spread of this vital public health problem (Figure 3.2).

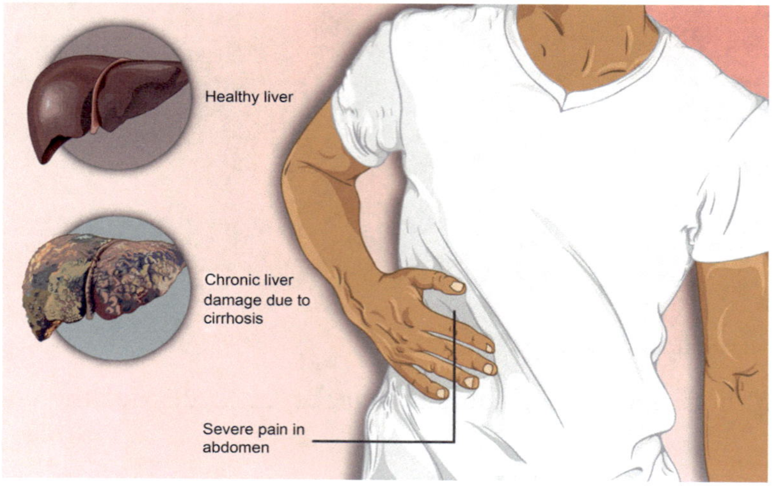

Figure 3.2. Person with cirrhosis and associated pain in the right upper region of the abdomen.

Source: https://upload.wikimedia.org/wikipedia/commons/thumb/3/39/Depiction_of_a_Cirrhosis_patient.png/1024px-Depiction_of_a_Cirrhosis_patient.png.

3.1. Causes of Cirrhosis

Many cases of cirrhosis begin with long-term liver damage from several causes, which leads to worsening scarring and finally causes the organ to fail. Alcohol consumption is one of the most widely recognized causes of cirrhosis, particularly alcoholic liver disease (ALD). Data suggest a significant increase in the incidence of alcoholic cirrhosis, which accounted for 50% of cases in Gothenburg, Sweden, compared to only 29% in Iceland, highlighting geographical disparities in alcohol-related liver damage (Gunnarsdóttir *et al.*, 2008). NAFLD has also become a common reason, mainly because of the increase in obesity. More and more people are developing cirrhosis because of NAFLD, which is related to the rise in metabolic syndromes and people leading less active lives. It is essential to know the many causes of cirrhosis to develop proper interventions and preventive plans. Hepatitis B and C viruses are major reasons for viral hepatitis, which often leads to cirrhosis globally. The change in demographics and disease causes is becoming evident; for instance, the proportion of patients with viral hepatitis has shown a decreasing trend while that of alcoholic cirrhosis has increased (Chalasani *et al.*, 2019). Constant viral infections may bring about inflammation, cell death, and scarring, which eventually develop into cirrhosis. It is most important in developing regions because many people there still lack access to vaccines and treatment for viral hepatitis. Furthermore, patients with hepatitis C cirrhosis display a markedly increased risk of hepatocellular carcinoma (HCC), presenting a dual challenge of managing both cirrhosis and its cancerous complications. For this reason, screening and treating viral hepatitis are very important for preventing cirrhosis. Some other important causes of cirrhosis are autoimmune liver diseases and genetic disorders, for example, hemochromatosis and Wilson's disease. If the immune system attacks liver cells by mistake, AIH results in liver inflammation and scarring. Many genetic disorders cause metals to build up in the liver, which makes the liver disease worse. As an example, people with hemochromatosis are much more likely to develop liver problems, including cirrhosis. Moreover, recent studies indicate an alarming rise in conditions related to non-alcoholic steatohepatitis (NASH), a more aggressive form of NAFLD, contributing significantly to the modern cirrhosis epidemic. The interplay of these diverse causes necessitates a multidimensional approach for prevention, diagnosis, and management strategies tailored to the specific etiologies, fostering better outcomes for individuals affected by cirrhosis and its related complications (Gunnarsdóttir *et al.*, 2008) (Figure 3.3).

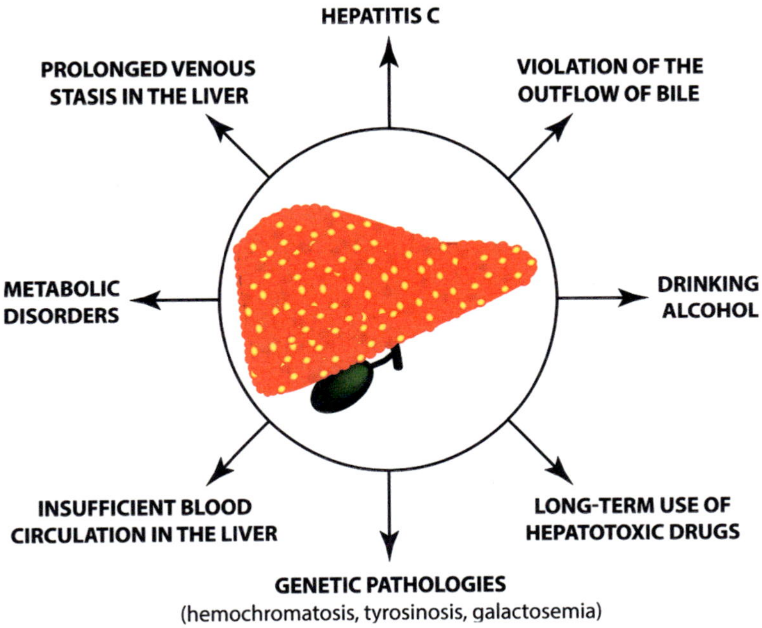

Figure 3.3. Causes of cirrhosis.

Source: https://cdn.vectorstock.com/i/1000v/57/34/causes-of-cirrhosis-infographics-vector-22645734.jpg.

3.1.1. Alcohol-Related Liver Disease

Alcohol-related liver disease (ARLD) is an important public health issue because excessive alcohol intake causes a range of liver abnormalities, the most extreme being cirrhosis. The evolution from alcohol use to severe liver disease progresses through several phases, and the process usually starts with fatty liver (steatosis) and may progress to alcoholic hepatitis and end with cirrhosis. The disparity between alcohol consumption and liver disease is particularly telling in patients with underlying illnesses, where even minimal drinking contributes to complications such as portal hypertension and liver failure. Importantly, alcohol use disorder is a significant cause of liver-related complications, and there is a need for targeted prevention interventions for not only the drinking behavior patterns of alcohol but also health determinants influencing drinking habits in different groups (Bonnefont-Rousselot *et al.*, 2022). The effects of cirrhosis in ARLD patients extend beyond liver damage, presenting in the form of advanced complications such as HCC. Cirrhotic individuals have an extremely increased risk of acquiring HCC, one of the leading cancer-related causes of mortality worldwide. Research has demonstrated that individuals with ALD are particularly vulnerable, with the incidence of HCC being significantly heightened among this population. Of importance, early detection of cirrhosis and treatment can significantly lower the risk of HCC development, but it is left to the majority of individuals to remain undiagnosed until their liver is severely impaired. This shows the very importance of regular screening and monitoring among individuals engaged in high-risk drinking behavior (Gunnarsdóttir *et al.*, 2008). Furthermore, the effect of alcohol consumption on other risk factors exacerbates liver morbidity among the affected individuals. For example, the co-existence of type-2 diabetes and ARLD has been found to increase the risk for progression of liver disease. A retrospective study identified that over half of the liver complications among patients with diabetes could be explained by the use of alcohol disorder. Based on these findings, health care professionals should adopt a combined approach in the treatment of ARLD, including consideration of metabolic comorbidities and tailored guidance regarding alcohol consumption to reduce the overall burden of liver disease. Alcohol moderation and lifestyle changes targeted public health interventions are essential in reducing the incidence of alcohol-related liver complications and promoting long-term liver health (Bonnefont-Rousselot *et al.*, 2022) (Figure 3.4).

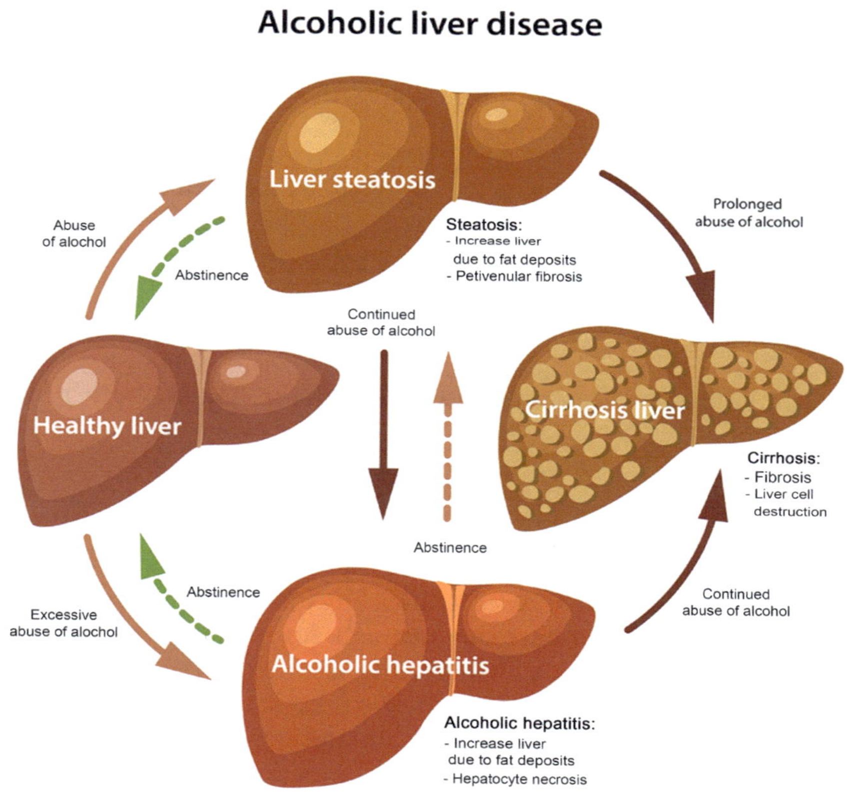

Figure 3.4. Alcohol-related liver disease (ARLD).

Source: https://www.expmedndm.ox.ac.uk/images/site_profiles/adobestock_275633332.jpeg.

3.1.2. Viral Hepatitis (Hepatitis B and C)

Viral hepatitis B and C are important in the process that leads to cirrhosis, which involves the liver being damaged and scarred until it fails. Hepatitis B virus (HBV) and hepatitis C virus (HCV) can cause both acute and chronic liver inflammation, with chronic infections being particularly insidious, often leading to cirrhosis over several decades. The CDC believes that many people in the United States have chronic hepatitis, and a lot of them are not aware of it. Because cirrhosis is a common complication of chronic hepatitis, patients are closely watched for HCC, which is much more likely to occur in those with significant liver damage. Because HCV is the main reason for CLD and cirrhosis in Western countries, its effects on public health are very significant. Many patients with cirrhosis eventually develop HCC, which is a cancer with a high rate of death. It highlights the need to have good screening and diagnostic methods for people with HCV. Recent studies suggest that serological determination of biomarkers, such as squamous cell carcinoma antigen-immunoglobulins M (SCCA-IgM), could play a vital role in monitoring liver disease progression among those infected with HCV. By identifying patients at risk for rapid disease advancement, healthcare providers can intervene early, potentially delaying the onset of cirrhosis and reducing associated complications, including HCC development (Fassina *et al.*, 2015). Hepatitis C, together with conditions like cryoglobulinemic vasculitis, makes the situation more complicated for patients with CLD. Cryoglobulinemic vasculitis, which causes cryoglobulins to form in the blood when it is cold, may worsen liver problems and affect kidney function, so it must be carefully watched. Having cryoglobulinemia in HCV patients along with hepatic disease points to the bodywide effects of viral hepatitis and its consequences. Interferon can help achieve remission, yet relapses are common, which makes it difficult to manage these diseases. These complexities highlight the necessity for comprehensive approaches to treat hepatitis B and C infections effectively, thereby minimizing the risks of cirrhosis and its severe complications (Boldeanu *et al.*, 2018) (Figure 3.5).

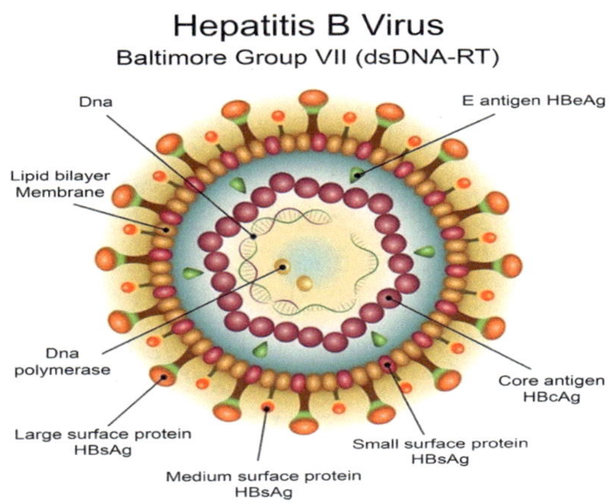

Figure 3.5. Hepatitis B virus.

Source: https://d2jx2rerrg6sh3.cloudfront.net/image-handler/picture/2019/8/shutterstock_173727872.jpg.

3.1.3. Non-Alcoholic Fatty Liver Disease (NAFLD)

NAFLD has emerged as a significant public health problem, particularly in industrialized nations where lifestyle-related concerns such as obesity and lack of physical activity are on the rise. NAFLD is a disease spectrum of liver diseases beginning with simple hepatic steatosis that progresses to NASH, which ultimately leads to advanced fibrosis and cirrhosis. In actuality, NAFLD is progressively recognized as the leading most frequent etiology of cryptogenic cirrhosis, contributing to significant liver morbidity and mortality in the current era (Campo *et al.*, 2018). The speedy increase of NAFLD is concurrently overlapping with that of obesity and IR, suggesting the obvious necessity for public health intervention in disease prevention and lifestyle modification. Genetic and epigenetic elements play a significant role in the pathogenesis of NAFLD, affecting susceptibility and disease progression. Studies identify the function of certain genetic polymorphisms, especially within the *PNPLA3* and *MBOAT7* genes, which are associated with the etiology of NAFLD. Moreover, epigenetic changes, including changes in DNA methylation patterns and histone status, can induce or suppress genes involved in lipid metabolism and inflammation. These interactions provide a platform upon which heritable risk factors and environmental inputs converge to influence a patient's disease trajectory (Campo *et al.*, 2018). Identification of these epigenetic and genetic components not only enhances our understanding of NAFLD but also opens novel possibilities for personalized medicine approaches to the management of liver disease. Treatment of NAFLD remains challenging, partly due to the fact that the disease may not be diagnosed until extensive liver damage has occurred. Weight loss and exercise, lifestyle modification, are now the cornerstones of therapy, both of which have been proven to reduce liver fat content and improve overall liver function. While the study continues, no approved drug therapy for NAFLD exists. This contrast underscores the urgency of further investigation into treatments, such as the exploration of circulating profiles of microRNA as a disease severity and progression biomarker (Abdelmalek *et al.*, 2009). Through awareness of the complexities of NAFLD and its progression to cirrhosis, health professionals can better prepare to manage this emerging public health issue and avoid its complications in infected populations.

3.2. Pathophysiology of Cirrhosis

The pathophysiology of cirrhosis is a complex interaction between cellular and biochemical events resulting in the progression of the normal architecture of the liver to fibrotic tissue. The sequence usually happens as a result of chronic liver injury, whose cause may be more than one etiology, like viral hepatitis, ALD, and NAFLD. With the progress of metabolic science, NAFLD has been reclassified as Metabolic Dysfunction-Associated Steatotic Liver Disease (MASLD) according to its association with diabetes and obesity, recognizing the multifactorial etiology of liver injury. As liver cells are repeatedly injured, regenerative nodules emerge between fibrotic bands, disrupting normal hepatic architecture and flow, leading to portal hypertension and liver failure. The overwhelming reality that almost one million deaths globally are related to cirrhosis complications underscores the need to recognize such pathophysiological changes more urgently (Reddy *et al.*, 2025). Furthermore, the inflammatory aspect of cirrhosis pathophysiology cannot be overemphasized, especially regarding the contribution of the liver's response to injury. Chronic inflammation is embedded in hepatic disease because recurrent injury induces an immune reaction with the activation of Kupffer cells and the release of pro-inflammatory cytokines. This cascade is followed by a cascade of adverse effects, such as apoptosis of the parenchymal cells and activation of hepatic stellate cells (HSCs), which proliferate and lay down extracellular matrix proteins, resulting in the maintenance of the fibrotic process. Additionally, drug abuse causes cirrhosis-inflammatory reactions to be significantly more severe by further impairing liver function through dysregulation of metabolism and oxidative stress. The findings regarding how various drugs—and alcohol—influence liver function explain the multifaceted nature of substance-induced liver disease, and furthermore, emphasize the necessity of holistic treatment measures to address both liver function and the problems of dependency (Mostafa *et al.*, 2023). Given the multifactorial etiology of cirrhosis, an understanding of its pathophysiology also offers a window of opportunity for research into novel therapeutic avenues aimed at inhibiting progression and complications. Early detection and treatment are paramount since progression to decompensated cirrhosis is more likely to herald life-threatening complications such as variceal bleeding, ascites, and HE. Various biomarkers have been discovered to have the potential to diagnose as well as track disease progression and thus enlighten therapeutic targets. Besides this, synthesizing traditional medical wisdom, such as concepts in Ayurveda for liver wellbeing, with modern diagnostic practice is sure to bring more culturally suitable approaches to the management of liver disease. With the use of conventional science coupled with new insights from past paradigms, we can augment knowledge and countermeasure cirrhosis and, consequently, reduce its morbidity and mortality (Reddy *et al.*, 2025) (Figure 3.6).

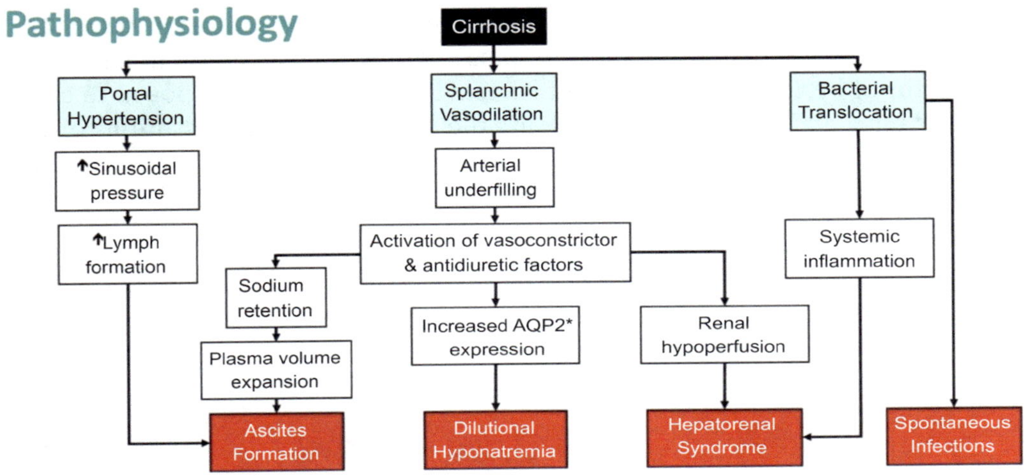

Figure 3.6. Cirrhosis pathophysiology.

Source: https://img.grepmed.com/uploads/11430/cirrhosis-hepatology-liver-pathophysiology-original.jpeg.

3.2.1. Mechanism of Liver Damage

The mechanisms of pathogenesis leading to liver damage are multifaceted and are closely linked to a number of pathological processes that eventually result in cirrhosis. Hepatocyte injury, a common cause, typically results from prolonged toxin exposure, chronic viral hepatitis, or metabolic illness. Initial injury initiates inflammatory responses, as white blood cells invade the liver and secrete cytokines that continue to cause injury. This chronic inflammation causes hepatocyte apoptosis and necrosis, whereas fibrogenesis occurs by the transformation of activated HSCs into myofibroblasts and deposition of surplus extracellular matrix components. This fibrotic tissue thereby replaces the normal architecture of the liver and causes impairment in hepatic function. Fibrotic tissue deposition also alters the portal blood flow, leading to elevated portal venous pressure, and causes the patient to have complications such as portal hypertension and esophageal varices. In liver resection surgery, for instance, mechanisms of liver damage can also be observed, namely in the context of postoperative complications like liver failure and biliary fistulae. In conjunction with the performance of the procedure itself, stringent control of hemostasis and biliostasis is paramount to prevent damage. Despite enhanced surgery, the intrinsic risk of post-resectional liver failure testifies to the fragility of liver function and identifies the role of surgical expertise in counteracting such risks. Although liver resection successfully reduces malignancies, underlying liver disease, whether chronic hepatitis or cirrhosis, continues to exert its harmful effects, ultimately influencing patient outcomes and survival. The interplay between surgical intervention and preoperative liver disease highlights an essential aspect of liver health: the importance of preoperative evaluation and optimization in optimizing postoperative recovery. Acute kidney injury (AKI) is another severe complication accompanying liver injury, especially following liver transplantation. Post-reperfusion syndrome (PRS) is one such classic example of this concomitance, where reperfusion-related ischemia-reperfusion injury during graft revascularization leads to renal dysfunction. The pathophysiology of AKI due to PRS is multifactorial and involves a cascade of inflammatory mediators, oxidative stress, and microcirculatory dysfunction. Underlying conditions, like a higher Model for End-stage Liver Disease score, heavily enhance the risk of AKI in the context of transplantation and also complicate the patient's management. The impact of AKI is considerable because it not only serves as a predictor of perioperative risk but also leaves recipients predisposed to chronic kidney disease in the long term and, in so doing, augments the multifaceted complications of cirrhosis and its treatment (Evison *et al.*, 2016). It is crucial to treat these mechanisms for improving outcomes and focused preventive interventions in liver disease management (Figure 3.7).

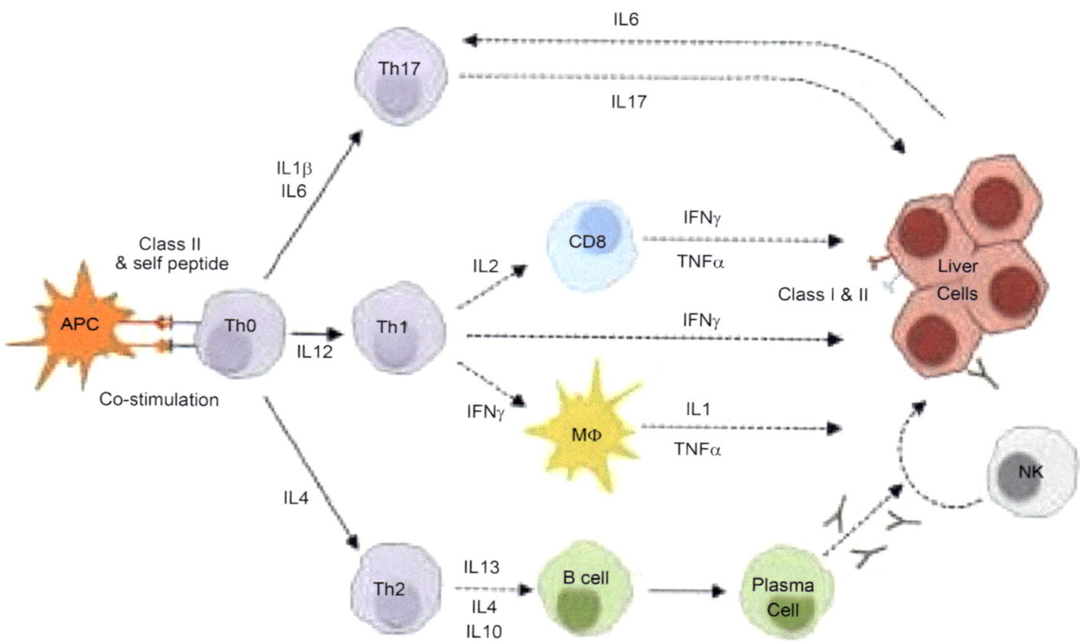

Figure 3.7. Mechanisms of liver damage.

Source: https://www.researchgate.net/profile/Giorgina-Mieli-Vergani/publication/302475250/figure/fig1/AS:614017592741895@1523404610197/Mechanisms-of-liver-damage-Liver-damage-is-initiated-by-the-presentation-of-a.png.

3.2.2. Fibrosis and Scar Tissue Formation

Formation of scar tissue and fibrosis is crucial in the advancement of cirrhosis. When the liver is injured over time, the body responds by forming too much scar tissue, which is called fibrosis. HSCs are important in this process because they become myofibroblasts, and immune cells such as macrophages are also involved by causing inflammation and helping to rebuild tissue. A pivotal finding in recent research underscored the role of macrophage metalloelastase (MMP-12), which is essential for the turnover of elastin within fibrous scars. This enzyme's activity, regulated by its inhibitor Timp-1, denotes a critical imbalance that can culminate in irreversible fibrosis, where tissue architecture is significantly altered and cannot revert to a healthy state (Pares *et al.*, 2012). Knowing about these mechanisms is important for designing strategies to stop fibrosis. The changes seen in advanced fibrosis show how scar tissue can be very complex. When fibrosis is irreversible, pluricellular scars develop, and these are marked by the extensive cross-linking of fibrillar collagen and elastin in the matrix. Because of this, the liver's structure is disturbed, and it cannot function properly, which may result in portal hypertension and liver failure. The extra elastin found in fibrotic tissues hints that the body is not remodeling properly, which can result in a chronic and harmful healing process. Some research suggests that if the main causes of chronic injury are handled, such as reducing exposure to harm or treating viral infections, in some cases, fibrosis will resolve on its own. However, this outcome is less likely in advanced stages, thus emphasizing the critical need for early detection and intervention (Pares *et al.*, 2012). In parallel with understanding the cellular dynamics of fibrosis, recent studies have explored the potential protective roles of certain bioactive compounds, such as virgin coconut oil (VCO), in mitigating liver damage and promoting healing. Some research suggests that VCO may help the immune system, which could affect the development of fibrosis. Specifically, it has been observed to increase the activity of superoxide dismutase (SOD) and facilitate lymphocyte proliferation, thereby enhancing the body's defense mechanisms against liver injury. Examining the treated subjects under a microscope found less leukocyte infiltration and better hepatocyte health, which suggests that VCO may help the immune system and also protect the liver and kidneys. This finding opens new avenues for adjunctive therapies in managing cirrhosis, emphasizing the importance of exploring alternative or complementary approaches in conjunction with traditional treatment strategies (Figure 3.8).

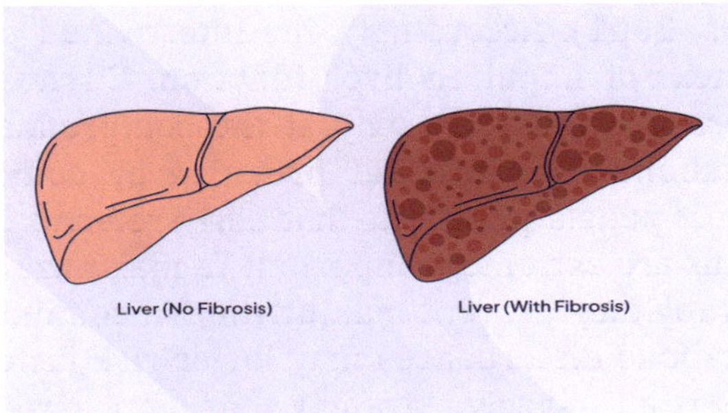

Figure 3.8. Fibrosis.

Source: https://www.health.com/thmb/PLKljsFYAo76hBRY_DUz2d-fZ1g=/1500x0/filters:no_upscale():max_bytes(150000):strip_icc()/HDC-What-You-Should-Know-About-Liver-Fibrosis-FINAL-1-1-b50fabad3d7c4d8d90139ee646a8f376.png.

3.2.3. Impact on Liver Function

Cirrhosis profoundly modifies liver function to cause numerous metabolic derangements and clinical sequelae that may additionally worsen the patient's overall health status. As progressively more liver tissue becomes fibrotic and is replaced by scar tissue, the functional ability of the liver is impaired. This impairment is made up of a reduced ability for detoxification, protein synthesis, and regulation of lipid and carbohydrate metabolism. The impacts of impaired liver function cascade into other systems in the body, frequently resulting in complications such as portal hypertension and HE. The intricately interdependent association between cirrhosis and liver function illustrates the organ as not just a metabolic hub but as the keystone to overall homeostasis in the body. Furthermore, the relationship between diabetes mellitus (DM) and cirrhosis illustrates the impact of liver function on metabolic health. Research has indicated diabetic conditions to be highly prevalent in the case of cirrhosis patients, adding to the dangers of the two diseases. Diabetic patients with cirrhosis, for instance, carry a high risk of facing complications following post-orthotopic liver transplantation (OLT). Study on cirrhotic liver transplant candidates identified that candidates with the requirement for pharmacologic therapy for DM had significant survival discrepancies with non-diabetic candidates. Notably, while their post-transplantation survival rates in the intermediate period may not be affected adversely, the metabolic cost of DM can jeopardize clinical outcome and complicate recovery in patients (Blanco *et al.*, 2001). Accordingly, the intertwined pathways of diabetes and cirrhosis signal the broader context of impaired liver function. Cirrhosis management practice needs a multi-dimensional approach aimed not only at the compromised architecture of the liver but also at the resulting metabolic abnormalities provided by comorbidities such as diabetes. Recommendations from expert panels point out that early referral for liver transplant and optimal control of nutritional status are extremely important to maximize outcomes (Burra *et al.*, 2018). Appropriate nutritional therapy may prevent malnutrition, a common complication in cirrhotic patients, and treatment of metabolic disturbances may lower risk factors for the development of subsequent complications. This is an inclusive strategy that emphasizes the need for a comprehensive model of care that is capable of monitoring not only hepatic function but also the interaction between metabolic health, demonstrating how cirrhosis subverts conventional paradigms of the management of liver disease (Figure 3.9).

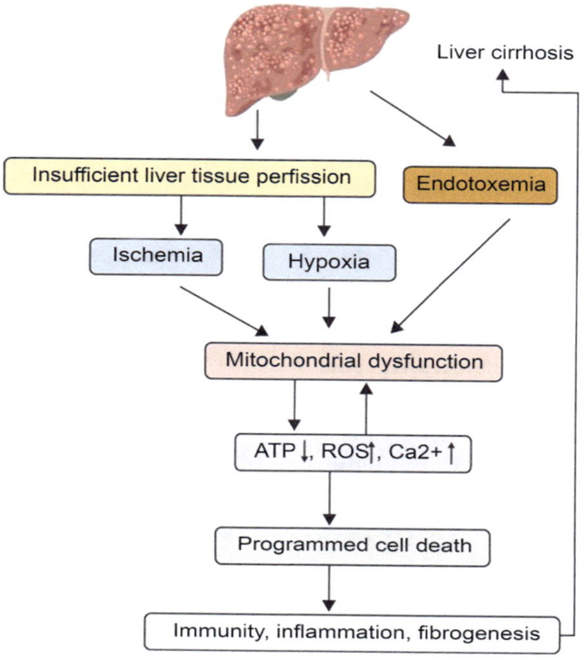

Figure 3.9. Mitochondrial dysfunction and liver cirrhosis.

Source: https://www.researchgate.net/publication/356162556/figure/fig4/AS:1089285352624128@1636717274034/Mitochondrial-dysfunction-and-liver-cirrhosis-In-liver-cirrhosis-stimuli-such-as.jpg.

3.3. Symptoms of Cirrhosis

The signs of cirrhosis are caused by a range of physical changes that show the liver is damaged. At the beginning of cirrhosis, a person may feel tired, weak, and notice their skin and eyes turning yellow, which is called jaundice. As the liver is damaged more and more, it has less ability to clear bilirubin, which causes jaundice. If the liver does not produce enough albumin, patients might get edema, which causes swelling in the lower body and abdomen. Anyone showing these signs should be checked further, since they usually mean the liver is not functioning properly and should be treated quickly. As cirrhosis becomes worse, patients might start to have more severe symptoms such as varices and ascites caused by portal hypertension. Varices are caused by high blood pressure in the portal circulation, which results in the veins in the esophagus and stomach swelling; this condition can be very dangerous because it increases the risk of severe bleeding. Besides, ascites, which is the buildup of fluid in the abdomen, both reduces quality of life and can cause serious infections such as spontaneous bacterial peritonitis. Such complications demonstrate that the liver is not functioning well and stress the importance of using a range of strategies to prevent further health problems and death from the disease. Cirrhosis is often linked to other issues in the body, such as HE, which can affect people besides the patient. Impaired liver function causes toxins to accumulate, which can lead to changes in the brain and cause confusion, altered mental states, and sometimes coma. CLD can also predispose patients to infections, as evidenced by its association with necrotizing fasciitis, particularly in individuals with compromised immune systems, such as those suffering from LC (Andronache *et al.*, 2020). Because these symptoms are so linked, finding and treating cirrhosis early can greatly improve both the outcome and daily life for those who have it. Furthermore, it is essential to recognize that inadequate screening for hepatitis C, a leading cause of cirrhosis, underscores the need for more proactive health care strategies to address this public health concern (Thompson *et al.*, 2015) (Figure 3.10).

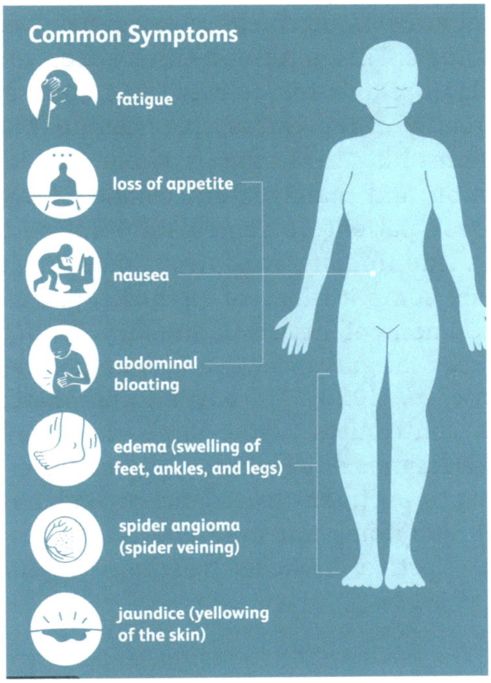

Figure 3.10. Common symptoms of cirrhosis.

Source: https://www.verywellhealth.com/thmb/9zkvvaobDJUOzUefRA52kQQMkDg=/1500x0/filters:no_upscale():max_bytes(150000):strip_icc()/cirrhosis-what-you-need-to-know-1759889_color3-5c454d94c9e77c0001b2bba8.png.

3.3.1. Early Symptoms (Fatigue, Weakness)

In cirrhosis, such symptoms as weakness and fatigue are vital markers of declining liver function and general well-being and are typically brought on by a myriad of causes, including metabolic dysregulation, accumulation of toxins, and nutrition deficiencies common with liver disease. With the liver's ability to metabolize and detoxify diminished by cirrhosis, patients will find that they have greater fatigue that affects daily activities. There will also be a weakness that is often combined with malnourishment and wasting away of the muscles. It is important to treat these symptoms early in the diagnostic phase because they will have a significant impact on the prognosis and the quality of life in the patients, highlighting the need for close monitoring by doctors. Weakness and fatigue not only reflect the physiologic price of cirrhosis but also have significant psychological implications. End-stage liver disease patients are frequently dominated by affective and cognitive impairment with a subsequent fatigue syndrome that is as much psychological as it is physiologic. This mind-body interaction complicates cirrhosis treatment, as patients can experience complaining and self-referent but apparently minor symptoms that severely disrupt motivation and quality of life. Successful treatment strategies must therefore attend not only to the somatic symptoms but also to the psychological concomitants of liver disease. As earlier studies identified, detection and management of such early manifestations can guide later treatment, leading to improved patient outcomes, all pointing to the intricacy of cirrhosis interventions (Yaman *et al.*, 2023). Additionally, weakness and fatigue, earlier symptoms, can be precursors to the evolution of some complications of cirrhosis, particularly as advanced levels are attained. For instance, the development of hepatopulmonary syndrome or portopulmonary hypertension can manifest as increased fatigue and weakness in general as the body strives to access its required oxygen needs (Chan *et al.*, 2020). Moreover, inflammatory responses within the body trigger additional fatigue, which contributes to the cirrhosis patient's complications. Therefore, timely identification and proper diagnosis reveal the significance of monitoring of these mundane but significant symptoms, leading to pertinent treatment regimens considering future complications. Anticipatory control of initial symptoms not only alleviates pain for the patient but also is an unavoidable component of an effective cirrhosis treatment regimen, ultimately contributing to better long-term health (Figure 3.11).

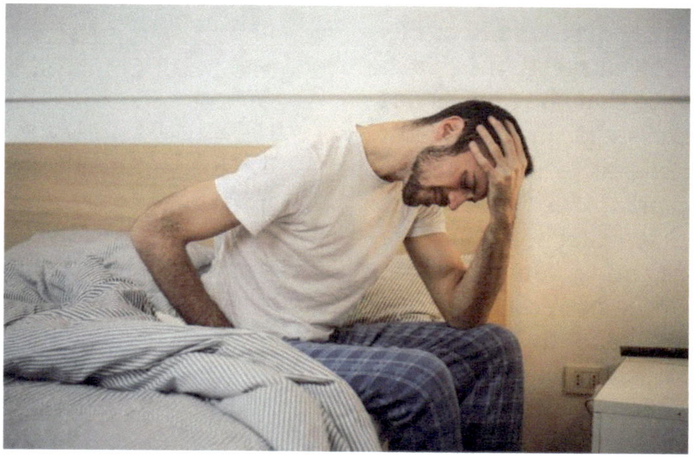

Figure 3.11. Symptoms of cirrhosis

Source: https://circledna.com/blog/wp-content/uploads/2023/08/content_images_assets.prenetics.com_blog.circledna.com_wp-content_uploads_2021_11_16003744_pexels-andrea-piacquadio-3771115_adobespark.jpg.

3.3.2. Advanced Symptoms (Jaundice, Ascites)

When cirrhosis becomes severe, patients often develop symptoms that have a big effect on their quality of life, such as jaundice and ascites. Jaundice happens when the liver cannot properly remove bilirubin, which is made when red blood cells break down. The yellowing of both the skin and the sclera is a sign that the liver is not working properly and indicates the severity of the liver's impairment. Besides, jaundice could be a sign that the condition is worsening, which may lead to other severe problems in decompensated cirrhosis. Jaundice is an indication of liver problems and is also linked to increased risk of health problems, which may call for closer care and possible medical actions to help the patient.

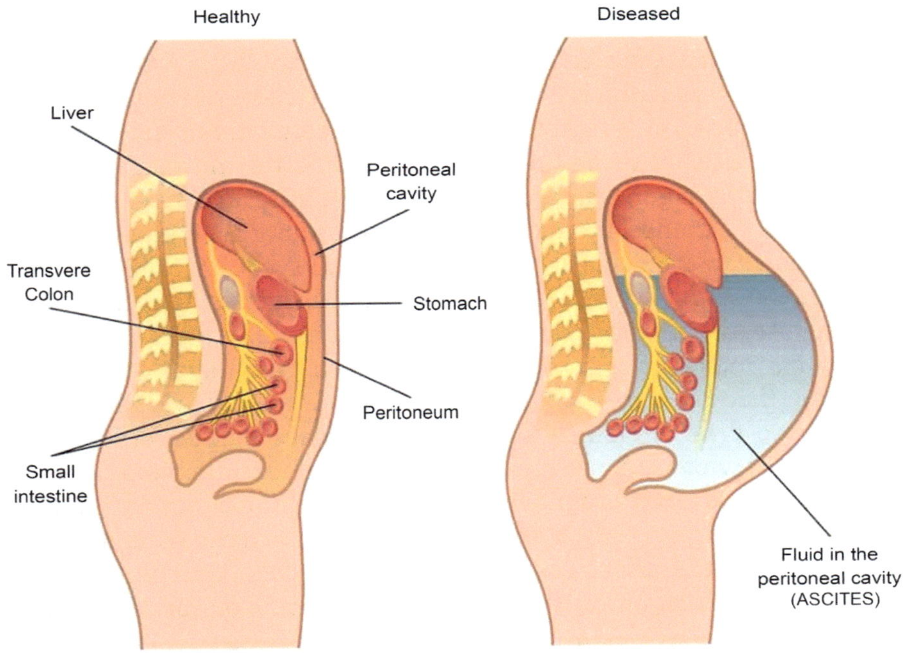

Figure 3.12. Ascites illustration.

Source: https://irp.cdn-website.com/91c80bfd/dms3rep/multi/ascites-illustration.jpg.

Besides jaundice, another serious complication of cirrhosis is ascites, which is the buildup of fluid in the abdomen. It mainly happens because of portal hypertension, and it can be severe for the patient. The fluid build-up can lead to abdominal distension, discomfort, and a myriad of complications, including renal impairment and spontaneous bacterial peritonitis (SBP)—a common infection in these patients. Studies have shown that albumin infusion can be beneficial in the management of ascites, as it helps in restoring intravascular volume and reducing the risk of paracentesis-induced circulatory dysfunction (Heybe *et al.*, 2024). But since ascites is present, surgery is difficult because patients are more likely to get umbilical hernias, and these hernias can cause additional health problems if they are not treated promptly. When jaundice and ascites are found together in someone with cirrhosis, it shows how seriously the liver is not working and how quickly medical action is required. Both symptoms can make each other worse, which results in a cycle that worsens the patient's health. An example is that increased pressure in the abdomen from ascites can reduce blood flow to the liver, which makes jaundice worse and aggravates the liver problem. For this reason, handling such advanced symptoms usually involves a team of specialists working together to address both the liver's functions and the complications that arise. Addressing these symptoms in tandem not only improves patient comfort but also significantly enhances the potential for better health outcomes in individuals suffering from cirrhosis (Figure 3.12).

3.3.3. Complications Related to Symptoms

Complications of cirrhosis symptoms can profoundly impact patients' lives and have a tendency to perpetuate a cycle of worsening health. One of the biggest consequences is increased hospitalization from symptoms such as HE and functional impairment. Studies utilizing health-related quality of life (HRQOL) measures have illustrated that cirrhotic patients commonly struggle with daily activities, founded on disabling fatigue and physical function loss. Further, PROMIS tool scores have indicated that decreased scores for daily function are linked to an increased risk of non-elective hospitalization, revealing the relationship between symptom severity and healthcare utilization in this group (Bajaj *et al.*, 2017). The consequences of these findings illustrate how symptoms of cirrhosis function as predictors and precipitants of a general decline in health status, further emphasizing the need for intervention to avoid such outcomes. Both depression and anxiety are frequent in cirrhotic patients, and both add another layer to the disease symptomatology. Psychological status has been found to have a significant influence on HRQOL, demonstrating that psychiatric conditions are not merely comorbidities but are integral parts of cirrhosis management. Emotional distress is usually added to the somatic symptoms and leads to further impairment in everyday functioning. Assessments of cirrhotic patients show that rates of psychiatric disease prevalence are quite overwhelming, and studies catch some of the diverse elements of mood disorders that adversely affect their quality of life (Bilzer *et al.*, 2002). Hence, treatment of these mood complications is a must as they are greatly intertwined with the overall prognosis and need a multidisciplinary intervention including physical health as well. The interrelation of the symptoms of cirrhosis is also illustrated by the way pain and functional status affect readmission to hospitals. Outcomes have indicated that pain management isn't merely significant in rendering patients comfortable but also in reducing hospitalization rates. The PROMIS pain domain similarly has been shown to predict highly the risk of re-hospitalization, implying that chronic pain should be a target for treatment within this population of patients (Bajaj *et al.*, 2017). Furthermore, those patients who experience substantial pain are also more likely to experience elevated levels of distress, which continues as a vicious cycle to exacerbate both their clinical condition and quality of life. Thus, care of cirrhotic patients must extend beyond the usual medical therapy to include pain management and psychological support interventions, and an understanding of the multifaceted complications of the condition.

3.4. Diagnosis of Cirrhosis

Diagnosing cirrhosis is not simple and requires using clinical, laboratory, and imaging methods at the same time. Initially, a thorough medical history (anamnesis) is crucial to identify potential risk factors such as alcohol consumption, viral hepatitis, and autoimmune disorders. Signs of liver dysfunction, for example, jaundice, ascites, or spider angiomata, may be found during a physical examination. LFTs and serologic markers, which are tested in the laboratory, provide helpful information for making a diagnosis. Even so, these tests are essential, but they do not always give a clear answer.

Thus, imaging studies, including ultrasound or CT scans, help visualize liver structure and function, allowing for the identification of complications like portal hypertension or nodular liver morphology, commonly associated with cirrhosis (Hendriani *et al.*, 2023). All these tests together give a clear picture of liver health, which is important for diagnosing cirrhosis. Confirming a diagnosis of cirrhosis often requires more invasive techniques, with liver biopsy (LBx) remaining the gold standard. This way, pathologists can directly look at liver tissue, which helps them see fibrosis, necrosis, and the regenerative nodules that characterize cirrhosis. The biopsy also provides insights into the etiology of the disease, which is critical for effective management (Hendriani *et al.*, 2023). In recent years, non-invasive methods such as transient elastography (FibroScan) have emerged as valuable alternatives, offering the ability to assess liver stiffness and estimate fibrosis levels without the associated risks of a biopsy. Such advances help lower the risk of discomfort and additional issues for patients while ensuring correct results. As a result, as we discover more about liver disease, we have more tools to diagnose cirrhosis, which means doctors should customize their assessments for each patient. Managing cirrhosis requires knowing about its complications, which are caused by the disease progressing. Those who have cirrhosis are likely to develop problems such as portal hypertension, ascites, HE, and HCC, which should be closely watched and treated when necessary. If ascites is present, paracentesis may be done to ease discomfort and avoid infection, and HE may require diet changes and drugs to control ammonia. This intricate web of complications necessitates timely diagnosis and a multidisciplinary approach to treatment, incorporating gastroenterologists, dietitians, and transplant surgeons when applicable (Mostafa and Nwidu, 2023). As such, the accurate and timely diagnosis of cirrhosis is not just pivotal for immediate management but also plays a crucial role in guiding long-term therapeutic strategies, ultimately influencing patient outcomes (Figure 3.13).

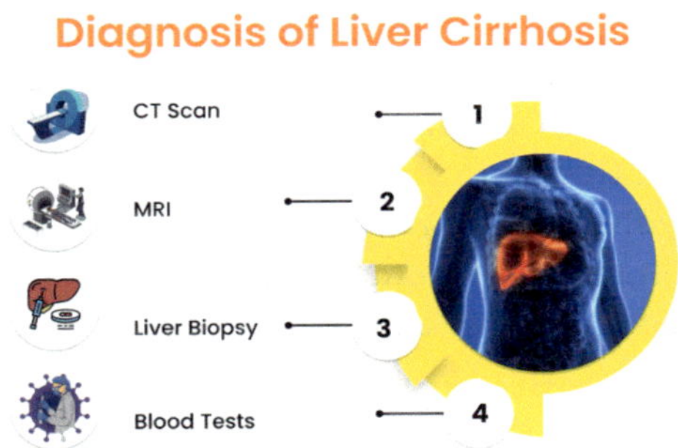

Figure 3.13. Diagnosis of liver cirrhosis.

Source: https://www.acegastrojaipur.com/wp-content/uploads/2022/06/imgpsh_fullsize_anim-59.png.

3.4.1. Medical History and Physical Examination

The role of medical history in assessing cirrhotic patients is overwhelming, for it provides an integrated model of liver disease etiology. A sufficient history not only encompasses the patient's alcohol intake and potential exposure to viral hepatitis but also conditions such as familial liver disease and metabolic disorders. In particular, the differences in the presentation of alcoholic hepatitis between ethnic groups are a reflection of the need for cultural competence in the taking of medical history. For instance, studies have shown that Latino patients experience ALD-related complications, including gastrointestinal bleeding and HE, at a higher frequency than their Caucasian counterparts (Durbin-Johnson *et al.*, 2017). Understanding of these nuances can have a large bearing on management plans and patient outcomes, and the significance of proper medical history in the case of cirrhosis and its complications cannot be overstated. Physical examination in patients with suspected cirrhosis is also a significant component of the overall assessment and can provide information that is critical to diagnosis and management. Key findings may include jaundice, ascites, and spider angiomata, which are indicative of portal hypertension and hepatic decompensation. Additionally, physical examination will most often manifest signs of systemic expressions of liver disease, i.e., HE or muscle wasting. For instance, asterixis—a tremor of hands that flaps—may reflect severe hepatic dysfunction (Hu *et al.*, 2006). Besides physical findings, observational evidence shows that certain populations are at increased risk for some cirrhosis complications, making it relevant to conduct a delicate physical examination. A detailed physical examination is therefore a foundation for early intervention and further investigation steps in the management of cirrhosis. Integration of history taking and physical examination is essential in the general management of cirrhosis, especially in the prophylaxis of possible complications. The relationship between the individual history of liver disease in a patient and the patient's presentation is useful to the clinician in developing a targeted plan of treatment. For example, identification of risk factors such as a history of admission for alcoholism or recurrent SBP is useful in developing anticipatory management plans. Also, determination of the systemic significance of cirrhosis, such as the risk of HCC among patients with chronic hepatitis C, highlights the importance of active surveillance and follow-up (Hu *et al.*, 2006). Through data integration from both medical history and physical examination, clinicians can better address the multidimensional complexity of cirrhosis and reduce its complications, thus improving patient outcomes.

3.4.2. Imaging Tests (Ultrasound, CT Scan)

To diagnose and treat cirrhosis and its complications, imaging tests are very important. Since it is available, inexpensive, and painless, ultrasound is usually the initial test doctors use. It makes it possible to observe the liver, find ascites, and check for complications, including PVT. With Doppler ultrasound, it is now easier to see the flow in the hepatic and portal veins, which supports the accurate diagnosis of PVT, which is being found more often with these new imaging methods. The lifetime risk of developing PVT is notable, particularly in patients with cirrhosis, underlining the importance of thorough ultrasonographic evaluation in this population to prevent further complications (Cuschieri *et al.*, 2013). Computed tomography (CT) scans serve as another critical imaging modality, particularly in evaluating complicated cases of cirrhosis. CT scans are very good at showing detailed sections of the liver, which helps find HCC and any related lesions. Contrast-enhanced CT scanning allows doctors to see tumors more clearly and check for vascular involvement, which helps with diagnosis. According to studies, CT is very effective in detecting HCC in cirrhotic patients, which is why it is an important tool for monitoring these patients. Moreover, the role of CT extends beyond mere diagnosis; it also assists in planning interventions such as radiofrequency ablation by accurately characterizing lesions and their relationship to surrounding structures (Bezzi *et al.*, 2009). Choosing between ultrasound and CT scans for cirrhosis is mostly determined by the patient's condition and what the doctor needs to find out. Usually, ultrasound is used to check and monitor liver problems at first, but CT scans may be done if more information about the liver is needed or if signs of advanced disease appear. Every imaging method brings different benefits, and using them together can improve patient diagnosis and treatment outcomes. Ultimately, a thorough understanding of the strengths and limitations of ultrasound and CT scans enables clinicians to make informed decisions, optimizing the management of patients with cirrhosis and its myriad complications (Figure 3.14).

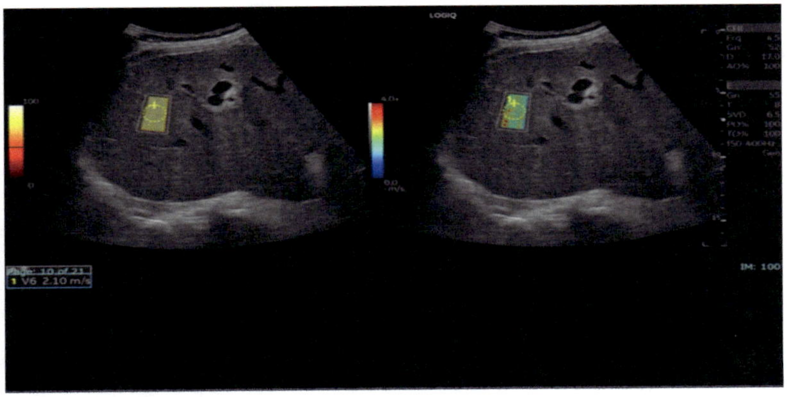

Figure 3.14. Abdominal ultrasound with a cirrhotic nodular appearing liver and moderate ascites.

Source: .https://prod-imagesstatic.radiopaedia.org/images/59633350/987649321aaf07531393b4b99b12e41a236ab42b411747e683a98bafdb2966d8_big_gallery.jpeg

3.4.3. Liver Biopsy and Laboratory Tests

The evaluation of the pathology of the liver usually involves the use of LBx in combination with several laboratory tests to ascertain the grade of cirrhosis and associated complications. LBx is an anchor diagnosis test, and it provides valuable histological information that can be used to differentiate various liver conditions, grade the severity of fibrosis, and diagnose other pathologies such as hepatitis or HCC. This critical evaluation not only aids in diagnosis but also in treatment planning. In conjunction with histological findings, laboratory tests such as serum transaminases and bilirubin are also essential in measuring liver function and the progression of disease. They can provide evidence of hepatic inflammation and dysfunction and help clinicians in their approach to managing patients who are diagnosed with cirrhosis and its complications. Execution of some laboratory tests is a crucial function in raising knowledge regarding liver illness, with certain tests to diagnose underlying conditions that may result in cirrhosis. As a case in point, the presence of HCV can be determined by serological testing for HCV antibodies and HCV RNA quantification. These tests not only present high sensitivity but also impact treatment since the response rates to antiviral treatment are significantly varied based on HCV genotype (Hu *et al.*, 2006). The results of these tests can also contribute to determining whether patients require treatment urgently or further monitoring. As diagnostic laboratory tests evolve, they form a critical component of true holistic management of cirrhosis tailored to the individual needs and risk factors of the patient. With LBx and laboratory tests, awareness of the prognostic significance of their results plays a critical role in optimal management of cirrhosis. The possibility of complications such as HCC or transplant candidacy largely lies with biopsy results, capable of identifying severe fibrosis or advanced cirrhosis. Furthermore, evidence shows that the severity of liver injury, as histologically determined, correlates with post-transplant outcomes, including graft survival and potential occurrence of complications (DiMartini *et al.*, 2001). This data is not only a guide for clinical decision-making but also highlights the requirement for thorough pre-transplant evaluation in an attempt to identify co-existent conditions which can further enhance morbidity and mortality in treatment subjects of ALD or other complications of cirrhosis (Figure 3.15).

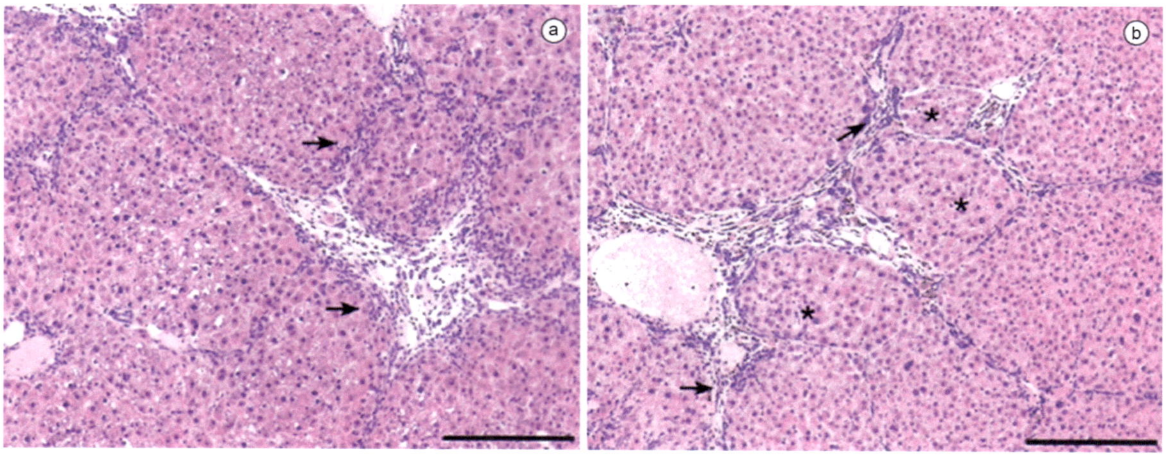

Figure 3.15. Photomicrography representing liver cirrhosis (a) Material collected at biopsy, just after induction of cirrhosis. (b) Material collected at euthanasia, 80 days after induction.

Source: https://www.researchgate.net/profile/Francisco-Javier-Hernandez-Blazquez/publication/269807257/figure/fig2/AS:408605372239872@1474430520184/Photomicrography-representing-liver-cirrhosis-a-Material-collected-at-biopsy-just-after.png.

3.5. Treatment Options for Cirrhosis

Treatments for cirrhosis depend on the cause and work to control the problems that come from the disease. One main approach is to deal with the causes of liver damage, which may involve antiviral medicines for viral hepatitis. The introduction of direct-acting antiviral (DAA) agents has revolutionized the management of HCV infection, leading to sustained virological response rates that significantly improve clinical outcomes. With these therapies, which are now the standard, it is possible to stop cirrhosis from worsening and lower the chances of people dying from it. Successful treatment can also diminish the need for liver transplantation and lower the incidence of HCC, especially among patients with advanced liver disease and chronic infections (Hu *et al.*, 2006). For this reason, it is very important to find candidates early by using serological and molecular tests to use the best treatment methods and prevent complications of cirrhosis. Along with antiviral drugs, managing cirrhosis usually involves taking care of symptoms and preventing complications. Many patients deal with ascites, HE, and variceal bleeding, which require special treatments to improve their quality of life. Fluid retention is managed with diuretics such as spironolactone, and lactulose helps to prevent or manage HE by reducing the amount of ammonia in the blood. Also, preventing variceal hemorrhage is important, and this is done with band ligation or sclerotherapy based on the size and risk factors of the varices. Since cirrhosis can cause many difficulties, it is important to keep monitoring and managing the condition, which highlights the need for overall care that looks after both the liver and its consequences. In addition, modifying lifestyle is essential in managing cirrhosis, especially for patients with alcoholic or nonalcoholic fatty liver disease. Having no alcohol and eating a balanced diet can greatly improve liver health and slow down the progression of diseases. Using strategies to help overweight and obese patients lose weight has been shown to lower hepatic inflammation and improve LFTs. Routine check-ups and teaching patients help them stick to their treatment, notice possible complications, and ask for help when needed. The multifactorial nature of cirrhosis requires an integrated approach, taking into account pharmacological interventions and lifestyle changes as complementary components of a robust treatment framework (Dumitru *et al.*, 2019). This comprehensive strategy aims not only to prolong survival but also to improve overall health and well-being in patients suffering from this chronic condition (Figure 3.16).

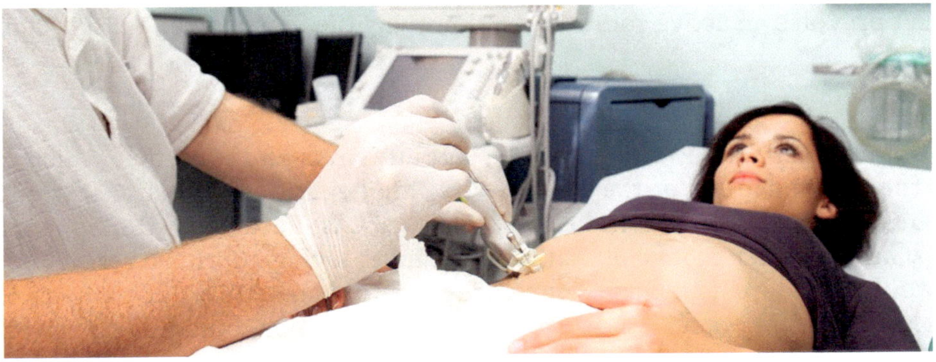

Figure 3.16. Abdominal ultrasound

Source: https://www.hopkinsmedicine.org/-/media/images/health/1_-conditions/liver-cancer/chronic-liver-disease-hero.jpg?h=500&iar=0&mh=500&mw=1300&w=1297&hash=BA095B82666F7E3AB7B76772783BEC65.

3.5.1. Lifestyle Changes (Diet, Alcohol Cessation)

The management of cirrhosis is significantly enhanced by dietary adjustments, particularly in diet and alcohol avoidance. Dietary adjustments are capable of decreasing the progression of liver disease and its associated complications. Healthy dietary intake containing fruits, vegetables, whole grains, and lean proteins provides the nutrients necessary for liver health as well as possibly enhancing overall metabolic function. Additionally, an adequate demand of fundamental vitamins and minerals, such as calcium and vitamin D, is crucial. These dietary reforms play a critical role in offering recovery and forming immunity against future liver damage, especially in those who abuse alcohol chronically, which is commonly the primary etiology of cirrhosis. With healthy eating habits, one can not only restore liver function but also treat other health conditions like osteoporosis, which is worsened by cirrhosis, as well as one's choice of living (Potashkin *et al.*, 2024). Abstinence from alcohol is still one of the pillars of cirrhosis management, immediately controlling the progression of the disease and risk of complications. Recurrent alcohol use in the context of liver disease has been shown to exacerbate liver injury, as in some research that shows alcohol's harmful effects being compounded when they are combined with conditions like diabetes (Gopinath *et al.*, 2024). Abstention from alcohol allows the liver to heal from such activities, thereby reducing inflammation and fibrosis. Further, studies have determined that those who are successful at avoiding alcohol experience a drastic decrease in morbidity and mortality due to cirrhosis. Therefore, those patients who undertake this life change not only improve the quality of their lives but also improve the chances of survival for an extended period of time, as well as reduce hospitalization due to liver disease. In addition to nutritional supplementation and alcohol withdrawal, the implementation of physical activity interventions can also enhance the management of cirrhosis. Weight and insulin sensitivity are kept optimal with regular exercise, and overall liver function is enhanced. Exercise has been shown to have a positive impact on bone health, which is especially beneficial in cirrhotic patients who may be at increased risk for developing osteoporosis. As one makes changes to their lifestyle by incorporating exercise along with diet change and cessation of alcohol intake, one gains a synergistic effect towards improving overall health. Not only does this general approach address the short-term complications of cirrhosis, but it also lays the foundation for long-term health benefits. Prioritizing these lifestyle changes in any individual who has cirrhosis is of the utmost importance, as it provides an active solution for improving the management of this complex disease.

3.5.2. Medications (Antivirals, Diuretics)

The treatment of cirrhosis often requires the use of antivirals and diuretics, which are important for managing the complications of the disease. Chronic hepatitis C infections, which often cause cirrhosis, are best treated with antiviral drugs, mainly DAAs. Because of DAAs, people living with hepatitis C now have a better chance of being cured and enjoying improved results from treatment. It is vital, however, to address potential drug-drug interactions (DDIs) as patients with cirrhosis frequently manage multiple medications for comorbid conditions and adverse events related to the virus.

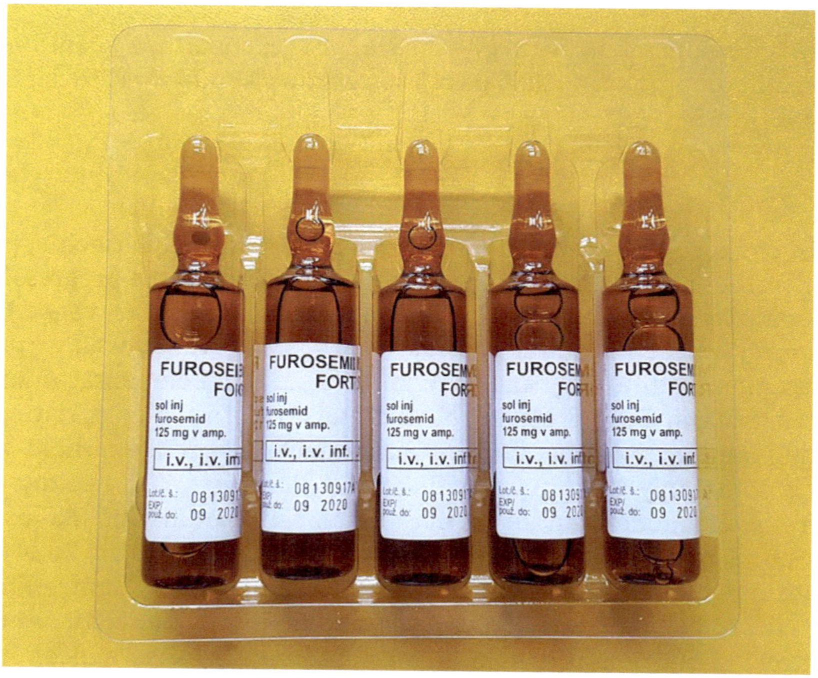

Figure 3.17. Furosemid 125mg/2ml ampule.

Source: https://upload.wikimedia.org/wikipedia/commons/thumb/2/27/Furosemid_125mg_vials_yellow_background.jpg/800px-Furosemid_125mg_vials_yellow_background.jpg.

Thus, understanding pharmacokinetics and the disposition of these drugs becomes critical for ensuring effective and safe treatment, particularly in patients already compromised by liver dysfunction (Erceg *et al.*, 2017). Doctors often give spironolactone and furosemide to help manage fluid buildup and swelling that happens due to cirrhosis-related portal hypertension. The medications help reduce the symptoms, which improves how patients feel. Still, it is necessary to carefully watch their use to prevent problems such as electrolyte problems and kidney damage in patients with cirrhosis. Doctors must be careful with the amount of diuretic given to avoid both benefits and side effects. It is also necessary to keep monitoring renal function and electrolyte levels since they can play a major role in deciding the right treatment. Furthermore, knowing how these diuretics interact with other medications, especially in the context of polypharmacy, heightens the necessity for comprehensive management approaches (Blumberg *et al.*, 2012). Using antivirals and diuretics together to treat cirrhosis shows how complicated managing this disease can be. Physicians can make better decisions about drugs by using available online interactive tools. Such platforms help doctors learn about possible interactions and decide how to change the patient's dose or monitor their treatment. Because cirrhosis treatment can be complex, it is important to use a team approach to improve how well medications work and reduce side effects. As clinical guidelines evolve, continuous education on the pharmacological management of cirrhosis is imperative, ensuring both healthcare providers and patients are well-informed about the intricacies of their treatment regimens (Erceg *et al.*, 2017) (Figure 3.17).

3.5.3. Surgical Interventions (Liver Transplant)

The severity of cirrhosis typically results in the necessity for urgent surgical intervention, primarily liver transplantation, which is a curative option for end-stage liver disease. The procedure is particularly important for patients who have undergone marked liver decompensation and for whom normal treatment measures are no longer effective. Timely referral to transplant centers is underscored by literature as essential in order to optimize outcomes and survival rates among candidates with advanced liver disease. For instance, a consensus panel of the Italian Association for the Study of the Liver has outlined determinants to decision-making for liver transplantation that entail identification of difficult-to-manage candidates and ensuring that referral mechanisms are effective (Burra *et al.*, 2018). This consensus is intended to emphasize multi-dimensional decision-making considerations in patient selection and the expertise in the effective management of complex liver cases. Among all complications of cirrhosis, the assessment of physical frailty has been seen to be a significant predictor for candidates waiting for a liver transplant. Recent evidence indicates that frailty, as detected through standardized tools such as the Fried Frailty Index, is present in a significant number of transplant-listed cirrhotic patients. Interestingly, almost 31.6% of such patients exhibit signs of frailty, statistically correlated with increased hospitalizations and risk of adverse outcomes (Dodge *et al.*, 2016). Signs like grip strength, gait speed, and activity level are crucial predictors of a patient's capacity to tolerate major surgery. Thus, frailty assessment not only plays an important role in the evaluation of possible transplant candidates but also guides preoperative optimization procedures that aim to reduce hospitalization rates. Results following liver transplant in cirrhosis can be significantly improved if preoperative frailty is addressed. Physical resilience can be enhanced through certain measures, such as nutrition therapy and physiotherapy, possibly with improved recovery and reduced complication risk during and following transplant surgery. Malnutrition treatment—a common condition in cirrhosis—remains further able to maximize patient outcomes because inadequate nutrition hastens frailty and post-operative risk. Furthermore, composite treatment protocols now facilitate the use of DAA agents for managing associated hepatitis infections, potentially maximizing transplant success (Burra *et al.*, 2018). As the nuances regarding surgery for cirrhosis continue to evolve, a concerted focus on frailty and operative fitness will continue to drive next-generation transplant protocols and patient care strategy (Figure 3.18).

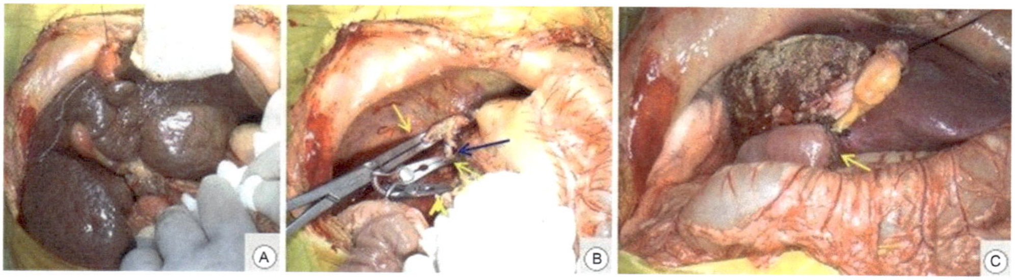

Figure 3.18. Liver transplantation procedures. (A) Naïve liver: enlarged liver with cirrhosis. (B) Anhepatic phase: inferior vena cava (IVC) was totally clamped. Yellow arrows show vascular clamp that was applied to the suprahepatic IVC and the intrahepatic IVC and a blue arrow indicates the IVC. An arrow head points to the bulldog clamp occluding the portal vein. (C) Engrafted left lateral section after reperfusion. Bile duct was reconstructed with Roux-en-Y hepaticojejunostomy. The yellow arrow indicates jejunum Roux limb.

Source: https://www.researchgate.net/publication/260684758/figure/fig2/AS:214278150856708@1428099300763/Liver-transplantation-procedures-A-Naive-liver-enlarged-liver-with-cirrhosis-B.png.

3.6. Complications of Cirrhosis

Cirrhosis brings with it many serious health issues that have a significant effect on how well patients do and how long they live. A major complication is portal hypertension, which happens when blood flow through the hepatic portal system becomes more resistant. Because of this condition, varices may form, mainly in the esophagus and stomach, and ruptures can cause dangerous bleeding inside the digestive tract. Besides, portal hypertension may result in ascites, a buildup of fluid in the abdomen, which raises the chance of developing SBP. Notably, studies indicate that varied access to healthcare resources may influence the complications experienced by different demographic groups, as evidenced by the higher rates of complications associated with alcoholic hepatitis in Latino patients compared to Caucasians, highlighting disparities in treatment and outcomes (Durbin-Johnson *et al.*, 2017). Because the liver cannot properly remove toxins, encephalopathy is a serious complication of cirrhosis, especially caused by ammonia. Sometimes, it results in brain dysfunction, changes in level of consciousness, and may lead to a hepatic coma. HE develops when neurotoxins build up and infections, changes in electrolytes, and kidney problems also play a role. When someone has cirrhosis, the treatment may involve managing the causes and using lactulose as well as making changes to their diet. The complexity of treating encephalopathy further complicates the overall management of cirrhosis, necessitating a comprehensive approach to minimize risk and optimize recovery (Burra *et al.*, 2018). In addition, many patients with cirrhosis often develop malnutrition, which is often missed. Problems with the liver can reduce the body's ability to absorb nutrients, which makes it more likely for muscles to waste and for the immune system to be weakened. Because of this lack of nutrition, patients are more likely to get infections and are less able to handle other complications. A nutritional assessment and dietary plan that fits the patient's needs are important in managing malnutrition in cirrhosis. Also, giving proper nutritional care is necessary to ensure the liver functions well and the patient's clinical outcomes improve. Given these interrelated challenges, the management of cirrhosis requires a multidisciplinary approach, integrating hepatology, dietetics, and patient education to counteract adverse complications (Burra *et al.*, 2018; Durbin-Johnson *et al.*, 2017).

3.6.1. Portal Hypertension and Varices

Portal hypertension, which is a direct consequence of cirrhosis, refers to high blood pressure in the portal venous circulation. This is caused primarily by the obstruction of blood flow through the liver, a physiological phenomenon in advanced CLD such as cirrhosis. The resulting elevated pressure can lead to a vast array of complications, including the formation of varices, which are dilated and deformed veins in areas such as the stomach and esophagus.

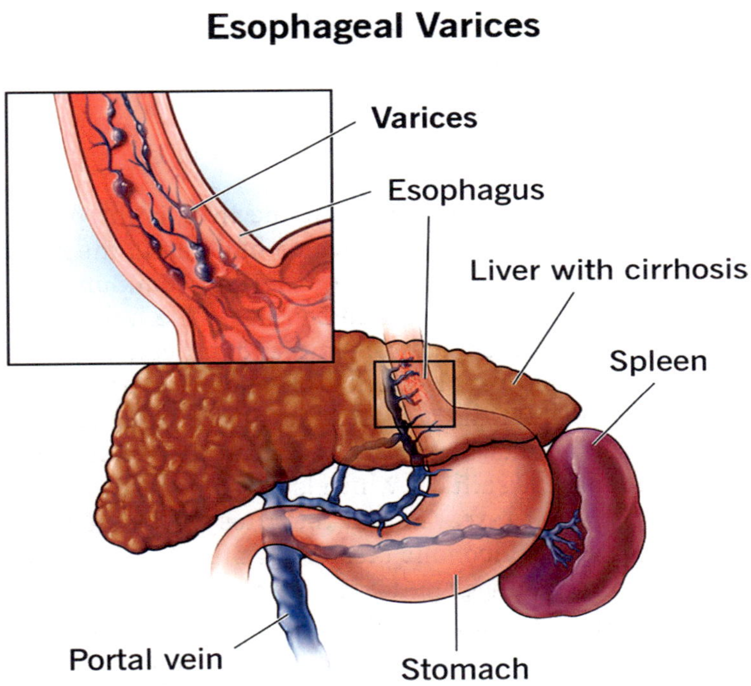

Figure 3.19. Esophageal varices.

Source: https://my.clevelandclinic.org/-/scassets/images/org/health/articles/15429-esophageal-varices.

Varices are a significant danger to patients since their rupture will cause lethal hemorrhages, which further complicate cirrhosis treatment and expend additional resources for the healthcare system. Knowledge of the pathophysiologic processes in portal hypertension is essential in designing prevention and management regimens to mitigate the severe effects of these complications (Foster *et al.*, 2020). Portal hypertension leads to the formation of varices as a direct consequence of collateral formation while attempting to circumvent the increased resistance within the liver.

Esophageal varices, in particular, are one of the best-described and most frequent complications in cirrhotic patients. Risk factors for determining the likelihood of variceal development include the severity of liver disease and portal hypertension, which often need close monitoring by endoscopy in cirrhotic patients. In some cases, non-invasive measures such as elastography can be useful in assessing liver stiffness and the risk of variceal development. This advanced thinking encourages early intervention, which is an important factor in preventing resultant esophageal hemorrhage and associated morbidity and mortality (Kim *et al.*, 2017). Portal hypertension and associated varices management essentially involves pharmacotherapy, endoscopic therapy, and, in advanced forms, surgery. Non-selective beta-blockers are often employed to lower portal pressure and reduce the risk of bleeding varices by lowering cardiac output and increasing splanchnic flow. If varices are detected, endoscopic band ligation is an effective technique to prevent hemorrhage. More intensive therapies, such as transjugular intrahepatic portosystemic shunt (TIPS), may be employed in non-responding patients. But these interventions themselves can carry risk for complications such as HE, and there is a need for ongoing patient monitoring and individualized care strategies in the treatment of portal hypertension and varices in the context of cirrhosis (Foster *et al.*, 2020) (Figure 3.19).

3.6.2. Hepatic Encephalopathy

Liver problems due to cirrhosis show how important the liver is for proper brain function. HE happens when the liver is unable to remove toxins, which build up in the blood and lead to various symptoms. As the liver fails in cirrhotic patients, the level of ammonia in the blood increases because the liver cannot change it into urea, which can harm the brain. HE usually starts subtly, and early signs are changes in mood, sleeping problems, and difficulties with thinking. As cirrhosis worsens, people may experience confusion, disorientation, and even coma, which greatly affects their daily lives and makes it harder to treat the disease. Tackling HE is essential, since it affects both the health and survival of these patients, so proper care and close observation are necessary. The characteristics of cirrhosis patients are shifting, which is causing more concern in the epidemiology of HE. It has been shown from recent research that the rates of cirrhosis are going up, especially due to alcoholic liver disease and nonalcoholic steatohepatitis. As noted, the demographic shifts, such as an increasing proportion of younger patients with alcoholic cirrhosis, require public health interventions focused on prevention and treatment modalities tailored to these specific populations (Chalasani *et al.*, 2019). Because older patients have a higher risk of liver-related complications, it is important to use personalized healthcare strategies for them. Being aware of these factors can guide doctors in screening, early diagnosis, and managing cirrhosis and its primary issue, HE. In cirrhosis, HE is managed by using a combination of medicines and non-medical methods. Common treatments for hepatic encephalopathy are lactulose, which stops ammonia from being absorbed, and rifaximin, an antibiotic that changes the bacteria in the gut to reduce ammonia production. Taking care of gastrointestinal bleeding, infections, and dehydration is very important to prevent HE from occurring. Importantly, demographic studies reveal disparities in healthcare access and outcomes related to HE, particularly among Latino populations, who exhibit higher rates of encephalopathy and complications associated with ARLD (Durbin-Johnson *et al.*, 2017). This disparity highlights the necessity for targeted healthcare initiatives that ensure equitable access to outpatient care and effective management strategies for all patients suffering from cirrhosis and its complications, especially those who are disproportionately affected (Figure 3.20).

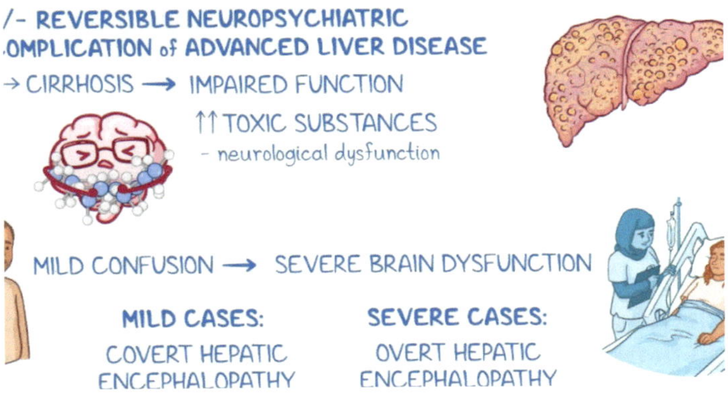

Figure 3.20. Hepatic encephalopathy.

Source: https://d16qt3wv6xm098.cloudfront.net/DOZDQloLTmqzGKqzImMiemboR7qdhfmS/_.jpg.

3.6.3. Liver Cancer Risk

The relationship between LC and risk of HCC development is also established, with considerable management implications for the patient. Because cirrhosis is the ultimate end point for most chronic liver diseases, its presence threatens to increase the risk of developing HCC highly. It is noted that cirrhotic patients have a 267-fold increased risk of developing HCC, particularly in those with underlying HCV infection or ALD. Specifically, nearly 19% of patients with HCV (hepatitis C virus) cirrhosis will become afflicted with HCC (hepatocellular carcinoma), highlighting the critical importance of vigilant surveillance in this population. Furthermore, the risk for other malignancies, such as cholangiocarcinoma and cancer of the gastrointestinal tract, is similarly elevated in cirrhotic patients relative to the general population, further emphasized by a broader oncological risk being present among CLD (Gunnarsdóttir *et al.*, 2008). Cirrhosis not only acts as a promoter for HCC but also produces a hypercoagulable state, which augments the risk for thromboembolic complications. Patients with HCC frequently present with complications of PVT, which dramatically alter their course of disease. Hemostatic balance in such patients is tilted towards a prothrombotic state, both due to the hepatic impairment secondary to cirrhosis and the tumor itself. Several interrelated mechanisms, including fibrinogen elevation and thrombocytosis, have been reported to be responsible for this hypercoagulable alteration. Therefore, management of the increased risk of thromboembolic complications is imperative for maximizing outcomes in HCC patients with cirrhosis. However, the lack of specific guidelines for thromboprophylaxis in this special group points to a need for further study and clinical attention (Burra *et al.*, 2018). Furthermore, the complications of LC extend beyond the risk of accelerated cancer and affect the general health and quality of life of patients. Gastrointestinal symptoms, minor cognitive impairment, and HE are common findings in advanced liver disease, complicating the clinical presentation. That portal hypertension also occurs with small bowel motility disorders implies a systemic reach of the effect. For instance, studies have shown that cirrhotic patients typically develop alterations in intestinal microbial flora secondary to motility alterations, which can further exacerbate liver dysfunction and complications. This coupled pathogenesis of cirrhosis-related factors emphasizes the necessity of multidisciplinary management options to decrease cancer risk and other secondary complications of this heterogeneous disease process, consequently leading to enhanced patient care and survival (Gunnarsdóttir *et al.*, 2008).

SUMMARY

In highlighting the intricacies involved in cirrhosis and its complications, it is clear that efficient management protocols are vital for enhancing patients' outcomes. Cirrhosis, as a condition with irreversible liver damage and fibrosis, tends to result in multi-dimensional complications involving heightened vulnerability to infections, HE, and deterioration of the overall function of the liver. Appreciation of these complications not only emphasizes the issue of early detection and intervention but also supports the issue of employing holistic treatment modalities. LC patients need to be handled with extreme care since their risk for the development of severe complications increases, hence the need for a subtle treatment approach both in the clinical and management contexts. The use of combined therapies such as long-term human albumin (HA) infusion has also been impressive, particularly in patients who have concomitant underlying conditions such as type 2 DM. Applying this has been linked with enhanced survival and reduction of complications associated with cirrhosis, such as overt HE and renal dysfunction. especially among patients with co-morbidities, certain treatment pathways can deliver stark clinical improvements, presenting crucial evidence in favor of personalized interventions among cirrhotic patients. Surprisingly, the data does suggest that enhanced overall survival is observed with adopting holistic treatment approaches (Pompili *et al.*, 2024), establishing a crucial correlation between personalized therapy and outcomes. Further, with the ongoing complicated patient management, advanced liver disease, and procedural risks such as those of Trans Arterial Chemo-Embolization (TACE) cannot be minimized. It is important to know the risk factors for hepatic decompensation following TACE since it will inform the choice of patient and clinical management. Identification of such critical markers as serum albumin and tumor size has a strong correlation with the post-TACE outcome, indicating that thorough patient evaluation should be performed to minimize adverse effects. Therefore, further research and clinical follow-up are warranted to evolve these treatment modalities and risk estimates in order to enable healthcare professionals cirrhosis and enhance the quality of life of affected individuals (El-Masry *et al.*, 2022).

Cirrhosis, being a chronic liver disease (CLD), leads to drastic physiological changes that determine the course of many complications. One of the foremost things to understand is the formation of liver fibrosis and its development into cirrhosis, characterized by the replacement of normal tissue in the liver with scar tissue. This disrupts the liver's capability to perform its essential functions, leading to complications such as portal hypertension, HE, and liver failure. The polyaspect of cirrhosis requires a comprehensive management plan that involves treating etiologic causes like alcohol consumption, viral hepatitis, and metabolic syndromes. Also, early diagnosis of cirrhosis signs and symptoms can be of crucial importance in facilitating timely intervention, patient outcome improvement, and survival. Another key consideration about cirrhosis is the challenge of managing associated complications. One of the most threatening of these complications is the esophageal varices, which pose the risk of life-threatening hemorrhage from increased portal hypertension. Prophylactic treatments and routine surveillance, such as the use of beta-blockers, can minimize these risks and make the patient safer. Control of the state of HE also needs to be scrupulous, with close monitoring of ammonia levels to prevent neurological decline. As also pointed out by the Italian Association for the Study of the Liver, other guidelines focus on early referral and proper cirrhotic patient management to ensure optimal outcomes of care, emphasizing the complexity of treating this illness (Burra *et al.*, 2018). Finally, liver transplant continues to be a prime consideration for advanced cirrhotic patients, especially those who have already developed complications such as HCC. Transplantation not only repairs the intrinsic defects pertaining to liver function but also has a very high impact on long-term survival. Liver transplantation, based on experiences, can achieve excellent prognosis in patients with end-stage liver disease, as indicated by survival rates of 89% at one year, five years, and ten years following transplant in certain groups of patients, such as primary biliary cirrhosis. Also, planning for the optimal timing of transplantation is necessary since delayed intervention will have adverse effects on outcomes. Incorporation of clinical data and prognosis scores in patient assessment is essential to enhance decision-making for transplantation candidacy and timing (Beuers *et al.*, 2000). Overall, knowledge of these most critical aspects of cirrhosis and its complications provokes effective management and care strategies.

CLOSER LOOK

PORTAL VEIN THROMBOSIS (PVT)

PVT is a condition where a blood clot blocks or narrows the portal vein, the major blood vessel that carries blood from the digestive system to the liver. This can lead to complications like portal hypertension and reduced blood supply to the liver.

The portal vein is a large vein that carries blood from the intestines, stomach, spleen, and pancreas to the liver. This blood is rich in nutrients absorbed from the digestive tract and carries it to the liver for processing (Figure 3.21).

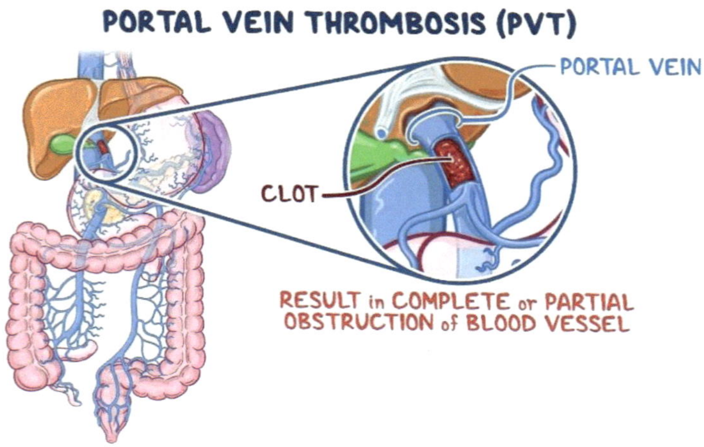

Figure 3.21. Portal vein thrombosis

Source: https://www.osmosis.org/_next/image?url=https%3A%2F%2Fd16qt3wv6xm098.cloudfront.net%2FF3cVIrc3RjiSHRpnEgHriPGgT2CIOeTb%2F_.jpg&w=3840&q=75.

What Happens in Portal Vein Thrombosis?

In PVT, a blood clot (thrombus) forms in the portal vein, obstructing or narrowing the blood flow. This can lead to several issues, including:

- **Increased Pressure in the Portal Vein (Portal Hypertension):** The clot blocks the flow, causing pressure to build up in the portal system.
- **Reduced Blood Flow to the Liver:** The clot can restrict blood flow, affecting liver function.
- **Potential Complications:** PVT can lead to complications like esophageal varices (swollen veins in the esophagus), ascites (fluid buildup in the abdomen), and splenomegaly (enlarged spleen).

Causes of Portal Vein Thrombosis:

PVT can be caused by various factors, including:

- ***Liver Disease*:** Cirrhosis (scarring of the liver) is a common cause, increasing the risk of clot formation.
- ***Other Medical Conditions*:** Abdominal malignancy, abdominal sepsis, pancreatitis, and certain blood-clotting disorders can also increase the risk.
- ***Inherited or Acquired Conditions*:** Some individuals may have inherited conditions that make them more prone to blood clots.
- ***Iatrogenic Causes*:** Rarely, PVT can be caused by medical procedures like bariatric surgery or radiofrequency ablation.

Symptoms of Portal Vein Thrombosis

PVT can be asymptomatic in some cases, and symptoms often appear when complications develop. Common symptoms may include:

- **Abdominal Pain:** Mild to severe pain, especially in the upper abdomen.
- **Swelling in the Abdomen (Ascites):** Fluid buildup in the abdominal cavity.
- **Vomiting Blood (Hematemesis) or Bloody Stools:** Indicative of esophageal varices or intestinal bleeding.
- **Jaundice:** Yellowing of the skin and eyes, indicating liver dysfunction.
- **Splenomegaly:** Enlarged spleen.

Diagnosis of Portal Vein Thrombosis

PVT is typically diagnosed through imaging tests, such as:

- **Ultrasound**: A non-invasive imaging technique that can visualize the portal vein and detect blood clots.
- **CT scan or MRI:** Provide more detailed images of the portal vein and surrounding structures.
- **Doppler Ultrasound:** A type of ultrasound that measures blood flow in the portal vein.

Treatment of Portal Vein Thrombosis

Treatment for PVT depends on the severity of the condition and the presence of complications:

- **Medications:** Blood thinners (anticoagulants) or thrombolytics (drugs that dissolve blood clots) may be used.
- **Surgical Procedures:** Thrombectomy (surgical removal of the clot) or a transvenous intrahepatic portosystemic shunt (TIPS) may be necessary in severe cases.
- **Other Treatments:** Treatment of underlying liver disease or other contributing factors may also be necessary.

References

1. Abdelmalek, M., Adams, L. A., Adams, L., Aithal, G. P., Albanis, E., Andrews, J. M., *et al.* (2009). *Pathogenesis of Non-Alcoholic Fatty Liver Disease.* https://core.ac.uk/download/pdf/19226.pdf.
2. Andronache, L. F., Bica, C., Gherghiceanu, F., *et al.* (2020). Diabetes mellitus and necrotizing fasciitis–a deadly combination; case report. https://core.ac.uk/download/304672921.pdf (accessed on 24 May 2025).
3. Bajaj, J. S., Fagan, A., Fuchs, M., *et al.* (2017). Symptom domain groups of the patient-reported outcomes measurement information system tools independently predict hospitalizations and re-hospitalizations in cirrhosis. https://core.ac.uk/download/84402872.pdf (accessed on 24 May 2025).
4. Beuers, U., Gerbes, A. L., Haller, M., *et al.* (2000). Liver transplantation in primary biliary cirrhosis: Risk assessment and 11-year follow-up. https://core.ac.uk/download/16432768.pdf (accessed on 24 May 2025).
5. Bezzi, M., Calliada, F., Cantisani, V., D'Ambrosio, U., *et al.* (2009). Is contrast-enhanced US alternative to spiral CT in the assessment of treatment outcome of radiofrequency ablation in hepatocellular carcinoma? https://core.ac.uk/download/54381315.pdf (accessed on 24 May 2025).
6. Bilzer, M., Ehrentraut, S., Gerbes, A. L., *et al.* (2002). Psychiatric and psychosocial outcome of orthotopic liver transplantation. https://core.ac.uk/download/16432271.pdf (accessed on 24 May 2025).
7. Blanco, J. J., Gomez-Manero, N., Herrero, J. I., *et al.* (2001). Liver transplantation in cirrhotic patients with diabetes mellitus: Midterm results, survival, and adverse events. https://core.ac.uk/download/83572434.pdf (accessed on 24 May 2025).
8. Blumberg, E., Hay, J. E., Lucey, M. R., *et al.* (2012). Long-term management of the successful adult liver transplant: 2012 practice guideline by the American Association for the Study of Liver Diseases and the American Society of Transplantation. http://deepblue.lib.umich.edu/bitstream/2027.42/95693/1/23566_ftp.pdf (accessed on 24 May 2025).
9. Boldeanu, L., Boldeanu, M. V., Caragea, D. C., *et al.* (2018). Clinical-evolutional particularities of the cryoglobulinemic vasculitis in the case of a patient diagnosed with hepatitis C virus in the predialitic phase. https://core.ac.uk/download/216808139.pdf (accessed on 24 May 2025).
10. Bonnefont-Rousselot, D., Bouam, S., *et al.* (2022). Burden of liver disease progression in hospitalized patients with type 2 diabetes mellitus. https://core.ac.uk/download/480394591.pdf (accessed on 24 May 2025).
11. Burra, P., Campello, E., Russo, F. P., *et al.* (2018). Cancer-associated thrombosis in cirrhotic patients with hepatocellular carcinoma. https://core.ac.uk/download/185557275.pdf (accessed on 24 May 2025).
12. Burra, P., Caraceni, P., Ferri, F., *et al.* (2018). Specific issues concerning the management of patients on the waiting list and after liver transplantation. https://core.ac.uk/download/159268374.pdf (accessed on 24 May 2025).

13. Campo, J. A. del, Gallego, P., Gallego-Durán, R., *et al.* (2018). Genetic and epigenetic regulation in nonalcoholic fatty liver disease (NAFLD). https://core.ac.uk/download/161254838.pdf (accessed on 24 May 2025).

14. Chalasani, N., Desai, A., Ghabril, M., Nephew, *et al.* (2019). Trends in characteristics, mortality, and other outcomes of patients with newly diagnosed cirrhosis. https://core.ac.uk/download/228066148.pdf (accessed on 24 May 2025).

15. Chan, S. L., El-Khoueiry, A., Galle, P. R., Meyer, *et al.* (2020). Diagnosis and management of toxicities of immune checkpoint inhibitors in hepatocellular carcinoma. https://core.ac.uk/download/323205689.pdf (accessed on 24 May 2025).

16. Cuschieri, S., Gauci, J., & Vassallo, M. (2013). Portal vein thrombosis: A case report and literature review. https://core.ac.uk/download/46602431.pdf (accessed on 24 May 2025).

17. DiMartini, A. M., Demetris, A. J., Jain, A., Balan, V., Bassendine, M., Becker, T., *et al.* (2001). Liver transplantation for alcoholic cirrhosis: Long term follow-up and impact of disease recurrence. https://core.ac.uk/download/12205555.pdf (accessed on 24 May 2025).

18. Dodge, J. L., Lai, J. C., Poltayskiy, E., *et al.* (2016). Frailty is independently associated with increased hospitalization days in patients on the liver transplant waitlist. https://core.ac.uk/download/323074083.pdf.

19. Dugas, M., Gavaler, J. S., Iwatsuki, S., *et al.* (1982). Liver transplantation in adults. https://core.ac.uk/download/12203903.pdf (accessed on 24 May 2025).

20. Dumitru, A., Popoiag, E., Micu, S. I., *et al.* (2019). The burden of Clostridium difficile infection in patients with liver cirrhosis. https://core.ac.uk/download/232440323.pdf (accessed on 24 May 2025).

21. Durbin-Johnson, B., Halsted, C. H., Medici, V., *et al.* (2017). Clinical features of alcoholic hepatitis in Latinos and Caucasians: A single center experience. https://core.ac.uk/download/323070371.pdf (accessed on 24 May 2025).

22. El-Masry, M., Abdel-Moez, F., Othman, M., Moussa, A. M., & Ismaiel, A. A. R. (2022). Analysis of risk factors for hepatic decompensation post trans arterial chemo embolization (TACE) for hepatocellular carcinoma (HCC) on top of cirrhotic liver. *The Egyptian Journal of Hospital Medicine*. https://www.semanticscholar.org/paper/0a8ed69034515c1a6badbb9ee767237867a54283 (accessed on 24 May 2025).

23. Erceg, D., Raguž-Lučić, N., & Steiner, S. (2017). Direct-acting antivirals (DAAs): Drug-drug interactions (DDIs) in the treatment of hepatitis C virus (HCV). https://core.ac.uk/download/322432848.pdf (accessed on 24 May 2025).

24. Evison, F., Ferguson, J., Gunson, B., *et al.* (2016). Acute kidney injury and post-reperfusion syndrome in liver transplantation. https://core.ac.uk/download/74320327.pdf (accessed on 24 May 2025).

25. Fassina, G., Gallotta, A., Martini, A., *et al.* (2015). Clinical applications of squamous cell carcinoma antigen-immunoglobulins M to monitor chronic hepatitis C. https://core.ac.uk/download/53529132.pdf (accessed on 24 May 2025).

26. Foster, K. (2020). Cirrhosis for the PCP. https://core.ac.uk/download/323270118.pdf (accessed on 24 May 2025).

27. Gopinath, V., Davis, A. M., Menon, T. K., & Raghavamenon, A. (2024). Alcohol promotes liver fibrosis

in high fat diet induced diabetic rats. *Journal of Basic and Clinical Physiology and Pharmacology*. https://www.semanticscholar.org/paper/e8b02cecbd7b04923de5effdc33864d303393577 (accessed on 24 May 2025).

28. Grazi, G. L. (2007). Liver resections: Complications and survival outcome. https://core.ac.uk/download/11162431.pdf (accessed on 24 May 2025).
29. Gunnarsdóttir, S. A. (2008). Liver cirrhosis—Epidemiological and clinical aspects. https://core.ac.uk/download/16315138.pdf (accessed on 24 May 2025).
30. Hendriani, A. D., Iswari, P. W. P., & Maharani, B. N. P. (2023). Liver cirrhosis: Pathophysiology, diagnosis, and management. https://core.ac.uk/download/599214433.pdf (accessed on 24 May 2025).
31. Heybe, M. A., & Mehta, K. J. (2024). Role of albumin infusion in cirrhosis-associated complications. *Clinical and Experimental Medicine*, 24. https://www.semanticscholar.org/paper/3c95fd75577e979196546b9aacc90c32fb9e02a1 (accessed on 24 May 2025).
32. Hu, K. Q., & Huang, R. H. (2006). A practical approach to managing patients with HCV infection. https://core.ac.uk/download/323075269.pdf.
33. Kim, S. K., Korenblat, K., Lee, K. A., *et al.* (2017). Comparison of transjugular intrahepatic portosystemic shunt with covered stent and balloon-occluded retrograde transvenous obliteration in managing isolated gastric varices. https://core.ac.uk/download/83101055.pdf (accessed on 24 May 2025).
34. Mostafa, M., & Nwidu, E. (2023). Liver function abnormalities among substance abusers: An in-depth examination. *Global Journal of Medical and Pharmaceutical Sciences*. https://www.semanticscholar.org/paper/71a17f03323862c8d162ed5c7aa233407a4baf4f (accessed on 24 May 2025).
35. Pares, A., Pellicoro, A., Sagir, A., Burt, A. D., Elsharkawy, A. M., Pellicoro, A., Leon, D. A., *et al.* (2012). *Reversibility of Liver Fibrosis*. https://core.ac.uk/download/pdf/8736939.pdf.
36. Pompili, E., Baldassarre, M., Iannone, G., Tedesco, G., Nardelli, S., Piano, S., Alessandria, C., *et al.* (2024). Long-term albumin improves the outcomes of patients with decompensated cirrhosis and diabetes mellitus: Post hoc analysis of the ANSWER trial. *Liver International: Official Journal of the International Association for the Study of the Liver*. https://www.semanticscholar.org/paper/c1ed063c21dadafcfe1ca7556c42d1092d58c79a (accessed on 24 May 2025).
37. Potashkin, J., & Kim, N. (2024). Reversal of bone mineral density loss through lifestyle changes: A case report. *American Journal of Lifestyle Medicine*. https://www.semanticscholar.org/paper/e4bf19839adc79be065ab01cee4a389f1f294a1a (accessed on 24 May 2025).
38. Reddy, B. L., Kanchan, G., & Devi, C. R. (2025). Critical analysis of Yakrit Vikara in Ayurveda in relation to non-alcohol fatty liver disease (NAFLD). *International Journal for Multidisciplinary Research*. https://www.semanticscholar.org/paper/fc67eb34b67cdfef67d9c698138e6825a5b16d38 (accessed on 24 May 2025).
39. Salasia, S. I. O., & Widianingrum, D. C. (2021). Immunomodulatory effect of virgin coconut oil in Wistar rats infected with *Staphylococcus aureus*. JITV Vol. 26 No. 1 Th. 2021: 31-38 https://core.ac.uk/download/389103437.pdf (accessed on 24 May 2025).

40. Thompson, J. A. (2015). Practices of nurse practitioners in screening for hepatitis C. https://core.ac.uk/download/162577448.pdf (accessed on 24 May 2025).

41. Yaman, M., & Syifa, M. (2023). Lung abnormalities in liver cirrhosis. https://core.ac.uk/download/591390054.pdf (accessed on 24 May 2025).

42. Yashfeen, M., & Thilakavathi, R. (2023). A case report of an ethanol-related decompensated chronic liver disease with complications. International Journal of Research in Medical Sciences Sep;11(9):3443-3446 https://core.ac.uk/download/588568130.pdf

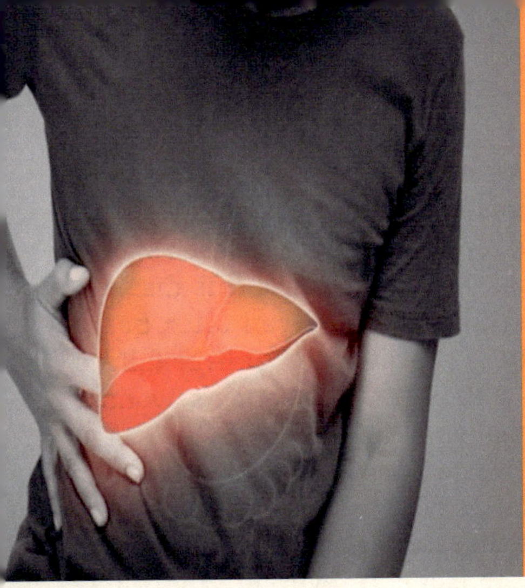

Chapter 4

LIVER FAILURE

Contents

Introduction

The pathogenesis of liver failure is a severe clinical condition that is characterized by the failure of the liver to perform its rudimentary metabolic, synthetic, and detoxification functions. It is a multifactorial condition that can be acute or chronic, resulting from various etiologies, including viral infections, autoimmune illnesses, and chronic exposure to hepatotoxic agents. CLD, such as hepatitis C and B, and diseases like ALD and NAFLD are high-performing etiologies of liver failure across the globe. Furthermore, etiologies such as genetic predisposition and rising obesity and diabetes incidence add to this public health problem, further highlighting the need for strict epidemiological research and prevention. In addition to the previously described causes of liver failure, new infections have been recognized to cause atypical yet severe presentations of the disease. An example is *Talaromyces marneffei*, an organism that causes systemic infection nearly exclusively in immunocompromised individuals. The clinical presentation provided by *Talaromyces marneffei* infection is unique; instances have reported acute deterioration of liver function in patients with no prior hepatic disease. In probing this condition, it is important to emphasize the necessity of early identification of differential diagnoses of immunocompromised patients. Galloping liver failure in these cases shows the necessity of early diagnosis and management because of the sudden evolution of this disease, as seen in the case history of a patient who succumbed due to this infection even after being subjected to standard therapies (Xia *et al.*, 2024). To the complexity of the situation of liver failure is added autoimmune hepatitis (AIH). This multifactorial illness almost entirely affects women and is triggered by an inflammatory process leading to liver damage. With such a broad range of clinical presentations ranging from asymptomatic elevation of liver enzymes to fulminant liver failure (FLF), the presentation heterogeneity of AIH calls for a high index of suspicion in healthcare practitioners' minds. AIH may often coexist with other autoimmune diseases, making diagnosis and treatment more difficult. That no treatment protocols have been established for overlap syndromes (OS), like AIH and primary biliary cholangitis (PBC), calls for a collaborative research investigation to establish appropriate treatment protocols. Ultimately, it is vital to comprehend these multiple presentations of liver failure to improve patient outcomes and guide clinical management (Batista *et al.*, 2024).

Definition of Liver Failure

Liver failure happens when the liver cannot do its main jobs, which are detoxifying the body, making proteins, and producing chemicals needed for digestion. It can manifest as either acute liver failure (ALF) or chronic liver failure, each characterized by distinct etiology and symptomology. ALF often develops rapidly, in a short period, usually in someone without previous liver disease, and is commonly caused by viruses, too much medication, or harmful substances. Unlike sudden liver failure, chronic liver failure happens slowly over months or years, usually because of ongoing liver diseases such as hepatitis, cirrhosis, or fatty liver disease. The differences in these terms point out the need to know the causes and act fast, which could involve liver transplantation in critical cases. The clinical manifestations of liver failure are diverse, often encompassing jaundice, coagulopathy, hepatic encephalopathy (HE), and ascites, among other symptoms. If the liver does not work properly, bilirubin builds up and causes the skin and eyes to turn yellow, which is known as jaundice. As a result of coagulopathy, the liver does not make enough clotting factors, which can cause the patient to bleed more easily. HE, which is a serious problem, can cause mental and behavioral changes from mild confusion to coma, because the liver cannot remove ammonia and other toxins that harm the brain. Ascites, or the buildup of fluid in the abdomen, happens when the portal vein pressure increases because of liver problems. Early diagnosis and understanding of these symptoms are critical, as timely intervention can significantly influence the prognosis and survival rates for affected patients, especially in the context of ALF reported in various studies, like that of Egyptian children, where hepatitis A was a predominant cause (Mansour *et al.*, 2024). Also, the factors that predict outcomes in liver failure are important for judging the seriousness of the condition and selecting the best treatment plan. For instance, higher levels of international normalized ratio (INR), total bilirubin, and creatinine in patients are indicative of poor outcomes, with studies suggesting specific cutoff values that can predict mortality risks (Mansour *et al.*, 2024). A good management strategy is to use these factors to get ready for liver transplantation as soon as it is required. In chronic cases, a concerted effort to prevent the progression of liver disease through medical therapy can also help mitigate the worsening of liver function, as noted in heart failure (HF) management, where guidelines are crucial for treatment. Understanding both the definition and the implications of liver failure not only aids healthcare providers in delivering timely and effective care but also contributes to improving patient outcomes significantly (Figure 4.1).

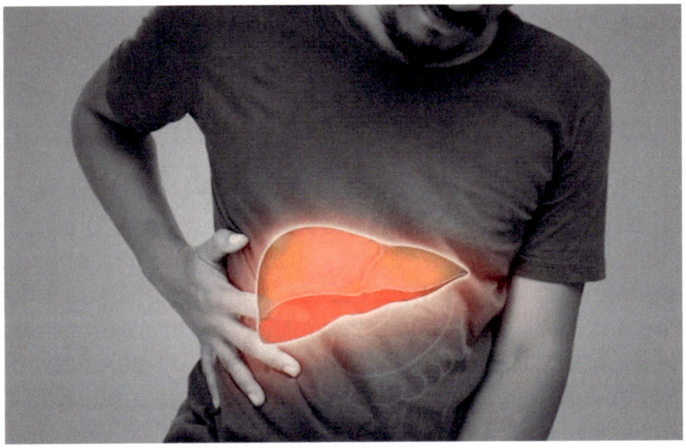

Figure 4.1. Abdominal Pain.

Source: https://www.metropolisindia.com/upgrade/blog/upload/23/12/Liver-Failure1703930383.webp.

Importance of the Liver in Bodily Functions

The liver is a vital organ with intricate functions that are required for the general well-being of an individual. It is a biochemical factory that produces proteins critical in blood clotting and various other metabolic processes. It includes the production of albumin to maintain osmotic pressure and nutrient transport within the circulatory system. In addition, the liver plays a crucial role in the detoxification of harmful substances such as drugs and alcohol by ensuring these toxins are metabolized to non-toxic metabolites or eliminated from the body. The liver's capacity to eliminate harmful substances is its defense against the risk of systemic harm, indicating its importance in protecting body functions and ensuring homeostasis, particularly in the event of metabolic changes that can lead to liver failure. Another critical function of the liver is nutrient metabolism, in which it acts as a clearinghouse for the metabolism of nutrients absorbed from the gut. Carbohydrates are metabolized to glucose, which can be utilized as an immediately available source of energy, and fats are metabolized and stored for future use as energy. This organ also facilitates the process of transforming excess glucose into glycogen, a polysaccharide that can be easily mobilized during fasting or prolonged exercise. The liver is also implicated in vitamin and mineral metabolism, rendering some nutrients appropriately processed and used by the body. The severe disruption of these metabolic activities due to liver failure can lead to severe nutritional deficiency and energy imbalance, further highlighting the liver's critical role in maintaining metabolic wellness. The liver also plays an auxiliary role in immunity with its production of inflammation-related proteins and immune cells that actively protect the body from pathogens. This organ harbors a unique reservoir of immune cells known as Kupffer cells that play the role of scavenging foreign pathogens from the blood and clearing them from the circulation. Immune activities of livers are quite relevant, especially in patients with liver failure, as dysregulated immune responses could predispose to infection and progression of disease. Research on the liver's immunological functions, such as the role of microRNAs in regulating the immune response, suggests potential therapies for maintaining liver function and immune healing in compromised patients (Condrat *et al.*, 2020). Thus, the radically critical function of the liver goes beyond metabolization and detoxification, with an important role in immunological well-being as well.

4.1. Types of Liver Failure

It is essential to know the different types of liver failure to choose the right treatment methods. Generally, liver failure can be categorized into acute liver failure (ALF) and chronic liver failure. The liver function in ALF deteriorates very fast, often within days or weeks, and is usually caused by viral hepatitis, DILI, or exposure to toxins. Because of this type of liver failure, patients experience HE and coagulopathy, which can be very dangerous and require quick medical attention. Chronic liver failure happens slowly, often starting with CLD caused by alcohol abuse, NAFLD, or chronic viral hepatitis. Knowing these differences helps with diagnosis and choosing the right treatment for the kind of liver failure present. The distinction between FLF and sub ALF shows that acute liver problems can be very complex. FLF usually develops very quickly, often within eight weeks, and does not start with any existing liver disease. Because jaundice, ascites, and HE start quickly, doctors may need to use aggressive treatments, which may involve transplanting the liver. Unlike ALF, Sub ALF is used when the disease lasts for a more extended period, anywhere from eight weeks to six months, and is usually found in people who already have liver problems. Stabilizing the liver and controlling symptoms are the main priorities in managing subacute cases, and a thorough evaluation is done to find out if surgery is required. Having a detailed awareness of these categories allows clinicians to predict problems and take early action. It is possible to classify liver failure by the reason for it; for example, metabolic liver failure is important in primary hyperoxaluria. Because of this rare disorder, oxalate builds up in the body, which causes kidney stones and slowly damages the kidneys. When the liver cannot handle some metabolites well, it can cause problems in the kidneys, as recent studies have shown. Common approaches in management are symptomatic treatment, heavy hydration, and transplantation of the liver and kidneys when the condition is very severe. In addition, gene therapy and RNA interference are showing how the management of metabolic liver failures is advancing. Overall, understanding these diverse types of liver failure is critical for optimizing patient outcomes and guiding clinical practice in the face of liver disorders (Audu *et al.*, 2023; Zhu *et al.*, 2024).

4.1.1. Acute Liver Failure (ALF)

ALF is a critical hepatological challenge that is actualized through the rapid loss of liver function. Though uncommon, it has severe complications like multi-organ dysfunction and death if not treated as an emergency. Its presentation is typically insidious, caused by varied etiologic factors such as viral hepatitis, drug toxicity, or alcohol overdose. Surprisingly, when an individual has a combination of risk factors such as dyslipidemia and a family history of diabetes or hepatitis, it considerably increases the risk of ALF. When scientists studied a group of people with different health histories, they saw that these independent risks are strongly correlated with the occurrence of ALF, indicating there is a requirement for proper screening and awareness of symptomatic presentation in high-risk patients (Ding *et al.*, 2022). The clinical impact of ALF is serious, and prompt intervention is required to avert long-term injury. Once diagnosed, patients are likely to experience an avalanche of systemic complications, ranging from HE to acute kidney injury. There is innovative promise in treating this fatal illness with bioartificial liver (BAL) therapy. In clinical settings, BAL therapy is already proving to be hopeful in supplementing liver function by supporting hepatic cell viability and minimizing systemic inflammation. The research discovers that when the BAL treatment was used on ALF models, there were notable survival rates and liver regeneration, which shows that this new strategy could provide significant relief to ALF patients (Weng *et al.*, 2021). Even with these advancements, the treatment of ALF is complex. These approaches currently employed are generally restrictive, such as variation in the response of the patient and the possibility of further damage to the organ. Knowledge of ALF mechanisms and their systemic consequences can help tailor effective treatment regimens. In addition, identification of vulnerable populations through health screens may help with timely interventions that improve outcomes. With breakthroughs in research, multimodal approaches' integration will play a key role in the treatment of the complexities of ALF, ranging from the time of initial diagnosis to therapeutic management integration, thus lowering mortality from the severe illness (Ding *et al.*, 2022; Weng *et al.*, 2021) (Figure 4.2).

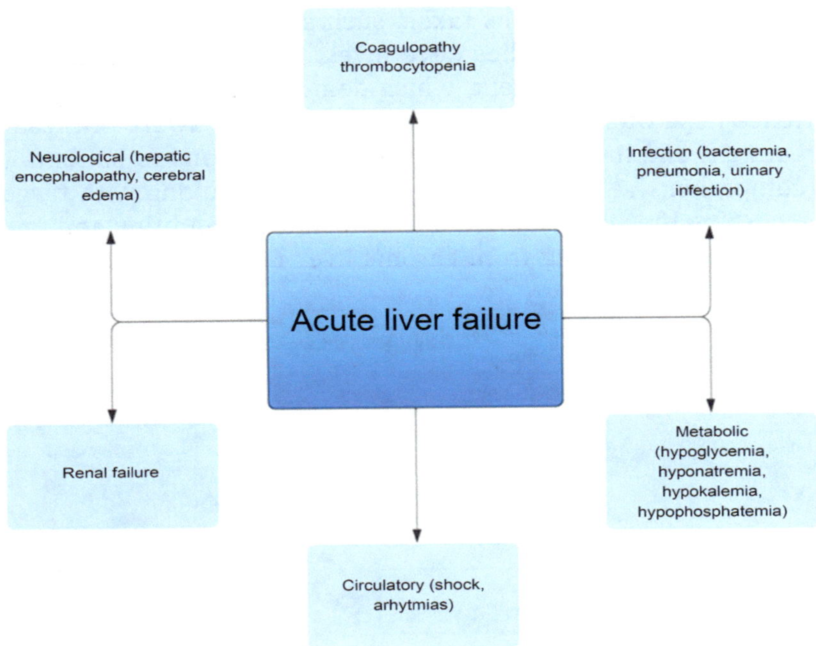

Figure 4.2. Acute liver failure (ALF).

Source: https://pub.mdpi-res.com/jcm/jcm-12-07451/article_deploy/html/images/jcm-12-07451-g001.png?1701655117.

4.1.2. Chronic Liver Failure

Liver failure that lasts for a long time is a major and complicated health issue marked by the gradual loss of liver function. Several reasons can cause this slow decline, such as chronic viral hepatitis, ALD, and NAFLD. With the liver's functions failing, such as detoxification, metabolism, and making vital proteins, patients may develop symptoms like tiredness, jaundice, ascites, and HE. Understanding why chronic liver failure happens is very important, since it guides the treatment plans doctors use to help patients recover and enjoy a better quality of life. It is very important to catch the disease early because it can progress without notice until it becomes serious, requiring thorough testing and treatment. Chronic liver failure has a major effect on both patients and the healthcare system. When the liver does not function well, it can cause serious illness and require patients to be hospitalized several times, which increases healthcare expenses. Chronic liver failure can cause many problems in patients, such as pain, weakness, and psychological issues, that may reduce their quality of life. It becomes very difficult to provide end-of-life care for these patients because many are not willing to go to the hospital as their condition worsens. Research has highlighted that advanced liver failure is often the most common cause of death among vulnerable populations, indicating the urgent need for tailored palliative care strategies that address both the physical and emotional suffering of patients (N/A, 2011). It includes treating pain, easing bothersome symptoms, and meeting the patients' psychological needs as they progress. In addition, it is very important to use preventive strategies and effectively manage chronic liver failure. It is important to regularly check LFTs in patients known to be at risk, so that any changes can be found early and appropriate actions taken, such as changing lifestyle or using medication to control the disease. For instance, studies have investigated the incidence of DILI, particularly in the context of anti-tuberculosis treatment, which demonstrates that a significant percentage of patients may experience hepatotoxicity (Joby *et al.*, 2011). Being aware of these risk factors helps doctors improve treatment and lower the chances of complications in patients with chronic liver failure. Ultimately, comprehensive education about liver health, along with targeted public health strategies, is vital in curbing the rising burden of this insidious condition and improving long-term clinical outcomes for patients suffering from chronic liver failure (Figure 4.3).

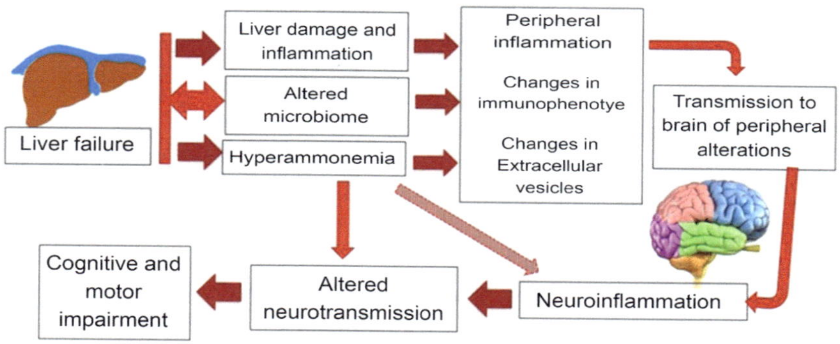

Figure 4.3. Main steps of the process by which chronic liver failure (mainly liver cirrhosis) leads to cognitive and motor impairment in MHE and HE.

Source: https://www.researchgate.net/publication/383345853/figure/fig1/AS:11431281288730379@1730862182719/Main-steps-of-the-process-by-which-chronic-liver-failure-mainly-liver-cirrhosis-leads.png.

4.1.3. Fulminant Liver Failure

FLF is a severe medical disorder involving acute liver failure with sudden onset of insufficiency of the liver, typically in a few days or weeks, in individuals whose liver had been normal beforehand. The disease could be preceded by various etiologies, including viral hepatitis, drug-induced hepatotoxicity, and metabolic disorders. One of the primary causes includes Wilson's disease, which is an autosomal recessive disorder. It results in copper accumulation in the liver and other vital organs. In acute presentation, such as in a previously healthy young female presenting with hemolytic anemia followed by acute liver failure, it is clear that there is a need for early diagnosis and treatment. Early detection of Wilson's disease is crucial, as with early treatment with chelating agents like penicillamine, mortality and morbidity due to FLF can be prevented to a large extent (Ghias *et al.*, 2024). Pathophysiology of FLF also typically involves extensive hepatocellular injury, resulting in lost liver function and resultant complications such as coagulopathy, encephalopathy, and multi-organ failure. In some cases, FLF not only results from intrinsic causes but also from extrinsic agents. For example, the combination of a pheochromocytoma crisis with the concurrent administration of Garcinia cambogia has been reported to induce acute hepatic failure in a patient. This case is evidence of the multifactorial character of FLF because it necessitates multidisciplinary diagnosis and treatment. Proper evaluation of the relationship between internal factors and external forces is necessary for the formulation of an effective treatment strategy, further evidence of the multidimensionality of liver diseases (Selim *et al.*, 2023). FLF treatment is multidimensional and is based on the underlying etiology and the degree of hepatic compromise. Supportive care in the form of monitoring of LFTs and management of complications is significant during the initial period of treatment. Liver transplantation is also thought to be a pivotal intervention in scenarios where conservative management fails or liver function worsens exponentially. Patient condition overall, as well as availability of donors, are, however, significant determiners of eligibility for transplantation. Even though FLF presents significant dangers to the healthcare practitioner, advances in medical treatment and surgery still improve the prognosis of the patient. The understanding of the heterogeneous etiology and pathogenesis of FLF is significant to the development of directed therapies, which can ultimately reduce the impact of this fatal condition (Figure 4.4).

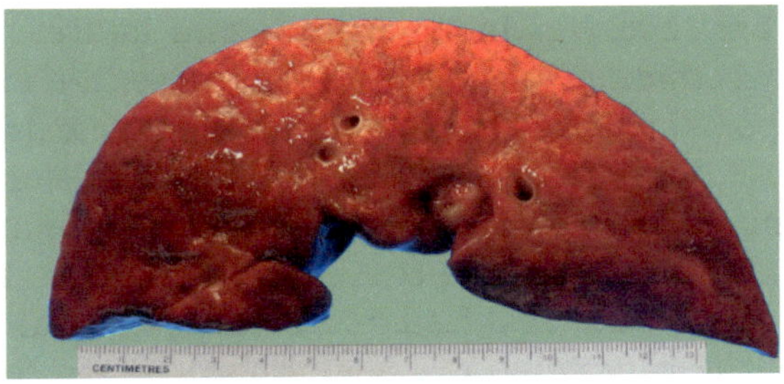

Figure 4.4. Gross photograph of a liver with fulminant hepatic failure.

Source: https://www.researchgate.net/publication/338896325/figure/fig1/AS:11431281255042543@1719383906605/Gross-photograph-of-a-liver-with-fulminant-hepatic-failure-Note-the-bosselated.tif.

4.2. Causes of Liver Failure

Many things can cause liver failure, and metabolic dysfunction has become a major factor in recent years. This phenomenon is often encapsulated in the term metabolic dysfunction-associated steatotic liver disease (MASLD), which links CLD with metabolic disorders such as obesity and type 2 diabetes. As fat accumulates in liver hepatocytes, exceeding 5%, it induces cellular stress that can escalate into more severe conditions like metabolic dysfunction-associated steatohepatitis (MASH). MASH causes the liver to become inflamed and fibrous, which gradually reduces blood flow and may result in cirrhosis or liver cancer. The complexity of

MASLD's pathophysiology reflects a myriad of influences, including dietary habits, sedentary lifestyles, and genetic predispositions, emphasizing the need for comprehensive strategies to address these multifactorial risks and prevent liver failure (Devasia *et al.*, 2025). Infections with viruses and especially HBV are still a major reason for liver failure. The progression from chronic HBV to acute-on-chronic liver failure (ACLF) is heavily influenced by immune dysregulation and metabolic disturbances, which can create a vicious cycle exacerbating liver damage. Many studies have found that HBV-related ACLF results in major mitochondrial problems and changes in liver energy production, which can cause extensive cell death in the liver. Such changes are not accidental; they are linked to the immune system, which causes more macrophages to enter and cytokines to be produced. By understanding these mechanisms, we can identify potential therapeutic targets to enhance treatment efficacy and address the metabolic factors that exacerbate liver disease progression (Zhang *et al.*, 2024). Also, the effects of substance abuse, mainly alcohol, are another important reason for liver failure. Chronic drinking too much alcohol can result in ALD, which may show up as fatty liver, alcoholic hepatitis, and cirrhosis. The liver cannot process much alcohol, which leads to oxidative stress and inflammation, which seriously injures the liver cells. When these risk factors are present together such as obesity or liver conditions, they can cause the liver to deteriorate at a faster rate. As the global incidence of liver failure continues to rise, especially in at-risk populations, a multifaceted approach that combines medical intervention with public health initiatives is crucial to mitigate the impact of alcohol-related liver disease (ARLD) (Devasia *et al.*, 2025) (Figure 4.5).

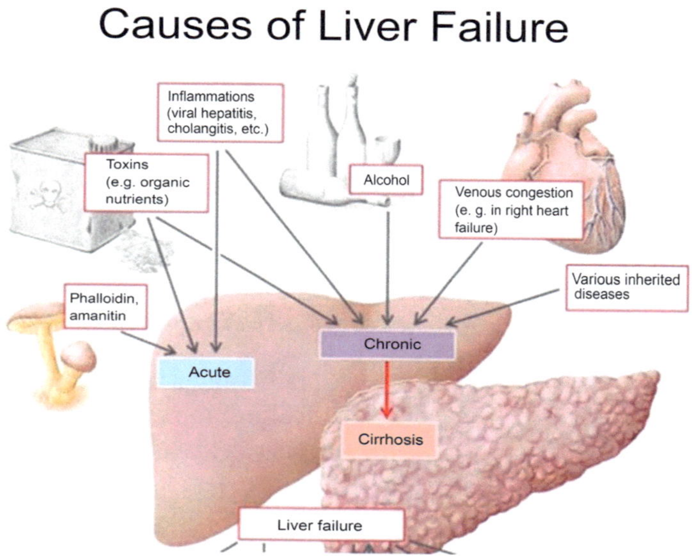

Figure 4.5. Liver failure causes.

Source: https://media.licdn.com/dms/image/sync/v2/D4E27AQHh2H8eY0Oa3g/articleshare-shrink_800/articleshare-shrink_800/0/1712329552859?e=2147483647&v=beta&t=onK8HKuW-fsmIlyZjbDGvRlT_BmxM2sxrdRQzTSvK6Y.

4.2.1. Viral Infections (Hepatitis)

Hepatitis virus infections are significant contributors to the global burden of liver disease, which eventually manifests as conditions such as liver failure. Hepatitis B and C viruses can cause CLD due to chronic inflammation and hepatic damage. The chronic damage will ultimately progress to cirrhosis, a condition where the liver is severely scarred and unable to function properly. The chronicity of these viral infections guarantees that many patients go undetected for years, raising the risk of the development of severe complications like HE, portal hypertension, and, in the majority of cases, liver failure. Notably, the virus strain and the host immune system can influence the course of the disease, thus necessitating early diagnosis and treatment to prevent severe hepatic complications. One significant region of hepatitis care is the evolution of DAAs, which have revolutionized the treatment of hepatitis C. They target particular viral components and record high SVR rates. However, a subset of patients is resistant to treatment, typically as a result of RASs in the virus. Studies have established that a higher proportion of treatment-failed patients exhibit baseline resistance-associated substitutions (RASs), indicating that such genetic mutations can significantly reduce the level of effectiveness of treatment (Fahnøe *et al.*, 2020). Moreover, the challenge is not only in the initial attempt at treatment but also in repeated attempts at retreatment due to the continued presence of the mutations, necessitating improved knowledge of viral genetics in order to optimize therapeutic intervention and patient recovery. The impact of hepatitis in vulnerable populations, such as pregnant females, illustrates the differential influence of viral infections on the well-being of the liver. Hepatitis E, in particular, endangers pregnancy with robust correlations of poor fetal and maternal outcomes. Research has indicated that pregnant women with hepatitis E can experience mortality rates of as high as 42.5%, intrauterine fetal losses, and HE being prevalent in these patients (Mishra *et al.*, 2019). The pathogenesis of the mechanism through which hepatitis E leads to liver injury remains unclear, thus calling for further research into the pathogenesis of the disease. Effective management is achieved through early diagnosis and multi-disciplinary teamwork to combat the devastating consequences of this infection in both the mothers and the unborn child, pre-empting the complex interaction between the viral infections and liver failure.

4.2.2. Alcohol Abuse

Alcohol abuse seriously affects the liver, and chronic drinking is a major reason for liver failure around the world. Too much alcohol can make the liver unable to remove harmful chemicals, which causes permanent damage. In the beginning, fatty liver disease occurs, marked by the buildup of fat, and this may lead to inflammation and, later on, fibrosis—the scarring of liver tissue that reduces its functioning. The severe condition of cirrhosis can appear, and it greatly reduces the liver's ability to function while also raising the risk of HCC. The strong link between alcohol and liver failure calls for public measures that encourage less alcohol use and help people understand its dangers, which can lower the number of liver-related disorders. Alcohol abuse and liver disease are connected, and this connection has consequences for the gut microbiome. Regular alcohol use changes the types of bacteria in the gut, which may lead to dysbiosis and worsen problems in the liver. Studies have indicated that this imbalance can promote inflammation and contribute to the progression of alcohol-associated liver disease (ALD) through mechanisms such as increased intestinal permeability and bacterial translocation. They can cause the body to become more inflamed and the liver to get injured, which only makes the liver damage from alcohol worse. Furthermore, emerging research suggests that strategies such as fecal microbiota transplantation (FMT) may hold therapeutic potential in reversing some of the alterations induced by alcohol on the gut microbiome, though much of this remains investigational (Wolstenholme *et al.*, 2024). Liver failure due to alcohol abuse should be managed by treating the alcohol problem and also focusing on liver health. Many providers are hesitant and do not know enough about effective interventions, which leads to underuse of pharmacotherapy for alcohol use disorder. Improving how healthcare providers are educated and increasing treatment access can help a lot in lowering the burden of ARLD. Also, following a healthy diet and having regular medical checkups are important for people who are at risk of liver problems. Ultimately, comprehensive strategies that tackle the multifactorial nature of alcohol abuse will be imperative in combating the increasing incidence of liver failure linked to alcohol consumption, addressing both prevention and treatment to achieve better patient outcomes (Wolstenholme *et al.*, 2024) (Figure 4.6).

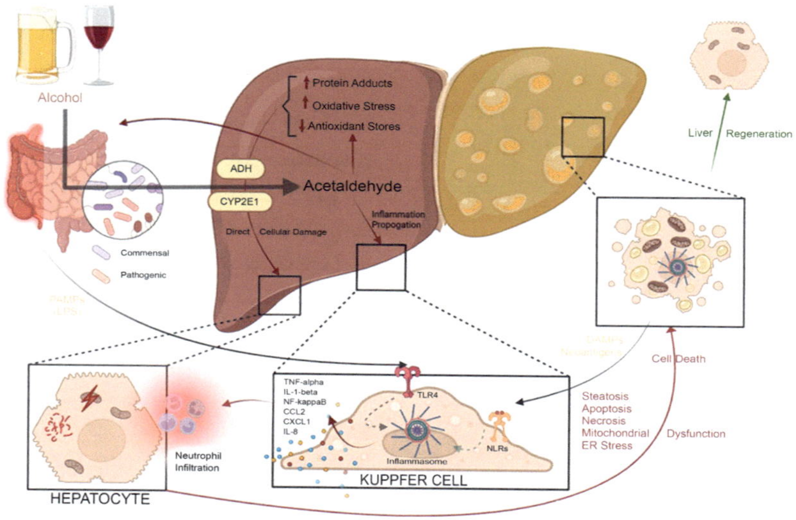

Figure 4.6. Pathophysiology of alcohol-induced liver damage alcohol consumption leads to both direct cellular damage and indirect injury via inflammation propagation.

Source: https://www.researchgate.net/publication/360588800/figure/fig1/AS:11431281173635974@1688999835857/Pathophysiology-of-alcohol-induced-liver-damage-alcohol-consumption-leads-to-both-direct.png.

4.2.3. Non-Alcoholic Fatty Liver Disease (NAFLD)

The global health landscape is increasingly taxed by NAFLD, a condition of having fat (NAFL) in the liver irrespective of alcohol consumption. Not only does the condition signify hepatic steatosis, but it also points towards a harbinger of severe liver conditions like NASH, fibrosis, and cirrhosis. The strong association of NAFLD with other metabolic conditions, such as obesity and type 2 diabetes, underscores the need to be aware of these associations. The clinical burden of NAFLD is also a public health challenge that would amplify liver-related morbidity and mortality if left untreated. Identifying effective therapeutic and preventative methods entails extensive research on the reason why NAFLDs develop and their relation to broader metabolic syndromes, as emphasized in recent publications. Recent studies have highlighted the central role of lifestyle modification in treating NAFLD, as these not only improve the liver but also prevent the risk of concomitant metabolic diseases. Large-scale interventions include dietary modifications, particularly those that guarantee gut microbiota diversity, which have been promising in the prevention of NAFLD risk. For instance, the Dietary Index for Gut Microbiota (DI-GM) has been inversely associated with reduced risks of NAFLD and liver fibrosis; as DI-GM scores increase, the risk of developing these conditions significantly decreases (Zheng *et al.*, 2025). These findings indicate that promotion of a healthy diet can be a central element in the prevention and management of NAFLD, which could slow the progression of the disease and enhance liver function. Multidisciplinary practices incorporating dietary therapy should thus be an essential component of clinical management in patients at risk of or with NAFLD.

The dynamic interaction between NAFLD and the onset of liver failure is the most critical concern that needs further investigation. When NAFLD progresses to its later stages, the risk of developing complications arising from the liver becomes more pressing, raising the stakes for timely action. This condition varies from benign hepatic steatosis to severe and potentially fatal disease, e.g., cirrhosis, and therefore early diagnosis and treatment are essential to prevent irreversible loss. Identifying the severity of liver injury associated with NAFLD is paramount in the development of targeted therapeutic interventions and the improvement of patient outcomes. Evidence shows that NAFLD not only impacts liver function but also is associated with increased cardiovascular risk, thereby requiring multifaceted care strategies (Bazargaliyev *et al.*, 2025). Understanding these dynamics is central to avoiding the progression of liver disease and preventing life-threatening consequences linked to liver failure.

4.3. Symptoms of Liver Failure

The beginning of liver failure is often noticed by a wide range of symptoms, showing how important the liver is for many body functions. Initial symptoms are often fatigue, nausea, and a feeling of being unwell, and these may be confused with milder health problems. When liver function worsens, the symptoms become more obvious, such as jaundice, which is seen as a yellowing of the skin and eyes because of high bilirubin. At the same time, ascites, which is a buildup of fluid in the abdomen, may result, making the patient feel uncomfortable and lowering their quality of life. Early symptoms are significant for diagnosis because they help doctors understand the liver problems and take action early, which may prevent the disease from becoming more serious. Liver failure can cause major neurological problems, which are most noticeable in the most severe cases. A significant problem is HE, which may lead to cognitive dysfunction, including personality changes, stupor, and coma. The buildup of toxic substances in the blood is the reason for this neuropsychiatric disturbance, which happens because the liver cannot detoxify properly. HE patients may have altered awareness and trouble with orientation, which are important symptoms for diagnosis. Such disturbances not only highlight the systemic ramifications of liver failure but also emphasize the need for rigorous clinical assessment and monitoring, particularly as the healthcare community recognizes the potential reversibility of this condition with appropriate treatment interventions as detailed in emerging research (Tejpal *et al.*, 2024). As well as neurological and physical problems, patients with liver failure may have changes in their metabolism, which make their condition more complicated. The liver is important for protein synthesis, so not enough albumin can cause serious problems such as edema and a higher risk of infections. Also, if the liver cannot make important clotting factors, patients may experience excessive bleeding. Besides, chronic liver failure usually causes problems such as portal hypertension and the buildup of collagen in liver tissue, which can result in fibrosis and cirrhosis. This progression is marked by significant symptoms, including malaise and abdominal pain, which may also be alleviated through innovative therapeutic approaches such as the CXCR4-targeted nano-system aimed at diagnosing and treating liver conditions (Wang *et al.*, 2024). Noticing these symptoms and how they relate is important for managing liver failure in individuals.

4.3.1. Jaundice

Jaundice is a clinical picture that is usually seen with liver dysfunction, characterized by an increase in blood bilirubin that leads to yellow discoloration of the skin and sclera. Jaundice may result from a variety of etiologies, including hemolysis, hepatocellular dysfunction, and cholestasis. In liver failure, the liver's ability to conjugate and excrete bilirubin is severely impaired, and unconjugated and conjugated bilirubin build up.

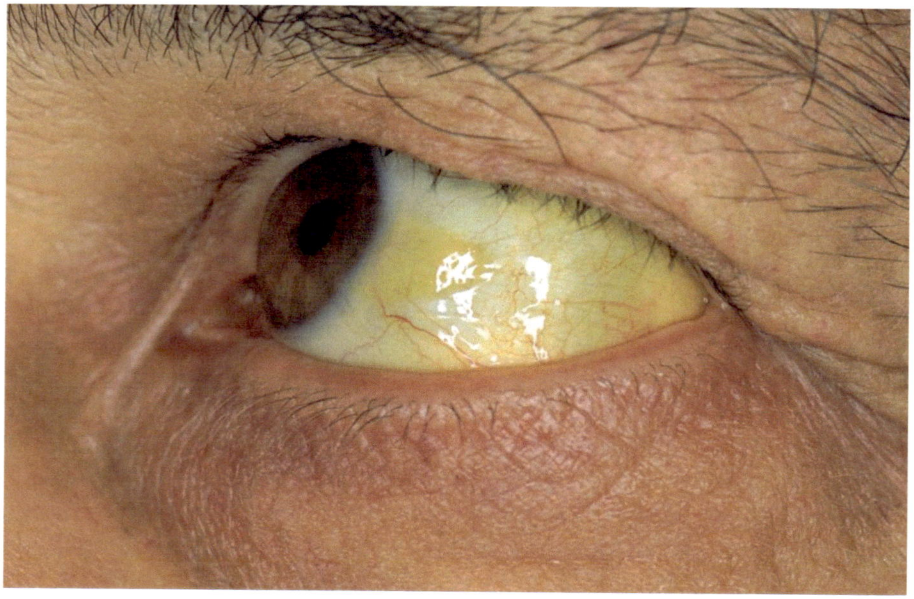

Figure 4.7. Jaundice.

Source: https://media.healthdirect.org.au/images/inline/original/jaundice-f55738.jpg.

Hence, jaundice is a major clinical sign that clinicians use to assess the degree of liver impairment and to guide diagnosis and management. Importantly, however, jaundice does not inherently signify ALF by itself; it can also signify CLD that has reached the point where they have produced widespread hepatic impairment, and thus its recognition is important to effective medical therapy in compromised patients. The jaundice course in liver-failure patients can often be preceded or associated with other physical symptoms and signs evidencing worsening liver function. For instance, jaundice is usually joined by hepatomegaly and ascites, as noted in cases documented in the literature, for instance, in a boy infant who presented with jaundice, abdominal distension, and severe liver dysfunction and subsequently liver failure (Lu *et al.*, 2024). This multiplanar presentation serves to illustrate the necessity for extensive clinical evaluation, even with imaging and laboratory tests, for determining underlying causes of liver failure. Furthermore, jaundice is not only responsible for symptomatology; it is also a significant feature of differential diagnosis, leading clinicians to consider varied causes—ranging from infectious processes through to metabolic disorders—when managing potential hepatic compromise. In liver failure, jaundice can also be caused by infectious pathogens that can induce hepatic injury. *Talaromyces marneffei* is a good example in this context because it has been reported to cause systemic fungal infection leading to ALF in patients without underlying liver disease (Xia *et al.*, 2024). These reports highlight the importance of including atypical infectious pathogens in the differential diagnosis of jaundice and liver failure, particularly in immunocompromised patients. An early and firm diagnostic testing for potential infectious etiologies is necessary to initiate proper treatment regimens in a timely fashion. Knowledge of the interaction between jaundice and liver failure is therefore important for physicians to create effective diagnostic and treatment protocols that address both symptom and etiology (Figure 4.7).

4.3.2. Abdominal Swelling

In liver failure, abdominal swelling or ascites is a usual symptom caused by portal hypertension and changes in how the body handles fluids. Patients with liver dysfunction have a greatly reduced ability for the liver to make albumin, which is important for oncotic pressure. The lack of fluid in the vascular system causes it to leak into the peritoneal cavity, resulting in the abdomen becoming distended. More pressure in the portal venous system also leads to fluid building up in the abdomen, which makes the swelling caused by liver problems worse. Being aware of these physiological changes is very important, especially in ALF, since quick actions may be required to handle severe symptoms and stop infections or peritonitis caused by ascites. As the liver fails, the belly tends to become swollen, which usually means the condition is more serious and is linked to HE and renal failure. Ascites causes more than just discomfort; it lowers the quality of life and often creates difficulties for managing the patient. An example is if fluid builds up too much, it may stop the diaphragm from moving properly, which can lead to breathing problems. A swollen belly may hide serious problems that should be treated quickly, which could cause delays in important medical actions. Ascites is a sign that hemodynamics are changing, which means the body's efforts to adjust are becoming more difficult. So, catching ascites early allows medical staff to understand how much the liver is affected and choose treatments that address both the symptoms and the cause of liver failure. Even with new treatments for liver problems, managing the challenging symptoms of abdominal swelling is still very important for liver failure patients. Although paracentesis helps by removing extra fluid from ascites, it cannot treat the main problem in the liver. New treatments are being developed to help patients, such as BAL, which aims to assist the liver and lessen the body's general inflammatory response. Using new techniques may help the liver recover and deal with problems outside the liver, such as those caused by ascites, since animal studies have shown that BAL therapy leads to better survival and health results. By continuing to investigate and develop targeted treatment modalities, clinicians can better manage the debilitating effects of abdominal swelling, ultimately leading to enhanced quality of life and improved prognoses for individuals suffering from liver failure (Malik *et al.*, 2023; Weng *et al.*, 2021) (Figure 4.8).

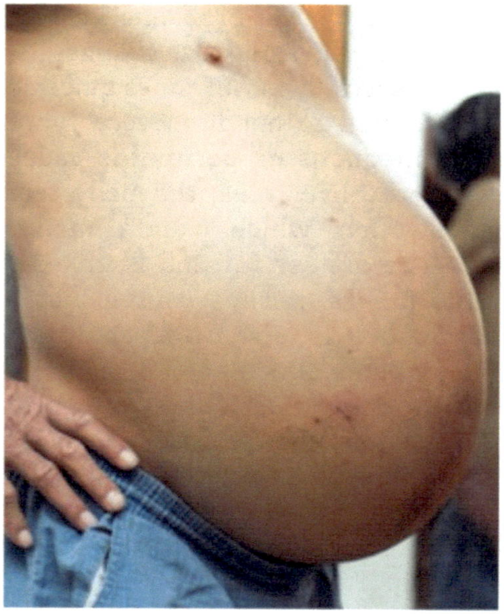

Figure 4.8. Abdominal swelling.

Source: https://www.carehospitalbti.com/Assets/images/services/Abdominal.jpg.

4.3.3. Confusion and Cognitive Changes

Cognitive alterations and confusion are prominent symptoms that arise as complications of liver failure, compromising the quality of life in patients. HE, which is a common condition occurring in liver failure, appears as a continuum of neuropsychiatric alterations from mild confusion to profound cognitive dysfunction. The defective detoxification processes characteristic of liver failure result in the build-up of neurotoxic compounds, most notably ammonia, which adversely compromises brain function. This biochemical derangement can result in disturbances in the thought process, ability to make decisions, and memory, all of which contribute to patient and caregiver burden. Thus, it is crucial to understand the subtleties of HE to develop effective treatment protocols aimed at preventing or reversing these cognitive deficits and improving outcomes. The role of nutritional deficiencies must also not be overlooked against the backdrop of liver failure, along with cognitive impairment. A number of studies suggest that a lack of essential nutrients, including thiamine, can produce neurological symptoms found in patients with liver dysfunction. Thiamine deficiency, for instance, has been associated with a variety of neurological complications, ranging from confusion and memory loss to insomnia, which can drastically alter a patient's mental terrain.

This deficit is particularly risky to the brain, which relies on efficient mitochondrial operation, thus highlighting the relevance of nutritional assessment to the clinic. Supplementation to this degree may potentially reverse some cognitive changes of liver failure, illustrating the importance of a multidisciplinary strategy for patient management that addresses both metabolic and nutritional needs in order to improve cognitive function. Studies investigating cognitive impact in at-risk populations further reveal the need for thorough assessment. Comparisons of cognitive performance in patients with chronic liver disease and healthy controls might reveal the degree of cognitive impairment often not assessed in clinical practice. Revealing the pathophysiology that supports these changes in cognition is essential, as it serves as the basis for prevention and treatment. For instance, knowing the link between cognitive decline and liver failure can inform anticipatory management. Furthermore, research into correlations between cognitive impairment and chronic conditions—such as those that concern neurotrauma—may illuminate common pathways of neurodegeneration that need to be elucidated. Finally, raising awareness and the use of specific cognitive interventions are key to making substantial enhancements in patient care approaches for those battling the deepening effects of liver failure on mental health and cognition.

4.4. Diagnosis of Liver Failure

Liver failure is diagnosed by using both medical examinations and laboratory tests. At first, healthcare providers look at the patient's history and perform a physical exam, paying attention to jaundice, ascites, and changes in mental state. Such clinical signs can be a sign that the liver is not working as well as it should. Laboratory tests are also very important for finding out if a person has liver failure. If liver enzymes, bilirubin, and prothrombin time are increased, it usually indicates some kind of liver dysfunction. Doctors may use imaging tests such as ultrasound and CT scans to check the liver's size, structure, and possible blockages. These first steps guide the diagnosis of liver failure, but often more investigation, such as LBx, is needed for a clear diagnosis in unclear cases. The study of liver tissue samples can be very helpful in diagnosing liver failure, mainly when it is due to alcoholic liver disease. Recent studies have highlighted specific histological features that correlate with acute-on-chronic liver failure (ACLF), a severe and often fatal complication of liver disease. For example, studies have shown that *ductular bilirubinostasis* is much more common in patients with ACLF than in those without, showing how important liver histology is for diagnosis. Clinical information should be used together with histological results to distinguish between the causes of liver dysfunction, for example, alcoholic hepatitis and NAFLD. Such comprehensive evaluations enable healthcare professionals to tailor treatment strategies effectively, addressing the underlying causes of liver failure while considering individual patient circumstances (Broekhoven *et al.*, 2024). Besides clinical and histological exams, new biomarkers and advanced diagnostic tools are improving the way liver failure is diagnosed. For instance, arterial lactate concentration levels have been proposed as an early predictor of post-hepatectomy liver failure (PHLF), with studies demonstrating that elevated lactate ratios can significantly correlate with postoperative complications. Spotting patients with these biomarkers makes it possible to treat them promptly, which may help avoid severe results of liver failure. Also, using these advanced tools along with traditional methods helps improve patient care. This holistic approach emphasizes the need for continuous research into liver function indicators, thereby refining existing diagnostic criteria and better informing clinical decisions in the management of liver failure (Wang *et al.*, 2024).

4.4.1. Blood Tests (Liver Function Tests)

Blood tests play a significant role in liver failure diagnosis and management, providing insight into the liver's functional status along with underlying causes. LFTs are most commonly done to evaluate for parameters like alanine aminotransferase (ALT), aspartate aminotransferase (AST), alkaline phosphatase (ALP), and bilirubin levels. Increased enzyme levels indicate hepatocellular injury, cholestasis, or obstruction of the bile duct and play an important role in determining the liver's viability. In other studies, for instance, an audit of St. Luke's Hospital in Malta, a significant proportion of congestive HF patients were observed to have LFTs performed (36%) as part of clinical evaluation, in accordance with the overlap between hepatic and cardiac health in the context of liver failure (Camilleri *et al.*, 2004). Therefore, routine blood examination is a crucial diagnostic method for clinicians to detect early liver insufficiency and monitor disease progression. In addition to LFTs, other laboratory investigations are useful in providing information about a patient's overall status in suspected liver failure. These tests may also include the measurement of the complete blood count (CBC), kidney function tests, and clotting profiles to aid in complications of liver disease, such as coagulopathy from impaired synthesis of clotting factors. For instance, in a case of primary sclerosing cholangitis (PSC) reported previously, lab results showed significant aberrations, such as anemia and platelet and white blood cell drops with increased liver enzyme levels, indicating severe liver impairment and requiring further diagnostic evaluation (Glaz *et al.*, 2022). These wide-ranging evaluations not only assist in confirming diagnosis but also guide therapeutic decisions and ongoing surveillance, attesting to the utility of adding blood testing to the management of liver failure. Ultimately, ongoing monitoring of blood work is priceless to the successful diagnosis and treatment of liver failure. Doctors make use of these tests to monitor changes over time, which in a great way can make a difference in the identification of advancement or recovery of liver-related conditions. Furthermore, information derived from the tests can direct treatment strategies, for instance, the application of pharmacological treatments or potential liver transplantation, especially in acute conditions where the liver is permanently damaged. In patients with deteriorating liver disease, blood tests, for example, in patients with chronic kidney disease such as PSC, may assist in functional monitoring at set intervals, allowing early treatment to limit complications, enhance functional outcomes, and promote quality of life (Glaz *et al.*, 2022). Therefore, not only does blood testing provide a critical window on the liver, but also it is an irreplaceable component of integrated management of liver failure (Figure 4.9).

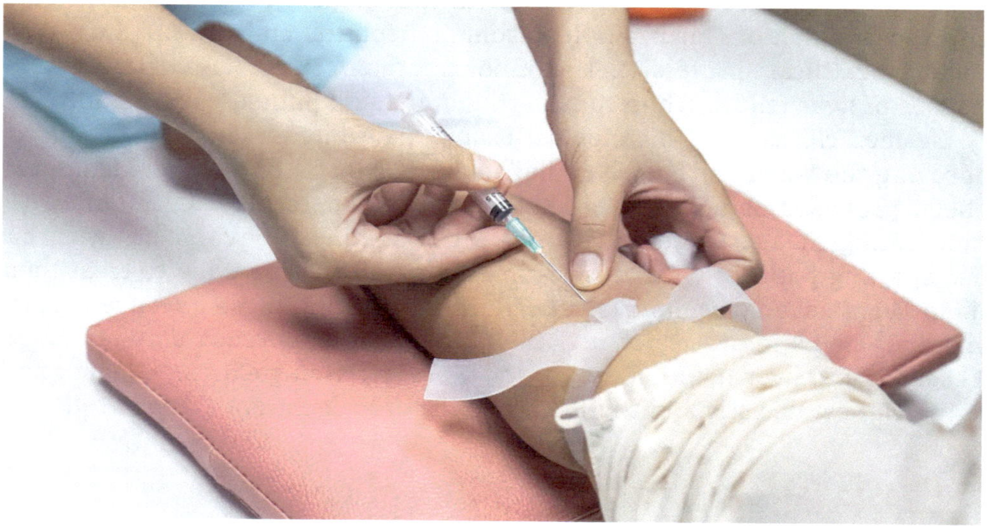

Figure 4.9. Liver- Function tests.

Source: https://pharmaceutical-journal.com/wp-content/uploads/2022/01/Liver-function-tests-Leadart-1.jpg.

4.4.2. Imaging Studies (Ultrasound, CT Scan)

Knowing the different imaging studies used to diagnose liver failure is very important for proper and swift management. Among these, nonenhanced computed tomography (NECT) serves as a foundational tool, offering clear visualization of hepatic structures and identification of abnormalities such as lesions or fluid accumulation. Even so, NECT is very good at spotting large anatomical differences, but it is less sensitive to smaller problems. In patients with liver failure, this problem can be very significant since the small differences in pathology may have a major impact on their treatment plan. It is important to be able to tell benign lesions apart from malignant ones, which is why better imaging methods are needed for assessing liver problems. In contrast, ultrasound (US) and, more specifically, contrast-enhanced ultrasound (CEUS) present significant advantages when evaluating liver pathologies.

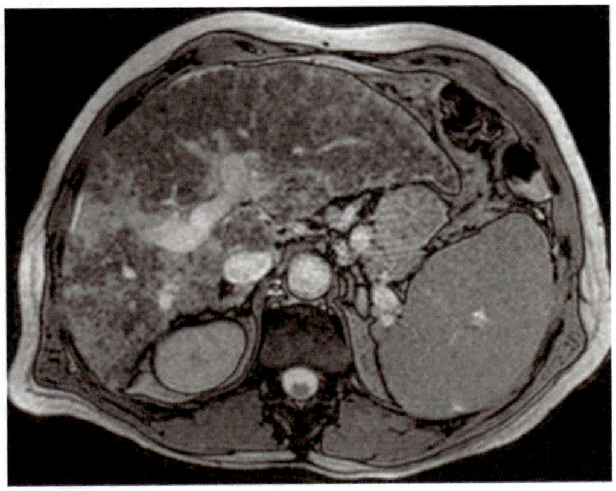

Figure 4.10. MR imaging.

Source: https://media.springernature.com/lw685/springer-static/image/art%3A10.1007%2Fs13244-010-0034-7/MediaObjects/13244_2010_34_Fig7_HTML.jpg.

Recent studies indicate that US, especially when used with CEUS, is better than NECT at detecting and defining hepatic conditions. Contrast agents make it easier to see blood flow and tissue perfusion in US, which helps doctors assess liver lesions more accurately. Evidence from research shows that CEUS is 100% sensitive in detecting liver problems, so it is very useful in clinical care when liver function is affected. Because of this, CEUS is widely used to diagnose liver problems, especially in those with kidney impairment, who may not be able to have CT scans due to the nephrotoxic agents used. Also, using imaging studies in the process of diagnosing liver failure points to the importance of a team approach in care. Although NECT and CEUS give a lot of information, this information is most useful when used together by radiologists, hepatologists, and the clinical team. By working together, doctors can review the images, symptoms, and test results together. Because of this, having set procedures for using these imaging tools can help doctors make more accurate diagnoses and benefit patients. By leveraging the strengths of various imaging techniques, clinicians can develop tailored management strategies that address the complexities associated with liver failure and its associated conditions, ultimately leading to more effective interventions and improved patient prognoses (Figure 4.10).

4.4.3. Liver Biopsy (LBx)

The LBx is an essential diagnostic tool in the diagnosis of liver diseases, particularly in the presence of suspected liver failure. By the aspiration of a tiny amount of liver tissue, physicians can assess the histopathological features of numerous disparate hepatic disorders. It is particularly valuable when LFTs are noncontributory or when the etiology of liver failure is unclear. A highly cautious examination of the biopsy will be capable of yielding significant information, such as the presence of inflammation, fibrosis, or malignancy. In cases where complications are reached, such as hemophagocytic lymphohistiocytosis (HLH), LBx can be utilized in reaching a diagnosis, ultimately resulting in the suitable therapeutic interventions (Decker *et al.*, 2016). Therefore, in liver failure, the role of LBx is not just limited to diagnosis but can provide information that can highly determine management interventions. The diagnosis of LBx results calls for a vast knowledge of liver pathology and its underlying disorders. Pathologists examine the tissue sample to identify characteristics that may indicate specific liver diseases, such as hepatitis, cirrhosis, or fatty liver disease. Further, the biopsy can be applied to analyze the extent of liver damage, which is critical in determining the prognosis and treatment required in patients with liver failure. The juxtaposition of tissue findings and clinical presentation necessitates a multidisciplinary approach towards treating liver disease. Furthermore, continuous research into immunological responses expounds on the complexities engaged by liver transplantation. Symbiotic interaction between implanted tissues and host immune responses highlights the new face of liver diagnostics and interventions (Demetris *et al.*, 1993). Thus, LBx not only serves a diagnostic purpose but also sharpens the overall understanding of liver pathophysiology. Although LBx is a very valuable tool in contemporary hepatology, it is far from riskless and has its own shortcomings. Side effects such as bleeding, infection, and pain are an eventual risk that must be weighed against the diagnostic benefit. Also, the invasive nature of the procedure can make some of these patients apprehensive, and adequate explanations about the need for the biopsy and potential outcomes are necessary. Non-invasive imaging technologies and serological markers are under active study but not always as precisely as a biopsy. As our understanding of liver disease evolves further, the use of LBx data in conjunction with other methods of diagnosis will become progressively crucial in optimizing our approach to liver failure. Ultimately, LBx will remain a valuable addition to the diagnostic repertoire, always directing therapy and improving results in the environment of liver failure (Figure 4.11).

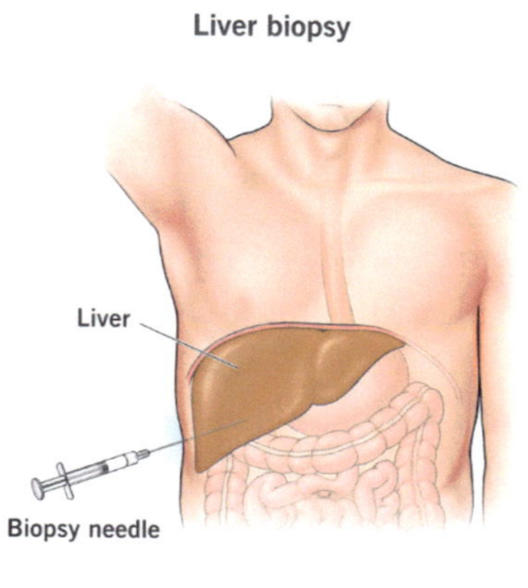

Figure 4.11. Liver biopsy.

Source: https://my.clevelandclinic.org/-/scassets/images/org/health/articles/9503-liver-biopsy.

4.5. Treatment Options

Treatment options for liver failure are chosen based on what is causing the failure and how severe it is. Treatment at first usually involves handling the factors that cause liver damage, such as controlling viral hepatitis or getting patients to stop drinking alcohol if they have ALD. Besides primary treatments, supportive care is very important for stabilizing patients and may consist of giving nutritional support, treating ascites, and correcting coagulopathies. If liver failure becomes severe, for example, in ALF or when the liver is at end-stage, more serious treatments are needed, and this may result in considering a liver transplant. This approach stresses that early care and good management can help patients with liver failure recover better. Treatment for patients with severe liver disease and ALF depends mainly on liver transplantation. Many recent studies have found that patients with acute hepatic failure often do not get the procedure in time, mainly because of either inadequate assessment or problems caused by other serious health conditions, such as renal failure. Managing pain after a liver transplant is a major concern, since giving enough pain relief can also increase the risk of adverse effects. The current literature points out that using a combination of approaches can help control pain after transplant, as opioids may cause trouble like HE and renal failure. By utilizing alternative analgesic strategies, there is an opportunity to enhance patient recovery and improve overall survival rates (Nicolini *et al.*, 2023). The risk of developing secondary complications, such as hepatorenal syndrome (HRS), further complicates the management of patients with liver failure. Because HRS often appears in people with advanced cirrhosis or ALF, it is important to identify and treat it as soon as possible. Even though several treatments are used, they are not very effective at fixing renal impairment and mainly help patients live longer until a liver transplant is available. Many studies have looked into the ways HRS occurs, which has helped improve how patients are managed. Improvements in this field suggest better results could be achieved, but also point to the need for a total approach that treats both liver and kidney problems. This highlights the evolving nature of liver failure management and the demands for continued research and development in therapeutic interventions (Hasan *et al.*, 2021).

4.5.1. Medications and Therapies

Liver failure treatment is generally based on the effective employment of drugs and treatments that are individually targeted based on the etiology of the disease. For instance, patients with complications of hepatitis C infection can derive tremendous advantage from the application of direct-acting antiviral agents (DAAs), which have revolutionized the treatment pattern. These drugs exhibit varying rates and modes of action that actively disrupt the viral life cycle directly, with consequent increased cure rates and overall effective reduction in liver disease burden. DAAs' efficacy is also compromised by patient-related factors such as advanced cirrhosis and comorbidities, which necessitate careful treatment protocol considerations. In addition, the expense of these treatments can restrict access, thus compounding health disparities across various patient groups (Bidell *et al.*, 2016).

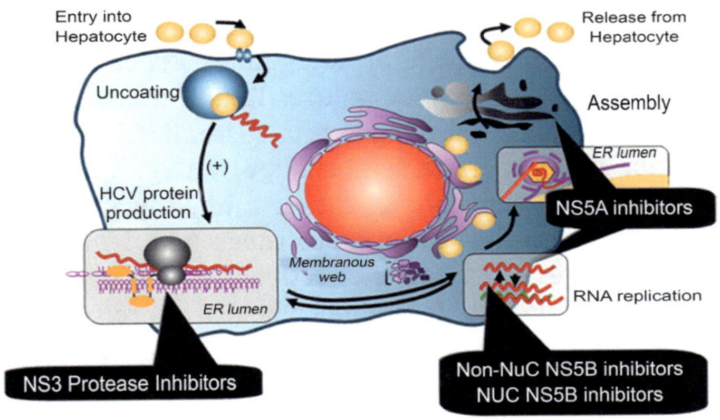

Figure 4.12. Specific targets of the direct acting antiviral agents.

Source: https://www.amjtransplant.org/cms/10.1111/ajt.12714/asset/043b74ea-68d4-4150-ac47-8aca0557f04e/main.assets/gr1_lrg.jpg.

Accordingly, although DAAs are an exciting development, albeit a pharmacologic one, in the treatment of liver failure, an evidence-based strategy is needed to maximize patient outcomes. In addition to antiviral treatment, treatment for liver failure usually involves symptomatic support to control complications due to liver insufficiency. Medications such as lactulose are usually employed for the treatment of HE, which is a serious mental impairment resulting from the accumulation of toxins that the impaired liver cannot eliminate. Lactulose causes excretion of ammonia and thus improves the mental status and well-being of those affected. Moreover, diuretics are frequently utilized in the treatment of fluid overload, which is one of the significant complications of liver failure that can contribute to the formation of ascites and other ensuing issues. Symptomatic therapy of this type is the gold standard for enhancing patient comfort and physiologic stability, but must be utilized with care in order not to precipitate increased liver morbidity. The intervention between treatment of the root cause of liver failure and regulation of its symptoms illustrates the holistic mode of treatment strategies in this multi-factorial disorder. New therapies also hold the promise for upgrading treatment paradigms in liver failure. New modalities such as gene therapy and cell-based therapies are being explored for the management of acute and chronic liver conditions. For instance, researchers are investigating the therapeutic promise of stem cell therapies in the restoration of liver tissue following injury, holding out a new hope for end-stage liver disease patients. Also, advances in drug therapy to inhibit inflammatory pathways may mitigate patients' symptoms of metabolic-associated fatty liver disease. Nevertheless, the bench to bedside bridge is still riddled with challenges, including regulatory burdens and the need for extensive clinical evidence. The growing understanding of liver pathophysiology and the promise of innovative therapies are announcing a dramatic era for managing liver failure, in which these innovative therapies become central components of the therapeutic arsenal against this fatal disease (Kay *et al.*, 2015) (Figure 4.12).

4.5.2. Lifestyle Changes and Dietary Modifications

Changing your lifestyle and eating habits is very important for managing the liver, especially when someone has liver failure. Because the liver is important for metabolism, any decline in its function requires both activity and dietary changes. People who have liver problems or are at risk, such as those with NAFLD, are usually recommended to manage their weight along with changes in their diet. Evidence suggests that low-carbohydrate or ketogenic diets can reduce fat in the liver, which may stop the disease from progressing to liver failure. Taking this step can support the liver and also help with overall metabolic health, showing how a customized diet is central to good lifestyle changes. Being physically active is an important change that greatly affects liver health. Doing physical activity on a regular basis can help maintain a healthy weight, lower IR, and improve liver function, mainly for people with liver failure. For those with NAFLD, exercise programs given by doctors can help dietary changes work more effectively, which supports weight loss and helps prevent the disease from advancing. Also, including physical exercise can help people feel better emotionally and stick to their new diet. For example, VITALISE shows that a well-organized digital platform can help patients reach their health targets by giving them useful information on both diet and exercise. This multifaceted approach acknowledges the complexity of liver conditions and tailors interventions to individual patient needs, enhancing feasibility and sustainability in managing liver health (Avery *et al.*, 2023). Strategies that focus on lifestyle changes and dietary adjustments help with immediate health problems and also focus on managing liver conditions long-term. Because diet, exercise, and liver health are related, those at risk of liver failure need to keep learning and receiving support. When we understand personalized treatment, patients benefit a lot, as it is important to address their unique symptoms and habits. When nutrition counseling, physical activity, and behavioral coaching are part of clinical care, patients feel more encouraged to look after their health. As research continues to uncover the intricacies of liver disease management, the emphasis on lifestyle changes will undoubtedly remain central to therapeutic strategies aimed at reinforcing liver function and preventing further decline (Namoosi *et al.*, 2024).

4.5.3. Liver Transplantation

Liver transplantation has become a central intervention for individuals undergoing liver failure, especially in the case of ALF. The disease is marked by acute liver dysfunction with serious complications and, in most cases, high mortality. The causes of ALF differ across the world; DILI, including acetaminophen toxicity, is the predominant cause in developed nations, while viral infections predominantly prevail in developing countries (McSteen *et al.*, 2024). Early recognition and treatment of ALF are crucial, since therapeutic success can significantly influence patient outcomes. In those instances, in which conventional therapies cannot stabilize the patient, liver transplantation not only becomes a life-saving procedure but most often becomes the only method by which hepatic function is reconstituted and survival is ensured.

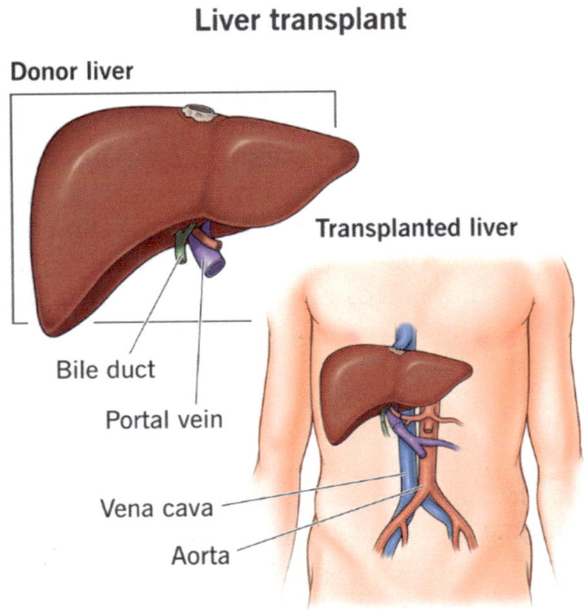

Figure 4.13. Liver transplant.

Source: https://my.clevelandclinic.org/-/scassets/images/org/health/articles/8111-liver-transplant.jpg.

Moreover, liver transplant is not limited to the acute case but also for CLD patients, including cholestatic liver diseases. These chronic conditions, which are characterized by impaired bile flow and liver injury, typically cause liver failure that cannot be effectively managed with conservative therapy alone. Transplantation, hence, becomes the only treatment option. As recent evidence has shown, transplantation has made significant strides in its eligibility, now extending to patients who may only express diminished quality of life due to cholestatic presentation. Consequently, liver transplantation significantly improves life expectancy and overall prognosis for health in patients suffering from conditions such as PSC and PBC (Hlavatý *et al.*, 2024). Post-transplantation comes with its own set of challenges, particularly regarding the management of immune-mediated complications. Patients undergoing liver transplantation due to conditions like cholestatic liver disease are typically at increased risk for recurrence of their original disease within the allograft, jeopardizing graft survival and quality of life. Specialized care after transplantation is necessary to avoid such risks and screen for complications, including the development of inflammatory bowel disease (IBD) among patients with PSC (Hlavatý *et al.*, 2024). Yet, long-term outcomes for liver transplantation in cholestatic liver disease remain excellent, typically achieving higher survival rates than in the other transplant recipient groups. This is a sign of the drive to optimize therapeutic strategies and constant monitoring to enhance post-operative care for liver transplant recipients (Figure 4.13).

4.6. Complications of Liver Failure

Many complications may result from liver failure, which can have a big impact on how the disease progresses. A serious complication is HE, which occurs when the liver can no longer remove toxins from the body. It causes problems with thinking and may advance to confusion, seizures, and coma. Ammonia poisoning is more common in people with acute-on-chronic liver failure because their livers cannot break down ammonia well. Data suggest that interventions like extracorporeal liver support systems may reduce the occurrence of HE, offering a survival advantage that is critical for effective management (Liu *et al.*, 2024). The new treatment methods should be discussed more, especially in terms of how they affect the pathways to encephalopathy and the patient's chances of survival. SBP, which is an infection of the fluid in the abdominal cavity, is another major problem connected to liver failure. The risk factors for SBP are closely linked to the severity of liver disease, often indicated by elevated model for end-stage liver disease (MELD) scores. Patients with advanced liver disease face a higher prevalence of these infections, which can complicate their clinical picture, leading to longer hospital stays and increased mortality rates (Chen *et al.*, 2024). In addition, early detection and proper treatment of SBP are critical because delays can cause the condition to worsen quickly and increase the chances of needing intensive care. Giving antibiotics to people at risk before surgery has become a good way to reduce risks and improve their chances of surviving. Another serious problem linked to liver failure is HRS, which happens when the kidneys rapidly deteriorate due to severe liver problems. Liver failure causes changes in how blood moves through the kidneys, which results in the kidneys narrowing their blood vessels and failing. The outlook for people with HRS is usually poor, and many of them must receive renal replacement therapy. Recent studies indicate that the use of specialized therapies, such as extracorporeal liver support systems, can potentially alleviate symptoms and improve survival rates in these patients (Liu *et al.*, 2024). Taking care of HRS calls for early detection, fast treatment of liver failure, and close observation of kidney health, which are all crucial for better results in patients with severe liver disease.

4.6.1. Hepatic Encephalopathy (HE)

HE is a neuropsychiatric condition with multifaceted pathophysiology as a result of liver failure, with cognitive dysfunction, alteration of consciousness, and in the most severe cases, coma. HE pathophysiology arises from the accumulation of neurotoxic agents, primarily ammonia, in the blood due to the liver's ineffective detoxifying mechanisms failing to eliminate the chemicals. HE usually arises in patients with CLD or acute, whose livers' compromised function is unable to clear the toxins. As hepatic function declines, the central nervous system becomes affected, and thus a spectrum of neurological dysfunction from minimal confusion to significant mental status change ensues. Treatment of HE in liver failure is crucial because it immediately impacts the patient's outcome and quality of life and, therefore, needs early recognition and treatment to prevent progression to more advanced forms of encephalopathy (Philippart *et al.*, 2024). Furthermore, the clinical manifestation of HE may be further subclassified into four stages, each characterized by characteristic neurological features. Stage I is characterized by minimal alterations in cognition and mood, while stages II to IV are characterized by progressively severe behavioral alterations, including asterixis, lethargy, and coma. Assessment and diagnosis of HE requires a comprehensive approach consisting of clinical evaluation by history-taking and neurological examination, accompanied by supportive laboratory tests to identify the etiology, e.g., elevated blood ammonia. Of significance is the identification of overt HE, which may go unnoticed and be missed, as it is important for effective management. Use of standardized assessment tools and neuropsychological tests can potentially assist clinicians in identifying early cognitive impairment, thus opening the door for early therapeutic interventions to manage symptoms and improve overall prognosis (Tanaka *et al.*, 2011). Management of HE is primarily based on addressing the underlying cause while providing supportive care to reduce ammonia levels and promote cognitive improvement. Lactulose is an unabsorbed disaccharide that can be used to stimulate ammonia excretion through the gut. Rifaximin, a gut flora-manipulated antibiotic, can also be utilized to help lower ammonia production further in the recurrent group. These interventions are crucial in the acute setting, especially for those who have signs of decompensated liver failure. While the gold standard for carefully evaluating patients with end-stage liver disease is undoubtedly liver transplantation, treatment of HE remains essential to optimize survival and prevent complications from liver failure. This approach highlights the importance of understanding the intricate interplay between neurology and the liver to best treat patients with HE (Philippart *et al.*, 2024). (Figure 4.14).

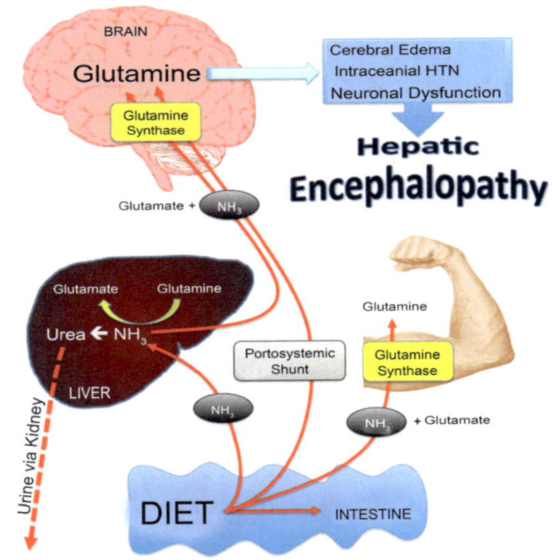

Figure 4.14. A schematic summary of pathophysiology of hepatic encephalopathy and ammoniogenesis in end-stage liver disease patients.

Source: https://www.researchgate.net/publication/338953586/figure/fig1/AS:961416378982412@1606230935506/A-schematic-summary-of-pathophysiology-of-hepatic-encephalopathy-and-ammoniogenesis-in.png.

4.6.2. Kidney Failure

Because the liver and kidneys are linked, the health of one can quickly affect the health of the other. When a patient's liver fails, AKI is often seen, and this happens because of several reasons, such as decreased blood flow to the kidneys and changes in blood pressure. Failure of the liver can cause changes in the body that affect kidney function, which makes the condition worse. The complex relationship is underscored by the pathophysiology of acute decompensated cirrhosis, wherein 10% to 20% of affected individuals face a high in-hospital mortality rate due to complications such as AKI (McPherson *et al.*, 2025). It is important to understand these links, since liver failure can seriously affect kidney function and call for a well-planned treatment plan. Managing kidney failure together with liver problems is very challenging for healthcare staff. Anemia, and especially anemia related to cirrhosis, adds to the difficulty of managing the patient's condition. It is very important to manage anemia, since it is common in patients with kidney disease and can worsen their quality of life and their ability to recover. The treatment may involve erythropoietin stimulants and iron supplementation, tailored to the underlying chronic disease, including liver failure, chronic kidney disease, and others (Orlova *et al.*, 2024). For patients to have better results, a team approach is required, which means specialists from different fields need to join forces to address the complex needs caused by these interconnected organ failures. With more research revealing the difficulties of liver failure and kidney dysfunction, it is obvious that preventing problems and acting early are important for patients. The British Society of Gastroenterology's care bundles signify a proactive stance in managing complications associated with acute decompensated liver disease, thereby indirectly benefiting renal outcomes through structured care protocols (McPherson *et al.*, 2025). Using standardized guidelines and protocols, healthcare centers can improve the care and results for patients suffering from kidney and liver failure simultaneously. Effective ways of handling these linked conditions, when made available to people, may help lower deaths and improve patients' chances of recovery. These efforts underscore the necessity for continued research and collaboration in treating these life-threatening conditions (Figure 4.15).

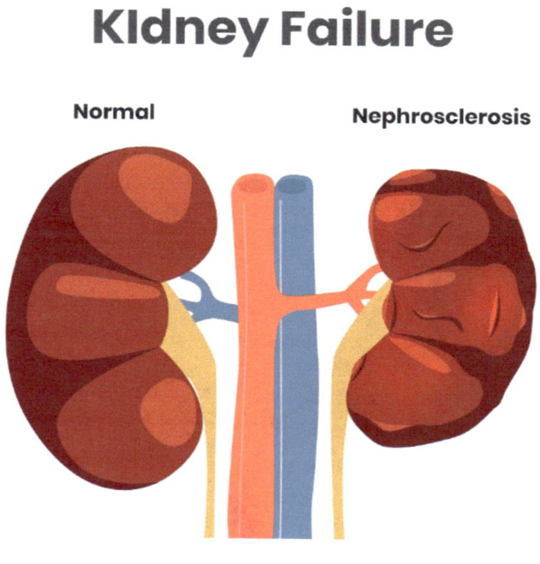

Figure 4.15. Kidney failure.

Source: https://images.squarespace-cdn.com/content/v1/633ba514bb0a7342b4a41bc8/aae77a5d-09d5-45bc-84e8-75f8a39f5441/The-Foundation-to-Advance-Vascular-Cures-Kidney-Failure-and-Vascular-Disease.jpeg.

4.6.3. Increased Risk of Infections

The state of increased risk of infection among patients with liver failure is largely attributed to the immunocompromised state, which ensues due to cirrhosis and other liver diseases. Liver failure disrupts the homeostatic role of the liver in the immune complex, which culminates in what, in a clinical setting, is referred to as cirrhosis-associated immune dysfunction (CAID). This disorder degrades both systemic and local immune competence, making the patients susceptible to any infections, including bacterial infections (BI) that may result in severe complications. Of most concern, BI is exceedingly prevalent in these patients, particularly in those awaiting liver transplantation, since they are exceedingly susceptible. These infections contribute to a significant amount of morbidity and mortality among this group of patients and are therefore an essential aspect of treating liver failure patients (Becchetti *et al.*, 2018). Among the plethora of infections faced by liver failure patients, Clostridium Difficile Infection (CDI) has emerged as an essential concern. The increased incidence of CDI in hospital patients is mainly responsible for the immune compromise of liver cirrhosis (LC). Contributing to this include recurrent hospitalization, antibiotic treatment for prophylaxis or therapy of SBP, and the administration of proton pump inhibitors (PPIs). These actions, although inevitable, inadvertently increase the vulnerability to CDI, already a prevalent cause of hospital-acquired diarrhea. The effect of CDI in patients with liver failure is widespread, as such infection not only results in a decline in overall health but also enhances 30-day mortality risk, and thus makes the already risky treatment of liver failure complicated (Dumitru *et al.*, 2019). The connection between liver failure and an increased risk of infection increases the need for comprehensive care approaches focused on prevention as well as prompt intervention. Proactive care entails constant monitoring for signs of infection, prompt antibiotic therapy when indicated, and judicious use of medication that may increase the risk of CDI. Additionally, the imposition of infection control within health facilities can be very effective in preventing the spread of resistant strains of bacteria, particularly in healthcare-associated settings. As the epidemiology of infections has evolved, particularly in the age of rising multidrug-resistant organisms, medical professionals are obliged to be vigilant and updated to achieve the optimal outcome in patients who are facing the multi-dimensional complexity of liver failure (Becchetti *et al.*, 2018; Dumitru *et al.*, 2019).

SUMMARY

The complicated and multidimensional character of liver failure is a testament to its recognition as a critical health issue necessitating ongoing research and intervention strategies. The liver is an invaluable organ tasked with the metabolism of materials, the regulation of blood composition, and the detoxification of harmful substances. Liver functions can be deranged by many factors, such as viral illness, alcohol consumption, and drug poisoning. Thus, liver failure not only leads to hepatic impairment but also causes systemic illness, making it imperative to understand the underlying mechanisms adequately. Medical professionals must understand current guidelines and clinical advice, as emphasized by the recent ESC/EAS Guidelines, which encourage well-informed clinical decisions in the face of evolving scientific evidence (Mach *et al.*, 2019). Liver failure requires an integrated management strategy that includes prevention, early detection, and proper management of the condition. Advances in the modalities of treatment, including progress in transplant surgery and pharmacotherapy, have improved outcomes. However, awareness about the risk factors for liver failure is equally important, particularly for drug-induced hepatotoxicity. For instance, acetaminophen, a commonly available analgesic, was identified as a major etiology of ALF, with severe mortality outcomes following transplantation (Chopyk *et al.*, 2019). Practitioners and patients must find risk factors and signs of liver damage to lower the risk of permanent damage and thus enhance the quality of life for the victim. Lastly, as the understanding of liver failure evolves, so too must the strategies used in its management and prevention. Continued research is imperative to uncover the complex interactions between lifestyle, environmental factors, and hepatic function, particularly regarding how substances like acetaminophen impact not only liver health but also intestinal integrity. The new evidence supports that hepatotoxicity's effects extend beyond the liver and require a holistic approach to patient management, including gut and overall physiology. Therefore, structuring healthcare resources toward education, diverse treatments, and interprofessional practices can ultimately result in better management of liver disease, an innovative strategy in addressing the burden of liver failure among populations (Chopyk *et al.*, 2019).

When the cause of liver failure is considered, one must be aware of the demography and the clinical characteristics of patients who develop ALF due to specific causes, e.g., viral infections. For example, a study of dengue fever indicates that even though hepatic involvement in the disease is common, the occurrence of ALF is uncommon. The population statistics recorded the age of patients as 38 years, which indicates a high occurrence among adults, particularly when there was an underlying health condition. This is a reflection of the need for early intervention and education among susceptible populations regarding the dangers of serious complications of dengue infection, particularly as ALF can become acute within a couple of days of symptom onset (Juneja *et al.*, 2024). The bear importance of this renders it critical in focusing the attention of healthcare providers towards early diagnosis and management strategies unique to these patients. Combining our insights into the mechanism of liver failure as well as presumed pathways sheds light on the intricacy of the disease. Recent research demystifies the role of various modes of cell death in acute-on-chronic liver failure (ACLF) with great emphasis on mechanisms such as pyroptosis, apoptosis, and necroptosis. This study into the PANoptosis pathway, which includes these types of cell death, is a complex comprehension of acute-on-chronic liver failure (ACLF) inflammatory processes. Bioinformatic analysis suggests these pathways to be extremely up-regulated, and inflammatory factors to exist, and interventions that target these regulated mechanisms of cell death to be potentially useful. Determining the key proteins involved in such processes, such as BAX and CASP, enables scientists to open avenues for future therapeutic measures that may prevent or buffer the progression of liver failure (Ye *et al.*, 2024). Further, clinical prognosis associated with liver failure highlights the imperative need for holistic care strategies. Patients who present with dengue infection showing signs of ALF might require intensive care interventions due to organ failures, with the neurological complications being particularly severe. One notable observation among the reported case series is that supportive therapy can prove successful in the majority of patients since most of them improved after getting appropriate medical treatment. However, organ support or transplantation among refractory patients also emerged as a deciding factor. The low mortality in patients of ALF caused by dengue says a lot about the extent of recovery when there is early diagnosis and appropriate management. This highlights the need for studies and clinical practice awareness to better manage those with liver failure (Juneja *et al.*, 2024).

CLOSER LOOK

BIOARTIFICIAL LIVER (BAL)

A BAL is a device that uses living liver cells in a bioreactor to perform some of the liver's functions, like filtering blood and producing essential substances. It's used as a bridge therapy for patients with liver failure, providing temporary support while a donor liver becomes available or the patient's liver recovers (Figure 4.16).

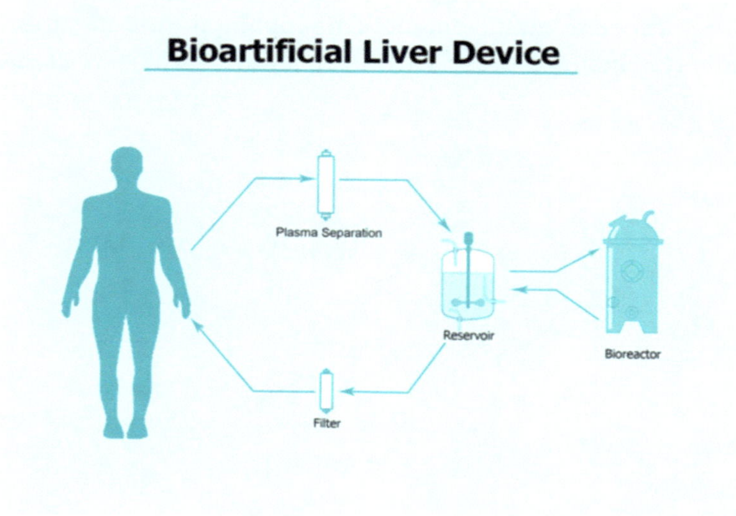

Figure 4.16. Bioartificial liver device.

Source: https://www.mdpi.com/cells/cells-09-00386/article_deploy/html/images/cells-09-00386-g003-550.jpg.

How It Works

BALs typically use a bioreactor where liver cells (usually hepatocytes) are cultured and maintained in a way that allows them to perform some of the liver's metabolic and detoxification functions. The patient's blood or plasma is circulated through the device, allowing the liver cells to process and filter the blood.

Purpose

BALs are primarily used to support patients with ALF or PHLF. They provide a temporary solution to help the patient survive until a liver transplant is possible or the patient's liver recovers.

Clinical Application

BALs have been used in clinical settings, with some studies showing promising results in improving patient survival rates and outcomes.

Potential Benefits

BALs offer a potential bridge to liver transplantation, allowing patients to survive longer and potentially improve their overall health. They also offer a non-transplant option for some patients who may not be eligible for transplantation or who may not have a suitable donor liver.

References

1. Audu, D., Patel, V. B., Petagine, L., Idowu, O. A., & Idowu, A. B. (2023). Repeated treatment with antimalarial agents causes *in vitro* liver toxicity. *Liver Research–Open Journal*. https://www.semanticscholar.org/paper/53e2372958624526b4b84e09481df239c9f7d2d2 (accessed on 24 May 2025).

2. Avery, L., Hallsworth, K., McPherson, S., Smith, A., *et al.* (2023). Feasibility and acceptability of an evidence-informed digital intervention to support self-management in people with non-alcoholic fatty liver disease: Protocol for a non-randomized feasibility study (VITALISE). https://core.ac.uk/download/564443449.docx.

3. Batista, M., Brito, P., Miranda, P., Barbosa, S., & Cotter, J. (2024). Liver failure in autoimmune hepatitis overlap syndrome with primary biliary cholangitis: A case report. *Cureus, 16*. https://www.semanticscholar.org/paper/97ae1fb7248fda3b5a8fa18dd65d30360f9e323d (accessed on 24 May 2025).

4. Bazargaliyev, Sh. Y., Madenbayeva, A. M., Kudabayeva, I. K., & Rysmaganbetov, S. S. (2025). Non-alcoholic fatty liver disease and its relationship with metabolic syndrome: Modern approaches to treatment and prevention. *Farmaciâ Kazahstana*. https://www.semanticscholar.org/paper/c38138d4f8d1b37b21e0f427b36febfdd5931c78 (accessed on 24 May 2025).

5. Becchetti, C., Burra, P., Ferrarese, A., Gambato, M., *et al.* (2018). Management of bacterial infection in the liver transplant candidate. https://core.ac.uk/download/154331081.pdf (accessed on 24 May 2025).

6. Bidell, M. R., Faragon, J., McLaughlin, M., Morse, A., *et al.* (2016). Desirable characteristics of hepatitis C treatment regimens: A review of what we have and what we need. https://core.ac.uk/download/323066109.pdf.

7. Broekhoven, A., Ostyn, T., Van Melkebeke, L., Verspaget, H. W., Van der Merwe, S. W., Verbeek, J., Coenraad, M., *et al.* (2024). Histological characteristics in patients admitted to the hospital with alcoholic hepatitis complicated by acute-on-chronic liver failure. *Scandinavian Journal of Gastroenterology, 59*, 577–583. https://www.semanticscholar.org/paper/592355a99741f5a1429612d31d5ca89052a3bc6a (accessed on 24 May 2025).

8. Camilleri, N., Sammut, D., & Schembri, S. (2004). An overview of the management of congestive heart failure in Malta. https://core.ac.uk/download/46601876.pdf (accessed on 24 May 2025).

9. Casali PG, Blay JY, Abecassis N, Bajpai J, Bauer S, Biagini R, Bielack S, Bonvalot S, Boukovinas I, Bovee JVMG, Boye K, Brodowicz T, Buonadonna A, *et. al.* Gastrointestinal stromal tumours: ESMO-EURACAN-GENTURIS Clinical Practice Guidelines for diagnosis, treatment and follow-up. Ann Oncol. 2022 Jan;33(1):20-33. doi: 10.1016/j.annonc.2021.09.005. Epub 2021 Sep 21. PMID: 34560242.

10. Nicolini Castellani , N., Belfiore, J., & Biancofiore, G. (2023). Multimodal pain management of liver transplantation: What is new? *OBM Transplantation*. https://www.semanticscholar.org/paper/f6cc9f936594345ebd16c0ec694dacca4713e0fd (accessed on 24 May 2025).

11. Chen, X., Gao, F., Pan, Q., Huang, C., Luo, R., Lu, X., Chen, X., *et al.* (2024). aCCI-HBV-ACLF: A novel predictive model for hepatitis B virus-related acute-on-chronic liver failure. *Alimentary Pharmacology & Therapeutics, 61*, 286–298. https://www.semanticscholar.org/paper/1f4d760bee923b153b455fad1262fb6479a95d3f (accessed on 24 May 2025).

12. Chopyk, D. M., Stuart, J. D., Zimmerman, M. G., Wen, J., Gumber, S., Suthar, M. S., Thapa, M., *et al.* (2019). Acetaminophen intoxication rapidly induces apoptosis of intestinal crypt stem cells and enhances intestinal permeability. *Hepatology Communications, 3*, 1435–1449. https://doi.org/10.1002/hep4.1406.

13. Condrat, C. E., Thompson, D. C., Barbu, M. G., Bugnar, O. L., Boboc, A. E., Crețoiu, D., Suciu, N., *et al.* (2020). miRNAs as biomarkers in disease: Latest findings regarding their role in diagnosis and prognosis. *Cells, 9*, 276. https://doi.org/10.3390/cells9020276.

14. Dhir S, Tarasenko M, Napoli E, Giulivi C. Neurological, Psychiatric, and Biochemical Aspects of Thiamine Deficiency in Children and Adults. Front Psychiatry. 2019 Apr 4;10:207. doi: 10.3389/fpsyt.2019.00207. PMID: 31019473; PMCID: PMC6459027.

15. Decker, K. A., Fix, O. K., Giard, J. M., Gill, R. M., *et al.* (2016). Acute liver failure secondary to hemophagocytic lymph histiocytosis during pregnancy. https://core.ac.uk/download/323073489.pdf.

16. Demetris, A. J., Fung, J. J., Ildstad, S., Kocova, M., *et al.* (1993). Cell migration and chimerism after whole-organ transplantation: The basis of graft acceptance. https://core.ac.uk/download/12204910.pdf (accessed on 24 May 2025).

17. Devasia, A. G., Ramasamy, A., & Leo, C. H. (2025). Current therapeutic landscape for metabolic dysfunction-associated steatohepatitis. *International Journal of Molecular Sciences, 26*. https://www.semanticscholar.org/paper/3d71a27d1b0c3ac9a353e1a6dc5a57c8117e3225 (accessed on 24 May 2025).

18. Ding, Z., Mai, Y., & Yuan, Y. (2022). Statistical investigation on potential triggering factors of acute liver failure. *Proceedings of SPIE, 12163*, 121630W–121630W-6. https://www.semanticscholar.org/paper/19a75faa53421f7ac20fad21f75119d2ae9188d4 (accessed on 24 May 2025).

19. Dumitru, A., Popoiag, E., Micu, S. I., Moraru, C., *et al.* (2019). The burden of Clostridium difficile infection in patients with liver cirrhosis. https://core.ac.uk/download/232440323.pdf (accessed on 24 May 2025).

20. Fahnøe, U., Pedersen, M. S., Sølund, C., Ernst, A., Krarup, H., Røge, B., Christensen, P., *et al.* (2020). Global evolutionary analysis of chronic hepatitis C patients revealed significant effect of baseline viral resistance, including novel non-target sites, for DAA-based treatment and retreatment outcome. *Journal of Viral Hepatitis, 28*, 302–316. https://www.semanticscholar.org/paper/bfcfbfb65ad116383266194f1717d1d0a97b65a2 (accessed on 24 May 2025).

21. Ghias, M., Sunzeri, L., Romero, L. J., Bogdansky, K., & Arevalo Marcano, C. (2024). Hemolytic anemia leading to fulminant hepatic failure as the initial presentation of Wilson's disease in a young female. *Cureus, 16*. https://www.semanticscholar.org/paper/ab0a96277890d8fd0324eb77769c4a60d0983fb5 (accessed on 24 May 2025).

22. Glaz, A., Kasztelan-Szczerbinska, B., Knop, K., Kochanowska, M., *et al.* (2022). Primary sclerosing cholangitis–an insidious enemy of the liver–case report. https://core.ac.uk/download/587245962.pdf (accessed on 24 May 2025).

23. Hasan, I., Rashid, T., Chirila, R., Ghali, P., & Wadei, H. (2021). Hepatorenal syndrome: Pathophysiology and evidence-based management update. *Romanian Journal of Internal Medicine, 59*, 227–261. https://www.semanticscholar.org/paper/65aa2c2c0cf58716904c681e9d41c9229520cf35 (accessed on 24 May 2025).

24. Hlavatý, M., Bajer, L., Fraňková, S., & Drastich, P. (2024). Liver transplantation for cholestatic diseases. *Gastroenterologie a hepatologie*. https://www.semanticscholar.org/paper/f78394b57ab4dc052df2bda7fa1697188060b060 (accessed on 24 May 2025).

25. Joby, A. (2011). Clinical profile, prognostic factors and outcomes in anti-tuberculous drug induced liver injury. https://core.ac.uk/download/235655160.pdf (accessed on 24 May 2025).

26. Juneja, D., Jain, R., & Nasa, P. (2024). Dengue induced acute liver failure: A meta summary of case reports. *World Journal of Virology, 13*. https://www.semanticscholar.org/paper/af0702c8dd96064e71c5add6b5f91c67c7b33963 (accessed on 24 May 2025).

27. Kay, K. A. (2015). *Relapsing-Remitting Multiple Sclerosis: Advances in Disease-Modifying Therapies* [Master's thesis, Boston University]. https://open.bu.edu/bitstream/2144/13960/10/Kay_bu_0017N_11509_WEB.pdf (accessed on 24 May 2025).

28. Liu, H., Yang, Z., Luo, Q., & Lin, J. (2024). Extracorporeal liver support systems in patients with acute-on-chronic liver failure: An updated systematic review and meta-analysis. *Artificial Organs, 49*, 762–777. https://www.semanticscholar.org/paper/5c47248be9580ab61a3daead47c77c64684be967 (accessed on 24 May 2025).

29. Lu, X. X., Lu, Y., Yang, L., Ma, Y. Y., & Wang, H. H. (2024). [A case of neonatal liver failure]. *Zhongguo Dang Dai Er Ke Za Zhi = Chinese Journal of Contemporary Pediatrics, 26*(2), 213–218. https://www.semanticscholar.org/paper/0b902adbd0c51f05f769f947b8fd0779fe59b8b6 (accessed on 24 May 2025).

30. Mach, F., Baigent, C., Catapano, A. L., Koskinas, K. C., Casula, M., Badimón, L., Chapman, M. J., *et al.* (2019). 2019 ESC/EAS guidelines for the management of dyslipidemias: Lipid modification to reduce cardiovascular risk. *European Heart Journal, 41*, 111–188. https://doi.org/10.1093/eurheartj/ehz455.

31. Malik, H., Malik, H., Uderani, M., Berhanu, M., Soto, C. J., & Saleem, F. (2023). Fulminant hepatitis A and E co-infection leading to acute liver failure: A case report. *Cureus, 15*. https://www.semanticscholar.org/paper/fd340d768f12c67f07324079febbe83b94fc7d69 (accessed on 24 May 2025).

32. Mandi, O., Silverii, M., Fattiroli, F., Burgisser, C., Valoti, P., Orso, F., Baldasseroni, S., Cappelli, F., Contiello, C., Lombardo, V., Agusto, S., D'Ambrosio, G., & Ungar, A. (2024). PARTIALLY REVERSIBLE DILATED CARDIOMYOPATHY ASSOCIATED WITH AMPHOTERICIN B THERAPY. European Heart Journal Supplements.. https://www.semanticscholar.org/paper/PARTIALLY-REVERSIBLE-DILATED-CARDIOMYOPATHY-WITH-B-Mandi-Silverii/3c84a0f4f1c647992d92c38c830b3fd664f1eb9b

33. Mansour, N. S., Behairy, B., Sira, A., Elkhadry, S., & Fouad, O. A. (2024). Epidemiology of acute liver failure in Egyptian children. *Egyptian Liver Journal, 14*, 1–8. https://www.semanticscholar.org/paper/94b8876ef926ed2d246b5c6bd7669f9ec9456882 (accessed on 24 May 2025).

34. McPherson, S., Abbas, N., Allison, M. E. D., Backhouse, D., Boothman, H., Cooksley, T., Corless, L., *et al.* (2025). Decompensated cirrhosis: An update of the BSG/BASL admission care bundle. *Frontline Gastroenterology*. https://www.semanticscholar.org/paper/a148d878ec78bb04d50944cb7786a7ea1cb635f6 (accessed on 24 May 2025).

35. McSteen, B. W., Ying, X., Lucero, C., & Jesudian, A. B. (2024). Viral etiologies of acute liver failure. *World Journal of Virology, 13*. https://www.semanticscholar.org/paper/9ea8ffb7d85c975a882a8be6277379b7689eb245 (accessed on 24 May 2025).

36. Metra, M., Tomasoni, D., Adamo, M., Bayés-Genís, A., Filippatos, G.S., Abdelhamid, M., Adamopoulos, S., Anker, S.D., Antohi, L.E., Böhm, M., Braunschweig, F., Gal, T.B., Butler, J., Cleland, J., Cohen-Solal, A., Damman, K., Gustafsson, F., Hill, L., Jankowska, E.A., Lainščak, M., Lund, L.H., McDonagh, T., Mebazaa, A., Moura, B., Mullens, W., Piepoli, M.F., Ponikowski, P., Rakisheva, A., Ristic, A., Savarese, G., Seferovic, P.M., Sharma, R., Tocchetti, C.G., Yılmaz, M.B., Vitale, C., Volterrani, M., von Haehling, S., Chioncel, O., Coats, A.J., & Rosano, G.M. (2023). Worsening of chronic heart failure: definition, epidemiology, management and prevention. A clinical consensus statement by the Heart Failure Association of the European Society of Cardiology. European Journal of Heart Failure, 25. https://www.semanticscholar.org/paper/Worsening-of-chronic-heart-failure%3A-definition%2C-and-Metra-Tomasoni/08d90f026e7c19b5e67d5c8a53d5ad74cb2e1c3b

37. Mishra, R., Nayak, A., & Mehendale, M. (2019). An observational study of maternal and fetal outcome in pregnant women with Hepatitis E. *International Journal of Reproduction, Contraception, Obstetrics and Gynecology*. https://www.semanticscholar.org/paper/7ff1429842e09576937e8d5dd6321379ea564e97 (accessed on 24 May 2025).

38. N/A. (2011). *Supporting Homeless People with Advanced Liver Disease Approaching the End of Life*. https://core.ac.uk/download/71364969.pdf (accessed on 24 May 2025).

39. Namoosi, R. (2024). *Study of Food Patterns Among Patients with Polycystic Ovarian Syndrome*. https://core.ac.uk/download/620847719.pdf (accessed on 24 May 2025).

40. Orlova, N., & Karseladze, N. D. (2024). Anemia of chronic diseases. *Medical Alphabet*. https://www.semanticscholar.org/paper/7c5713b9cb7afb251ecca0ca4e307060f98a9b30 (accessed on 24 May 2025).

41. Pelliccia, A., Sharma, S., Gati, S., Bäck, M., Börjesson, M., Caselli, S., Collet, J. P., *et al.* (2020). 2020 ESC guidelines on sports cardiology and exercise in patients with cardiovascular disease. *European Heart Journal, 42*, 17–96. https://doi.org/10.1093/eurheartj/ehaa605.

42. Philippart, M., Mesland, J. B., Haufroid, V., Collienne, C., & Hantson, P. (2024). Unconjugated hyperbilirubinemia in acetaminophen-related acute liver failure. *The American Journal of Case Reports, 25*, e942703-1–e942703-4. https://www.semanticscholar.org/paper/ac2b37173fe7b241eddf35a33a7b946d268fa3fd (accessed on 24 May 2025).

43. Sage, M. (2018). *Neurocognitive Findings in Adults Who Played Youth Football* [Master's thesis, Boston University]. https://open.bu.edu/bitstream/2144/33032/5/Sage_bu_0017N_14075.pdf

44. Sawhney, S., & Wilson, S. R. (2017). Can ultrasound with contrast enhancement replace nonenhanced computed tomography scans in patients with contraindication to computed tomography contrast agents? *Ultrasound Quarterly, 33*, 125–132. https://doi.org/10.1097/ruq.0000000000000271.

45. Selim, M., Weierstahl, K., Eriksen, C., Pearson, T., & Woehlck, H. (2023). Liver transplantation for fulminant hepatic failure precipitated by pheochromocytoma crisis in the setting of using Garcinia cambogia weight loss supplement: A case report. *Cureus, 15*. https://www.semanticscholar.org/paper/92e56f2f67140bf8fd083d884c3dea3c29d3eb15 (accessed on 24 May 2025).

46. Tanaka, T., Ishizaka, Y., Mitushima, T., Tani, M., Toda, A., Toda, E., Okada, M., *et al.* (2011). Plasma amino acid profile is altered by visceral fat accumulation and is a predictor of visceral

obesity in humans. *Nature Precedings*. https://www.semanticscholar.org/paper/27efa46e7ccf7c91390f368aca9c9f4a6accdeda (accessed on 24 May 2025).

47. Tejpal, S., Sharma, S. K., Sharma, A., & Sharma, S. (2024). A comprehensive review on hepatic encephalopathy: Pathophysiology, symptoms, epidemiology, classification, diagnosis and treatment. *Journal for Research in Applied Sciences and Biotechnology*. https://www.semanticscholar.org/paper/b3eeaacd427663e3f6923f0d6f557e39b0d066e2 (accessed on 24 May 2025).
48. Wang, D. D., Dong, M. M., Xie, Y., Xu, F. Q., Fu, T. W., Wu, Y. C., Zhang, Z., *et al.* (2024). Effect of early peri-operative arterial lactate concentration level ratios on post-hepatectomy liver failure. *Discover Oncology, 15*. https://www.semanticscholar.org/paper/f5cf5ad0e65f16a6ba92621c810da212b89f6910 (accessed on 24 May 2025).
49. Wang, L., Zhou, J., Wang, J., Wang, X., Dong, H., Zhao, L., Wu, J., *et al.* (2024). Hepatic stellate cell-targeting micelle nanomedicine for early diagnosis and treatment of liver fibrosis. *Advanced Healthcare Materials, 13*. https://www.semanticscholar.org/paper/785385aeb3f9cd168377c04f904676648898dfda (accessed on 24 May 2025).
50. Weng, J., Han, X., Zeng, F., Zhang, Y., Feng, L., Cai, L., Liang, K. Y., *et al.* (2021). Fiber scaffold bioartificial liver therapy relieves acute liver failure and extrahepatic organ injury in pigs. *Theragnostic, 11*, 7620–7639. https://www.semanticscholar.org/paper/6fce345d2c31dca0ae37d0020c90b760769a4ec0 (accessed on 24 May 2025).
51. Wolstenholme, J. T., Duong, N., Brocato, E. R., & Bajaj, J. (2024). Gut-liver-brain axis and alcohol use disorder: Treatment potential of fecal microbiota transplantation. *Alcohol Research: Current Reviews, 44*. https://www.semanticscholar.org/paper/f7de8b529fb764ae3d0aba240699624162345f60 (accessed on 24 May 2025).
52. Xia, Y., Liao, F., Yang, Y., Luo, J., Zuo, L., Xia, A., & Ma, X. (2024). Can *Talaromyces marneffei* infection cause acute liver failure? A case report. *Hepatitis Monthly*. https://www.semanticscholar.org/paper/6c0adb17e9e2846633e64080363e060168bd7c38 (accessed on 24 May 2025).
53. Ye, Q., Wang, H., Chen, Y., Zheng, Y., Du, Y., Ma, C., & Zhang, Q. (2024). PANoptosis-like death in acute-on-chronic liver failure injury. *Scientific Reports, 14*. https://www.semanticscholar.org/paper/f665b480cf4cf715b86ea0af8915ce2cd1b7caa2 (accessed on 24 May 2025).
54. Zhang, Y., Tian, X., Li, J., Wu, D., Li, Q., & Chen, B. (2024). Mitochondrial dysfunction affects hepatic immune and metabolic remodeling in patients with hepatitis B virus-related acute-on-chronic liver failure. *World Journal of Gastroenterology, 30*, 881–900. https://www.semanticscholar.org/paper/4351531b2c31790f1518e00bac4b77e25627874a (accessed on 24 May 2025).
55. Zheng, C., Qi, Z., Chen, R., Liao, Z., Xie, L., & Zhang, F. (2025). The association between the dietary index for gut microbiota and non-alcoholic fatty liver disease and liver fibrosis: Evidence from NHANES 2017–2020. *BMC Gastroenterology, 25*. https://www.semanticscholar.org/paper/39616e9fb680c56fbb2edad621240dec49c0b9fb (accessed on 24 May 2025).
56. Zhu, X., Cheung, W. W., Zhang, A., & Ding, G. (2024). Mutation characteristics of primary hyperoxaluria in the Chinese population and current international diagnosis and treatment status. *Kidney Diseases, 10*, 313–326. https://www.semanticscholar.org/paper/d573caa3b23c5e4f25703076911ecaa5919c3bbe (accessed on 24 May 2025).

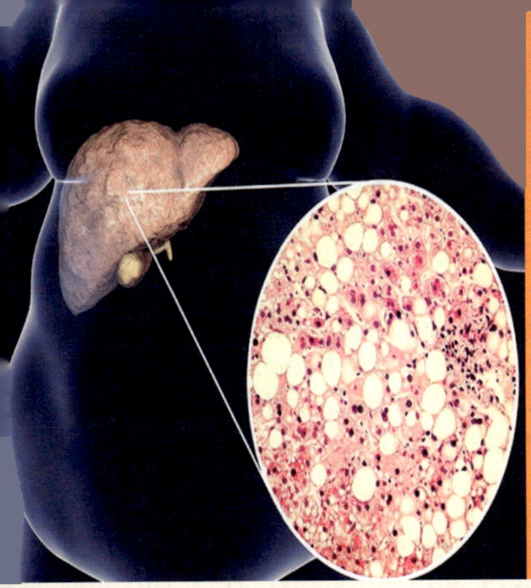

Chapter 5

NON-ALCOHOLIC FATTY LIVER DISEASE (NAFLD)

Contents

Introduction

Non-alcoholic fatty liver disease (NAFLD) is a global emerging public health issue due to its increasing incidence, affecting almost 25% of the world population. The disease is multifactorial and challenging and may vary from mild steatosis with lipid accumulation in the liver without significant inflammation to more severe types like non-alcoholic steatohepatitis (NASH), which may progress to fibrosis and cirrhosis. Early detection cannot be overestimated, as early diagnosis can transform the course of the disease and limit the potential for permanent liver damage. Traditional methods of diagnosis, such as LFTs and liver biopsy, are prone to fail due to their invasive nature and lowered sensitivity, and once again highlight the need for new non-invasive technologies. The finding of new biomarkers matters since these can be utilized to improve the diagnostic accuracy and facilitate stage differentiation between NAFLD patients (Veldi *et al.*, 2025). The latest on the identification of NAFLD has trended towards non-invasive biomarkers, which have promise in identifying and categorizing the disease without the constraint of traditional approaches. These biomarkers include microRNAs (miRNAs), lipidomic profiles, and metabolomic data, which all provide information about the cellular environment of the liver and the development of disease. For instance, miR-122 and miR-21 are identified as potential indicators of the severity of NAFLD, whose diagnostic effectiveness is greater compared to conventional methods. Similarly, lipidomics has been shown to target individual lipid species, such as diacylglycerols and ceramides, which are implicated in NASH incidence and liver inflammation extent. Through the inclusion of these new diagnostics in clinical management, clinicians shall gain a better understanding of NAFLD, potentially allowing for more constrained and advantageous treatment interventions in patients (Veldi *et al.*, 2025).

Furthermore, the overlap of systemic conditions such as periodontal disease can provide further significance to the etiology and outcomes of NAFLD. There has been an established relationship between periodontal disease and NAFLD with a high odds ratio, suggesting a potential correlation between the two conditions. This association highlights the common pathway of chronic inflammation as a potential mechanism that might exacerbate both conditions. Because systemic inflammation and pro-inflammatory markers can influence the pathophysiology of diseases, studies examining the interaction between oral disease and liver disease are crucial to creating a complete understanding of a patient's condition. Additional studies need to be done in order to clarify these interactions, and hopefully, they will lead to enhanced early diagnosis and treatment protocols for NAFLD, thus improving patient outcomes across various aspects of health.

Definition of Non-Alcoholic Fatty Liver Disease

NAFLD is a condition caused by too much fat in the liver, and it affects people who drink little or no alcohol. NAFLD is mainly divided into simple steatosis and NASH, and it can lead from harmless fat buildup to serious liver problems such as inflammation and scarring. Although the exact causes of NAFLD are being studied, it is commonly thought that IR, obesity, and dyslipidemia are important factors in its development. During the early stages, NAFLD usually does not cause symptoms, which makes it hard to find and treat. The wide range of the disease means it needs careful study, particularly because its prevalence is rising due to the global obesity epidemic, which makes it a major health concern. Researchers in global studies are concerned about the high prevalence of NAFLD, which is present in about 25% of the population. The condition is not only found in adults; its occurrence in children and adolescents is rising, mainly in those who are overweight. A study on NAFLD knowledge among different groups found that many people do not understand the risks and complications of the disease; for instance, 10.8% of respondents thought that people with fatty liver did not experience any symptoms, and over 80% were unaware of good treatment options. Since patients may not know about NAFLD, this could cause the disease to worsen, since early treatment is very important. Therefore, improving public and clinical awareness of NAFLD is essential, as it may directly influence screening processes and promote healthier lifestyle choices among at-risk populations (Hegazy *et al.*, 2024). There are not many therapies for NAFLD, and the main approach is to change lifestyle habits. Eating differently, being active, and losing weight can greatly lower liver fat and improve how the liver works. Emerging research has begun to explore pharmacological interventions, such as vitamin E and pioglitazone; a randomized controlled trial demonstrated that vitamin E was more effective than pioglitazone in managing NAFLD in certain populations (Fazal *et al.*, 2024). Still, there is not enough knowledge about NAFLD among professionals and the public, which is a major obstacle. Addressing these misconceptions is crucial for fostering better patient education and prevention strategies, ultimately reducing the global burden of this increasingly prevalent condition (Figure 5.1).

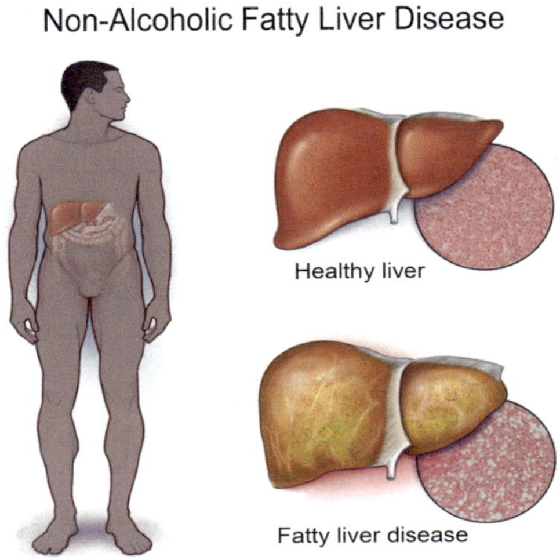

Figure 5.1. Non-alcoholic fatty liver disease.

Source: https://fundahigadoamerica.org/wp-content/uploads/2023/09/22437-non-alcoholic-fatty-liver-disease.webp.

Prevalence and Significance in Public Health

The prevalence of NAFLD is a public health priority, and its increasing impact on the global population places it in the priority category. Epidemiological studies document that NAFLD has been one of the most common liver diseases, with estimates suggesting that it affects approximately 25% of the global adult population. This growing prevalence has a close relation with growing rates of obesity, diabetes, and metabolic syndrome, all being etiologies of the disease pathophysiology. Also growing, the shift to sedentary lifestyles and unhealthy dietary habits boosts the trend and emphasizes the necessity for public health interventions aimed at informing groups about risks encompassing NAFLD. These programs are not only essential in the prevention of disease but also in its complications, such as LC and risk of increased mortality, as emphasized through critical reflection on world trends of liver disease, for example, in Sri Lanka, where NAFLD is the leading cause of the highest hospital mortality (Aslam *et al.*, 2017). The public health significance transcends the mere individual effect of NAFLD and affects society at large. The healthcare cost of managing NAFLD is rising with the progression of the disease, particularly with regard to the possibility of severe complications. As indicated in the literature, NAFLD patients are at risk for silent cirrhosis progression, prompting early identification and intervention to reduce healthcare expenditure. Moreover, the potential link between NAFLD and other chronic conditions, such as cardiovascular disease, adds a further degree of complexity to the public health problem. The interconnectedness highlights the necessity of an integral approach that not only addresses liver wellness but also integrates strategies for preserving metabolic syndrome and risk factor attenuation, the key to optimizing population-level health outcomes (Fox *et al.*, 2017). Finally, management of the prevalence of NAFLD at the public health level consists of innovative strategies aimed at education and community action. Current guidelines are largely based on diet and exercise interventions as protective factors against the risk factors for NAFLD. However, studies into alternative therapies such as vitamin D supplementation continue to offer hope for new forms of intervention. There is evidence that low levels of serum vitamin D are linked to NAFLD hepatic damage, so vitamin D is an appealing adjuvant treatment. This low-cost and simple intervention may significantly influence public health interventions against NAFLD, particularly in those who have socioeconomic barriers to adhering to lifestyle changes. Thus, expanding our understanding of the prevalence and consequences of NAFLD reinforces the imperative to prioritize public health action (Fox *et al.*, 2017).

5.1. Pathophysiology of NAFLD

Understanding the pathophysiology of Non-Alcoholic Fatty Liver Disease (NAFLD) requires a comprehensive examination of its multifactorial origins, which primarily revolve around metabolic dysregulation. An excess of fatty acids in hepatocytes is the main feature of NAFLD, which happens mostly because of IR and its related metabolic conditions like obesity and type 2 diabetes. Liver cells become overloaded with lipids, which starts a chain of events that causes inflammation and damage to the liver cells. As the disease progresses, some individuals develop non-alcoholic steatohepatitis (NASH), which is marked by significant hepatic inflammation and liver cell damage.

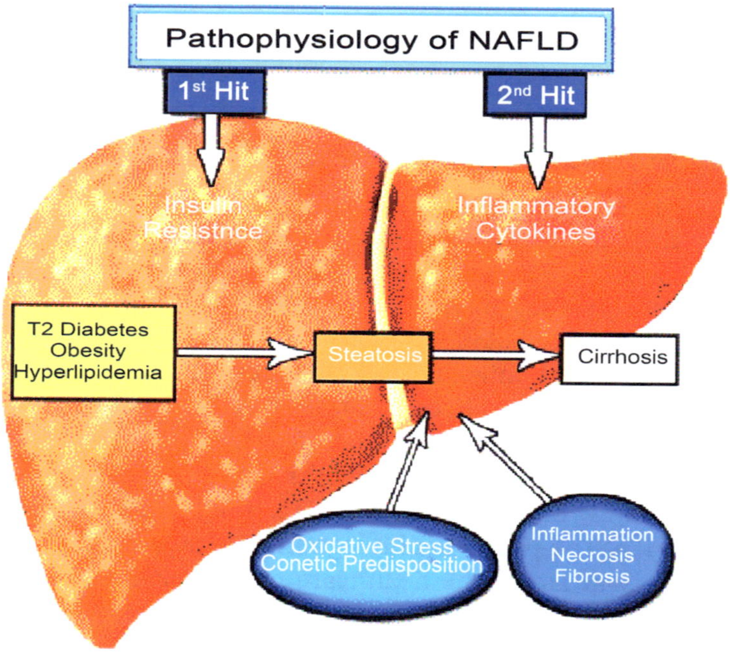

Figure 5.2. Pathophysiology of non-alcoholic fatty liver disease (NAFLD).

Source: https://www.researchgate.net/profile/Hassan-El-Sayyad/publication/308903742/figure/fig1/AS:414230462386176@1475771646523/Pathophysiology-of-non-alcoholic-fatty-liver-disease-NAFLD-Two-models-illustrated-the.png.

This complex interplay between lipid metabolism, insulin signaling, and the inflammatory response underscores the need for a detailed understanding of the disease's progression. It highlights the potential for targeted therapeutic interventions that address underlying metabolic dysfunctions (Rinella *et al.*, 2023). Oxidative stress plays a key role in the development of inflammation in the liver, which is important in NAFLDs. Hepatocytes exposed to excess fatty acids experience mitochondrial dysfunction, which amplifies the production of reactive oxygen species (ROS). As a result of oxidative stress, liver cells are further damaged, and the body starts an inflammatory response by releasing cytokines and attracting inflammatory cells. Because of these events, there is more oxidative stress and worsening of fatty liver, which can eventually lead to fibrosis and cirrhosis. Recent studies have elucidated the interconnectedness of oxidative stress, inflammation, and coagulation dysfunction, suggesting that this triad of pathophysiological events plays a pivotal role in the progression of NAFLD (Robea *et al.*, 2023). The way NAFLDs are understood has led to changes in how they are diagnosed and how they are treated. The recent shift from the traditional NAFLD nomenclature to metabolic dysfunction-associated steatotic liver disease (MASLD) reflects an acknowledgment of the underlying metabolic syndromes contributing to the disease. By doing this, the system gives more importance to dealing with risk factors like obesity, diabetes, and dyslipidemia than just looking at the liver tissue. Clinicians should remember that NAFLDs are diverse in their symptoms, which is important for choosing the right treatment plan for each patient. They can consist of changing one's lifestyle, using medications to correct metabolism, and, for the most severe cases, doing a liver transplant. By bridging the gap between pathophysiological insights and clinical practice, a more comprehensive approach to NAFLD can be realized, ultimately enhancing patient outcomes and reducing the global burden of this prevalent liver condition (Rinella *et al.*, 2023) (Figure 5.2).

5.1.1. Mechanisms of Fat Accumulation in the Liver

The intricate mechanisms of lipid accumulation in the liver are central to NAFLD pathogenesis. Metabolic impairment, characterized by obesity, type 2 diabetes, and IR, is a central mechanism in the pathogenesis. IR disturbs lipid metabolism and enhances hepatic lipogenesis, facilitating a disturbance between lipid deposition and clearance within the liver. With constant metabolic disturbances, the caloric excess intake of fatty acids and triglycerides causes hepatic steatosis. This is compounded by alterations in dietary patterns and physical inactivity, resulting in increased calories and decreased energy expenditure. Therefore, an understanding of how metabolic derangement works at the cellular level becomes paramount to comprehending fat storage pathways in the liver and new therapeutic targets in NAFLD (Sakurai *et al.*, 2021). Furthermore, IR involvement is not only restricted to lipid metabolism because IR influences inflammatory pathways and disease progression in the liver. In an IR state, there is increased entry of free fatty acids into the liver, which has the potential to induce cellular stress and subsequently trigger inflammation. Such inflammation can lead to hepatocyte injury, further contributing to lipid loading and propagating a damage-regeneration cycle. Notably, studies have discovered that genetic vulnerabilities are also likely to play a substantial role in the deposition of fat in the liver and the occurrence of fibrosis, potentially complicating NAFLD's clinical presentation. Typically, the complexity of such processes highlights the necessity for interdisciplinary studies and clinical practices in addressing the complexity of liver fat deposition (Tillman *et al.*, 2020). In addition to metabolic derangement and inflammation, gut microbiota changes have also been found to be contributory in the pathogenesis of fatty liver deposition. Dysbiosis or gut microbial network disruption can impact lipid metabolism and increase intestinal permeability, causing spillover of endotoxin into the circulation and increasing liver inflammation. The gut-liver axis is increasingly recognized as a significant pathway through which nutrition contributes to hepatic fat accumulation. For instance, intake of high-fat diets has been demonstrated to alter microbial content, favoring the expansion of microbial groups that are pro-fatty acid storage over lipid-oxidizing groups. Synergy between these factors creates a cycle where fat deposition in the liver promotes metabolic derangement, creating a vicious cycle. This insight into the gut-liver axis emphasizes the importance of holistic treatment strategies that consider both hepatic and gastrointestinal health in the therapy of NAFLD (Sakurai *et al.*, 2021) (Figure 5.3).

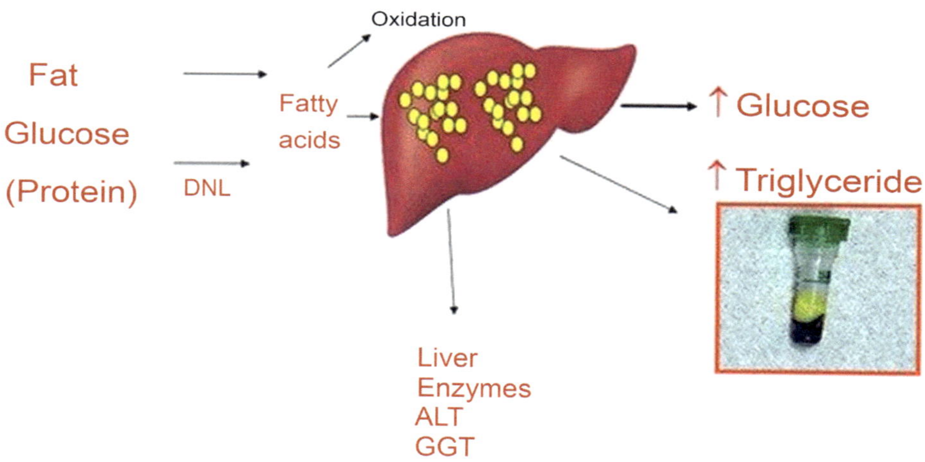

Figure 5.3. Fat accumulation in liver.

Source: https://www.researchgate.net/profile/Naveed-Sattar/publication/265095961/figure/fig3/AS:202671597330448@1425332082516/Biochemical-findings-supporting-excess-liver-fat-This-simple-figure-signals-the-link.png.

5.1.2. Role of Insulin Resistance (IR)

There are many ways in which IR is involved in the development of NAFLD, and this has attracted a lot of research attention. IR increases the amount of fat stored in the liver, which is one of the main ways it contributes to NAFLD. If cells in the body become insulin-resistant, taking in glucose becomes a problem, which causes insulin levels to increase. Because of hyperinsulinemia, the liver starts to increase lipogenesis, which turns carbohydrates into fatty acids and lipids. Therefore, the liver is overwhelmed with fat, leading to steatosis, which is usually the starting point for NASH and other serious liver problems. Understanding this association between IR and lipid metabolism is crucial, especially as NAFLD prevalence continues to rise in the global population, reflecting growing metabolic syndrome rates (Kozak, 2024). As well as causing lipid buildup, IR speeds up the development of liver fibrosis in those with NAFLD. Studies reveal that individuals with NAFLD and concomitant IR exhibit significantly higher liver stiffness, a marker for fibrosis, compared to those with isolated NAFLD (Kozak, 2024). It seems that the inflammatory and fibrosis-related effects of IR worsen the damage to the liver. Elevated markers of liver dysfunction, such as alanine aminotransferase (ALT) and aspartate aminotransferase (AST), are often observed alongside increased IR, indicating a direct linkage between metabolic dysregulation and liver health. Notably, advanced fibrosis has been identified as a predictor of worse clinical outcomes in NAFLD, reinforcing the need for early interventions targeting IR to mitigate liver damage and improve overall patient prognosis (Kozak, 2024). Also, recent studies suggest that the inflammatory cytokines linked to IR are important in the development and progression of NAFLD, mainly in children. Studies have found that children with NAFLD have higher levels of certain inflammatory substances, such as IL-6 and TNFα, and also have higher HOMA-IR scores. They are linked to obesity and fat distribution in the body, which shows that inflammation due to IR is involved in causing hepatic steatosis and its problems. By observing this inflammation, doctors can tell how much damage the liver has, and it may help identify various types of NAFLD. As the understanding of IR continues to evolve, it becomes increasingly apparent that addressing IR is imperative for the effective management and prevention of NAFLD and its associated morbidities (Figure 5.4).

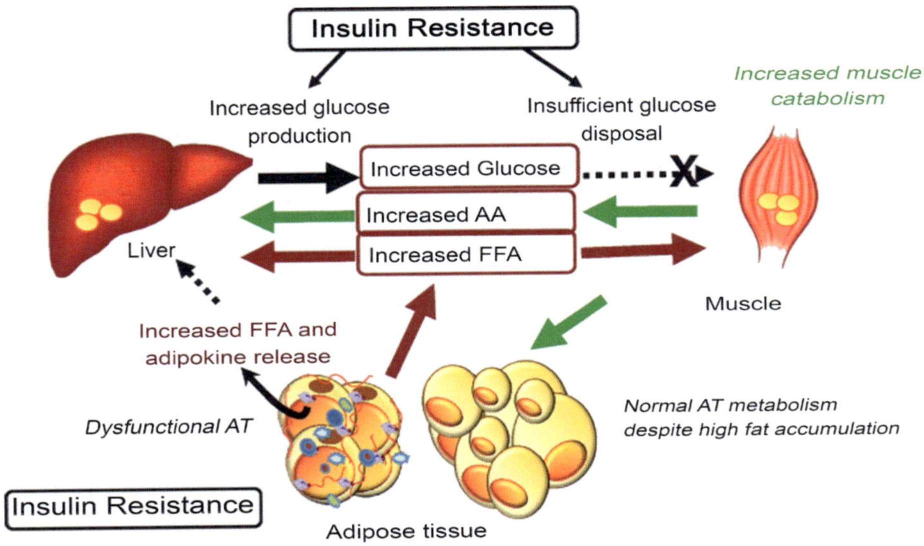

Figure 5.4. NAFLD and insulin resistance.

Source: https://media.springernature.com/lw685/springer-static/image/chp%3A10.1007%2F978-3-319-95828-6_4/MediaObjects/453534_1_En_4_Fig1_HTML.png.

5.1.3. Progression from Simple Steatosis to Non-Alcoholic Steatohepatitis (NASH)

Evolution to NASH from simple steatosis is a significant evolution within the spectrum of NAFLD. Simple steatosis, which is characterized by fat deposition in liver cells in the absence of related inflammation or injury, poses relatively minimal risk for serious complications at presentation. However, as metabolic disturbance continues to increase, often brought about by factors of obesity, IR, and related metabolic disturbances, the disease may evolve into NASH. This stage is not only characterized by the presence of hepatic steatosis but also by inflammatory processes and liver cell injury, which are critical precursors to more severe liver disease, including cirrhosis and HCC. Understanding these intermediate stages is necessary for the creation of effective prevention and intervention strategies in high-risk populations, highlighting the need for early diagnosis and management of NAFLD (Gato *et al.*, 2024). Etiologies of steatosis advancement to NASH are multifactorial and incredibly intricate. Among these, diet, genetic predisposition, and comorbidities such as type 2 diabetes and obesity play important roles. Increased liver lipid levels have been found to render individuals more susceptible to the development of NASH-like inflammatory responses. This inflammatory process becomes significant as it can potentially lead to hepatocyte injury and the onset of fibrogenesis, where liver tissue becomes replaced with scar tissue. This consequent fibrosis can disrupt further liver function, contributing to systemic complications. With the rise in NAFLD prevalence globally, it increasingly becomes important for scientists and clinicians to have insights into molecular and cellular mechanisms driving this advancement in a bid to curtail the public health burden of advanced liver disease (Awad *et al.*, 2024). Additionally, the clinical significance of progressing from simple steatosis to NASH suggests that one needs to start intervening early. Current studies highlight the importance of using non-invasive tests such as the Fibrosis-4 Index (FIB-4) to differentiate patients experiencing simple steatosis from those likely to transition into the more complicated NASH stage. Non-invasive tests used to determine the health of the liver can reduce reliance on invasive methods such as liver biopsies and so yield patient-friendlier and more accessible diagnosis and monitoring. Particularly in NAFLD populations with very high prevalence, effective screening and risk stratification practices can guide therapy, lifestyle change, and patient education. Ultimately, greater insight into the pathway from steatosis to NASH can guide public health strategies and emphasize prevention as a key component of NAFLD management (Awad *et al.*, 2024; Gato *et al.*, 2024) (Figure 5.5).

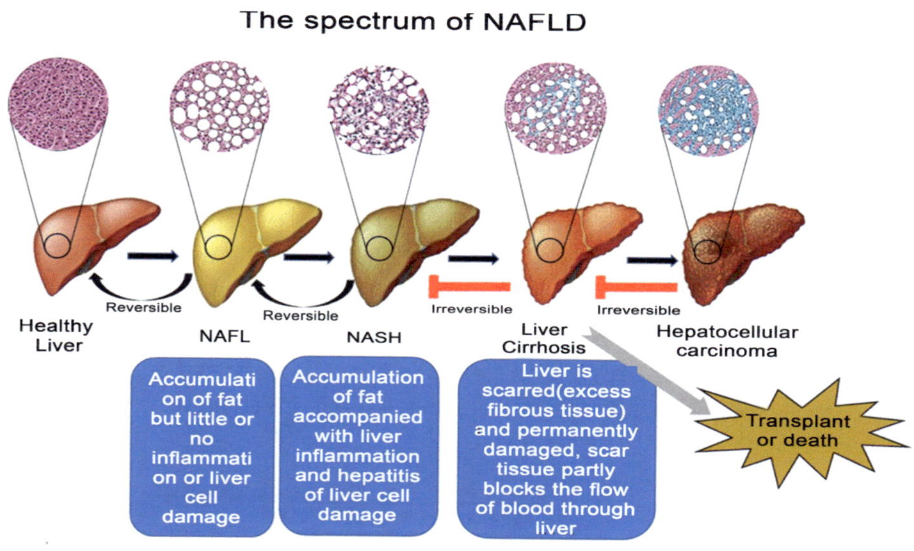

Figure 5.5. Spectrum of NAFLD progression. The development of NAFLD is divided into four stages: simple steatosis (or NAFL), NASH, liver cirrhosis, and eventually HCC.

Source: https://www.researchgate.net/publication/340611620/figure/fig2/AS:963249365348363@1606667953573/Spectrum-of-NAFLD-progression-The-development-of-NAFLD-is-divided-into-four-stages.png.

5.2. Risk Factors

Knowing the risk factors for NAFLD is important for handling this condition, which is becoming more common. Studies have pointed out that obesity, diabetes, hypertension, and dyslipidemia are major factors that lead to NAFLD. Notably, a study examining non-obese patients with schizophrenia found a NAFLD prevalence rate of 25%, indicating that even individuals without elevated body mass index (BMI) can be at significant risk. It was found that age, BMI, metabolic indices, and liver enzyme levels like ALT are related to NAFLD in non-obese patients. Therefore, a comprehensive understanding of these risk factors allows for earlier identification and intervention, particularly in populations that may traditionally be considered at lower risk due to their weight status (Yi *et al.*, 2024). Another critical aspect of NAFLD risk factors involves their role as precursors to other severe health conditions, particularly cardiovascular diseases (CVDs). The relationship between NAFLD and HF shows that this liver disease can affect many parts of the body. A study done in retrospect found that patients with NAFLD are much more likely to develop heart failure within ten years than those without the condition. The report showed that NAFLD patients have a 34% higher chance of getting HF, regardless of being male or female, and their age. This finding emphasizes that NAFLD should not only be viewed as a liver-centric ailment; it inherently involves broader metabolic and cardiovascular implications that necessitate a multidisciplinary approach to patient care and risk management (Roderburg *et al.*, 2023). Also, being aware of new risk factors for NAFLD is important for creating effective public health strategies. NAFLD is becoming more common because of a sedentary lifestyle, eating a lot of refined carbs and saturated fats, and having certain genes. It is especially worrying that a poor lifestyle, such as less exercise and more junk food, can cause the liver to accumulate fat. Noticing these factors early can guide strategies to reduce the chances of NAFLD in people who are more at risk. As the evidence surrounding these risk factors continues to evolve, health practitioners must remain vigilant and adopt proactive screening measures to address NAFLD before it leads to more severe health complications (Yi *et al.*, 2024).

5.2.1. Obesity and Metabolic Syndrome

The cross-link between NAFLD and obesity defines an inner component of metabolic syndrome that mirrors the polyphonic character of such diseases. Obesity represents an inborn cause of metabolic disturbance, setting the stage for fat storage in the liver, a pathognomonic characteristic of NAFLD. With progressive accumulation of visceral fat, it amplifies IR, further accentuating hepatic steatosis. In particular, patients with metabolic syndrome, which comprises a cluster of disorders like obesity, hypertension, and dyslipidemia, are particularly vulnerable to the development of NAFLD. The synergy of these components suggests that the decrease in obesity not only enhances the liver but also inhibits the overall effects of metabolic syndrome on health. Thus, targeted weight loss interventions may be linked with improved liver function and decreased metabolic risks based on metabolic syndrome. Additional evidence supports poor muscle quality as a primary risk factor for advanced liver fibrosis in patients with NAFLD, ultimately linking muscle health to obesity and metabolic syndrome. Recent studies demonstrate that individuals with greater proportions of non-contractile muscle mass have a substantially increased risk for liver fibrosis, and thus measure muscle composition in addition to standard indicators of health such as BMI. Muscle echo-intensity measurement by ultrasonography has been identified as a useful, non-invasive method of assessing muscle quality and detecting at-risk individuals who are likely to develop severe disease. This evolution offers the potential to delineate the relationship between muscle health and liver disease more clearly. Through the development of muscle quality through exercise and nutrition, it is possible that risk factors for both metabolic syndrome and NAFLD progression could be minimized, offering an opportunity for integrative health interventions (Oshida *et al.*, 2024). Besides, the cardiovascular impacts of NAFLD cannot be separated from the obesity epidemic, which highlights the significance of worldwide management of metabolic syndrome. NAFLD patients typically are found to exhibit increased risk factors for CVDs, including hypertension and dyslipidemia, diseases that are prevalent along the continuum of metabolic syndrome. The chronic inflammation of NAFLD has also been proven to be involved in endothelial dysfunction, thereby raising the risk of atherosclerosis and cardiovascular complications. Thus, there exists a profound interrelation wherein obesity not only contributes to liver pathology but also establishes serious cardiovascular complications. Improvement of these interrelated factors through the implementation of life-style modifications, pharmacologic treatment, and education could enhance cardiovascular outcomes in patients with NAFLD and metabolic syndrome. This combined approach puts strong emphasis on the necessity of considering overall metabolic health, where optimization in one area can be interpreted as improved performance in multiple facets of health (Karshina *et al.*, 2024) (Figure 5.6).

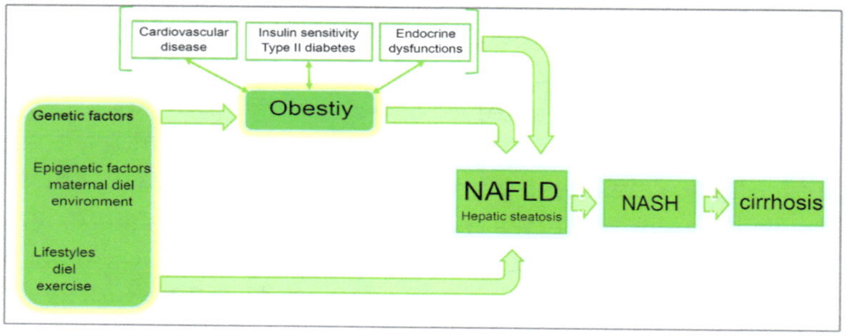

Figure 5.6. Obesity and Non-Alcoholic Fatty Liver Disease (NAFLD).

Source: https://www.researchgate.net/publication/304005574/figure/fig1/AS:373716149129216@1466112281322/Obesity-and-Non-Alcoholic-Fatty-Liver-Disease-NAFLD-Abbreviations-NAFLD-nonalcoholic.png.

5.2.2. Genetic Predisposition

Knowing about genetic predisposition in NAFLD is very important for understanding this condition. Genetics is very important in deciding how likely someone is to get NAFLD, mainly because of its effects on metabolism and liver function. It has been found that certain gene variants, for example those affecting lipid handling and insulin response, greatly increase the chance of NAFLD. People with these genetic predispositions may not show typical risk factors like obesity or diabetes, which is why we must examine how genes and lifestyle factors interact. By combining genetic knowledge with other aspects of NAFLD, it becomes possible to assess risk and provide personalized care, so research into the genetics of the disease should continue. In addition, seeing many cases of NAFLD in the same family points to a strong hereditary aspect, so more genetic research is needed to identify the inherited factors. It has been observed that populations with a higher prevalence of certain genetic markers, including the Pattin-like phospholipase domain-containing protein 3 (PNPLA3) gene variant, are at a greater risk of NAFLD and its progression to more severe liver conditions. Also, genetic factors usually overlap with ethnicity and location, which makes the epidemiology of these diseases more complex. Since genetics has many interactions, it requires integrating knowledge from genetics, biochemistry, and clinical practice. Knowing these predispositions helps doctors group patients according to their risk and choose the best treatment, which benefits those at genetic risk for NAFLD. Considering genetic predisposition in the treatment of NAFLD may lead to the creation of new approaches to care. A genetic predisposition can be spotted, which helps doctors make lifestyle and medication changes to prevent the disease from advancing. It has been found through research that weight loss and metabolic interventions may not work the same for everyone, which suggests that general strategies could be less successful. Also, new gene-based therapies may one day help in treating NAFLD, as scientists study the role of genes in influencing these diseases. As our understanding of the genetic underpinnings of NAFLD evolves, the potential for developing precision medicine approaches becomes increasingly realistic, offering hope for improved management and better patient outcomes in this prevalent liver disease (Devi *et al.*, 2024; Jadhav *et al.*, 2024).

5.2.3. Lifestyle Factors, Including Diet and Physical Activity

Lifestyle determinants, particularly diet and physical activity levels, play a central role in NAFLD progression and development. The ongoing epidemic of obesity, closely related to the increased intake of ultra-processed foods and the decline in the intensity of physical activity, has contributed to the growing prevalence of NAFLD. This connection shows how lifestyle forces can impact liver well-being since individuals who are of lower socioeconomic status often face dietary restrictions, subjecting them to poor diets. Understanding these lifestyle forces matters since they can be improved with significant changes in liver health. Of particular interest, since there is no absolute medical treatment for NAFLD, lifestyle modifications play a pivotal role in managing and potentially reversing the disease process (Aerts *et al.*, 2024). A review of the impact of a healthy lifestyle factor score (HLS) in NAFLD risk provides yet another insight into the impact of lifestyle factors. The research highlights that eating habits like adhering to a healthy diet, being at a healthy weight range for the body, adhering to regular physical activity, and not smoking significantly reduce the incidence of developing NAFLD. Individuals with greater HLS scores had a significant decline in the likelihood of being diagnosed with the condition, emphasizing the protective role that healthy living has to provide. Specifically, adherence to dietary regimes, i.e., alternate healthy eating index (AHEI), was associated with reducing incidence rates of NAFLD. These findings underscore the importance of health professionals promoting lifestyle interventions as a prevention measure for at-risk populations (Jahromi *et al.*, 2023). Incorporating sustainable lifestyle modifications not only advantages liver health but is also important in enhancing overall health. Patient education regarding their condition and the implications of choices in diet and exercise provides them with a feeling of control, leading them to become more responsible for their health. Greater adherence to advice can lead to improved disease outcomes, as those patients who are informed about NAFLD make favorable lifestyle modifications. Teleconsulting, a trend that escalated during the COVID-19 pandemic, offers an innovative way to ensure ongoing patient engagement and support for lifestyle modification. By integrating knowledge of healthful lifestyle practice into daily care, healthcare providers can help reduce the disease burden of NAFLD as well as the carbon imprint of recurrent in-person consultations (Aerts *et al.*, 2024).

5.3. Symptoms and Diagnosis

It is important to know the symptoms and how NAFLD is diagnosed to manage the disease well. Most people with NAFLD do not have symptoms at first, which makes it hard to identify in the early stages. As the disease worsens, patients may feel tired, lose weight, have abdominal pain, and notice their liver is larger than normal, which can be found during a physical checkup. Such nonspecific symptoms are also common in those who have obesity or type 2 diabetes, which can add to the difficulties in diagnosis. The absence of symptoms in the early stages emphasizes the need for proactive screening in high-risk populations, particularly those with metabolic syndrome and systemic diseases that predispose them to liver conditions, including NAFLD (Jeong *et al.*, 2022). A diagnosis for NAFLD usually requires looking at the patient's history, doing a physical exam, and running specific laboratory tests. Blood tests may show that the liver enzymes are high, though these markers can be unreliable and usually do not reflect the actual severity of liver steatosis. To confirm the diagnosis, imaging studies, such as ultrasound, CT, or magnetic resonance imaging (MRI), are frequently used to visualize liver fat accumulation. Among these imaging modalities, ultrasound is the most widely utilized due to its availability and cost-effectiveness, while MRI offers higher sensitivity and specificity (Moon *et al.*, 2020). If the diagnosis is not clear, an LBx may be done to check the liver for steatosis, fibrosis, or inflammation. It is important to identify and address the risk factors that can lead to NAFLD. NAFLD is often caused by obesity, IR, and metabolic syndrome, which is why it is important to review the patient's overall metabolic health. Also, identifying NAFLD is important because it can suggest other cardiometabolic problems. Watching for these risk factors helps both with the correct diagnosis and the choice of treatment for each patient. Clinicians must remain vigilant for the implications of NAFLD on overall health, especially given its significant correlation with disorders such as cardiovascular disease and type 2 diabetes that present parallel challenges for management and intervention (Jeong *et al.*, 2022).

5.3.1. Common Symptoms Associated with NAFLD

The presentation of NAFLD clinically is generally mild and highly variable with respect to symptomatology. A high percentage of patients are asymptomatic during the initial presentation of the disease and, therefore, may be late presenters for treatment. As the condition progresses, some of the potential symptoms include tiredness, malaise, and non-specific abdominal discomfort. These presentations, while not unique to NAFLD, may trigger further testing that reveals elevated liver enzymes and imaging study abnormalities. Symptomatic subjects should be identified early in the management of NAFLD since early treatment can reverse the abnormality of the histology and arrest the advancement of the disease (Gao, 2024). It is therefore necessary for clinicians to be aware of these common symptoms to facilitate early screening and effective patient care strategies. Besides gastrointestinal manifestations, NAFLD also typically presents with systemic metabolic disorders. NAFLD patients also typically have comorbid conditions such as obesity, type 2 diabetes, and dyslipidemia that raise the worldwide risk of CVDs. The association of NAFLD with metabolic components significantly worsens patient management. Abdominal obesity and IR are typical of NAFLD patients, and they are also compromised in terms of quality of life. The new term NAFLD, now redefined as metabolic (dysfunction) associated fatty liver disease (MAFLD), emphasizes the need for a comprehensive management approach considering these associated conditions (Rong *et al.*, 2023). Therefore, detection and treatment of these comorbid symptoms are crucial to effective management and reduction in the global health risk of NAFLD. The chronic course of NAFLD can cause severe pathologies of the liver, like NASH, which are responsible for more severe symptoms like jaundice and severe liver impairment. Patients can also present hepatic-related symptoms like pruritus, a sign of liver involvement, especially in cases leading to cirrhosis. Some patients also report complications like portal hypertension or liver complications, which indicate the disease's severity. This transformation emphasizes a dire need for regular monitoring and assessment of liver function in NAFLD patients to allow early interventions and lifestyle changes. Comprehensive management by means of diet, exercise, and, in some instances, pharmacotherapy targets the improvement of liver function and minimizes the dangers of such severe presentation (Gao, 2024). By addressing these symptoms, health care professionals are able to better plan their approach to maximizing patient outcomes in the scenario of NAFLD (Figure 5.7).

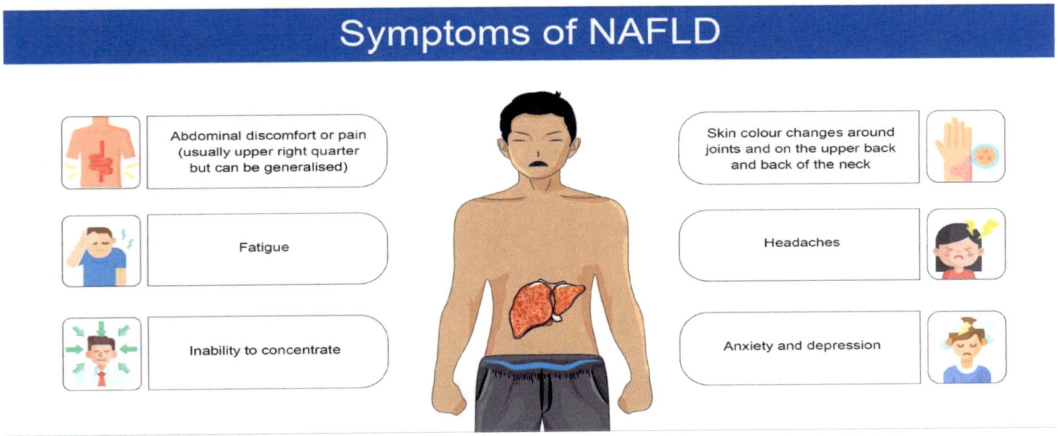

Figure 5.7. Symptoms of NAFLD.

Source: https://www.manipalhospitals.com/uploads/image_gallery/symptoms-of-nafld.jpg.

5.3.2. Diagnostic Imaging Techniques

In the assessment and diagnosis of NAFLD, which affects many people around the world, diagnostic imaging techniques play a crucial role. Traditional imaging methods such as ultrasound, CT, and magnetic resonance imaging (MRI) have been integral in identifying hepatic steatosis, the hallmark of NAFLD. Ultrasound is preferred because it is non-invasive, widely available, and inexpensive, which makes it easy to see any fatty infiltration in the liver. Even so, ultrasound is not very good at telling the difference between simple fat accumulation and the more serious NASH. This diagnostic challenge underscores the need for advanced imaging techniques or complementary diagnostic methods to enhance the accuracy of NAFLD assessments, especially in light of the disease's rising prevalence and associated systemic complications, as noted in (Khan *et al.*, 2025). Improvements in diagnostic imaging techniques are trying to overcome the problems of traditional approaches. Fibro scan, which makes use of transient elastography, is a safe way to check liver stiffness and assess the progression of fibrosis in NAFLD. Furthermore, magnetic resonance elastography (MRE) non-invasively assesses liver stiffness with higher accuracy and offers detailed visualization of liver anatomy, making it valuable for diagnosing and staging fibrosis. Also, new imaging technologies such as computer-aided diagnosis have shown potential to make diagnoses more accurate. For example, studies that combine deep learning algorithms, ultrasound, and biomarker data have shown excellent accuracy in identifying NAFLD. These technological advancements are vital, as they potentially reduce the need for invasive liver biopsies while improving patient outcomes in NAFLD management, as highlighted by the studies referenced in Geetha *et al.* (2024). Because the diagnostic approach to NAFLD is constantly progressing, using multiple imaging tools and advanced computer methods is important for a thorough assessment of the liver. The combination of traditional imaging with modern methods such as machine learning (ML) could facilitate earlier detection and more accurate differentiation between simple fatty liver and NASH, thus informing appropriate treatment strategies. By using this approach, physicians can be more certain about the diagnosis, which also fits with the idea that NAFLD is linked to metabolic syndrome. Because NAFLD is leading to more health problems, healthcare providers should use new imaging techniques to help patients and guide their treatment. Ultimately, the ongoing research and development in diagnostic imaging techniques hold significant promise for advancing the management of NAFLD as it continues to rise in prevalence across diverse populations, thereby addressing the critical need for reliable identification and staging methods, as noted in (Khan *et al.*, 2025) (Figure 5.8).

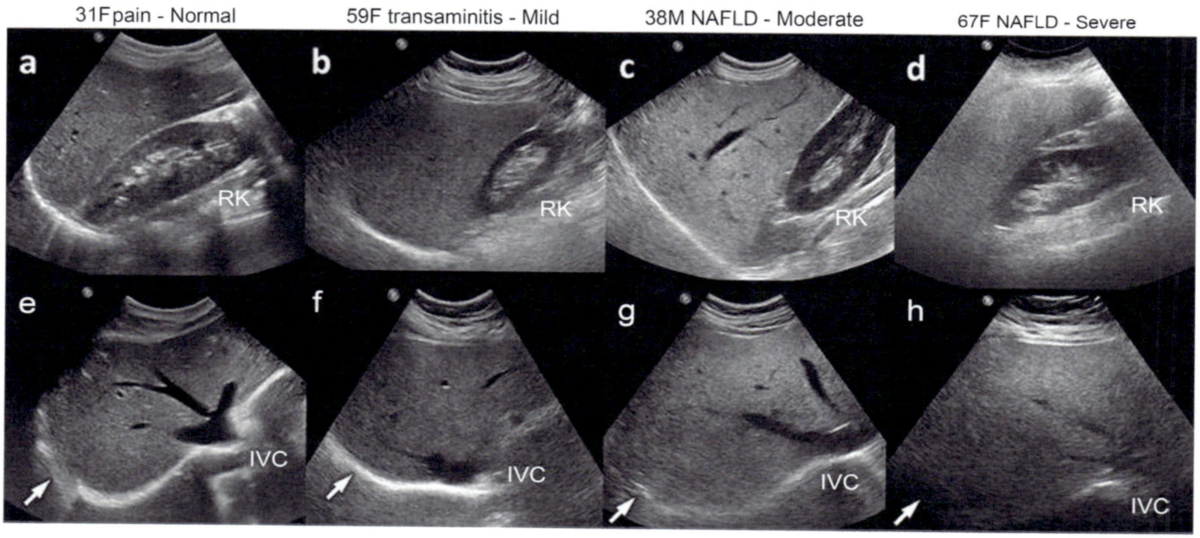

Figure 5.8. Ultrasound of NAFLD — examples. Longitudinal ultrasound images of the right haptic lobe and right kidney (a–d) and transverse images at hepatic venous confluence (e–h) in four patients are shown. In normal liver, the liver parenchyma is slightly more echogenic (i.e., brighter) than the right kidney (a). Posterior structures are well seen, including diaphragm (e). In the steatotic liver, the parenchyma becomes increasingly more echogenic than the kidney (b–d) and deep structures, including the diaphragm (arrow), which become progressively blurred (f–h).

Source: https://www.researchgate.net/publication/293170195/figure/fig6/AS:961411417112586@1606229752429/Ultrasound-of-NAFLD-examples-Longitudinal-ultrasound-images-of-the-right-haptic-lobe-and.jpg.

5.3.3. Liver Biopsy and Its Role in Diagnosis

LBx has long been regarded as the gold standard for NAFLD diagnosis and assessing the severity of liver injury, including fibrosis. The test permits direct histological inspection of liver tissue, making absolute diagnosis and grading of NAFLD, ranging from simple steatosis to NASH and severe fibrosis, feasible. While its key function, the invasive nature of LBx, is a concern in terms of patient safety and the likelihood of complications like bleeding and infection. Secondly, sampling variability could lead to diagnostic errors, whereby the biopsy, will not represent the overall liver status due to its small size. With these limitations in view, the medical community continues to look for non-invasive modes that can offer comparable diagnostic capability without the complications associated with biopsy procedures, thereby improving patient care without risking complications of invasive diagnostics. Non-invasive diagnostic tests (NITs) have emerged in the role of evaluating liver pathology in patients with NAFLD, where LBx continues to be an essential but less favored option. Notably, the acoustic radiation force impulse (ARFI) elastography has been adequately proven to diagnose liver fibrosis with a diagnostic accuracy likely superior to conventional serum biomarkers such as the aspartate aminotransferase-to-platelet ratio index (APRI) and the NAFLD fibrosis score (NFS) (Kang *et al.*, 2024). In a retrospective study of 136 patients, ARFI had an AUROC that was significantly higher compared with APRI and FIB-4 indices, highlighting its future promise as a non-invasive, reliable diagnostic test. With the advancement of technology, ARFI and other similar technologies can reduce the reliance on LBx, and the paradigm can shift towards more efficient and safer diagnostic pathways for NAFLD. Additionally, serum markers have been effective adjuncts in NAFLD assessment, identifying severity and disease progression without invasive processes. For instance, studies indicate that serum adiponectin and chemerin correlate with the disease spectrum, indicating NAFLD pathophysiology (Seleem *et al.*, 2023). They are found to have predictive significance in distinguishing between simple steatosis, NASH, and even cirrhosis. The dramatic rise in serum chemerin and fall in adiponectin levels in NAFLD patients alludes to them as non-invasive diagnostic biomarkers. If employed in combination with techniques like point shear wave elastography, patient prognosis may be enhanced through a better comprehension of the disease process. The future of NAFLD diagnosis will likely be in bringing together such non-invasive modalities to facilitate easier management of patients while minimizing risks linked with LBx (Figure 5.9).

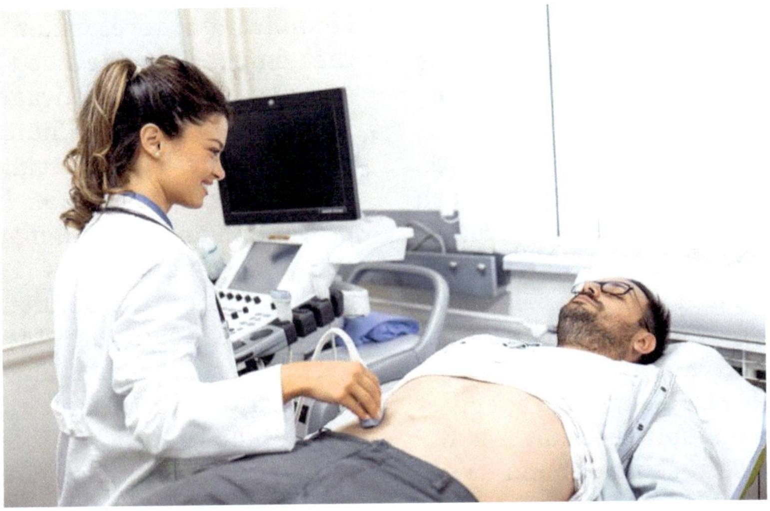

Figure 5.9. Diagnosis of liver disease

Source: https://phdiagnostics.ae/wp-content/uploads/2017/10/ARFI-th.jpg.

5.4. Complications of NAFLD

The difficulties linked to NAFLD play a major role in its significance in clinical care. If hepatic steatosis worsens, it might result in NASH, which involves inflammation and fibrosis. As a result, NASH may cause more serious liver problems, for example, cirrhosis and HCC. A number of things can cause the progression from simple fatty liver to NASH, including IR, obesity, and metabolic syndrome. Finding out the mechanisms behind this progression is necessary for designing targeted treatments. Research indicates that bioactive components, such as those found in Nankun Mountain Mao tea, may possess anti-steatosis properties and can mitigate inflammation within the liver, highlighting the potential for dietary interventions in managing the complications of NAFLD (Zhang *et al.*, 2024). NAFLD also has effects on many systems outside the liver. Patients with NAFLD often have comorbid conditions such as cardiovascular disease and type 2 diabetes mellitus (T2DM). All three conditions are linked to obesity and not being active, which makes the complications of NAFLD worse. Because NAFLD, T2DM, and CVDs are linked, it is important to manage them with various approaches, especially by encouraging healthy eating and exercise. Incorporating high-intensity interval training (HIIT) has been shown to enhance metabolic health, demonstrating superior outcomes in areas such as liver fat reduction and inflammatory marker improvements compared to moderate-intensity continuous training (MICT) (Chintapula *et al.*, 2024). The results show that doing the right kind of physical activity can help reduce many complications from NAFLD. Long-term effects of NAFLD can result in many serious changes in the body that may cause serious illness and death. Developing cirrhosis greatly raises the chance of complications like portal hypertension and liver failure, which are the main concerns in managing patients with liver disease. Also, the possibility of HCC in those with advanced liver disease can be very serious. As NAFLD advances, it is crucial to check liver health regularly, mainly in people who are more likely to develop the disease. Treatments that match a person's metabolic needs might help decrease these complications and increase their quality of life. Continuous research and evidence-based strategies are essential for minimizing the impact of NAFLD's complications, highlighting the necessity for an integrative approach in both clinical practices and public health policies focused on metabolic wellness (Zhang *et al.*, 2024).

5.4.1. Development of Liver Fibrosis and Cirrhosis

The development of fibrosis and cirrhosis of the liver in the context of NAFLD is a significant health issue. Because NAFLD itself is a spectrum of liver disease, ranging from simple steatosis to NASH, the potential for progression to more advanced liver damage is greatly enhanced. IR, one of the features common to metabolic syndrome patients, has been demonstrated to be a significant contributor to this development. T2D patients usually show a faster rate of progression of fibrosis and an increased risk of cirrhosis and complication development. This is a pattern that emphasizes the need for early detection and therapy because advanced liver fibrosis is a significant prognostic indicator of liver-related health status. Thus, revealing the mechanisms behind such progression is significant in the prevention and optimal management of NAFLD and its advanced stages (Park *et al.*, 2025). In recent studies, the incidence of liver adverse events in patients with NAFLD has increasingly been reported, once again indicating the need for proper management procedures. The development of fibrosis advances at a scary rate, with an incidence rate of 49.0 events per 1,000 person-years in those affected. Once the fibrosis advances, there is a marked increase in the risk of advancing to cirrhosis and HCC. Second, biopsy-proven NASH patients have a greater incidence of HCC than non-NASH patients. This association underscores the urgent need to follow up NAFLD patients, particularly those with clinical evidence of NASH, in order to allow for initiation of early treatment interventions to avoid further disease progression. The bitter truth is that the complications from the liver would be ready to outpace usual mortality in this group in the near future, and awareness and education about NAFLD and its impacts are thus of utmost importance (Le *et al.*, 2024). Modification of lifestyle and early medical intervention are preventive measures required to prevent the risk of fibrosis and cirrhosis in NAFLD patients. An integrated approach, which is centered on weight reduction, dietary changes, and exercise, can significantly reduce the incidence of adverse outcomes associated with liver disease. Second, health professionals need to apply non-invasive procedures in order to evaluate the status of liver fibrosis and NASH in the outpatient care system, thereby enabling early detection and individualized treatment strategies. Although existing treatments for NAFLD are not extensive, investigators are looking at an array of agents, both antioxidants and other pharmacologic therapies, which, in combination with lifestyle changes, could provide synergistic effects. Working together with patients to create holistic care plans that target both hepatic and extra-hepatic forms of NAFLD ultimately is a proactive measure in minimizing the burden of liver cirrhosis and fibrosis in patient populations (Park *et al.*, 2025) (Figure 5.10).

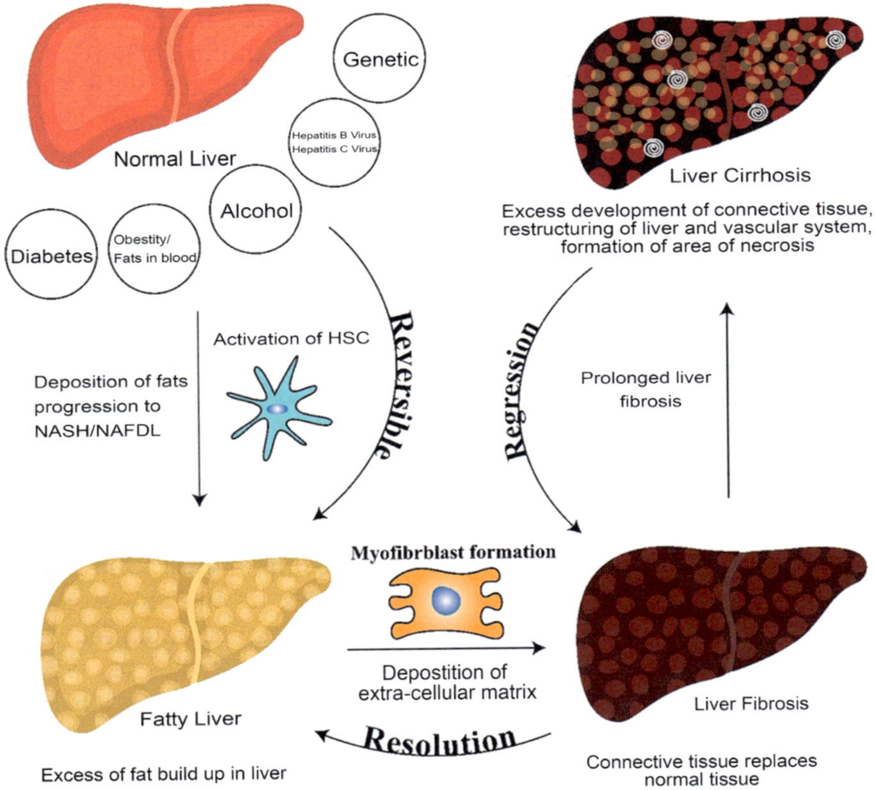

Figure 5.10. Schematic diagram of the progression of liver fibrosis.

Source: https://www.researchgate.net/publication/367528569/figure/fig1/AS:11431281122773306@1677525643784/Schematic-diagram-of-the-progression-of-liver-fibrosis.ppm.

5.4.2. Increased Risk of Hepatocellular Carcinoma (HCC)

It has become a major concern in modern medical research that NAFLD is linked to HCC. When NAFLD changes from steatosis to NASH, the risk of getting serious liver problems such as cirrhosis and HCC increases. Many times, this progression happens because of obesity and type 2 diabetes, which increase the risk of liver cancer by causing more damage to the liver. While the overall risk of liver-related complications in individuals with NAFLD may be relatively low, the increasing prevalence of this condition raises alarms about the potential future burden of HCC, particularly as metabolic syndromes become more widespread in developed nations like Korea, where NAFLD has become the most common liver disorder (Park *et al.*, 2025). HCC is most worrying for patients with advanced fibrosis, which is a usual result of living with NASH for a long time. It is clear from studies that people with progressive liver disease are much more likely to get HCC, which confirms the link between NAFLD and cancer. Also, having high cholesterol, which is part of metabolic syndrome, is known to increase the risk of the disease getting worse. Research has shown a strong association between elevated serum cholesterol levels and the presence of NAFLD, which reinforces the concept that metabolic dysregulation serves as a driver of liver disease pathology (Abbasi *et al.*, 2024). Because of this global link, it is important to carefully watch and manage patients with NAFLD, paying special attention to those showing signs of advanced fibrosis, to reduce the risk of HCC. Since NAFLD raises the risk of HCC, it requires a combination of changes in lifestyle and medical care. Taking care of one's weight and diet can help slow the progression of liver disease and reduce the risk of HCC, which shows how early intervention for metabolic issues is important. Although there are not many treatments for NAFLD, drugs that target metabolic pathways are promising, which suggests that more than one drug may be required to manage the disease. Continuous research is essential to understand the underlying mechanisms of NAFLD progression to HCC, as this knowledge could lead to more effective treatment strategies and ultimately reduce the burden of liver-related morbidity and mortality associated with NAFLD (Park *et al.*, 2025).

5.4.3. Association with Cardiovascular Diseases

The relationship between NAFLD and CVDs has drawn significant attention in recent research. It has been found that NAFLD patients are at greater cardiovascular risk. A comprehensive meta-analysis referred to the fact that NAFLD patients tend to exhibit reduced flow-mediated dilation (FMD) and increased serum asymmetric dimethylarginine (ADMA), both of which are strongly correlated with endothelial function and vascular disease. These physiological changes could be the cause of subclinical atherosclerosis, and NAFLD is therefore not only a predictor for hepatic disease but also for cardiovascular morbidity. The ensuing increase in carotid intima-media thickness (CIMT) and carotid plaque prevalence in NAFLD patients also underscores the importance of this association, confirming an intriguing connection between liver and vascular well-being deserving of clinical practice and public health attention (Mladenova *et al.*, 2025). Beyond direct cardiovascular impact, NAFLD's relationship to metabolic disorders may further potentiate its influence on heart health. The condition is accompanied by obesity and IR, both of which are already well-documented risk factors for CVDs. There has been a recent study that has underlined how evaluation of dietary patterns using models like the Healthy Eating Index-2015 identifies significant associations between nutrition and cardiovascular risk in patients with NAFLD. Outcomes show that participants with lower diet quality scores are at risk of increased hepatic steatosis and metabolic abnormalities, which may result in adverse cardiovascular effects. Cross-sectional comparison of the NAFLD group showed considerable differences in lipid profiles and other metabolic factors based on diet quality, and therefore avoidance of these lifestyle factors could be of key importance in hindering cardiovascular risks in NAFLD (Hosseini *et al.*, 2024). Therefore, management involving both hepatic and cardiovascular risk is required in the case of NAFLD-affected patients. The clinician must stay watchful of the patient's cardiovascular status, keeping an eye out for increased morbidity from this liver condition. Furthermore, preventive strategies like dietary adjustments and lifestyle modifications could be beneficial not just for the recovery of the liver but also for cardiovascular health in general. By assigning a priority to the intensive awareness of the NAFLD-CVD relationship, physicians can utilize prevention and treatment modalities more effectively, thereby causing improvement in the prognosis of patients battling the predicaments of these linked conditions. The high predictive accuracy of NAFLD for CVDs reveals a strong rationale for including cardiometabolic screening as part of the routine evaluation of involved patients (Mladenova *et al.*, 2025) (Figure 5.11).

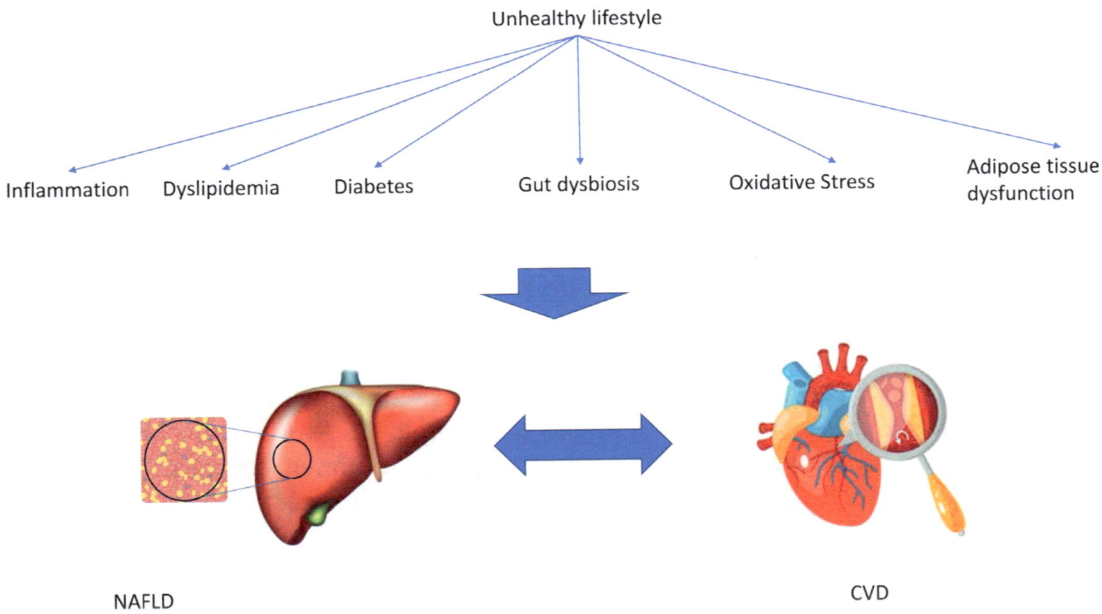

Figure 5.11. Several possible mechanisms have been proposed that might explain the association between non-alcoholic fatty liver disease (NAFLD) and cardiovascular disease (CVD).

Source: https://www.mdpi.com/jcm/jcm-10-00467/article_deploy/html/images/jcm-10-00467-g002.png.

5.5. Treatment and Management

Treating and managing NAFLD calls for knowledge of its many causes and the related metabolic problems. Most of the time, changing lifestyle habits is the main part of successful intervention. Changing one's diet and exercising more has been found to improve liver tissue in people with NAFLD greatly. A small amount of weight loss, such as 5-10%, can greatly improve liver fat and reduce inflammation. Patients are encouraged to eat foods from the Mediterranean diet, which contains antioxidants and may help with oxidative stress related to NAFLD. Because metabolic syndrome is related to PCOS, managing comorbidities such as obesity, diabetes, and dyslipidemia is very important for positive results. Treatments with medicines for NAFLD are being studied, mainly to help manage NASH, which is the more severe type of the disease. Vitamin E is one of the agents that has been studied, and it is thought to help non-diabetic, non-cirrhotic adults with active NASH; however, its recommendation is mainly supported by limited, but promising, clinical trial findings. Other treatments being studied are resveratrol, silybin, L-carnitine, and pentoxifylline, which try to reduce the effects of oxidative stress and inflammation in the liver. Even with these progresses, additional studies are needed to confirm that these treatments are safe and effective for people with NAFLD in the long run. Since there are no clear standardized protocols, the way treatments are given is still complex, so more clinical trials are needed to find the best methods for management. NAFLD in children is also very important to address because it may influence their long-term health. It seems that the prevalence of CLD in children is rising, which may lead to cirrhosis and HCC in adults. Noticing this condition early on is very difficult since the symptoms are often absent or unclear. For this reason, it is vital for healthcare providers to focus on regular screening and to stay aware. Recent progress in understanding how liver diseases develop has revealed new treatment options. Having a team of dietitians, liver specialists, and pediatricians helps create strategies that prevent issues and support health. The goal of this treatment approach is to raise the quality of life and health for children with NAFLD, helping them stay healthy as they grow into adults.

5.5.1. Lifestyle modifications and Dietary Changes

NAFLD management is very much based on lifestyle and dietary modification, and these interventions form central treatment modalities. Evidence indicates that a Mediterranean-style diet, high in whole grains, vegetables, fruits, lean meats, and good fats, can significantly enhance liver function and reduce the deposition of hepatic fat. In a research that employed NAFLD participants, they noted that adherence to this diet, together with a regular exercise regimen, led to notable recovery of the levels of liver enzymes, which indicated reduced liver inflammation and fat deposition. Of significant note was the observation that median ALT and AST levels were significantly lowered, indicating the efficacy of these lifestyle changes in managing the disease (Uqaili *et al.*, 2025). Therefore, dietary changes play not only a central role in optimizing liver function but are also of paramount significance in the management of NAFLD's metabolic disorders. Physical exercise is another essential element of lifestyle adjustment in NAFLD patients. The inclusion of a minimum of 150 minutes of moderate-intensity exercise per week can contribute to weight loss and optimization of the metabolic profile, hence minimizing liver fat content. Research indicates that these physical activities can cause a dramatic alteration in hepatic fat grading and that the majority of patients will experience improved liver health results. As NAFLD bears a strong correlation with diseases like obesity as well as metabolic syndrome, promoting an active life becomes a preventive as well as curative measure. As underscored, successful NAFLD control is inextricably bound with a person's willingness to implement these changes, suggesting that inherent motivation is the portal to the challenge of breaking this disease (Lv *et al.*, 2024). Lastly, lifestyle change and dietary modifications are not adjuncts alone but integral to the holistic management of NAFLD. With improved pharmacological treatment, the role of non-pharmacological interventions must attract more attention from medical professionals. Existing literature asserts that weight loss can delay the progression of NAFLD and promote global health. Patients employing profound lifestyle interventions display a higher quality of life and prolonged survival, which suggests the effect of these interventions. Synergistic combination of culturally adapted diet regimens with personalized exercise protocols may lead to highly significant improvements in liver function and metabolic profile, entrenching lifestyle interventions as the first-line treatment of NAFLD and emphasizing the need for individually adapted patient care strategies supported by ongoing investigations (Uqaili *et al.*, 2025) (Figure 5.12).

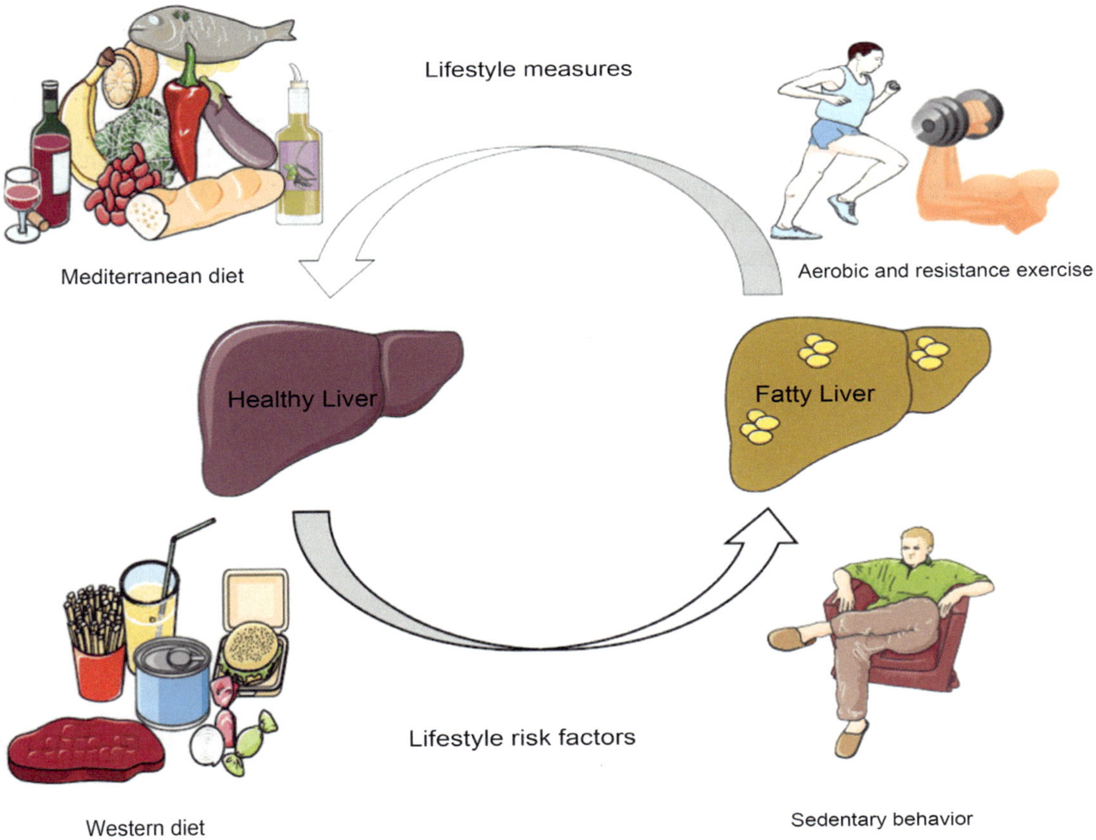

Figure 5.12. Lifestyle modifications and diet.

Source: https://encrypted-tbn0.gstatic.com/images?q=tbn:ANd9GcRPqBNdJ-CDDNcI6K0ZWACkTTJOsaDAs5bhKw&s.

5.5.2. Pharmacological Interventions

Treatments with medicines are very important for managing NAFLD, which is becoming more common. Several studies have found that some pharmacotherapies are more effective than just making lifestyle changes. For instance, pioglitazone and liraglutide (LG) have consistently demonstrated significant reductions in liver enzyme levels and weight among patients (Virk *et al.*, 2025). They show that while changing habits is key, using medicine in addition may be more effective for those with higher body mass indices and older people. It is clear from the results that different age and BMI groups respond differently, which means that pharmacotherapy may play a key role for some patients. Using both medicines and changes in lifestyle seems to improve the outcomes of people with NAFLD. Studies indicate that combining medications with lifestyle changes leads to better results, which shows why using various strategies is important. Both parts of this approach are designed to reduce weight and also handle issues that affect the liver. For example, intermittent fasting regimens, such as Alternate-Day Fasting and 5:2 interventions, have shown moderate benefits on various metabolic markers (Castillo *et al.*, 2024). Using lifestyle changes and pioglitazone together, clinicians can improve how patients address NAFLD. They play a major role in managing the disease, which demonstrates the importance of customized care for each patient. New drugs are being studied for how they may help manage NAFLD. Various new treatments, such as GLP-1 receptor agonists and other insulin-sensitizing drugs, are being studied for their effects on the liver as well as on related cardiometabolic factors. Current research emphasizes the importance of long-term studies to assess the safety and efficacy of these agents in diverse populations experiencing varying stages of NAFLD (Castillo F *et al.*, 2024). Because the field of medicine continues to change, using medications may help improve the treatment for this liver disease. Ongoing investigations into the long-term impacts of these agents will be critical in defining their roles within comprehensive management strategies for NAFLD, ensuring that patients receive the most effective and holistic care possible (Figure 5.13).

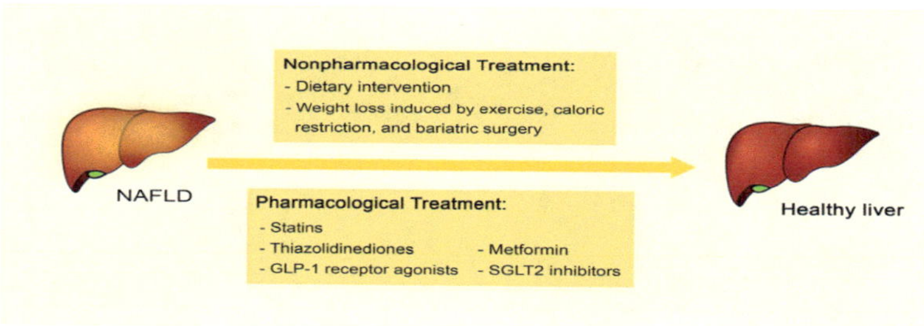

Figure 5.13. Current treatments for NAFLD.

Source: https://www.researchgate.net/publication/367073305/figure/fig2/AS:11431281187240889@1694158395462/Current-treatments-for-NAFLD-The-treatments-of-NAFLD-can-be-divided-into.tif.

5.5.3. Role of Regular Monitoring and Follow-Up

Regular monitoring and follow-up are critical factors in NAFLD management, primarily due to the insidious nature of the disease. NAFLD can range from mild steatosis to advanced disease, including NASH and cirrhosis. Patients will inevitably develop the complications of the disease that could go unnoticed until advanced stages if left under unmonitored circumstances. The incorporation of systematic follow-up protocols enables healthcare providers to assess trends in liver illness over time, making it possible for them to conduct early interventions. They may include changes to lifestyle, pharmacological treatment, or more invasive measures, when necessary, thus improving outcomes for patients and quality of life. Having a protocol for periodic assessments is aimed at holistic management of NAFLD, fostering an active strategy to patient health (Jennison *et al.*, 2023). The advent of non-invasive methods (NIMs) of liver health evaluation has revolutionized the clinical setting of patients with NAFLD. Such include serum biomarkers and physical means to quantify liver stiffness that are alternatives to invasive liver biopsy. NIMs have particular advantages when it comes to disease progression measurement and therapeutic interventions. Their sensitivity in diagnosing severe fibrosis or end-stage liver disease is of special interest to patient follow-up personalization, considering that these patients' risks of complications such as HCC and portal hypertension are higher. However, interpretation of these tests requires a proper account of the quality criteria suggested and a clinical setting appropriate to determine valid results. The prognostic value of NIMs also puts their usefulness in day-to-day monitoring into perspective, enabling clinicians to anticipate risks of NAFLD and adjust management strategies accordingly (Hiriart *et al.*, 2017). Follow-up not only aids in disease monitoring but is also an arena for patient education and active involvement in one's medical care. By opening up lines of communication between healthcare providers and patients, patients are better able to understand the importance of their diagnosis and the importance of adopting lifestyle changes. These types of changes, including diet, exercise, and other measures of prevention, can play a significant role in halting or even reversing disease. Informed patients are more likely to adhere to long-term follow-up guidelines and recommended interventions, facilitating collaborative care. Regular monitoring allows clinicians to facilitate patient empowerment via education, thereby ensuring a sustainable management strategy for NAFLD that is not just conducted in the clinical setting but rather in the everyday lives of patients (Jennison *et al.*, 2023).

5.6. Current Research and Future Directions

New studies have revealed that NAFLD is not simple, and this has led experts to focus on new ways to treat it. A notable area of exploration involves the role of cytokines, particularly Interleukin-22 (IL-22), which has demonstrated significant potential in mitigating liver inflammation and fibrosis. IL-22, which helps control lipid metabolism and improves liver function, is being seen as a potential treatment for NAFLD. Researchers are investigating how IL-22 acts to protect the body and how it impacts different metabolic pathways, which could help manage NAFLD. However, the challenges in translating these findings into clinical applications remain, indicating that further investigation is essential to understand fully how IL-22 can be integrated into broader therapeutic strategies for NAFLD treatment (Pan *et al.*, 2025). Besides cytokine research, phytotherapy is being used more often to support the management of NAFLD. Because the diseases have multiple causes, using herbal extracts and plant-based compounds can be a safe and unique way to treat them. Several recent studies have pointed out that silymarin and curcumin have hepatoprotective effects. They can reduce inflammation in the liver, make insulin work better, and have strong antioxidant properties which help fight the oxidative stress that leads to NAFLD. As more research shows that these natural remedies work, it is clear they could be important parts of managing NAFLD. Future directions should prioritize rigorous clinical trials that standardize dosages and evaluate long-term safety and efficacy in diverse populations (Ghosh *et al.*, 2025). Moving forward, it is essential to address NAFLD with multiple research methods. Because the number of cases is rising worldwide, future research should focus on all the genetic, metabolic, and environmental factors that contribute to the disease. Moreover, using genomics, proteomics, and metabolomics could help identify new biomarkers and therapeutic targets which would support precision medicine in NAFLD. Working together, researchers, clinicians, and regulatory groups will be necessary to help new therapies reach patients quickly. Using various methods and perfecting existing treatments can help patients with NAFLD, which would improve public health and lower the costs of liver disease.

5.6.1. Emerging Therapies and Clinical Trials

The therapeutic environment for NAFLD has revolutionized in the last decade with a shift towards better comprehension of the underlying pathophysiology. NAFLD management traditionally relied on lifestyle therapy using diet and weight reduction. There has been a strong surge in clinical trials assessing pharmacological intervention since the introduction of the metabolic dysfunction premise pertaining to NAFLD. Notably, the recent FDA clearance of resmetirom as a treatment targeted specifically at metabolic dysfunction-associated steatohepatitis (MASH) marks an important turning point in the treatment model, offering promise to those patients previously relegated to lifestyle modifications alone (Kim *et al.*, 2025).

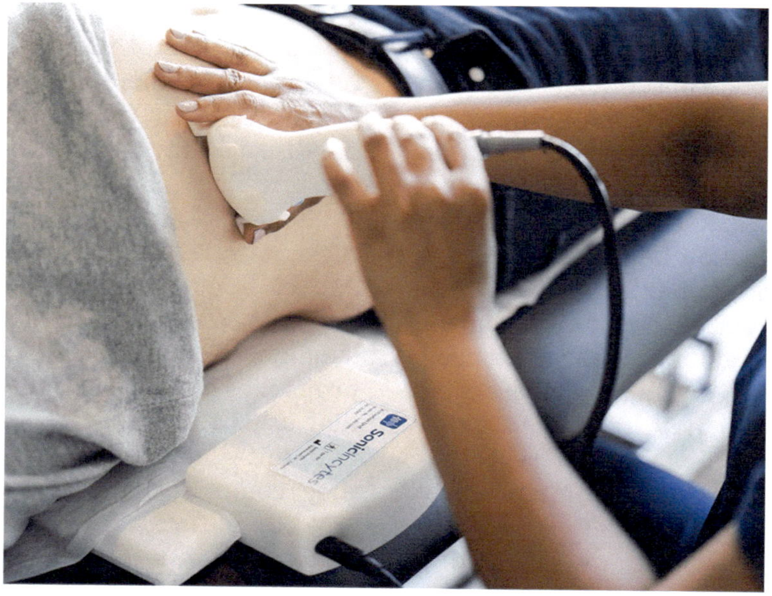

Figure 5.14. New therapies

Source: https://inovait.ca/wp-content/uploads/2023/11/Procedure_Product_13_Resized-min.png.

This paradigm shift emphasizes the demand for increased drug development that is supported by robust clinical evidence, as the necessity for successful treatment only increases with the global burden of NAFLD. Emerging therapies under investigation are diverse and possess a range of mechanisms of action involved in the pathogenesis of the diseases. Antagonists of lipid synthesis, insulin sensitizers, and anti-inflammatory and anti-fibrotic drugs are some of them. Research has identified various biomarkers and pathways that have the potential to be targets for upcoming pharmacotherapies (Prikhodko *et al.*, 2022). Clinical trials are the ones driving the research in this area, testing the safety and efficacy of various experimental drugs. For instance, some of the trials aim for drugs that activate mitochondrial activity or stimulate lipophagy, thereby targeting the steatosis aspect of the disease directly. With findings from these trials imminent, these will have the potential to inform clinical guidelines, providing clinicians with additional options with which to effectively treat this complex disease. As the clinical trials progress, the identification of patient populations most likely to benefit from new treatments is more critical. Individualized treatment according to patient factors, such as metabolic profile, comorbidities, and severity of disease, will improve treatment outcomes for NAFLD. Continued debate concerning the prioritization of liver-directed therapies must exist, particularly in light of the powerful effects of drug treatment being found (Kim *et al.*, 2025). This necessitates an integrative approach, with the utilization of multidisciplinary teams in order to assess and introduce new findings into practice. Challenges exist in the form of eliminating side effects of potential treatments, making novel treatments accessible, and finding their long-term impact on patient health. Therefore, NAFLD treatment in the future will have to incorporate innovative therapies as well as confluence frameworks to ensure progression is translated in an effective way into practice (Figure 5.14).

5.6.2. Understanding the Microbiome's Role in NAFLD

The importance of the microbiome has grown quickly in explaining different health conditions, like NAFLD. The gut microbiome, which is made up of many microorganisms in the gut, has many more functional genes than the human genome.

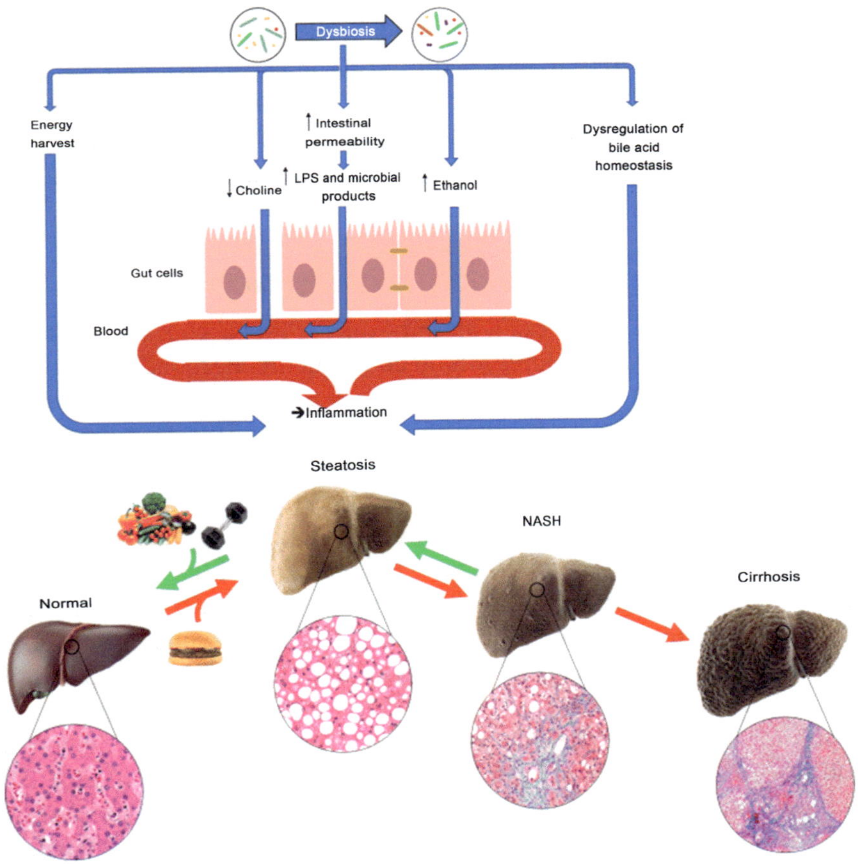

Figure 5.15. The mechanisms linking the microbiome to NAFLD development.

Source: https://www.researchgate.net/publication/330642220/figure/fig1/AS:941347691298816@1601446187026/The-mechanisms-linking-the-microbiome-to-NAFLD-development-Perturbation-in-the.png.

The microbes in the gut help to break down food, and their bioactive metabolites can have a direct effect on the health of the host. Accordingly, disturbances in the composition of the microbiome have been linked to a range of CLD, particularly NAFLD, suggesting that a better understanding of these microbial changes could provide insights into disease pathways and therapeutic targets (Alisi *et al.*, 2018). Recent studies have shown that certain groups of bacteria in the gut microbiome are linked to the development of NAFLD. In children with obesity and NAFLD, studies have revealed that the presence of helpful bacteria can vary significantly. For example, *Bifidobacterium spp.* are more common among healthy controls, which suggests they may help prevent NAFL from progressing to NASH. In contrast, *Lactobacillus spp.* were found to be more abundant in individuals with NAFLD, indicating a possible positive correlation between these microbes and the disease's progression (Alisi *et al.*, 2018). This shows that the microbiome is involved in many ways with the host's metabolism and that altering gut bacteria may be a way to help with liver disease. Studying the role of microbiomes in NAFLD helps discover ,the underlying mechanisms of the disease, and creates new options for treatment. Researchers are trying to use certain gut bacteria to develop probiotics that might protect the liver from damage. The gut-liver axis is showing that microbial metabolites can play a role in liver health, which supports the use of targeted probiotics. Furthermore, interventions aimed at restoring a healthy microbiome composition may help in reversing NAFLD and improving metabolic outcomes (Lynch *et al.*, 2019). As the research progresses, a deeper comprehension of the microbiome could ultimately lead to more effective, tailored approaches to managing this prevalent liver disease (Figure 5.15).

5.6.3. Potential for Personalized Medicine Approaches

The increasing prevalence of NAFLD has been an impetus for researchers to explore new therapeutic approaches, particularly within the era of personalized medicine. Personalized medicine personalizes the treatment modalities based on individual characteristics of each patient, considering the genetic, environmental, and lifestyle factors. As the pathogenesis of NAFLD is multi-factorial with genetic predisposition, IR, and lipid metabolic changes, personalized medicine can offer a better therapeutic paradigm. Combining genomic and metabolic profiling can potentially allow the identification of patients at higher risk of disease progression and guide the application of targeted therapies. These techniques embrace the beauty of individual patient profiles as opposed to the one-size-fits-all philosophy of conventional methods, which could serve the treatment outcomes of NAFLD patients. Research into traditional Chinese medicine (TCM) represents a fascinating convergence with personalized medicine in the treatment of NAFLD. TCM emphasizes a holistic concept of health, with treatment in consideration of patient symptoms and underlying conditions. This is particularly relevant for NAFLD as the pathogenesis of the disease is driven by multifactorial mechanisms, including inflammation and liver injury. Based on principles of TCM, including syndrome differentiation, can enhance western treatments and enhance patient outcomes. For instance, as noted in some recent reviews, certain Chinese herbal drugs have been clinically shown to be effective by intervening through complicated mechanisms that result in NAFLD. This approach is in alignment with the personalized medicine paradigm, in that integrating TCM with personalized intervention can potentially yield improved care for patients with this complex condition (Ding *et al.*, 2024). Further, the potential of personalized medicine in NAFLD justifies the requirement for ongoing research into biomarkers and treatment response. As noted in a number of studies, the inconsistently variable responses to pharmacotherapy serve to underscore the significance of understanding the variably individual metabolic profiles and their role in NAFLD progression (Liu *et al.*, 2024). By applying advanced approaches such as pharmacogenomics, physicians can predict which patients are most likely to benefit from specific treatments and therefore make the best therapeutic regimens. This type of information can advance in shaping a tailor-made approach so that clinicians preventively treat adverse effects and optimize treatment outcomes through optimizing medication regimens tailored to individual biochemical pathways. This level of individualization is not only able to improve patient outcomes but also possibly reduce overall healthcare costs associated with end-stage NAFLD.

SUMMARY

NAFLD comprehension demands a multi-faceted approach that tackles both clinical relevance and progressive research regarding efficacious diagnostics and therapeutic options. As NAFLD continues to increase in incidence worldwide, underscored by relevant epidemiological data, the necessity to employ sophisticated imaging modalities becomes increasingly evident. The master's thesis on MRI techniques demonstrates how such a non-invasive technique can play a crucial role in quantifying liver fat percentages for enhancing the diagnostic accuracy and research insight. All these advancements not only allow early diagnosis but also lead to the possibility of pharmacological intervention, subjecting the entire process to incredible scrutiny of the efficacy of treatment in diverse patient populations (Kavanaugh *et al.*, 2017). Apart from that, without a present consensus regarding pharmacological treatment for NAFLD, lifestyle modification remains the cornerstone of effective treatment. Intervention trials, such as the incorporation of the Mediterranean diet, have been found to impart great health benefits by reducing the risk factors for metabolic syndrome, hence mitigating the symptoms of NAFLD. The antioxidant and anti-inflammatory effects of this diet render it a probable weapon in the prevention of the progression of liver disease. The overall evidence points towards practitioners providing more focus towards lifestyle intervention along with ongoing pharmacological research for enhancing patient outcomes (Anania *et al.*, 2018). Finally, the complexity of NAFLD demands continued research into its pathophysiology along with treatment. Future studies must define more clearly the effectiveness of various types of diets, especially in heterogeneous age groups, and investigate novel pharmacologic therapies according to patient conditions. By broadening our knowledge of the pathophysiology of NAFLD and the determinations of aggregated clinical data, scientists can provide input into an improved approach for tackling this increasingly prevalent liver disorder. In the end, it will take cooperation among scientists, clinicians, and patients to reduce the burden of NAFLD and optimize public health outcomes.

In NAFLD, current studies focus on drug and natural treatments to enhance the condition. A deep exploration of dexamethasone (DXM) initiates its association with the onset of NAFLD, primarily through dysregulation of genes involved in lipid metabolism. The study highlights DXM's influence on gene expression of central genes FASN and CD36, critical in enabling the deposition of fat in the liver. In addition, LG's therapeutic utility against such side effects has been realized in the sense that it appears to mitigate DXM-induced metabolic dysregulation by enhancing p-AMPK levels and reducing gene expressions related to toxic lipids. Thus, the combination of DXM and LG is a major nexus in understanding NAFLD pathology (Selim *et al.*, 2025). Besides, the beneficial role of nutritional supplements against NAFLD has been debated extensively, particularly through the perspectives of oleuropein (OLE). The results show that OLE supplementation reduces body weight and liver weight in high-fat diet-induced NAFLD models, as well as enhances liver function via increased serum lipid levels. By regulating peroxisome proliferator-activated receptor alpha (PPARα), OLE is a significant regulator of lipid metabolism and inflammation in the liver. The OLE's metabolic role is further delineated by liver metabolomics analysis, which shows that this compound mediates desirable changes in liver metabolites required for lipid homeostasis. Therefore, OLE emerges as a possible natural therapy for enhancing the undesirable effects of NAFLD (Zhou *et al.*, 2024). The application of pharmacological and nutritional therapy in NAFLD illustrates the multifaceted strategy required for the efficient management of the disease. DXM, despite clinical significance, also requires consideration of side effects and NAFLD induction potential, thereby necessitating complementary interventions such as liraglutide (LG) to counter its shortcomings. Similarly, data on OLE suggest that natural products can provide protective action that would augment standard pharmacotherapy. This overlap of evidence not only continues to elucidate the pathophysiology of NAFLD but also highlights the value of a multidisciplinary treatment regimen that includes lifestyle modification and dietetics as well as pharmacologic therapy. Thus, the identification of these therapeutic targets will be key in developing appropriate strategies for the treatment and ultimately the prevention of NAFLD's effects (Selim *et al.*, 2025; Zhou *et al.*, 2024).

CLOSER LOOK

FIBROSIS-4 INDEX (FIB-4)

The FIB-4 index is a non-invasive, simple tool used to assess the degree of liver fibrosis (scarring). It's calculated using readily available blood test results and is particularly useful in situations where more invasive diagnostic methods like liver biopsies are not readily available. The index helps categorize individuals into low, indeterminate, or high risk for advanced fibrosis, aiding in patient management and decision-making (Figure 5.16).

FIB-4 Score	Degree of Fibrosis	Interpretation
< 1.45	Minimal to no fibrosis	Normal range
1.45 - 3.39	Significant fibrosis	Intermediate range
≥ 3.4	Advanced fibrosis or cirrhosis	High range

Figure 5.16. Fibrosis Index

Source: https://images.drlogy.com/assets/uploads/img/admin/health_blog/editor-img/fib-4-score-normal-range-drlogy-3.webp.

What It Is

The FIB-4 index is a score calculated from age, platelet count, and levels of AST and ALT. It was initially developed for patients with HIV/HCV coinfection and later validated in HCV-monoinfected individuals. It's a non-invasive alternative to LBx for assessing liver fibrosis.

How It Works

- The formula for FIB-4 is: (Age (years) x AST level (U/L) / (Platelet count (10/L) x $\sqrt{\text{ALT}}$ (U/L).
- Based on the calculated score, individuals are categorized into:
  - Low risk: <1.30, suggesting less advanced fibrosis.
  - Indeterminate risk: 1.30–2.67, requiring further assessment.
  - High risk: >2.67, indicating a higher likelihood of advanced fibrosis.

When It's Used

- **Screening for Liver Fibrosis:** FIB-4 can be used to screen individuals with suspected liver disease, particularly those with viral hepatitis (HCV, HBV) or NAFLD.

- **Monitoring Disease Progression:** It can help monitor the progression of fibrosis over time.
- **Decision-Making Regarding Treatment:** FIB-4 scores can guide treatment decisions, such as the need for antiviral therapy or further investigations.
- **Predicting Complications:** High FIB-4 scores have been linked to an increased risk of liver-related complications like cirrhosis, HCC, and liver-related mortality.

Strengths

- **Non-Invasive**: It avoids the need for invasive procedures like liver biopsies.
- **Easy to Calculate:** The formula is simple and readily available online or in medical software.
- **Cost-Effective:** It uses routinely performed blood tests, making it a relatively inexpensive assessment.

Limitations

- **Not always Accurate:** FIB-4 can have false positives and negatives, particularly in certain populations or with different liver diseases.
- **Limited in Some Situations:** It may not be as accurate in patients with alcoholic liver disease or those with other underlying conditions.
- **Not a Substitute for a Clinical Assessment:** FIB-4 scores should be interpreted in conjunction with other clinical information and patient history.

References

1. Abbasi, S., Sadiq, S., Haleem, N., Shazia, S., Jadoon, S., & Israr, M. (2024). Hypercholesterolemia as a causative risk factor for non-alcoholic fatty liver disease. *Journal of Ayub Medical College, Abbottabad: JAMC, 36*(3), 573–577. https://www.semanticscholar.org/paper/a52b2ab50d78456a7c15370dab03d00f20819d42 (accessed on 24 May 2025).

2. Aerts, M., Rosseel, Z., & de Waele, E. (2024). The evolution in non-alcoholic fatty liver disease patients' profile and the associated sustainable challenges: A multidisciplinary perspective. *Nutrients, 16*. https://www.semanticscholar.org/paper/e36c70541a1f03265c3129d98a4ace1ea156f7eb (accessed on 24 May 2025).

3. Albanese, F., Angelico, F., Baratta, F., Del Ben, M., *et al.* (2015). Oxidative stress: New insights on the association of nonalcoholic fatty liver disease and atherosclerosis. https://core.ac.uk/download/54528474.pdf

4. Alisi, A., Alterio, A., Della Corte, C., Mosca, A., *et al.* (2015). Pediatric liver diseases: Current challenges and future perspectives. https://core.ac.uk/download/84688423.pdf (accessed on 24 May 2025).

5. Alisi, A., De Chierico, F., Cucchiara, S., Drago, L., *et al.* (2018). Bifidobacteria and lactobacilli in the gut microbiome of children with non-alcoholic fatty liver disease: Which strains act as health players? https://core.ac.uk/download/188825679.pdf (accessed on 24 May 2025).

6. Anania, C., Chiesa, C., Perla, F. M., Olivero, F., *et al.* (2018). Mediterranean diet and nonalcoholic fatty liver disease. https://core.ac.uk/download/158328031.pdf (accessed on 24 May 2025).

7. Aslam, F., & Kulasena, H. (2017). To identify and examine the different causes of liver disease in Sri Lanka. https://core.ac.uk/download/293755106.pdf.

8. Awad, E., Ali-Eldin, Z., Allam, A., & Mahmoud, M. I. (2024). Diagnostic role of non-invasive risk scores in prediction of simple steatosis versus non-alcoholic steatohepatitis. *QJM: An International Journal of Medicine*. https://www.semanticscholar.org/paper/09ad3c67b8b04c6bb2c58f2d60ab25b82835a3e5 (accessed on 24 May 2025).

9. Castillo, M. F., Salgado-Canales, D., Arrese, M., Barrera, F., & Mikhailidis, D. P. (2024). Effect of intermittent fasting on lipid profile, anthropometric and hepatic markers in non-alcoholic fatty liver disease (NAFLD): A systematic review. *Current Vascular Pharmacology*. https://www.semanticscholar.org/paper/3030aa119c566a329530d47446de9f570e5013ff (accessed on 24 May 2025).

10. Chintapula, N., & Senthil, V. S. (2024). The effects of exercise intensity on metabolic health in patients with NAFLD and type 2 diabetes: A comparative study. *International Journal of Advanced Research*. https://www.semanticscholar.org/paper/4922e38df8af32cddb6681f959679b2c4dd091dd (accessed on 24 May 2025).

11. Devi, S., Sahu, S., Vennala, V. L., Panigrahi, M. K., & Behera, K. K. (2024). Comparison of clinico-biochemical and transient elastography findings among diabetic and non-diabetic patients with non-alcoholic fatty liver disease. *Series of Endocrinology, Diabetes and Metabolism*. https://www.semanticscholar.org/paper/5bd80a0513b9d5f62c0d76242617df8033fc37e9 (accessed on 24 May 2025).

12. Ding, X., He, X., Tang, B., & Lan, T. (2024). Integrated traditional Chinese and Western medicine in the prevention and treatment of non-alcoholic fatty liver disease: Future directions and

strategies. *Chinese Medicine, 19*. https://www.semanticscholar.org/paper/5b2fb34210f316a6c1ff81e40a7ff148b9537523 (accessed on 24 May 2025).

13. Fazal, M. O., Tahir, G. A., Yaqoob, Y., Zeeshan, A., Sharif, R., & Musharraf, M. U. (2024). Efficacy of vitamin E versus pioglitazone in treating non-alcoholic fatty liver disease (NAFLD) without diabetes: "Decoding the exodus of liver health." *The Professional Medical Journal*. https://www.semanticscholar.org/paper/3444791944bbc0b0c16954eb88a51c2627808d66 (accessed on 24 May 2025).

14. Fox, R. (2017). Vitamin D to reduce liver fibrosis in non-alcoholic fatty liver disease. https://open.bu.edu/bitstream/2144/26591/5/Fox_bu_0017N_13167.pdf (accessed on 24 May 2025).

15. Fuentes-Barría, H., Klahn-Acuña, B., Sepúlveda-Toro, D., Galaz-Cáceres, N., Aguilera-Eguía, R., & Alarcón-Rivera, M. (2024). Non-alcoholic fatty liver and periodontal disease in the adult population: Overview of systematic reviews. World of Journal Hepatology. World J Hepatol 2015 June 8; 7(10): 1325-1336 https://www.semanticscholar.org/paper/48a7dc7ca5184f7b56ddeb700373421bce8ccf57

16. Gao, R. (2024). Traditional Chinese medicine health management program for the common urban disease non-alcoholic fatty liver disease. *Journal of Clinical Medicine Research*. https://www.semanticscholar.org/paper/f32a2fc594539be6a4ba1b5e8b9de5935551d0b3 (accessed on 24 May 2025).

17. Gato, S., García-Fernández, V., Gil-Gómez, A., Rojas, Á., Montero-Vallejo, R., Muñoz-Hernández, R., & Romero-Gómez, M. (2024). Navigating the link between non-alcoholic fatty liver disease/non-alcoholic steatohepatitis and cardiometabolic syndrome. *European Cardiology Review, 19*. https://www.semanticscholar.org/paper/5fdc39a0c8244003dd7aa88a32cf71168e5ecd68 (accessed on 24 May 2025).

18. Geetha, R., Rani, D. J., & Anbarasu, K. (2024). Applying deep learning methods to non-alcoholic fatty liver disease management. In *2024 5th International Conference on Circuits, Control, Communication and Computing (I4C)*. https://www.semanticscholar.org/paper/57869e5db46971d258731e10bcd86028db2ea617 (accessed on 24 May 2025).

19. Ghosh, D., Pahan, A., Maity, C., Dey, M., Mondal, R., & Mondal, S. (2025). Phytotherapy for non-alcoholic fatty liver disease: A review of mechanisms, efficacy, and future directions. *Natural Therapy Advances*. https://www.semanticscholar.org/paper/a64105396570ea2e0dcd8e70162e87aedb881203 (accessed on 24 May 2025).

20. Hegazy, M. A., Elshafei, A., Salem, M. R., Ashoush, O., & Abdelghani, A. (2024). Non-alcoholic fatty liver disease related knowledge among a sample of Egyptians: An exploratory cross-sectional study. *Frontiers in Public Health, 11*. https://www.semanticscholar.org/paper/e545295a5972fdbf971a530c5897b1ed8cc5d6b9 (accessed on 24 May 2025).

21. Hiriart, J., & Ledinghen, V. (2017). Non-invasive methods for liver fibrosis assessment. *24*, 49–63. https://www.semanticscholar.org/paper/222f332b77a202fb7842c7a56e643b9a00dba65b (accessed on 24 May 2025).

22. Hosseini, S. A., Shayesteh, A., Hashemi, S. J., Rahimi, Z., Saki, N., Behbahani, H. B., Cheraghian, B., *et al.* (2024). The association between healthy eating index-2015 with anthropometric, cardiometabolic and hepatic indices among patients with non-alcoholic fatty liver disease. *BMC Gastroenterology, 24*. https://www.semanticscholar.org/paper/67b2ccb5344942b60e9f6ded4b6416c044c14430 (accessed on 24 May 2025).

23. Jadhav, P. A., Thomas, A. B., Chopada, V. M., Bokaria, P. V., Deokate, S. B., Chougule, P. S., Chavan, P. N., *et al.* (2024). Correlation of non-alcoholic fatty liver disease and neurodegenerative disorders. *Egyptian Liver Journal*. https://www.semanticscholar.org/paper/715dfc6464a7a535c906e813012f935c0e2636a2 (accessed on 24 May 2025).
24. Jahromi, M. K., Daftari, G., Farhadnejad, H., Tehrani, A., Teymoori, F., Salehi-Sahlabadi, A., & Mirmiran, P. (2023). The association of healthy lifestyle score and risk of non-alcoholic fatty liver disease. *BMC Public Health, 23*. https://www.semanticscholar.org/paper/3b3e68fa5c17376c002d1f50c2d5cfa363052b40 (accessed on 24 May 2025).
25. Jennison, E., & Byrne, C. (2023). Recent advances in NAFLD: Current areas of contention. *Faculty Reviews, 12*. https://www.semanticscholar.org/paper/c1343b349db84fe5672e45bbfa51c4dc97b216c7 (accessed on 24 May 2025).
26. Jeong, H. G., & Park, H. (2022). Metabolic disorders in menopause. *Metabolites, 12*, 954. https://doi.org/10.3390/metabo12100954.
27. Kang, Y., Baek, Y., Lee, J. H., Roh, Y. H., Kwon, H., Moon, S., Son, M., *et al.* (2024). Assessing the utility of acoustic radiation force impulse in the evaluation of non-alcoholic fatty liver disease with severe obesity or steatosis. *Diagnostics, 14*. https://www.semanticscholar.org/paper/54be699b7d7d839fbd7e22300e2a655baa96b481 (accessed on 24 May 2025).
28. Karshina, O., Sabirov, I., Kundashev, U., Mohammad, E., Inarkiev, R., & Fazilova, S. (2024). Association between cardiovascular risk and non-alcoholic fatty liver disease. *Bulletin of Science and Practice*. https://www.semanticscholar.org/paper/82e26a053e7a31e9c22c165acc7cd6197d9ce50b (accessed on 24 May 2025).
29. Kavanaugh, R. (2017). *MRI Overview for Fat Quantification in Non-Alcoholic Fatty Liver Disease in The Clinical and Research Settings* [Master's thesis, Boston University]. Boston University OpenBU. https://open.bu.edu/bitstream/2144/24022/5/Kavanaugh_bu_0017N_12875.pdf.
30. Khan, N., Khan, A., Naseer, S., Umar, Z., Abbas, S., Bashir, A., Ahmad, F., *et al.* (2025). Non-alcoholic fatty liver disease and its progression: Impact of metabolic syndrome and future treatment strategies. *Indus Journal of Bioscience Research*. https://www.semanticscholar.org/paper/a469fcfd1b6358d8cbbfe1144cd872d68e80c702 (accessed on 24 May 2025).
31. Kim, H. Y., & Rinella, M. (2025). Emerging therapies and real-world application of metabolic dysfunction-associated steatosis liver disease treatment. *Clinical and Molecular Hepatology*. https://www.semanticscholar.org/paper/f7f98ed0c083460a4d7d32a54fe46813eb0d13a0 (accessed on 24 May 2025).
32. Kozak, O. (2024). Evaluating liver fibrosis: The role of elastography and Fibro Test in patients with non-alcoholic fatty liver disease and insulin resistance. *Inter Colleges*. https://www.semanticscholar.org/paper/62b25881697b21f6bdc46155c754eec972f3016e (accessed on 24 May 2025).
33. Le, M., Le, D., Baez, T. C., Dang, H., Nguyen, V., Lee, K., Stave, C., *et al.* (2024). Global incidence of adverse clinical events in non-alcoholic fatty liver disease: A systematic review and meta-analysis. *Clinical and Molecular Hepatology, 30*, 235–246. https://www.semanticscholar.org/paper/01f08ce9e3f0f21eea8087c1abe395aaea9f2baf (accessed on 24 May 2025).
34. Liu, Y., Fan, Y., Liu, J., Liu, X., Li, X., & Hu, J. (2024). Application and mechanism of Chinese herb medicine in the treatment of non-alcoholic fatty liver disease. *Frontiers in Pharmacology,*

15. https://www.semanticscholar.org/paper/19373e8c7dd4d88ec0a5baaf4307dd6aa4eb434d (accessed on 24 May 2025).

35. Lv, H., & Liu, Y. (2024). Management of non-alcoholic fatty liver disease: Lifestyle changes. *World Journal of Gastroenterology, 30*, 2829–2833. https://www.semanticscholar.org/paper/010a475cd2fbc429911742f0eff82190752b3ac9 (accessed on 24 May 2025).

36. Lynch, S. V., Sharpton, S. R., Terrault, N. A., Yong, E., *et al.* (2019). Gut microbial metabolism and nonalcoholic fatty liver disease. https://core.ac.uk/download/323065660.pdf.

37. Mladenova, I. L., Tan, E. F., Ng, J. Y., & Sharma, P. (2025). Non-alcoholic fatty liver disease (NAFLD) and its association to cardiovascular disease: A comprehensive meta-analysis. *JRSM Cardiovascular Disease, 14*, 20480040251325929. https://www.semanticscholar.org/paper/e6609970f3239f6b0e785c140a5d13af5e9d3f15 (accessed on 24 May 2025).

38. Moon, A. M., Webb, G. J., Aloman, C., Armstrong, M. J., Cargill, T., Dhanasekaran, R., Genescà, J., *et al.* (2020). High mortality rates for SARS-CoV-2 infection in patients with pre-existing chronic liver disease and cirrhosis: Preliminary results from an international registry. *Journal of Hepatology, 73*, 705–708. https://doi.org/10.1016/j.jhep.2020.05.013.

39. Oshida, N., Oh, S., Kim, B., Miura, I., Hasegawa, N., Komine, S., Isobe, T., *et al.* (2024). Muscle quality as a potential diagnostic marker of advanced liver fibrosis in patients with non-alcoholic fatty liver disease. *Journal of Obesity & Metabolic Syndrome, 33*, 143–154. https://www.semanticscholar.org/paper/44f2ba7a309d50a772cd786e7312be71ac317f23 (accessed on 24 May 2025).

40. Pan, Y., & Yu, Z. (2025). Progress and prospects of interleukin-22 in the treatment of non-alcoholic fatty liver disease. *Journal of Contemporary Medical Practice*. https://www.semanticscholar.org/paper/baaacdc1f6efaf5ce84367b3f30e46de040c65d8 (accessed on 24 May 2025).

41. Park, Y., Ko, K. S., & Rhee, B. (2025). Non-alcoholic fatty liver disease (NAFLD) management in the community. *International Journal of Molecular Sciences, 26*. https://www.semanticscholar.org/paper/bcebb0cd742ebed2f7a189d737132b3a0ad0ee7f (accessed on 24 May 2025).

42. Prikhodko, V., Bezborodkina, N., & Okovityi, S. (2022). Pharmacotherapy for non-alcoholic fatty liver disease: Emerging targets and drug candidates. *Biomedicines, 10*. https://www.semanticscholar.org/paper/a85414677e599f3bef09d5ffa04f1f8ec19af3ed (accessed on 24 May 2025).

43. Rinella, M. E., & Sookoian, S. (2023). From NAFLD to MASLD: Updated naming and diagnosis criteria for fatty liver disease. *Journal of Lipid Research, 65*, 100485. https://doi.org/10.1016/j.jlr.2023.100485.

44. Robea, M. A., Balmuș, I. M., Gîrleanu, I., Huiban, L., Muzîca, C., Ciobîcă, A., Stanciu, C., *et al.* (2023). Coagulation dysfunctions in non-alcoholic fatty liver disease—Oxidative stress and inflammation relevance. *Medicina, 59*, 1614. https://doi.org/10.3390/medicina59091614.

45. Roderburg, C., Krieg, S., Krieg, A., Vaghiri, S., Mohr, R., Konrad, M., Luedde, M., *et al.* (2023). Non-alcoholic fatty liver disease (NAFLD) and risk of new-onset heart failure: A retrospective analysis of 173,966 patients. *Clinical Research in Cardiology, 112*, 1446–1453. https://www.semanticscholar.org/paper/aa59e4a9349dfab18995d22facd12b19893ae07c (accessed on 24 May 2025).

46. Rong, L., Zou, J., Ran, W., Qi, X., Chen, Y., Cui, H., & Guo, J. (2023). Advancements in the treatment of non-alcoholic fatty liver disease (NAFLD). *Frontiers in Endocrinology, 13*. https://www.semanticscholar.org/paper/51256c66ccc54f148963e726bdf2d89f3f97ba04 (accessed on 24 May 2025).

47. Sakurai, Y., Kubota, N., Yamauchi, T., & Kadowaki, T. (2021). Role of insulin resistance in MAFLD. *International Journal of Molecular Sciences, 22*, 4156. https://doi.org/10.3390/ijms22084156.

48. Seleem, H., El Lehleh, A., Elkhayat, M., El Abd, O., Badr, E., ElMezein, E. F., & Teima, A. (2023). Study of serum adiponectin and chemerin in patients with non-alcoholic fatty liver disease. *Menoufia Medical Journal*. https://www.semanticscholar.org/paper/a469ebc8f26e2e7627a72f8fb374c44f1e798cf6 (accessed on 24 May 2025).

49. Selim, D. H. H., Mokhlis, H., Elsayed, A. M., Shatat, A. S., Salama, S. A., & Ismail, R. S. (2025). Liraglutide mitigates dexamethasone-induced fatty acid synthase (FASN) and the cluster of differentiation 36 (CD36) expression: A potential treatment for glucocorticoid-induced non-alcoholic fatty liver disease (NAFLD). *Naunyn-Schmiedeberg's Archives of Pharmacology*. https://www.semanticscholar.org/paper/28cf94c30b72a8dca9079ce48ab8b089477b2519 (accessed on 24 May 2025).

50. Stepanov, Y., Zavhorodnia, N., Tatarchuk, O.M., Klenina, I.A., Konenko, I.S., & Petishko, O. (2022). Pathogenetic role of inflammation and insulin resistance in non-alcoholic fatty liver disease in obese children. Zaporozhye Medical Journal. https://www.semanticscholar.org/paper/Pathogenetic-role-of-inflammation-and-insulin-in-in-Stepanov-Zavhorodnia/aa6c30d6577f7ed2b1bcd00784d099d2e0de870b

51. Tillman, E. J., & Rolph, T. (2020). FGF21: An emerging therapeutic target for non-alcoholic steatohepatitis and related metabolic diseases. *Frontiers in Endocrinology, 11*. https://doi.org/10.3389/fendo.2020.601290.

52. Uqaili, A., Chang, A., Ali, S., Amjad, M., Samejo, M., & Tagar, M. (2025). Impact of lifestyle modifications on liver function, hepatic fat, and metabolic parameters in non-alcoholic fatty liver disease: A culturally adapted intervention study. *Pakistan Journal of Pathology*. https://www.semanticscholar.org/paper/a5f1743d871abe41aab366160d28f8cc2c4001ed (accessed on 24 May 2025).

53. Veldi, V. D. K., Gangahar, A., Kodapaka, L. N., Angara, S. S. P., Kaur, H., Sunil, A., Peela, S. T., *et al.* (2025). Emerging biomarkers in non-alcoholic fatty liver disease: A comprehensive narrative review of miRNA, lipidomic, and metabolomics for early detection and diagnosis. *Journal of Biomedical and Pharmaceutical Research*. https://www.semanticscholar.org/paper/98cf112aaebe31c25eb8996ed859c1a4d7dd289d (accessed on 24 May 2025).

54. Virk, G. S., Ray, R., Ullah, I., Rahman, S., Rashad, E., & Hassan, M. S. (2025). Efficacy of lifestyle intervention versus pharmacotherapy in the progression of non-alcoholic fatty liver disease: A systematic review and meta-analysis. *Journal of Advances in Medicine and Medical Research*. https://www.semanticscholar.org/paper/0f16542b6763512d5c261516a7ce4407110d1250 (accessed on 24 May 2025).

55. Yi, W., Wu, H., Fu, W., Feng, H., Huang, J., Li, H., Song, Z., *et al.* (2024). Prevalence and risk factors of non-alcoholic fatty liver disease (NAFLD) in non-obese patients with schizophrenia: A retrospective study. *Diabetes, Metabolic Syndrome and Obesity, 17*, 841–849. https://www.

semanticscholar.org/paper/97fbfdbb17be02092a8197a84be86b69ae2c5e0a (accessed on 24 May 2025).

56. Zhang, W., Feng, L., Li, P., Wang, A., Dai, C., Qi, Y., Lu, J., *et al.* (2024). Effects of Mao tea from Nankun Mountain on nonalcoholic fatty liver disease in mice. *Food & Function*. https://www.semanticscholar.org/paper/316dd585832fd36ebc47202f85070131662cd674 (accessed on 24 May 2025).

57. Zhou, W., & Du, Z. (2024). Oleuropein mitigates non-alcoholic fatty liver disease (NAFLD) and modulates liver metabolites in high-fat diet-induced obese mice via activating PPARα. *Journal of the Science of Food and Agriculture*. https://www.semanticscholar.org/paper/f123691925042b084d2bf9abbdec6b2444528d6d (accessed on 24 May 2025).

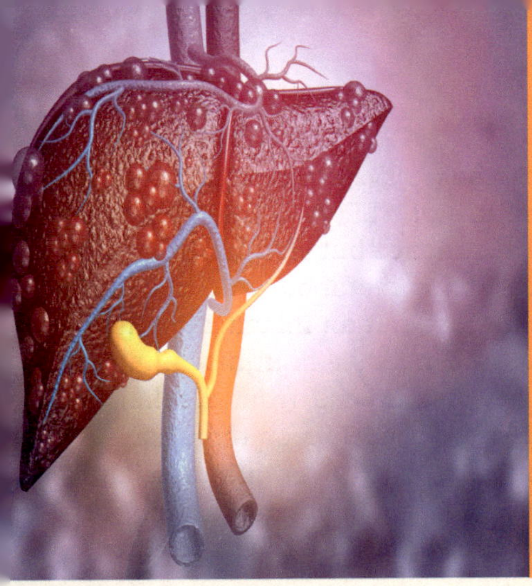

Chapter 6
ALCOHOLIC LIVER DISEASE

Contents

Introduction

Alcoholic Liver Disease (ALD) is a spectrum of liver disease that occurs as a result of chronic alcohol consumption. ALD is an illness with multiple stages, from hepatic steatosis to alcoholic hepatitis to cirrhosis. The pathologic features of ALD are primarily a result of the hepatotoxicity of alcohol and its metabolites on liver cells, leading to inflammation, cell damage, and liver dysfunction. Epidemiologically, ALD remains a worldwide public health issue, with millions of individuals affected, and knowledge of its etiology and effects is crucial. Moreover, awareness of the social and economic effects of ALD can guide prevention and intervention strategies for curbing its occurrence and enhancing patient outcomes. The pathogenesis of ALD is characterized by heterogeneous immunological and metabolic responses, typically complicated by genetic components and comorbidities such as viral hepatitis or obesity. Alcohol's interaction with these diseases can potentially increase cell destruction and inflammation, leading to more severe liver disease. There is evidence that patients with chronic alcohol use disorder develop an alteration of gut microbiota, which causes systemic inflammation and greater liver damage. By focusing on the multi-dimensional nature of ALD, it is important to create comprehensive treatment plans that not only address alcohol abstinence but also consider the general well-being of the patient, potentially with interventions addressing metabolic and immune function. These multi-dimensions turn ALD into not only a hepatic disease but an instance of more general lifestyle and health disturbances. Maximum management of ALD needs a multidisciplinary approach with the integration of clinical and supportive measures. Abstinence from alcohol is the first measure because abstinence is necessary to stop further progression of the disease. Nutrition and lifestyle changes also have indispensable roles in enhancing liver function and health. Treatment is with corticosteroids for severe alcoholic hepatitis and behavior therapy or counseling programs to manage the underlying alcohol use disorder. Prevention education about the harms of drinking excessive amounts of alcohol and the long-term consequences of ALD is the most important element in the implementation of preventive strategies. As awareness about this disease continues to spread, continuing research and public health action will be crucial to mitigating the effects of ALD on society and individuals alike, raising awareness, and encouraging healthier lifestyles.

Definition of Alcoholic Liver Disease

You need to know the different stages of ALD, which begin with simple fatty liver and can lead to alcoholic hepatitis and cirrhosis. ALD is a range of liver problems that are caused by drinking alcohol, and how much and how long the alcohol is consumed matters most. Drinking alcohol for a long period causes fat to build up in the liver cells, which then causes inflammation and damages the cells. As time goes on, these reactions may result in severe liver damage, shown by fibrosis and cirrhosis, which greatly raises the risk of death and illness from liver disease. The presence of this condition makes it clear how harmful alcohol abuse is and highlights the importance of strong public health steps to prevent and treat it early. Emerging research highlights the growing importance of accurately classifying liver diseases that evolve from fatty liver to conditions such as metabolic-associated fatty liver disease (MAFLD), which often coexist alongside ALD. Because of their relationship, it becomes more difficult to manage patients and requires doctors to understand their underlying causes. The shift from the term non-alcoholic fatty liver disease (NAFLD) to metabolic-associated fatty liver disease (MAFLD) reflects a broader understanding of liver pathology, particularly in patients with obesity and metabolic syndrome. This new way of naming the diseases better shows how complex they are and the different ways they can develop. As alcohol and metabolic factors intertwine, recognizing the implications of this overlap is crucial for individualized treatment approaches (Vaz *et al.*, 2023; Vimalesvaran *et al.*, 2024). ALD is affected by factors such as age, gender, and the level of income, which makes the disease more or less common in various populations. Men have traditionally drunk more alcohol, which puts them at greater risk, but recent trends show that women are now facing similar dangers. In addition, factors in society, including cultural views on drinking and the availability of healthcare, play a big role in how ALD appears and is diagnosed. It is important to know about these components to help both people with the disease and to create better public health policies. By identifying high-risk groups and tailoring interventions, the healthcare community can more effectively combat the rising tide of ALD and improve overall liver health within diverse populations (Figure 6.1).

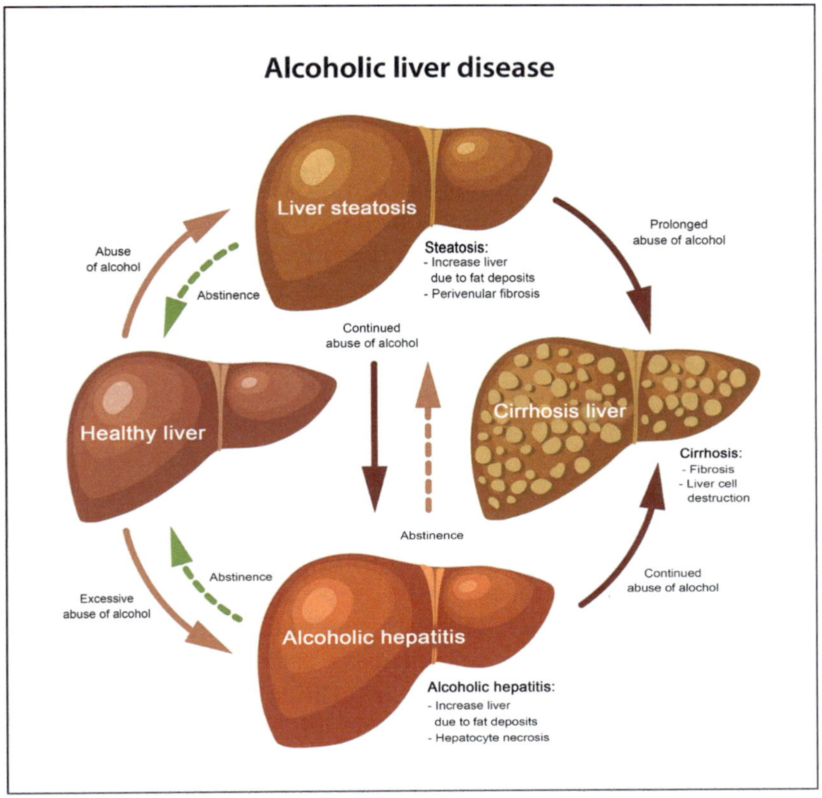

Figure 6.1. Alcoholic liver disease (ALD).

Source: https://continentalhospitals.com/uploads/mceu_86332911011700211281434.jpg.

Importance of the Topic in Public Health

The epidemiology of ALD is a critical aspect of public health issues, particularly as alcohol consumption continues to be an entrenched custom among most cultures worldwide. One must realize the severity of ALD to develop practical prevention programs that address lifestyle elements responsible for its occurrence. Studies indicate that individuals above 40 years are disproportionately affected by ALD, with an estimated odds ratio of 3.2, which warrants specially targeted public health campaigns to spread awareness about the risks of excessive alcohol consumption among older age brackets. Moreover, the long-term effects of ALD in producing chronic liver failure and even liver cancer raise the necessity of early intervention. Through raising awareness and promoting responsible drinking, public health agencies can mitigate the burden of this disease on the healthcare system and reduce alcohol abuse morbidity (Dudinskaya *et al.*, 2024). The interplay between socioeconomic status and ALD incidence further underscores its implication in public health discourse. People of lower socioeconomic status tend to suffer from higher levels of ALD, primarily because they have very little access to healthcare and are not informed about the risks of alcohol to their health. This is what attests to the critical importance of public health policy that not only targets educational programs but systemic inequalities themselves that create health disparities. Wide-scale screening campaigns, coupled with community-level interventions within vulnerable groups, can play a key role in controlling the transmission of ALD. In addition, these measures can lead to collaboration between healthcare providers, policy makers, and local leaders to formulate a combined framework focusing on reversing the root causes of alcohol misuse and its adverse health impacts (Dudinskaya *et al.*, 2024). The applicability of liver function evaluation through biochemical indicators, such as the Deritis ratio, also reflects the prognostic and diagnostic aspects of ALD in public health. Findings suggest that a raised AST/ALT ratio may serve as an early indicator of ALD, enabling interventions that can have significant effects on patient outcome. As ALD often does not manifest with symptoms in its early stages, increased monitoring in liver function tests (LFTs) within at-risk populations can provide useful insights into disease progression. Incorporation of these types of biomarkers into regular health screenings would enhance early detection as well as the capacity to start early medical interventions. Lastly, liver health investment in the broader context of public health might find its culmination in better planning towards ALD management, which in turn will decrease its long-term impact on people and the health care system (Shabnam *et al.*, 2023).

6.1. Causes of Alcoholic Liver Disease (ALD)

The development of alcoholic liver disease (ALD) is primarily influenced by the excessive and prolonged consumption of alcohol, which leads to liver inflammation and damage. The liver is where most alcohol is broken down, and this process creates acetaldehyde, which is toxic and causes metabolic problems and stress in cells. Long-term exposure to high alcohol levels changes how liver cells work, causing fat to build up in the liver, which is called alcoholic fatty liver disease. Failing to control this accumulation can result in more serious forms of ALD, for example, alcoholic hepatitis and cirrhosis, which highlights the importance of understanding how alcohol causes harm in the liver. Genetics can make a person more likely to develop ALD, and alcohol can make these risks even greater. How genes work in alcohol metabolism, inflammation, and the repair of the liver can greatly impact a person's response to drinking alcohol. For example, certain polymorphisms in the alcohol dehydrogenase (ADH) and aldehyde dehydrogenase (ALDH) genes can affect the efficiency of alcohol processing, thereby increasing the risk of liver damage. In addition, having a poor diet and other health conditions like obesity and metabolic syndrome can make the liver problems caused by alcohol worse, as these conditions raise inflammation and oxidative stress in the liver, which may result in more complications from ALD. Besides genes and behavior, the level of income and education in a person's life greatly affect the chances and severity of ALD. Lower socio-economic groups may be more likely to become alcohol dependent because they face stress from poverty, not having access to healthcare, and fewer educational opportunities. Difficulties in the social and economic sectors can stop or reduce disease prevention and treatment, which causes more disease. In addition, the attitudes in society and culture about drinking alcohol can greatly affect how people drink, which can make it more difficult for public health to deal with ALD. Because the world is always changing, it is vital to address these factors together to prevent and manage ALD well.

6.1.1. Mechanism of Alcohol Metabolism in the Liver

The liver is the principal organ that metabolizes alcohol, employing a sequence of enzyme-catalyzed reactions to metabolize alcohol into less harmful substances. The principal enzyme is ADH, which catalyzes the conversion of ethanol to acetaldehyde, extremely toxic in nature. Importantly, acetaldehyde is also converted by aldehyde dehydrogenase (ALDH) to acetate, which is much less toxic and easily secreted by the body. This metabolic pathway is important because acetaldehyde accumulation may lead to hepatic oxidative stress as well as to cellular damage and play a major role in the pathogenesis of ALD. Moreover, long-term alcohol consumption can lead to the upregulation of these enzymes, which not only accelerates metabolism but also enhances the generation of reactive oxygen species (ROS) and exacerbates liver damage and inflammation. In addition to ADH and ALDH, the microsomal ethanol oxidizing system (MEOS), predominantly cytochrome P450 2E1, plays a part in alcohol metabolism, particularly in chronic drinking. The MEOS occurs when the amount of alcohol is greater than the liver's capacity to metabolize it through the ADH mechanism. The system is linked to the production of free radicals and resulting hepatocellular injury. Excessive alcohol consumption will disrupt the normal redox balance of reactions within hepatocytes and is an essential part of healthy liver function. Also, ethanol metabolism via MEOS has been associated with the generation of pro-inflammatory mechanisms that activate cytokine generation and exacerbate injury to the liver. These mechanisms underscore the complexity of the action of alcohol on liver function and contribute to our knowledge of ALD pathogenesis. Recent research highlights the interaction between alcohol metabolism and changes in gut microbiota, suggesting that shifts in microbial composition may influence ALD development. For instance, treatments such as *pueraria* extract have shown potential in controlling gut microbiota, thereby reducing alcohol-induced inflammation and liver injury. Experiments confirm that the therapeutic action of *pueraria* is facilitated by the inhibition of ADH1 expression and the decrease in levels of acetaldehyde, implying a direct action on ethanol metabolism. The application of postbiotics, like thermally inactivated *Levilactobacillus brevis* PDD-2, has also been associated with enhanced oxidative stress equilibrium within the liver, and these microbial derivatives are able to modulate alcohol-related metabolic processes. This new field of research also suggests that microbiota-directed therapy can improve the alcohol metabolism risks and pathophysiologic effects of ALD, contributing to an all-around treatment approach (Liu *et al.*, 2024; Wu *et al.*, 2024) (Figure 6.2).

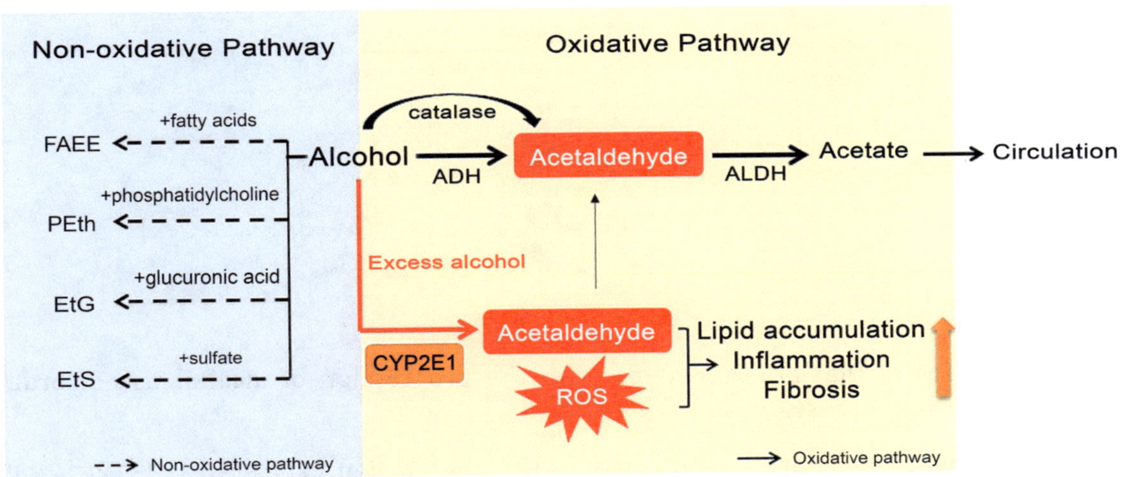

Figure 6.2. Scheme for alcohol metabolism in the liver.

Source: https://www.mdpi.com/ijms/ijms-22-05717/article_deploy/html/images/ijms-22-05717-g001.png.

6.1.2. Risk Factors Contributing to the Disease

Because ALD has many aspects, it is important to know the risk factors that can lead to it. The main factor here is how much and how often alcohol is consumed, because drinking too much over a long period can harm the liver. Long-term alcohol use causes fatty liver, inflammation, and fibrosis, which can lead to worse liver diseases. Even so, not all people who drink alcohol end up with ALD, which suggests that genes and the environment are also important. The way alcohol metabolism enzymes work in people can increase their risk of ALD, which shows that the disease is not simple and requires careful prevention and treatment. Besides the way someone drinks, having metabolic syndrome is important for understanding the risk of ALD. Obesity, diabetes, and hypertension can make liver damage caused by alcohol worse. Individuals with elevated body mass index (BMI) and waist circumference are particularly at risk, as fat accumulation in the liver can compound the effects of alcohol. Studies have found that NAFLD is strongly linked to body weight, as having a higher BMI increases the chances of liver injury from alcohol consumption, so metabolic health is important in assessing ALD risk. Furthermore, elevated liver enzymes such as alanine aminotransferase (ALT) and aspartate aminotransferase (AST) serve as indicators of liver damage, providing valuable information for clinicians in managing patients at risk of ALD, thus accentuating the need for early intervention strategies. Men are found to have a higher risk of alcohol-related liver damage than women, which is a significant risk factor in ALD. Physiological factors such as body type, hormones, and how alcohol is processed might be the reason for this difference. Because women have less body water than men, they get higher blood alcohol levels after drinking the same amount. At the same time, what we eat and how much we move play a role in gender-related differences in metabolic health, which can make both men and women more likely to get liver diseases at the same time. Understanding these nuances is essential for tailoring prevention and treatment strategies for ALD, ensuring they effectively address the unique risk profiles of diverse populations, while also highlighting the need for further research into gender-specific interventions (Amini-Salehi *et al.*, 2023; Liao *et al.*, 2023) (Figure 6.3).

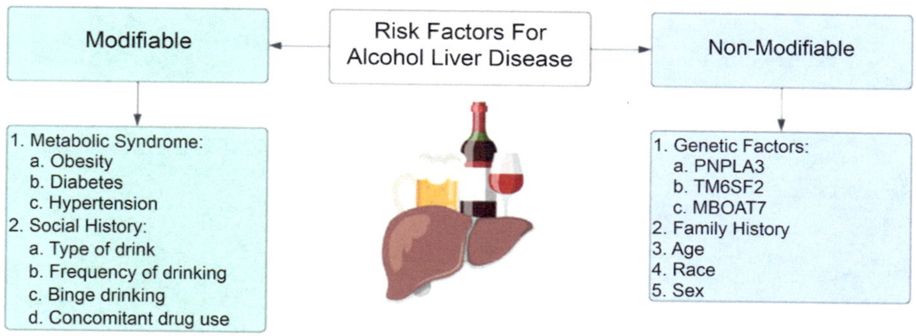

Figure 6.3. Risk factors that are associated with the progression of alcohol use disorder into alcohol-associated liver disease.

Source: https://www.researchgate.net/publication/385588612/figure/fig1/AS:11431281288914127@1730910108293/Risk-factors-that-are-associated-with-the-progression-of-alcohol-use-disorder-into.png.

6.1.3. Genetic Predisposition and Its Role

Genetic predisposition plays a critical role in understanding the multifactorial etiology of ALD. Certain genetic variants in patients can increase the risk of alcohol-induced liver injury. The susceptibility can be through metabolic pathways used in modulating alcohol metabolism and the resultant toxicities to liver cells. Studies have identified the key genetic factors influencing the metabolism of alcohol by the liver, that is, enzyme polymorphisms of alcohol metabolism. Consequently, genetic predisposition not only raises the susceptibility to liver damage but also influences variation in the clinical presentation and outcome of ALD in patients, calling for individualized prevention and management plans. The interaction of lifestyle factors with genetic susceptibility also further modifies the risk of ALD development. Patients with a genetic susceptibility to liver disease are thought to be significantly helped by dietary modification towards the reduction of this risk. For example, adherence to a healthy diet has been shown to reduce NAFLD incidence in patients at risk, something also applicable to ALD. Patients at high genetic risk with a healthy diet may even have diminished liver injury despite alcohol consumption, indicating that lifestyle interventions may partially counteract genetic predisposition. This connection is reflective of the need to couple genetic screening with lifestyle guidance in the total care of ALD at-risk patients. Furthermore, genetic susceptibility can accompany several health conditions and enhance the risk of ALD occurrence. As in studies involving cohorts with existing conditions like CVDs, genetic predisposition can enhance the effects of unhealthy lifestyle patterns such as excessive drinking. For example, patients recovering from myocardial infarction who are also genetically predisposed towards liver disease can face distinctive challenges when their liver health is involved and alcohol use is in the picture. Recognizing these interactions is important, as they both demonstrate the need for individualized treatment protocols that consider both genetic predispositions and environmental factors for the successful management of ALD. Finally, continued research into genetic predisposition will enhance our ability to predict and prevent ALD in various patient populations (Heerkens *et al.*, 2024; Yang *et al.*, 2024).

6.2. Stages of Alcoholic Liver Disease (ALD)

Understanding ALD is easier when you look at its stages, which are fatty liver, alcoholic hepatitis, and alcoholic cirrhosis. Fatty liver or steatosis is the first stage that happens when fat accumulates in the liver. Many times, this condition does not show symptoms, but it leads to more serious damage in the liver. After a long period of drinking, the liver may become inflamed, which is called alcoholic hepatitis. At this point, jaundice and abdominal pain may appear, which suggests the condition needs urgent medical care. Understanding these stages is crucial, as timely intervention during the initial phases can significantly alter disease outcomes and potentially prevent progression to more severe liver damage, such as cirrhosis, which presents irreversible complications and elevates the risk of liver failure and hepatocellular carcinoma (HCC). As ALD gets worse, from simple fatty liver to more severe forms, biomarkers help determine how severe it is. Finding liver fibrosis early on is very important because the liver can repair itself well if the problem is found early. Non-invasive serum biomarkers, such as hyaluronic acid and metalloproteinases, have been proposed to evaluate the stages of liver fibrosis and assess the progression of ALD (Maroto-García *et al.*, 2023). Also, systems that consider clinical factors have become important tools for grouping patients by their risk. These include the Fibrosis-4 (FIB-4) index and the Enhanced Liver Fibrosis (ELF) test. The presence of such biomarkers can guide clinicians in deciding when to start treatment or monitor the patient, which can improve outcomes for people with ALD. When ALD leads to cirrhosis, the liver's structure is greatly damaged, which causes many different medical problems. At this point, the liver is badly damaged and cannot heal, which leads to complications such as portal hypertension, liver failure, and more infections. Non-invasive biomarkers are still essential because they help track liver harm and identify possible problems such as HCC. Despite some inconsistencies in their predictive value for advanced liver disease, studies have shown that serum ferritin levels can serve as a valuable biomarker for assessing stages of liver disease progression in various contexts, including NAFLD (Wang *et al.*, 2022). Overall, recognizing and understanding the stages of ALD is crucial, as it provides direct insights into appropriate therapeutic interventions and informs clinicians about the prognosis of affected individuals (Figure 6.4).

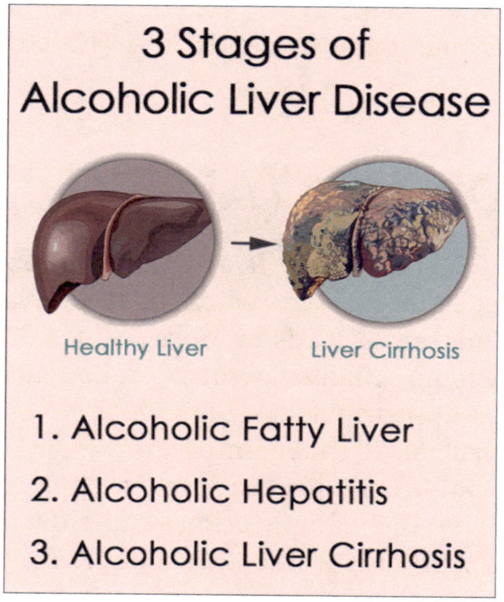

Figure 6.4. 3-stages-of-alcoholic-liver-disease.

Source: https://summitmalibu.com/wp-content/uploads/2023/04/3-stages-of-alcoholic-liver-disease-624x767.jpg.

6.2.1. Fatty Liver (Steatosis)

Fatty liver disease, particularly ALD, is a significant disorder globally. Fatty liver disease involves the accumulation of excess fat within the liver, resulting in liver enlargement and potential interruption of normal liver physiology. The pathogenesis of fatty liver results from complex interplays between chronic alcohol consumption, metabolic disturbance, and inflammation. When the liver is working under stress from alcohol, it prioritizes ethanol metabolism over fatty acid oxidation, and this leads to fat accumulation. It may develop asymptotically, with most individuals not presenting symptoms initially. However, as fatty liver progresses, it may lead to more severe issues like alcoholic steatosis, which is a milestone in the disease process. It is crucial to understand what the implications of this condition are because it forms the groundwork for more severe liver diseases like alcoholic hepatitis and cirrhosis. The connection of fatty liver disease with other illnesses cannot be overemphasized. Fatty liver exposes the person to a higher risk of IR development, a disorder that is normally associated with metabolic syndrome. This interaction emphasizes lifestyle care, i.e., diet and physical exercise, in managing fatty liver disease. The interaction of nutrient deficiency with hepatic fat accumulation further complicates the scenario. For instance, iron overload, as recognized in the various studies, is correlated with the advancement from simple steatosis to complex conditions such as NASH and could be causative of enhanced liver damage by ferroptosis mechanisms. Thus, understanding of these dynamics is critical to developing intervention measures aimed at the reversal or prevention of alcohol consumption-induced liver injury while promoting overall metabolic health. Fatty liver disease, while insidious, provides an avenue for prevention and early intervention.

Non-invasive diagnostic compounds, such as FibroScan liver elastography, also constitute new methods of measuring liver fat content, enabling clinicians to monitor the severity of disease without invasive biopsies. Dietary modifications, such as eating a healthy diet and increased physical activity, usually constitute effective ways of managing fatty liver and can have a very positive impact on liver function. Along with this, newer research has found the therapeutic value of certain micronutrients and supplements that may restore liver function as well as inhibit the accumulation of fat. As the incidence of fatty liver disease is on the rise, there will be a need for holistic management methods to not only treat the health of livers but also the overall well-being of the patients. The recognition and adaptation of life stages in combination with advanced therapies will be essential to combat the course of ALD and its complications (Filgueira *et al.*, 2014; Torshin *et al.*, 2024) (Figure 6.5).

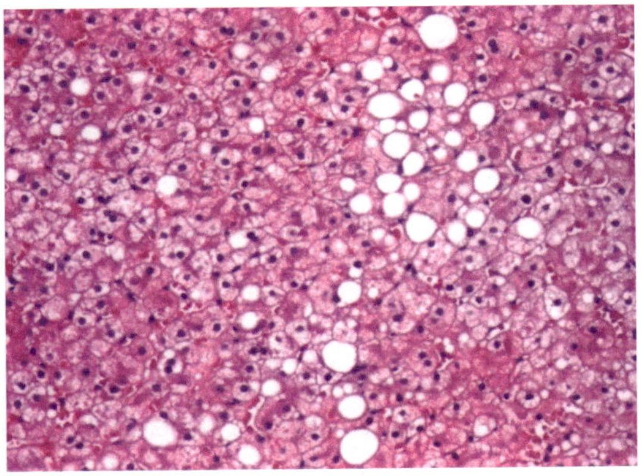

Figure 6.5. Microscopic image of moderate steatosis.

Source: https://www.researchgate.net/profile/Ion-Efrem/publication/306322296/figure/fig1/AS:614330601074708@1523479237964/Microscopic-image-of-moderate-steatosis-HE-staining-200.png.

6.2.2. Alcoholic Hepatitis

The major concern in alcoholic liver disease is alcoholic hepatitis, which shows how the liver responds to heavy alcohol use. This problem in the liver appears as inflammation, damage to liver cells, and different levels of liver dysfunction. Symptoms may be as simple as mild ones or as serious as jaundice and ascites, and patients usually have abdominal pain and feel generally unwell. A lot of people with alcoholic hepatitis suffer from serious health problems and may die, especially if they continue to drink alcohol. Usually, the seriousness of the disease is determined by applying well-known prognostic scoring systems that consider both clinical and laboratory factors, which guide the right management and interventions. Refraining from alcohol is very important for people with liver disease to prevent further harm and improve their health. Managing alcoholic hepatitis usually requires input from several specialists who look at both the body and mind. A study done recently pointed out that various drugs can be used, and basic support such as a healthy diet and avoiding alcohol, is important for improving patients' health and life quality. Most patients in the study (95.3%) pointed out that quitting alcohol was very important for stopping the disease from progressing. It is also very important to have hepatologists and addiction specialists collaborating to create complete treatment plans. Patients may be prescribed ursodeoxycholic acid and antibiotics, and they also receive support to help them avoid relapse. Such treatments are necessary to handle the problems of alcoholic hepatitis and help people with the disease live longer, since, if ignored, the disease may progress to more serious liver conditions. If alcohol consumption does not stop, the outcomes for patients with alcoholic hepatitis can become very serious, as shown in many case studies. One case report detailed the progression from alcoholic hepatitis to liver cirrhosis (LC) and, ultimately, HCC, underscoring the dire consequences of continued drinking. The patient's situation made it clear that continued alcohol use leads to more liver damage, which underlines the need for early detection and good management. Stopping alcohol consumption for a long time greatly reduces the chances of getting complications such as cirrhosis and liver cancer from ALD. Also, FibroScan and the Maddrey Discriminant Function are important in finding patients who may have liver problems and providing them with the right care. Through these measures, healthcare providers can improve the prognosis for individuals diagnosed with alcoholic hepatitis, potentially averting the dire transitions to cirrhosis and cancer (Figure 6.6).

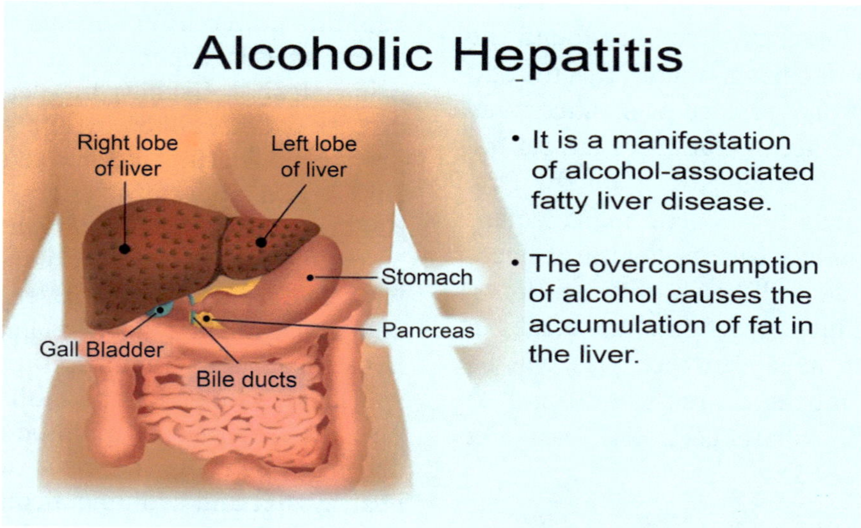

Figure 6.6. Alcoholic hepatitis.

Source: https://www.verywellhealth.com/thmb/CvmxyOHdInJ1yZsu9RxDED8KFVE=/750x0/filters:no_upscale():max_bytes(150000):strip_icc():format(webp)/AlcoholicHepatitis-StagesSignsCuttingAlcohol-final-3b31011ecc284ccf9111f5c081fa642e.png.

6.2.3. Alcoholic Cirrhosis

The progression of ALD to alcoholic cirrhosis is an important problem in the area of hepatology. Alcoholic cirrhosis results from ongoing heavy alcohol intake, leading to irreversible liver injury with scarring and fibrosis. The pathogenesis involves a multifactorial interplay of metabolic, inflammatory, and fibrogenic processes sensitized by continuous alcohol use. Particularly, acute alcoholic hepatitis may be a prodrome to cirrhosis, with inflammation and dysfunction of the liver. Even with improved comprehension of liver injury mechanisms, therapy is limited, and corticosteroids remain the cornerstone treatment despite differential rates of effectiveness in controlling disease symptomatology. The need for research into new treatment methods is underscored by the extent of problems surrounding the treatment of alcoholic cirrhosis, as evidenced by the prevalence of this condition among CLD patients (Enciu *et al.*, 2025). Alcoholic cirrhosis is not only a late complication of liver disease but is also associated with severe risks to patients, especially the risk of acquiring complications like HCC and liver failure. In cirrhosis, the liver is no longer able to perform essential functions like protein synthesis, metabolism and detoxification. Complications of this disturbed hepatic function contribute to morbidity and mortality. In epidemiological statistics, there is a strong correlation between long-term alcohol use and development of liver disease, and therefore, an early diagnosis and intervention are needed. Furthermore, with the health burden imposed by alcoholic cirrhosis on the health system, efficient public health measures are required that will reduce alcohol consumption and enhance awareness of liver health. There is a need for multifaceted management strategies to prevent long-term sequelae of liver damage and enhance patient outcomes (Enciu *et al.*, 2025). Alcoholic cirrhosis's complex problems require coordinated approach with both lifestyle and medical intervention. There are a few important aspects of management that involve abstinence from alcohol, nutritional supplementation, and carefully monitoring for complications. Nutritional interventions, not traditionally accorded much importance, play significant roles in supporting the liver and general health in the afflicted individuals. In addition to that, the promotion of lifestyle changes like weight control can have a great impact on the course of liver disease and decrease related risks. Multidisciplinary care models involving hepatologists, nutritionists, and psychiatrists are crucial in managing the disorder in an integrated manner. These strategies gain more importance as the prevalence of alcohol-related liver disease (ARLD) keeps rising, and new management paradigms are needed to cure the acute inflammatory phases and reverse the chronic effects of alcoholic cirrhosis (Figure 6.7).

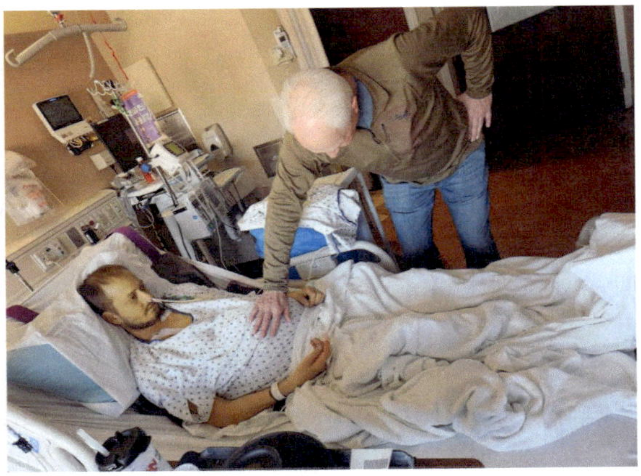

Figure 6.7. A patient with alcoholic cirrhosis.

Source: https://www.sdnewswatch.org/content/images/2024/07/20240327_160731.jpg.

6.3. Symptoms and Diagnosis

The symptoms that appear with ALD vary significantly based on the progress of the disease. At the beginning, patients might have symptoms like tiredness, a general feeling of sickness, abdominal pain, and changes in their appetite. As the disease progresses, more severe manifestations may emerge, including jaundice, ascites, and hepatic encephalopathy (HE). Jaundice, which makes the skin and eyes yellow, occurs when the liver does not break down bilirubin properly. Ascites, which is the buildup of fluid in the abdomen, can cause discomfort and breathing difficulties. These clinical features underscore the importance of early detection and diagnosis, as timely intervention can significantly alter the disease's trajectory and improve patient outcomes (Moon *et al.*, 2020). A doctor will usually use clinical evaluation, laboratory tests, and imaging to diagnose ALD. A complete patient history, especially about alcohol use and its risks, is very important. Tests in the laboratory typically check liver function by measuring serum aminotransferases, alkaline phosphatase, and bilirubin, which might suggest a problem with the liver. Advanced imaging techniques such as ultrasound, CT, or magnetic resonance imaging (MRI) can reveal structural changes in the liver, including fatty infiltration or fibrosis. Notably, the presence of certain markers, such as elevated gamma-glutamyl transferase (GGT), can also suggest alcohol-related liver injury. Clinicians may also utilize the Model for End-Stage Liver Disease (MELD) score to further assess the severity and prognosis of liver impairment in affected patients (Ji *et al.*, 2020). Using several medical specialties is important in diagnosing ALD for proper management. Since alcohol use disorders and liver disease are closely related, hepatologists, primary care physicians, and mental health professionals should work together. A thorough assessment may involve psychosocial evaluations to find patients who could be helped by addiction treatment that addresses the root of their condition. Studies done recently have discovered links between the severity of liver disease and markers like the Child-Pugh classification, which shows how well patients with cirrhosis can function. By integrating these diagnostic tools and treatment modalities, healthcare providers can create tailored management plans that encompass both the physical and psychological aspects of ALD, ultimately serving to enhance patient care and improve outcomes (Moon *et al.*, 2020).

6.3.1. Common Symptoms Associated with the Disease

Presentations of ALD consist of a spectrum of symptoms corresponding to different severities of liver pathology. If the disease takes its full course, individuals can experience abdominal pain and changes in bowel habits such as diarrhea or constipation. The early presentation of mild symptoms can be very insidious and can consist of fatigue, loss of appetite, and nausea, commonly prompting patients to underreport the severity of their condition. Worth mentioning, however, is fat buildup in the liver, or steatosis, which can exist without significant inflammation, underscoring the need for regular monitoring among individuals with excessive alcohol consumption.

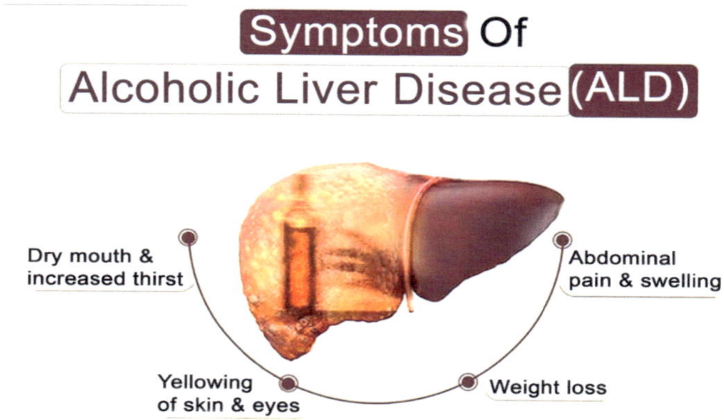

Figure 6.8. Symptoms of alcoholic liver disease (ALD).

Source: https://encrypted-tbn0.gstatic.com/images?q=tbn:ANd9GcTWBdFf4008-EKkEqLJRZErKMOq3LRbkuRgkg&s.

The spectrum of ALD symptoms is not fixed but instead changes as the disease advances, usually progressing to more severe manifestations that require immediate medical care. Therefore, recognition of such early warning signs is especially crucial in bringing about earlier medical consultation and intervention with the potential to reverse disease progression and outcome. As ALD advances, patients may begin to present with more severe symptoms indicative of liver failure. Jaundice, when the eyes and skin turn yellow, results from the liver's inability to break down bilirubin. Additionally, pruritus, or intense itching, can result from bile salt accumulation in the blood. Continued deterioration of liver function may cause such complications as ascites, or a collection of fluid in the abdominal cavity, resulting in a great deal of pain and limiting movement. HE, or mental impairments, is another serious consequence, where toxins accumulate in the blood since the liver is not functioning optimally, leading to confusion and altered mental status. These symptoms are not merely uncomfortable; they are a turning point in the disease process that must be carefully managed medically to maximize quality of life and prevent further decline in health. In severe liver disease, patients can have a constellation of uncomfortable symptoms that greatly diminish overall well-being. According to studies, acute liver failure tends to cause unbearable physical and psychological suffering, ultimately leading to a high rate of mortality among victims. As it reaches its terminal stage, patients may develop intense fatigue, loss of weight, and an inability to carry out normal daily activities. Moreover, the psychological load may develop in the shape of depression or anxiety, further aggravating the condition of the patient. Notably, the medical professionals are also capable of missing these symptoms as indicators of impending death, so that the families and caregivers do not prepare themselves for the loss (N/A, 2011). This low awareness serves to emphasize the importance of improved awareness and communication regarding the terminal phase of ALD and the necessity for palliative care in order to manage the complexity of terminal phase symptoms and enhance the quality of the remaining lifespan of the patients (Figure 6.8).

6.3.2. Diagnostic Tests and Procedures

A variety of tests and procedures are used in ALD to find out the degree of liver damage and decide on the best treatment approach. Tests used to diagnose liver disease are usually serological markers, imaging studies, and liver biopsies. Blood tests usually check liver enzymes, bilirubin and GGT to find out how the liver is functioning and if it has been damaged. Imaging techniques like ultrasound, computed tomography (CT), and magnetic resonance imaging (MRI) provide valuable insights into liver morphology and can help identify complications such as fatty liver or cirrhosis. They give a general idea of the patient's liver condition which makes it easier to act promptly. While these initial diagnostic tools are crucial, the invasive liver biopsy (LBx) remains the gold standard for defining the extent of fibrosis or cirrhosis in patients with ALD. However, due to its invasive nature and associated complications, there is an increasing interest in exploring non-invasive liver tests (NILTs) as alternatives to biopsy.

They are used to find out how stiff the liver is and to measure other signs linked to the amount of fibrosis, which can be safer and less costly than other methods. According to recent evidence, NILTs, such as elastography, can be particularly beneficial in assessing patients with CLD, including ALD, as they provide reliable diagnostic accuracy while minimizing patient risk (Alisi *et al.*, 2015). However, the use of these tests in clinical practice is still being examined, mainly because their cost is not always lower than that of a biopsy. Comprehending the disease and the differences in patient reactions is important for choosing the best way to diagnose ALD. With the progress in this field, NILTs might help doctors identify patients who are likely to get advanced liver disease, which can lead to better outcomes by allowing timely actions such as changing lifestyle and using medicines. More research is needed to confirm that these methods are effective and reliable for people from different backgrounds. Additionally, integrating these diagnostic procedures into clinical practice requires careful consideration of individual patient factors, including the likelihood of abstinence from alcohol, which profoundly influences the disease course (Alisi *et al.*, 2015). A flexible, evidence-based strategy tailored to each patient's unique context will enhance diagnostic accuracy and therapeutic efficacy in managing alcohol-related liver conditions (Figure 6.9).

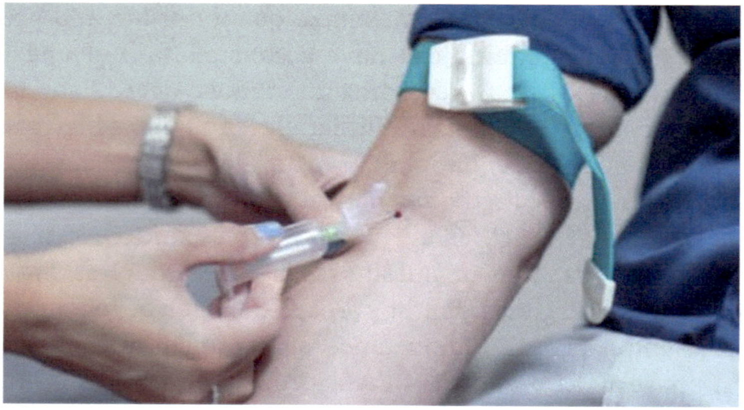

Figure 6.9. Diagnostic Tests

Source: https://cloudfront-eu-central-1.images.arcpublishing.com/irishtimes/Y5TGQ2ZXHPHIOLMOKXNYQJ36LU.jpg.

6.3.3. Importance of Early Detection

The role of early detection in the management of ALD cannot be overstated, as it critically influences treatment and prognosis overall. Early diagnosis enables clinicians to initiate selective interventions, which have the potential to halt the evolution of the disease to advanced stages like cirrhosis and HCC. Early ALD patients are typically without any suggestive symptoms, thereby leading to a lethal delay in diagnosis and management. Recognition of risk factors such as chronic alcoholism and metabolic syndromes allows for early intervention, hence prevention of more invasive methods of intervention such as liver transplant. Also, effective early detection can reduce health costs by preventing complications of end-stage disease. Early detection works since evidence shows the relationship between biomarkers and liver function. For instance, it has just been established that there are certain ratios, like the adiponectin-leptin ratio, that are of use as predictors of liver disease in the early stages, including lean NAFLD, in the context of heavy alcohol use and metabolic impairment (Chia-Lu *et al.*, 2023). Biomarkers of this sort play an important part in risk stratification to allow clinicians to tailor prevention and treatment to the risk level. By diagnosing those at heightened risk of ALD with straightforward blood tests, clinicians are able to treat or very significantly extend the disease early on. Screening for such risks routinely and raising awareness of them may influence better lifestyle choices and reduce the incidence of ALD among the population. Finally, the adoption of these techniques of early detection into day-to-day clinical practice has the power to revolutionize the management of ALD. Current treatment approaches lean toward intervention in the late stages, yet it is equally important to move towards a prevention model. Since HCC has a tendency to arise as an extension of CLD, risk factor information associated with ALD becomes relevant (Suresh *et al.*, 2020). With the implementation of evidence-based guidelines that place greater priority on the early screening and education of patients, healthcare systems can significantly enhance the opportunities for patients who are at risk of acquiring advanced liver disease. Early detection and treatment of ALD not only save lives but also improve long-term quality of life for individuals who suffer from this ravaging disease.

6.4. Treatment Options

Treating ALD involves handling the liver complications and the alcohol addiction at the same time. The first thing to do is to stop drinking alcohol, which protects the liver from further harm. Usually, doctors have to help patients in this stage by detoxifying them and giving them benzodiazepines to ease withdrawal symptoms. Also, nutritional advice and parenteral nutrition can be offered to address the malnutrition that often occurs in chronic alcoholism. It is very important to include psychological support in rehabilitation, since it enhances the effects of any medicines given for restoring liver function. Besides abstinence and counseling, drugs are important in treating ALD. Alcoholic hepatitis patients may be given corticosteroids to reduce inflammation, and pentoxifylline is given to protect the liver from damage.

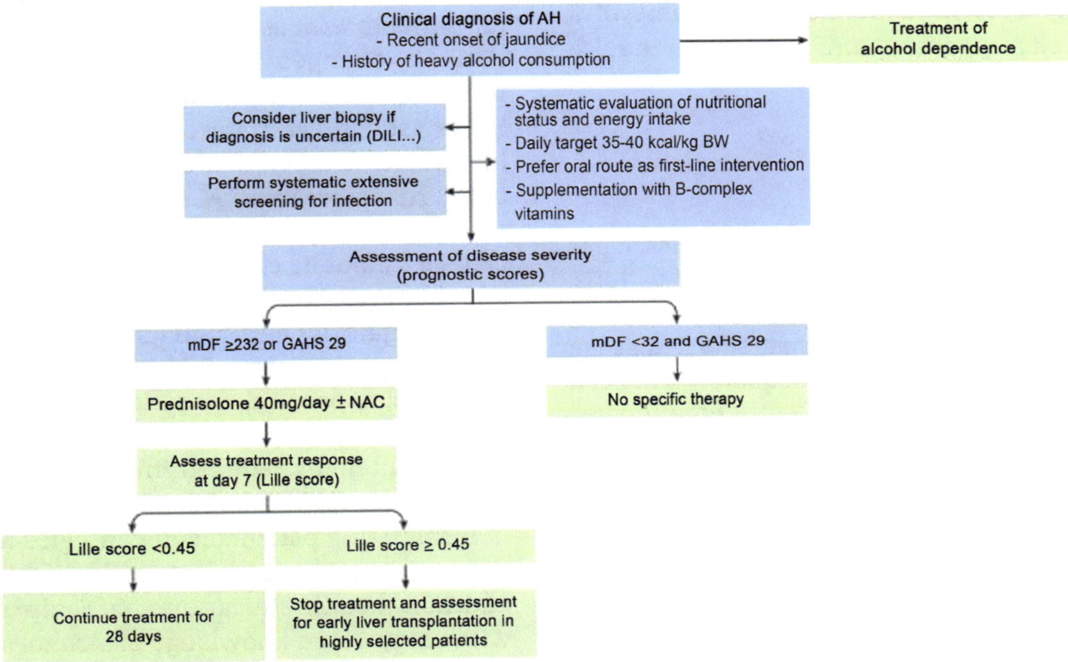

Figure 6.10. Treatment algorithm for the treatment of patients with alcoholic hepatitis.

Source: https://www.researchgate.net/profile/Vetriselvan-Subramaniyan-2/publication/349488439/figure/fig3/AS:994760533753859@1614180801461/Treatment-algorithm-for-the-treatment-of-patients-with-alcoholic-hepatitis-Particularly.png.

Recent research shows that drugs often used for other diseases could be helpful for people with ALD. As an example, therapies that focus on metabolic problems, based on NAFLD research, suggest patients modify their lifestyle by losing weight and changing their diet. Such strategies aim not only to improve liver health but also to mitigate associated risks, including cardiovascular complications inherent to liver disease (Linero *et al.*, 2024). So, a combination of lifestyle changes and drugs is important for improving the outcomes of ALD patients. In addition, as research progresses, new treatment options are becoming more popular in handling ALD. Agents that help decrease oxidative stress and improve insulin sensitivity are being studied for their potential effects.

For instance, studies evaluate the impact of antioxidants on liver histology and functionality in patients with ALD, drawing parallels with findings in NAFLD (Ktenopoulos *et al.*, 2024). More treatment choices allow healthcare providers to create individualized care plans for patients that consider their specific health problems and other medical conditions. The complexity of ALD requires an adaptable treatment strategy that prioritizes continuous monitoring and interdisciplinary collaboration, ultimately fostering a more effective framework for patient recovery and long-term health (Figure 6.10).

6.4.1. Lifestyle Changes and Dietary Modifications

In the management of ALD, the best potential lies in lifestyle changes and dietary modifications. Research has for a long time indicated adopting healthier eating habits to manage liver disease effectively. Incorporating an adequately balanced diet high in fruits, vegetables, whole grains, and lean proteins can provide the nutrients that support the liver in its functionality. Besides, limiting the intake of saturated fats, refined carbs, and highly processed foods is required because such food exacerbates the pathology caused by excessive alcohol consumption. Such dietary modifications not only avoid the advancement of liver disease but also enhance the overall health, enhancing resistance to secondary metabolic disorders. This emphasis on diet is further underscored by the observation that many patients with liver disease also have concurrent dyslipidemia, underlining the relevance of broader dietary strategies for improving clinical outcomes as reported in studies with dietary intervention and lipid analysis (Alazraki *et al.*, 2018). Lifestyle modification, more than diet, has been addressed using a multidisciplinary approach, with physical exercise and weight reduction being central to ALD management. Daily exercise can significantly improve insulin sensitivity and aid in weight loss, which is particularly beneficial for ALD patients who may also suffer from metabolic disorders such as obesity. Aerobic exercise, as well as strength training combined has proven to be useful in curing and improving the health of the liver by increasing its metabolic activity. Furthermore, maintaining a healthy weight also lightens the workload on a damaged liver to function and recover effectively. Combined with dietary modification, such as changes outlined in lipid control plans for patients with associated dyslipidemia, these lifestyle changes form a robust framework to facilitate effective disease management. Synergistic interactions of the changes offer an integrated strategy that can reverse or halt the deleterious impact of ALD (Pirola *et al.*, 2017). Lastly, the psychological aspect of lifestyle change cannot be circumvented since emotional and behavioral support play a fundamental role in guiding individuals through dietary and lifestyle changes. Counseling and support groups can provide essential encouragement and accountability to individuals confronting ALD challenges. Identifying the emotional trigger cues for alcohol consumption is critical in formulating personalized strategies for long-term abstinence and improved lifestyles. In addition, health education can equip patients with empowered knowledge of alcohol's impact on their health to promote a proactive self-care orientation. By addressing both the physical and psychological dimensions of lifestyle change, individuals stand a better chance of managing ALD and improving their overall quality of life, highlighting the need for the incorporation of multidimensional support systems alongside diet modification and physical activity (Pirola *et al.*, 2017).

6.4.2. Medications and Their Effectiveness

Treating ALD calls for using different medications together to improve patient outcomes. Taking corticosteroids and pentoxifylline is effective for people with severe alcoholic hepatitis in reducing inflammation and fibrosis of the liver. Improvements in liver function markers often happen when corticosteroids inhibit cytokines and inflammatory pathways, which is important for patient recovery. Pentoxifylline may also help by modulating angiogenesis and the process of liver regeneration, which could make it a useful addition to treating ALD. Still, the success of these drugs is affected by when they are given and how much the liver is damaged, which means doctors should adjust treatment plans according to each patient. Along with traditional drugs, new ways of treating illnesses, especially with herbal remedies, are becoming more popular. Plants that contain secondary metabolites could be very helpful in treating the causes of liver diseases such as ALD. Using these substances can help treat ALD by supporting the liver and reducing inflammation, which can be useful along with other treatments. Certain botanical compounds might prevent lipid peroxidation and oxidative stress which can cause liver damage.

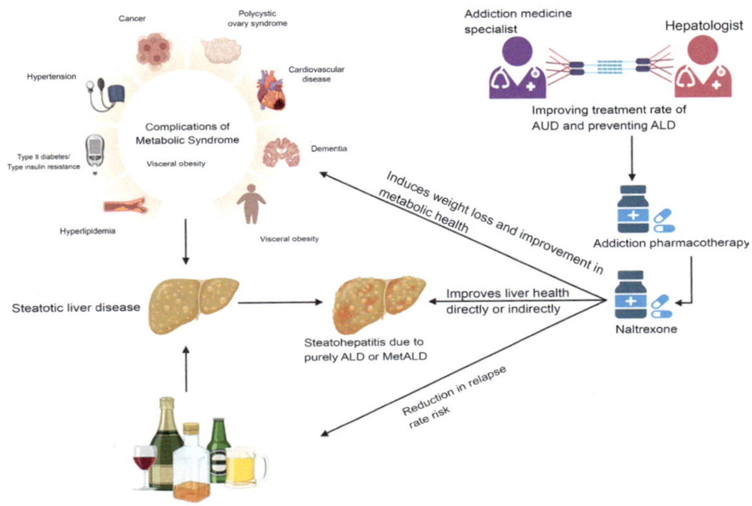

Figure 6.11. A proposed model for improving management of ALD Intensive multidisciplinary treatment of AUD alongside follow-up and management of ALD is proposed to improve liver disease-related morbimortality. AUD, alcohol use disorder; ALD, alcohol-associated liver disease; MetALD, metabolic dysfunction associated steatotic liver disease with concurrent increased alcohol intake.

Source: https://www.researchgate.net/publication/381909533/figure/fig1/AS:11431281276362494@1725630409026/A-proposed-model-for-improving-management-of-ALD-Intensive-multidisciplinary-treatment-of.tif.

As noted in current research, the integration of herbal remedies in treatment regimens could lead to improved efficacy and fewer side effects compared to standard medication protocols (Nucera *et al.*, 2023). Looking into plant-based therapies suggests a change in focus towards using natural options to fight ALD. Also, the presence of hyperuricemia shows how different metabolic disorders are linked with ALD. Taking medications to lower uric acid levels can be important for preventing issues linked to ALD, because high uric acid is related to several metabolic diseases. Studies indicate that ethylenediaminetetraacetic acid (EDTA) chelation therapy may present a novel intervention for patients whose conditions do not respond favorably to traditional uric acid-lowering drugs (Lee *et al.*, 2024). It stresses the need to watch for and control other health problems in people with ALD and also indicates that more medications may be helpful in treating this condition. Thus, a comprehensive approach that incorporates diverse treatment modalities is essential in effectively managing ALD (Figure 6.11).

6.4.3. Role of Liver Transplantation

Liver transplantation has become a significant component of the treatment of ALD since this life-threatening illness progresses in severity among the affected individuals. Liver transplantation offers the promise of recovery as well as improvement in the quality of life for end-stage liver failure patients. A method has been tried in recent years to select suitable candidates for transplantation from ALD patients. Recommendations stipulate that the patients must demonstrate a desire to be and stay sober and engage in rehabilitation therapy, as evidence points out that relapse rates can influence patient survival after transplant. This reflects the complex interaction between transplant candidacy and addiction treatment, which requires comprehensive evaluations by multidisciplinary teams to offer the optimal results for the patients (Maestri *et al.*, 2023). Moreover, the impact of liver transplantation goes beyond the physiological assessments of liver function; it also affects the psychological and social dimensions that are associated with ALD. Post-transplant patients most often receive intensive follow-up management, such as surveillance for psychiatric complications, such as depression or anxiety, which are commonly met in patients with a history of alcoholism. The post-transplant process may encompass a number of challenges, including the need for lifelong immunosuppressive therapy, which can also make recovery more difficult. The said challenges are thus advantaged by ensuring supportive interventions that aim at facilitating sustained psychological well-being and foster compliance with medication. This synergistic treatment addresses not only the physical complications of ALD but also emphasizes the significance of psychological health in the overall recovery process (Yang *et al.*, 2022). It also demands consideration of the wider implications of liver transplantation to include ethical debate concerning ethical issues regarding organ allocation in ALD patients.

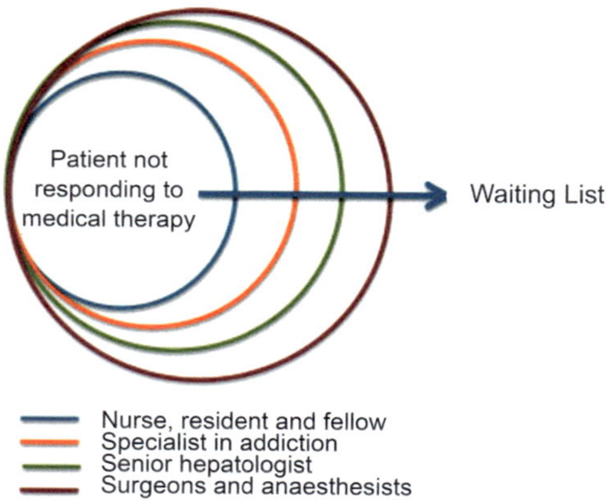

Figure 6.12. Selection process for liver transplantation of patients with alcoholic hepatitis not responding to medical therapy according to the four decision-making circles.

Source: https://www.researchgate.net/profile/Florent-Artru/publication/291553488/figure/fig2/AS:321238154137601@1453600552156/Selection-process-for-liver-transplantation-of-patient-with-alcoholic-hepatitis-not.png.

The perception of alcohol-related illness as self-induced raises ethical issues regarding whether or not it is ethical to prioritize such patients for transplantation. Disparities in access to transplantation can become intense, especially when they are viewed in terms of health and socioeconomic differences among them. Interventions to streamline transplant eligibility criteria without violating ethical standards are necessary to provide equitable access to liver transplantation. This emerging literature emphasizes the need for ongoing research and policy development that recognizes both medical and ethical complexities inherent in ALD care and the promise of transplantation as a therapeutic option (Maestri *et al.*, 2023) (Figure 6.12).

6.5. Complications of Alcoholic Liver Disease (ALD)

The problems caused by ALD usually show up as hepatic and extrahepatic conditions that increase both the sickness and the death rate. A very serious result is LC, in which the normal liver tissue is replaced by scar tissue, which reduces the liver's ability to function properly. HCC is more likely to occur in patients with cirrhosis, which makes managing their care more difficult. Also, the build-up of neurotoxic substances such as ammonia can cause HE to develop. People with this condition may become confused, lose consciousness, or even fall into a coma, which reveals how critical ALD is and requires immediate treatment. Because these problems are so varied, it is clear that alcohol, liver health, and the body's overall health are closely linked, so treatment should focus on both liver and systemic health concerns. Besides the other complications of ALD, those with the condition are at greater risk for CVDs. Such a relationship is likely because ALD patients often have IR and dyslipidemia, which are metabolic issues. Because of the inflammation and scarring in the liver, the risk of hypertension and coronary artery disease can increase significantly. In addition, people with metabolic syndromes together with liver disease have a harder time, since these diseases can work together to impair liver function and increase the risk of NAFLD. The overlap between ALD and cardiovascular disease accentuates the critical role of a holistic approach to treatment, where managing lifestyle factors, such as diet and physical activity, is emphasized to mitigate the risk of systemic complications associated with ALD (Bagriy *et al.*, 2021; Wilkhoo *et al.*, 2024). In addition, people with ALD often have psychiatric disorders as complications. It has been found through research that drinking alcohol for a long period can cause depression and anxiety. Alcohol dependency tends to be a repeating problem, which makes it harder for people to manage themselves and follow treatment plans. Some patients drink more alcohol to reduce psychological stress, which only makes their liver problems and other health issues worse. Consequently, mental health support becomes integral to holistic management. When counseling and social support are part of treatment, the results for people with ALD may be better. Taking care of both the body and mind is very important for helping patients recover and reducing the chance of future complications from ALD.

6.5.1. Risk of Liver Cancer

The relationship between ALD and the progression of liver cancer is a critical one to research because chronic alcohol consumption is a leading cause of liver disease development. Chronic alcohol consumption can lead to NAFLD and cirrhosis, both of which are known to be precursors for HCC, or hepatocellular carcinoma, the most common form of liver cancer. Epidemiological studies show that patients with cirrhosis, especially alcohol-related cirrhosis, are at a very high risk of developing liver cancer in the long term. Chronic inflammation and cellular damage cause an environment that is permissive to cancer development, so it is worth exploring the complex nature of alcohol consumption and oncogenesis in the liver. Nutritional factors bring another level of complexity to ALD and susceptibility to liver cancer. Current studies have indicated that dietary habits may influence the onset of liver ailments, including cirrhosis and later-stage HCC. Individuals following a Western dietary pattern—high in red meat and processed food intake—are said to be at a significantly elevated risk of contracting these ailments. Notably, participants in the high tertile of a Western-type dietary pattern scored high for a heightened risk, as findings revealed an 18% increased risk of liver cancer compared to those with more healthful diets. In contrast, high prudent dietary intake characterized by large amounts of cereals and fruits was associated with low incidence of cirrhosis, thus potentially lowering the risk of liver cancer (Guo *et al.*, 2022). Furthermore, the role of NAFLD in cancer risk cannot be overemphasized. Though it is mostly linked to metabolic syndrome and obesity, NAFLD has been proven to be a huge risk factor for various types of cancers, including liver and pancreatic cancer. It was revealed by a nationwide cohort that those diagnosed with NAFLD had an increased risk of pancreatic cancer, with potential for similar associations between NAFLD and liver cancer. The connection points to the liver disease as a condition of high health complexity that is multifactorial. Here, eating habits, obesity, and chronic liver inflammation come together to enhance cancer risk (Joo-Park *et al.*, 2022). These findings necessitate an overall process in prevention and early intervention strategies to stem both liver disease and cases of carcinoma.

6.5.2. Development of Portal Hypertension

The development of portal hypertension is very important in ALD, since it happens when the liver damage worsens. Because drinking alcohol causes liver inflammation, fat to build up, and finally leads to cirrhosis, these changes within the liver make it hard for blood to flow normally. Because of this increased resistance, the portal veins become hypertensive, which is a dangerous condition. In particular, the changes in the body due to portal hypertension may make liver problems worse and raise the risk of complications like variceal hemorrhage and ascites. Because of this relationship, it is important to catch and address portal hypertension early to avoid these harmful outcomes which demonstrates its main role in ALD. Besides the high pressure in the portal system, portal hypertension also influences the gut-liver axis which consists of both the liver and the gastrointestinal system. A common feature of advanced liver disease is increased permeability of the intestines, which lets bacteria and toxins move from the gut to the blood, making the liver disease worse. If chronic liver injury worsens due to portal hypertension, there is a higher risk of bacteria moving from the gut to the blood, which can cause SBP.

This close relationship points out that portal hypertension in ALD is complex, highlighting the need for treatments that improve the liver and the gastrointestinal tract, which supports better care and results for patients. Managing portal hypertension and its related problems is now given more importance in current medical practice. New diagnostic tools now help detect portal hypertension and cirrhosis early, which makes it possible to treat the disease early and potentially slow its progression. In addition, new medicines designed to manage the changing blood flow in the liver are giving hope for better care of portal hypertension. Treating the cause of ALD, which is too much alcohol, is important for patients to see improvement in their cirrhosis and portal hypertension. As research continues to evolve in this area, the emerging understanding of the relationship between gut health and liver function, alongside innovative treatment modalities, provides a pathway for more effective management of the complications of portal hypertension, ultimately enhancing patient health outcomes in ALD (Berzigotti, 2017; Nicoletti *et al.*, 2019).

6.5.3. Impact on Mental Health and Social Well-Being

The connection between ALD and mental health is profound, and increasingly, there is evidence indicating that those diagnosed with ALD tend to have severe mental health problems. Such problems can be depression, worry, and heightened stress levels due to the physical alteration and compromised well-being arising from extended consumption of alcohol. The ongoing worry of health deterioration, coupled with the stigmatizing effect of alcohol abuse, contributes to the emotional burden faced by victims. Additionally, neurobiological changes related to dysfunctions of the liver are responsible for mood and cognitive disturbances, further making it difficult for affected individuals to socialize and maintain relationships.

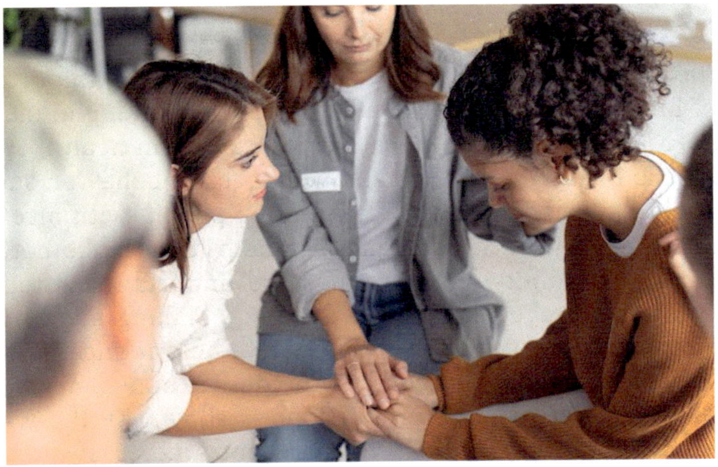

Figure 6.13. Support

Source: https://sunhouston.com/wp-content/uploads/2023/12/signs-of-liver-damage-from-alcohol.jpg.

As noted by research, such a connection between the health of the liver and mental well-being calls for a type of therapy that addresses both physical and psychological aspects of ALD towards ensuring comprehensive rehabilitation. Social well-being is also impacted by the effects of ALD, primarily due to the stigma and social rejection experienced by persons with this disorder. The cultural perspective of alcoholism will lead to exclusion and the loss of support from peers and community institutions. Alienation can cause shamefulness and worthlessness, further exacerbating the psychological impairment characteristic of the disease. Beyond that, social impact extends into family dynamics as relationship tension can lead to conflict, communication disruptions, and eventually a breakdown of family relationships. Social support, in this case, is an important factor for their rehabilitation, but individuals afflicted with ALD are likely to be isolated from healthy social interaction, again draining their mental capacity (Hou *et al.*, 2022). Detection of these factors is crucial to meaningful interventions that not only treat the physical state but also increase the scope of social contact and support networks. The interdependent nature of social well-being, mental health, and ALD emphasizes multidisciplinary care. Treating these interrelated issues requires healthcare providers to establish settings that foster open discussion about mental health in relation to liver health. By incorporating mental health services into standard medical treatment of ALD, healthcare providers can significantly improve the quality of life of those with these disorders. It must involve counseling, support groups in the community, and education on coping strategies unique to each patient's challenges. In addition, stigma awareness reduction campaigns can promote a more hospitable environment, allowing communities to embrace and comprehend. As is reflected in the majority of research, controlling mental health conditions that accompany ALD not only enhances the outcomes for patients but also contributes to more integrated and effective treatment strategies (Visseren *et al.*, 2021) (Figure 6.13).

6.6. Prevention Strategies

Various methods are used to stop ALD, such as individual actions, community efforts, and changes in policies to address the risks of drinking too much alcohol. It is very important for each person to learn about the risks of binge drinking and the advantages of drinking in moderation. Educational campaigns can highlight how drinking too much alcohol can harm health, especially the liver, and how important it is to make healthy choices. Making changes in behavior, such as setting drinking limits and joining support groups, can be very helpful for people with alcohol dependency. Also, helping at-risk people through outreach programs can help them make better choices and lower the number of ALD cases. Community-based actions are important in stopping ALD by making sure there are places that encourage responsible drinking. Making more events without alcohol and providing better mental health support have proven to help reduce how much alcohol people consume. Also, joining efforts with local healthcare providers to spot signs of alcohol misuse allows for early action. The value of these community actions is shown by the way alcohol use relates to many health issues. For instance, findings from recent studies suggest that conditions like NAFLD often correlate with excessive alcohol consumption, highlighting a need for comprehensive approaches to prevention that address multiple health issues simultaneously (Bazargaliyev *et al.*, 2025). If community leaders, local businesses, and healthcare providers are involved, the message can spread further and help the community change for the better. Strategies made at the policy level are important for handling the factors in society that lead to alcohol consumption and ALD. Tougher alcohol advertisement rules, higher taxes on alcohol, and setting minimum drinking ages have all been successful in cutting down alcohol use in different groups. Also, it is important to have integrated prevention programs that help people change their lifestyles. These programs should aim to address the rising incidence of comorbidities, such as obesity and metabolic syndrome, which are linked to alcohol misuse and liver disease (Demarquoy, 2025). Promoting healthcare policies that stress the role of the liver and the dangers of drinking alcohol can greatly reduce the number of ALD cases and enhance general public health.

6.6.1. Public Health Initiatives and Education

Effective public education and programs are critical to the prevention of ALD, in large measure, through heightened awareness of the risks of alcohol abuse. Through designated campaigns, clinicians can disseminate vital information regarding alcohol consumption and its effect on one's health with regard to possible harm to the liver, through evidence-based strategies, such as mass media and community workshop interventions, public health professionals can address different populations. These initiatives, apart from sensitizing individuals to the dangers of ALD, also encourage healthier lifestyles through education on restricted alcohol consumption and the need for alcohol addiction assistance. These initiatives strive to create an informed population that has knowledge of the relationships between life patterns and illnesses, especially with the rising incidence of fatty liver disease, such as Alcoholic Fatty Liver Disease (AFLD). In addition, health education in the public sphere must tackle the overall social determinants of ALD. The understanding that alcohol consumption is usually linked with socioeconomic status, cultural values of drinking, and mental disorder is required when designing effective interventions. The community leaders and the public health professionals must collaborate to create programs tailored to the values and beliefs of the community towards alcohol consumption. Also, such programs must be aimed at younger ages due to the staggering rate of increasing diagnosis among young adults and adolescents, as estimated in Zhang M *et al.* (2025). By creating an atmosphere of healthy discussion on alcohol consumption, families can play a crucial role in shaping youths' attitudes and behavior towards drinking. Constant production and utilization of culturally appropriate educational materials are imperative for prevention as well as perhaps stopping the development of ALD in high-risk groups. Incorporation of prevention interventions into public health programs is important in reducing the prevalence of ALD among the general population. Screening programs can be coordinated in the primary care centers and community health fairs to identify high-risk individuals and refer them to appropriate interventions. In addition, educational materials that outline the symptoms and complications of ALD can enable patients to seek medical care early, which is essential for proper treatment and management. To complement these efforts, medical professionals need to be trained on the warning signs of ALD as well as how to brief patients who have unhealthy drinking patterns. By implementing a multi-component response of education, screening, and tailored support, public health initiatives can effectively counteract the impact of ALD and improve liver health outcomes in many individuals, ultimately leading to an improved population.

6.6.2. Role of Support Groups and Counseling

Being part of a support group or receiving counseling is very important for recovery and better patient outcomes in ALD. These programs give people facing the effects of alcohol use a caring group where they can discuss what they go through and how they manage it. Support groups allow people to feel less alone, be more responsible, and follow their treatment plans. Participation in these groups seems to help patients stay sober, which is important for ALD because many patients experience depression and anxiety as a result of their condition. Hence, including support systems in treatment plans helps patients deal with their disease and gradually improve their lives. Counseling services add to the support groups by giving specific therapy that helps with the emotional and psychological side of addiction. Professionals with training can help patients manage their alcohol use and choose better ways to cope. Counseling can also assist people in handling any feelings of guilt, shame, or loss related to ALD, which can slow down their recovery. According to studies, having both peer support and professional counseling helps patients deal with the physical and emotional aspects of ALD treatment. Using this dual method helps patients recover faster and become stronger, so they have the skills to handle any setbacks and avoid relapses. In healthcare as a whole, including support groups and counseling in the management of ALD, is very important. Even though doctors and nurses pay attention to the liver and nutrition, the psychological part of the disease should not be ignored. For instance, as highlighted in Ford *et al.* (2007), vulnerable populations facing co-occurring challenges, such as mental health disorders, may benefit profoundly from community support and structured counseling programs. They are vital for improving traditional healthcare and handling the many needs of patients. Ultimately, fostering a network of support can lead to improved health outcomes, thereby reinforcing the importance of holistic treatment approaches in effectively managing ALD (Figure 6.14).

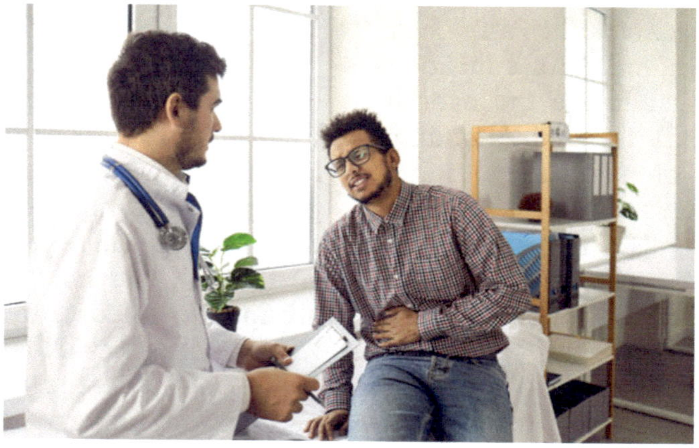

Figure 6.14. Counseling play a crucial role in fostering recovery and enhancing patient outcomes.

Source: https://t4.ftcdn.net/jpg/06/33/44/99/360_F_633449968_FEKhuguJjo7fLbqIj0XP6bZobzS05UdW.jpg.

6.6.3. Importance of Responsible Drinking

Moderate consumption is a vital factor in minimizing the risk of ALD. Consumption of alcohol, as it is practiced in most cultures, can have significant health effects if excessively consumed. Liver disease is estimated to be responsible for approximately two million deaths annually, and this points to the serious connotations that come with excess consumption of alcohol (Devarbhavi *et al.*, 2023). The liver also metabolizes alcohol, and excessive intake can lead to diseases such as alcoholic hepatitis and cirrhosis, which are generally not reversible. With moderate drinking, the risk of such fatal diseases can be effectively reduced. Apart from that, awareness campaigns promoting moderation can also induce a shift in the social norm toward drinking, promoting a culture of valuing health over social pressure. Comprehending the far-reaching effect of responsible drinking goes beyond one's personal health; it also accounts for societal and family welfare. Excessive drinking not only impairs the personal drinker but disproportionately burdens families and healthcare systems as well. Heavy drinking is more likely to lead to higher healthcare spending on the treatment of ALD, thus overloading public resources, particularly in healthcare institutions that are already strained in dealing with increasing numbers of liver complications (Devarbhavi *et al.*, 2023). Further, the resultant social stigma associated with heavy drinking is likely to hinder family relationships and lead to a culture of disregard for mental well-being. Through encouraging responsible drinking, communities can address the incidence of these problems, creating a ripple effect that maximizes overall societal health and robustness. In addition, gender and biological considerations also have an important role to play in determining alcohol's influence on people, calling for a sophisticated strategy for responsible drinking. Research indicates that differences in sex and gender have a profound effect on both the consequences of alcohol consumption and alcohol-related disease development, including liver diseases. For instance, women metabolize alcohol differently from men and, therefore, are at higher risk of acquiring liver damage with equal consumption of alcohol.

Thus, education and campaigns should be planned in a manner such that these disparities are considered, so that both men and women understand their risks. Highlighting responsible alcohol consumption considering these disparities, we can ensure a more holistic strategy that suits the heterogeneous needs of people, creating a culture of responsibility in the context of alcohol use and its impact on liver function.

SUMMARY

The study of ALD does depict a dynamic interaction between alcohol consumption and the liver's detoxification capacity for poisons. Awareness of heavy drinking effects is the prevention and treatment of ALD. As found in medical literature, recent studies emphasize lifestyle modification, including reduced alcohol consumption, as a means of lowering disease progression risk. In addition, new pharmacotherapeutic agents could potentially be beneficial for the treatment and reversal of liver injury in vulnerable populations, and it is thus indicated that the condition, though grave, is not impossible to overcome. The results highlight the importance of continuous education and awareness initiatives, as a change in behavior alone would go a long way in determining the course of ALD. More recent investigations have also clarified the association of several lifestyle conditions and the risk of developing ALD. For instance, the rising trend of NAFLD and alcohol conditions indicates a broader spectrum to study in liver health. Besides alcohol, obesity and food consumption are also implicated in liver pathologies. The multifactorial etiology of the diseases necessitates an integrated model of practice in clinical care and in public health interventions. Understanding how various factors like sleep habits highlighted in studies linking daytime napping with metabolic disorders affect liver health can be utilized to guide intervention strategies aimed at restricting ALD cases, and this presents a need for integrated approaches to care that integrate nutrition, lifestyle guidance, and prophylactic measures (Hegazi *et al.*, 2024; Qiao *et al.*, 2024). Overall, addressing ALD requires collaboration between healthcare workers, patients, and policymakers. There is a critical need for additional funding to research efforts that will further illuminate the mechanisms and probable therapeutic targets of ALD. Interdisciplinary collaborations can lead to the development of effective treatment modalities and prevention measures that are evidence-based. Moreover, reaffirming the importance of public health campaigns in targeting the dangers of heavy drinking and promoting better lifestyle choices will play an important role in confronting the epidemic of ALD. Moving forward, the ongoing dialogue for ALD will need to remain dynamic, incorporating new data from studies and addressing the evolving challenges posed by this incapacitating disease.

The controversy over ALD exhibits a multifactorial interplay among many factors that determine the course and management of the disease. Foremost among these is the recognition of ALD as a spectrum of liver damage from fatty liver to cirrhosis and HCC. The etiology of the disease is primarily alcohol excess, but genetic predisposition, malnutrition, and co-morbid liver diseases contribute significantly to its development. Knowledge of the pathophysiological mechanisms, such as the contribution of inflammation and oxidative stress, is key to successful disease management. Prognostic data regarding patient demographics, such as age, sex, and comorbid conditions, underscores the need for tailored intervention strategies to correlate with individual risk profiles for improved treatment outcomes. In addition, the ethical challenges of liver transplantation allocation underscore a pivotal area of concern in ALD. The decision-making process for candidates for transplant is controversial, as it involves not only medical need but also lifestyle preference, particularly in patients with alcohol use disorder. This challenges such fundamental tenets of fairness and justice in the health system. As can be seen in the NHS Blood and Transplant authority's policies, the selection process must play on urgency and ethics simultaneously, inclining towards showing inherent biases against patients with diseases due to presumed individual choices, such as alcoholism. This brings a pertinent debate about whether healthcare systems can be moral when they are under-resourced, challenging ultimately whether a just assessment process can be guaranteed at all. Lastly, the creation of non-invasive biomarkers and diagnostic devices for ALD is an encouraging advance in treating liver disease. Utilizing new and innovative imaging modalities, including those that use hyperpolarized [$^{1-13}$C] dehydroascorbic acid (HP DHA) to quantify liver oxidative stress, represents a welcome shift from biopsies. These approaches provide greater room for observing disease evolution and response to treatment, thereby redefining patient management practices. However, with all these advances in technology, addressing core behavioral issues related to ALD, such as alcohol dependence, remains of paramount concern. A holistic strategy that includes medical, psychological, and supportive therapies is essential for long-term remission and improved quality of life in patients with ALD.

CLOSER LOOK

ALCOHOL DEHYDROGENASE (ADH)

ADH is a family of enzymes that catalyze the interconversion of alcohols and aldehydes or ketones, primarily involved in alcohol metabolism. ADHs are found in various organisms, including humans, and play a crucial role in breaking down alcohol and other compounds, including some drugs (Figure 6.15).

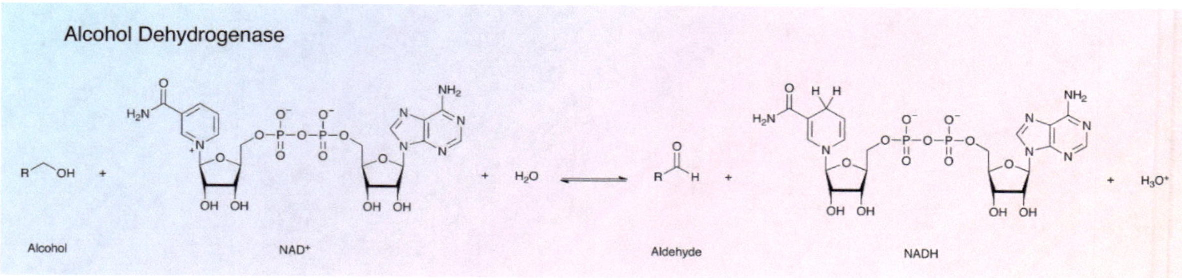

Figure 6.15. Alcohol Dehydrogenase

Source: https://www.worthington-biochem.com/sites/default/files/2022-02/ADH_reaction.jpg.

Key Functions of Alcohol Dehydrogenase

- **Ethanol Metabolism:** ADHs, particularly ADH1, are essential for metabolizing ethanol in the body, converting it to acetaldehyde, a toxic substance.
- **Drug Metabolism:** ADHs also play a role in the metabolism of various drugs and other chemicals containing alcohol functional groups.
- **Biotechnological Applications:** ADHs are of interest in biotechnology due to their ability to catalyze reversible oxidation and reduction reactions of alcohols, aldehydes, and ketones.
- **Detoxification:** ADHs are involved in the detoxification of ethanol and other potentially toxic alcohols, protecting the body from damage.
- **Fermentation:** In yeast, ADH is involved in the final step of alcoholic fermentation, converting acetaldehyde to ethanol.

Mechanism of Action

- ADHs catalyze the oxidation of alcohols to aldehydes (or ketones) by transferring a hydride ion from the alcohol to NAD^+ (nicotinamide adenine dinucleotide), converting it to NADH. This reaction can be reversed, allowing ADHs to also reduce aldehydes and ketones to alcohols.

Different Classes of ADHs

There are different classes of ADHs, with varying properties and substrate preferences, some of which are:

- **Class I ADHs:** These are found in the liver and are primarily involved in ethanol metabolism.
- **Class II ADHs:** These are found in the stomach and are less active in ethanol metabolism.
- **Class III ADHs:** [1-^{13}C] These are involved in the metabolism of other alcohols and drugs.

Clinical Significance

- **Alcohol Intolerance:** Genetic variations in ADH and aldehyde dehydrogenase (ALDH) genes can affect an individual's ability to metabolize alcohol, leading to symptoms like flushing, nausea, and alcohol intolerance.
- **Alcohol-Related Diseases:** ADH variants can influence an individual's susceptibility to developing alcohol-related diseases.
- **Antidote for Alcohol Poisoning:** ADH inhibitors are being explored as treatments for poisoning by methanol and ethylene glycol, which can be toxic byproducts of alcohol metabolism.

References

1. Alazraki, A., Jain, A. K., Wells, A., Hernandez, A., Towbin, A., Mencin, A., Sternberg, A., *et al.* (2018). Clinically actionable hypercholesterolemia and hypertriglyceridemia in children with nonalcoholic fatty liver disease. https://core.ac.uk/download/228066177.pdf (accessed on 24 May 2025).
2. Alisi, A., Alterio, A., Della Corte, C., Mosca, A., *et al.* (2015). Pediatric liver diseases: Current challenges and future perspectives. https://core.ac.uk/download/84688423.pdf (accessed on 24 May 2025).
3. Amini-Salehi, E., Hassanipour, S., Joukar, F., Daryagasht, A., Khosousi, M., Aleali, M. S., Ansar, M., *et al.* (2023). Risk factors of non-alcoholic fatty liver disease in the Iranian adult population: A systematic review and meta-analysis. *Hepatitis Monthly*. https://www.semanticscholar.org/paper/db521da8d598706d2e42eb6fbac0837310e3669b (accessed on 24 May 2025).
4. Andrezza Filgueira, C., & Liz Marjorie Batista, D.F. (2024). Relationship between non-alcoholic fatty liver disease and hepatocarcinoma: An integrative review. Archives of Clinical Gastroenterology.
5. Babu, D.S. (2025). Assessment of Pharmacological Interventions of Chronic Alcoholic Liver Disease and Their Clinical Outcomes. International Journal for Research in Applied Science and Engineering Technology. https://www.semanticscholar.org/paper/Assessment-of-Pharmacological-Interventions-of-and-Babu/f37a5aa83de5f28045ade7f1de7b5815e2e70965
6. Bagriy, A., Zubov, A., Khomenko, M., Mikhailichenko, E. S., Pylaeva, E., Khaustova, N. A., & Bryukhovetskaya, E. V. (2021). Patient management in non-alcoholic fatty liver disease and type 2 diabetes mellitus. *Russian Journal of Gastroenterology, Hepatology, Coloproctology*. https://www.semanticscholar.org/paper/8592e43f6e426e8bb554c9ba2f964c24fcfb6d49 (accessed on 24 May 2025).
7. Bazargaliyev, Sh. Y., Madenbayeva, A. M., Kudabayeva, I. K., & Rysmaganbetov, S. S. (2025). Non-alcoholic fatty liver disease and its relationship with metabolic syndrome: Modern approaches to treatment and prevention. *Farmaciâ Kazahstana*. https://www.semanticscholar.org/paper/c38138d4f8d1b37b21e0f427b36febfdd5931c78 (accessed on 24 May 2025).
8. Berzigotti, A. (2017). Advances and challenges in cirrhosis and portal hypertension. *BMC Medicine, 15*. https://doi.org/10.1186/s12916-017-0966-6.
9. Bok, R., Carroll, V., Di Gialleonardo, V., Keshari, K. R., *et al.* (2017). Hyperpolarized 13C spectroscopic evaluation of oxidative stress in a rodent model of steatohepatitis. https://core.ac.uk/download/323063388.pdf.
10. Cherkassky, L. (2011). The secret world of liver transplant candidate assessment. https://core.ac.uk/download/46170702.pdf.
11. Cho, N., Bae, H., & Lee, N. (2024). 15-Year Long-Term Follow-Up on the Progression to Liver Cancer in a Patient with Alcoholic Hepatitis Who Continued Drinking: A Case Report and Clinical Approach. The Journal of Internal Korean Medicine.
12. Demarquoy, J. (2025). Exploring the links between gallstone disease, non-alcoholic fatty liver disease, and kidney stones: A path to comprehensive prevention. *World Journal of Gastroenterology, 31*. https://www.semanticscholar.org/paper/d6fdb1dd6d0413576ff6e0870dd68bc41f7e4a79 (accessed on 24 May 2025).

13. Devarbhavi, H., Asrani, S. K., Arab, J. P., Nartey, Y. A., Pose, E., & Kamath, P. S. (2023). Global burden of liver disease: 2023 update. *Journal of Hepatology, 79*, 516–537. https://doi.org/10.1016/j.jhep.2023.03.017.

14. Dudinskaya, E. N., & Onuchina, Y. (2024). Non-alcoholic fatty liver disease and osteoporosis: A bi-directional association. *Problems of Geroscience*. https://www.semanticscholar.org/paper/9a6a164cef13be89452251d963a81e16c248ce71 (accessed on 24 May 2025).

15. Enciu, V., Ologeanu, P., Constantinescu, A., & Fierbinţeanu-Braticevici, C. (2025). Latest insights in alcohol-related liver disease and alcoholic hepatitis. *Romanian Journal of Internal Medicine = Revue Roumaine de Médecine Interne*. https://www.semanticscholar.org/paper/3c54418d8a44307d3d32670bfdadbedd6b1db1b0 (accessed on 24 May 2025).

16. Ford, J., & Cheong-Lee, C. (2007). The role of hepatology nurse in the difficult-to-treat hepatitis C population. *Canadian Journal of Gastroenterology, 21*(6), 353–354. https://www.semanticscholar.org/paper/064085cb34f9b875826545869742df174f9f44c9 (accessed on 24 May 2025).

17. Fuentes-Barría, H., Klahn-Acuña, B., Sepúlveda-Toro, D., Galaz-Cáceres, N., Aguilera-Eguía, R., & Alarcón-Rivera, M. (2024). Non-alcoholic fatty liver and periodontal disease in the adult population: Overview of systematic reviews. *Salud, Ciencia y Technology*. https://www.semanticscholar.org/paper/48a7dc7ca5184f7b56ddeb700373421bce8ccf57

18. G. Santos, E.R.R. Figueira, L.A.C. D'Albuquerque, P.B. Lisboa, M.D. de Almeida, N.A. Filgueira, et al. Ann Hepatol, 23 (2021), Evaluation of drug-induced liver injury as etiology for acute liver failure in Brazil. https://www.sciencedirect.com/science/article/pii/S1665268121000090

19. Guo, W., Ge, X., Lü, J., Xu, X., Gao, J., Wang, Q., Song, C., *et al.* (2022). Diet and risk of non-alcoholic fatty liver disease, cirrhosis, and liver cancer: A large prospective cohort study in UK Biobank. *Nutrients, 14*, 5335. https://doi.org/10.3390/nu14245335.

20. Haber, P., Liangpunsakul, S., & McCaughan, G. W. (2016). Alcoholic liver disease in Asia, Europe, and North America. https://core.ac.uk/download/141923190.pdf

21. Heerkens, L., Geleijnse, J., & van Duijnhoven, F. V. (2024). Dietary and genetic determinants of non-alcoholic fatty liver disease in coronary heart disease patients. *European Journal of Nutrition, 63*, 1847–1856. https://www.semanticscholar.org/paper/b423df0c779b5882b457436e5f304dc402c9b99c (accessed on 24 May 2025).

22. Hegazi, O. E., Alalalmeh, S. O., Shahwan, M., Jairoun, A., Alourfi, M., Bokhari, G., Alkhattabi, A., *et al.* (2024). Exploring promising therapies for non-alcoholic fatty liver disease: A ClinicalTrials.gov analysis. *Diabetes, Metabolic Syndrome and Obesity, 17*, 545–561. https://www.semanticscholar.org/paper/fc7caccb777ab99e2a63f6fce35c8764870ade80 (accessed on 24 May 2025).

23. Hou, K., Wu, Z. X., Chen, X. Y., Wang, J. Q., Zhang, D., Xiao, C., Zhu, D., *et al.* (2022). Microbiota in health and diseases. *Signal Transduction and Targeted Therapy, 7*. https://doi.org/10.1038/s41392-022-00974-4.

24. Ji, D., Qin, E., Xu, J., Zhang, D., Cheng, G., Wang, Y., & Lau, G. (2020). Non-alcoholic fatty liver diseases in patients with COVID-19: A retrospective study. *Journal of Hepatology, 73*, 451–453. https://doi.org/10.1016/j.jhep.2020.03.044.

25. Ktenopoulos, N., Sagris, M., Gerogianni, M., Pamporis, K., Apostolos, A., Balampanis, K., Tsioufis, K., *et al.* (2024). Non-alcoholic fatty liver disease and coronary artery disease: A

bidirectional association based on endothelial dysfunction. *International Journal of Molecular Sciences, 25.* https://www.semanticscholar.org/paper/79ee42b977e8a6f7933b6f951ff4310207cac74f (accessed on 24 May 2025).

26. Lee, H. R., Lee, S., & Joo, N. S. (2024). Efficacy of chelation therapy in hyperuricemia patients unresponsive to oral uric acid lowering agent. *Korean Institute for Functional Medicine.* https://www.semanticscholar.org/paper/f59001260506abf2bc3e2a601b3d9d1c68ebbdab (accessed on 24 May 2025).
27. Liao, Y., Liu, L., Yang, J., Zhou, X., Teng, X., Li, Y., Wan, Y., *et al.* (2023). Analysis of clinical features and identification of risk factors in patients with non-alcoholic fatty liver disease based on Fibro Touch. *Scientific Reports, 13.* https://www.semanticscholar.org/paper/92f06d4aa8615c6a4d40eab78cb66d6b8424d8c4 (accessed on 24 May 2025).
28. Liu, M., Jiang, X., Zeng, X., Guo, Y., Zhang, T., Fan, X., Xu, J., *et al.* (2024). A protective mechanism of heat inactivation to enhance *Levi lactobacillus brevis* PDD-2 against alcohol-induced chronic liver disease based on proteomic analysis. *Food & Function.* https://www.semanticscholar.org/paper/f3d58e97321e4267b79e4ab1aabb2c20472bd0a5 (accessed on 24 May 2025).
29. Lu, C. W., Yang, K. C., Chi, Y. C., Wu, T. Y., Chiang, C. H., Chang, H., Huang, K. C., *et al.* (2023). Adiponectin–leptin ratio for the early detection of lean non-alcoholic fatty liver disease independent of insulin resistance. *Annals of Medicine, 55,* 634–642. https://doi.org/10.1080/07853890.2023.2179106.
30. Luque Linero, P., & Castilla-Guerra, L. (2024). Management of cardiovascular risk in the non-alcoholic fatty liver disease setting. *European Cardiology Review, 19.* https://www.semanticscholar.org/paper/96af489a321edfa52863bb217468af115eda720b (accessed on 24 May 2025).
31. Maestri, M., Santopaolo, F., Pompili, M., Gasbarrini, A., & Ponziani, F. R. (2023). Gut microbiota modulation in patients with non-alcoholic fatty liver disease: Effects of current treatments and future strategies. *Frontiers in Nutrition, 10.* https://doi.org/10.3389/fnut.2023.1110536.
32. Maroto-García, J., Moreno Álvarez, A., Sanz de Pedro, M. P., Buño-Soto, A., & González, Á. (2023). Serum biomarkers for liver fibrosis assessment. *Advances in Laboratory Medicine, 5,* 115–130. https://www.semanticscholar.org/paper/2f56735826847fbc819426ab55a5b7888a21e3b6 (accessed on 24 May 2025).
33. Mauvais-Jarvis F, Bairey Merz N, Barnes PJ, Brinton RD, Carrero JJ, DeMeo DL, De Vries GJ, Epperson CN, Govindan R, Klein SL, Lonardo A, Maki PM, McCullough LD, Regitz-Zagrosek V, Regensteiner JG, Rubin JB, Sandberg K, Suzuki A. Sex and gender: modifiers of health, disease, and medicine. Lancet. 2020 Aug 22;396(10250):565-582. doi: 10.1016/S0140-6736(20)31561-0. Erratum in: Lancet. 2020 Sep 5;396(10252):668. doi: 10.1016/S0140-6736(20)31827-4. PMID: 32828189; PMCID: PMC7440877.
34. Mayr, H.L., Kostjasyn, S., Campbell, K.L., Palmer, M., & Hickman, I.J. (2020). Investigating Whether the Mediterranean Dietary Pattern Is Integrated in Routine Dietetic Practice for Management of Chronic Conditions: A National Survey of Dietitians. Nutrients, 12. https://www.semanticscholar.org/paper/Investigating-Whether-the-Mediterranean-Dietary-Is-Mayr-Kostjasyn/61936ce90e90560e05626aa5c91a11925344804d
35. Moon, A. M., Webb, G. J., Aloman, C., Armstrong, M. J., Cargill, T., Dhanasekaran, R., Genescà,

J., *et al.* (2020). High mortality rates for SARS-CoV-2 infection in patients with pre-existing chronic liver disease and cirrhosis: Preliminary results from an international registry. *Journal of Hepatology, 73*, 705–708. https://doi.org/10.1016/j.jhep.2020.05.013.

36. N/A. (2011). *Supporting Homeless People with Advanced Liver Disease Approaching the End of Life*. https://core.ac.uk/download/71364969.pdf (accessed on 24 May 2025).

37. Nicoletti, A., Ponziani, F. R., Biolato, M., Valenza, V., Marrone, G., Sganga, G., Gasbarrini, A., *et al.* (2019). Intestinal permeability in the pathogenesis of liver damage: From non-alcoholic fatty liver disease to liver transplantation. *World Journal of Gastroenterology, 25*, 4814–4834. https://doi.org/10.3748/wjg.v25.i33.4814.

38. Nucera, S., Bulotta, R. M., Ruga, S., Caminiti, R., Serra, M., Bava, R., Castagna, F., *et al.* (2023). Natural products for the treatment of non-alcoholic fatty liver disease: A comprehensive review. *Scientia Pharmaceutica*. https://www.semanticscholar.org/paper/6f2e0ed25afc5a773ad4b9001237e248ccf1c3ce (accessed on 24 May 2025).

39. Park, J. H., Hong, J. Y., Han, K., Kang, W., & Park, J. K. (2022). Increased risk of pancreatic cancer in individuals with non-alcoholic fatty liver disease. *Scientific Reports, 12*. https://doi.org/10.1038/s41598-022-14856-w.

40. Partsafa, M., & Panagiotakos, D.B. (2024). Non-alcoholic fatty liver disease and cardiovascular disease; from epidemiology to clinical and nutrition management: A narrative review. Journal of Atherosclerosis Prevention and Treatment. https://www.semanticscholar.org/paper/Non-alcoholic-fatty-liver-disease-and-disease%3B-from-Partsafa-Panagiotakos/a4dc3fa51045abdd736765279847ee40934c8223

41. Pirola, C. J., & Sookoian, S. C. (2017). Cell-free DNA methylation as liquid biopsy for the assessment of fibrosis in patients with nonalcoholic steatohepatitis: A gap between innovation and implementation. https://core.ac.uk/download/161784223.pdf (accessed on 24 May 2025).

42. Qiao, X., Wang, X., Guo, L., & Pan, Q. (2024). Excessive daytime napping increases the risk of non-alcoholic fatty liver disease: A meta-analysis and a Mendelian randomization study. *Nature and Science of Sleep, 16*, 1067–1074. https://www.semanticscholar.org/paper/c7ec27204bbd0f2edc485399da14438551bd4508 (accessed on 24 May 2025).

43. Robea, M.A., Balmuș, I.–., Gîrleanu, I., Huiban, L., Muzica, C.M., Ciobîcă, A.S., Stanciu, C., Cimpoeșu, C.D., & Trifan, A.V. (2023). Coagulation Dysfunctions in Non-Alcoholic Fatty Liver Disease—Oxidative Stress and Inflammation Relevance. Medicina, 59. https://www.semanticscholar.org/paper/Coagulation-Dysfunctions-in-Non-Alcoholic-Fatty-and-Robea-Balmu%C8%99/cfb7006c7edbb03d0e484ca6015ad8933db934a9

44. Savzikhanova, R.R., Subkhangulova, D.O., & Khazova, E.V. (2024). Hepatocardial relationships in non-alcoholic fatty liver disease: issues of epidemiology, diagnosis, prognosis. Kazan medical journal.https://www.semanticscholar.org/paper/Hepatocardial-relationships-in-non-alcoholic-fatty-Savzikhanova-Subkhangulova/7df28ddf57942543f6b9615696aa324718f59ff9

45. Shabnam, M., Venkateswarlu, M., & Vijayasree, A. P. (2023). The significance of transaminases and Deritis ratio for predicting alcoholic liver disease. *International Journal of Scientific Research*. https://www.semanticscholar.org/paper/28faa3ba286a7e8e14f678e67db249e4ba25cc3d (accessed on 24 May 2025).

46. Suresh, D., Srinivas, A. N., & Kumar, D. P. (2020). Etiology of hepatocellular carcinoma:

Special focus on fatty liver disease. *Frontiers in Oncology, 10*. https://doi.org/10.3389/fonc.2020.601710.

47. Torshin, I., Gromova, O., & Bogacheva, T. E. (2024). Systematic analysis of the relationship between non-alcoholic fatty liver disease and tissue iron overload: Promising areas for the use of polypeptide therapy. *Experimental and Clinical Gastroenterology*. https://www.semanticscholar.org/paper/8c96f8cf3e104c677d66305fed72097d58cf9c57 (accessed on 24 May 2025).
48. Vaz, K., Clayton-Chubb, D., Majeed, A., Lubel, J., Simmons, D., Kemp, W., & Roberts, S. K. (2023). Current understanding and future perspectives on the impact of changing NAFLD to MAFLD on global epidemiology and clinical outcomes. *Hepatology International, 17*, 1082–1097. https://www.semanticscholar.org/paper/a48400f594b4c93f3eab8ab0bfa08a0149a2f1db (accessed on 24 May 2025).
49. Vimalesvaran, S., Vajro, P., & Dhawan, A. (2024). Pediatric metabolic (dysfunction)-associated fatty liver disease: Current insights and future perspectives. *Hepatology International, 18*, 873–883. https://www.semanticscholar.org/paper/bd3f1099b9fe8ae7de34d0f8aac80a98df80f033 (accessed on 24 May 2025).
50. Visseren, F. L. J., Mach, F., Smulders, Y. M., Carballo, D., Koskinas, K. C., Bäck, M., Bénétos, A., *et al.* (2021). 2021 ESC guidelines on cardiovascular disease prevention in clinical practice. *European Heart Journal, 42*, 3227–3337. https://doi.org/10.1093/eurheartj/ehab484.
51. Wang, H., Sun, R., Yang, S., Ma, X., & Yu, C. (2022). Association between serum ferritin level and the various stages of non-alcoholic fatty liver disease: A systematic review. *Frontiers in Medicine, 9*. https://www.semanticscholar.org/paper/d70504d2bf5feb1921a680a866d37c2e9b40d1fd (accessed on 24 May 2025).
52. Wilkhoo, H. S., & Wilkhoo, H. S. (2024). Non-alcoholic fatty liver disease and its cardiovascular complications: Comprehensive analysis of its pathophysiology and management. *International Journal of Health Sciences and Research*. https://www.semanticscholar.org/paper/9265a9dd65e3f489933fb265ca4cdd9e3434decd (accessed on 24 May 2025).
53. Wu, Q., Li, P., Li, X., Ma, L., Chen, K., & Man, S. (2024). Pueraria extract ameliorates alcoholic liver disease via the liver-gut-brain axis: Focus on restoring the intestinal barrier and inhibiting alcohol metabolism. *Journal of Agricultural and Food Chemistry*. https://www.semanticscholar.org/paper/a05523800b344c4a4b306de3868e3b1954fe462d (accessed on 24 May 2025).
54. Yang, H., Ou, F., Chang, Q., Jiang, J., Liu, Y., Ji, C., Chen, L., *et al.* (2024). Physical frailty, genetic predisposition, and the risks of severe non-alcoholic fatty liver disease and cirrhosis: A cohort study. *Journal of Cachexia, Sarcopenia and Muscle, 15*, 1491–1500. https://www.semanticscholar.org/paper/3f7a0d29300c1c704378bbf6ba55d8ccaf21211c (accessed on 24 May 2025).
55. Yang, M., Liu, S., & Zhang, C. (2022). The related metabolic diseases and treatments of obesity. *Healthcare, 10*, 1616. https://doi.org/10.3390/healthcare10091616.
56. Zamani, D.A., & Syed, D.A. (2024). Pseudo-thrombocytopenia: A Comprehensive Overview with a Case Study of a 21-Year-Old Female with Non-Alcoholic Liver Disease. Scholars Journal of Medical Case Reports. https://www.semanticscholar.org/paper/Pseudo-thrombocytopenia%3A-A-Comprehensive-Overview-a-Zamani-Syed/ce130d405f52e75f64242a5f4cea72ffa277775d.

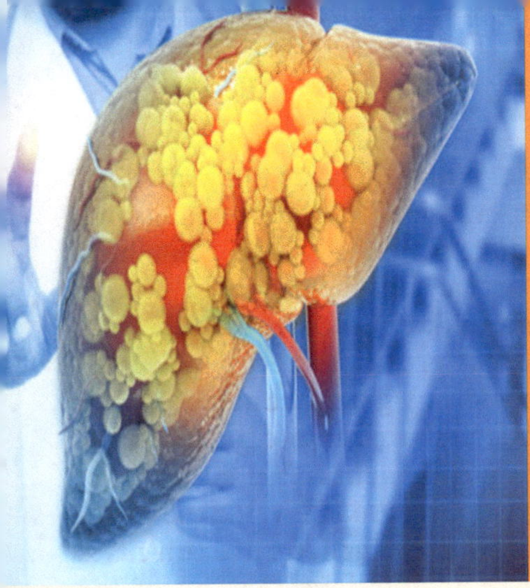

Chapter 7
METABOLIC AND GENETIC LIVER DISORDERS

Contents

Introduction

The complex interaction between metabolic and genetic disorders has gained increased interest in the background of liver pathology. As the liver plays a significant role in maintaining metabolic homeostasis, any form of disruption to its function can trigger a series of health complications like diabetes, fatty liver disease, and HE. Among the metabolic disorders, Type 2 Diabetes Mellitus (T2DM) is singular for its multifactorial nature of etiology caused by both inherited predispositions and environmental influences. The disruption of insulin signaling is particularly important, as highlighted in recent research, insulin metabolism abnormalities can have direct effects on liver function and intensify metabolic disturbances towards T2DM and other liver conditions. It is significant to understand these complex interactions in order to establish preventive as well as therapeutic interventions that can mitigate the risks of such conditions, and thus, research on metabolic and genetic liver disorders is not only significant but crucial. Moreover, genetic predispositions play a strong role in the etiology of liver disorders because they determine susceptibility to metabolic disorders at the individual level. Genetic mutations may interrupt the liver's metabolic activity and lead to several disorders, such as hemochromatosis and Wilson's disease, that may worsen disorders like IR and contribute to T2DM pathogenesis. The convergence of metabolic and genetic variables provides a unique setting for the understanding of the progression of liver disease and treatment. Current guidelines by the European Society of Cardiology and the European Atherosclerosis Society (ESC/EAS) accentuate the application of personalized risk assessments considering genetic and metabolic markers in formulating therapeutic plans. The integration of genetic research into clinical care is therefore imperative to address the complexity of liver health care management in the situation of metabolic disorder, which underscores the importance of an integrative approach. With the latest advances in genetics and molecular biology, the investigation of metabolic and genetic liver diseases has offered new avenues for study and therapeutic intervention. With our investigation of the multifactorial causation of these disorders, environmental factors as well as genetic determinants are no longer separable in the aetiology of these disorders. This convergence is not only the cause of the expression of symptoms but also for divergence of disease mechanisms among populations. Growing acceptance of these interconnected factors calls for a shift in the paradigm under which clinicians approach liver disease—focusing on prevention and individualized treatments informed by genetic factors.

Definition of Liver Disorders

A good grasp of the definitions of liver disorders is needed, since they cover a wide range of conditions that can seriously affect metabolism. Liver disorders are mainly either acute or chronic, and each type is further split by the different mechanisms that cause them. Most acute liver disorders happen rapidly because of viral infections, exposure to toxins, or problems with the immune system, and they can be treated effectively. However, chronic liver problems that develop over a long period might be caused by viral hepatitis, drinking alcohol, or metabolic syndromes, causing liver damage and possible complications like cirrhosis or HCC. Thus, knowing about liver disorders is necessary, both for treating each case and for the impact these conditions have on the health of the public, mainly related to metabolic and genetic factors that influence the liver. Genetics and the body's metabolic system meet at the point of metabolic liver disorders. Conditions such as non-alcoholic fatty liver disease (NAFLD) and hemochromatosis exemplify the influence of metabolic imbalances and genetic susceptibilities in liver pathophysiology. NAFLD, which means too much fat in the liver, is closely associated with obesity, IR, and dyslipidemia. In hemochromatosis, a disorder passed through families, too much iron is absorbed, which might harm the liver cells. According to studies, both disorders may influence cardiovascular and systemic health, and often the genetic background is the same. Understanding these metabolic liver disorders is essential since they illuminate the interplay between environmental factors, genetic makeup, and clinical manifestations, prompting the need for targeted therapies and interventions in affected populations (van der Meer *et al.*, 2024). Genetic liver disorders are another important group, and they are caused mainly by inherited problems in how the liver functions and metabolizes substances. Lysosomal storage disorders (LSDs), such as mucopolysaccharidosis, exemplify this group, arising from enzyme deficiencies that disrupt normal metabolic processes. Such errors in the liver can result in the buildup of toxic substances, which may cause the organ to not function properly and result in different health problems. As in other genetic diseases, early detection using genomic sequencing can discover the responsible variants, which may lead to new therapies for the gene.

New studies have found new genes and mutations responsible for lysosomal storage disorders, which underlines the importance of thorough genetic testing in different groups. By understanding the etiology and consequences of genetic liver disorders, healthcare providers can better devise management strategies and improve the long-term outlook for affected individuals (Gul *et al.*, 2023) (Figure 7.1).

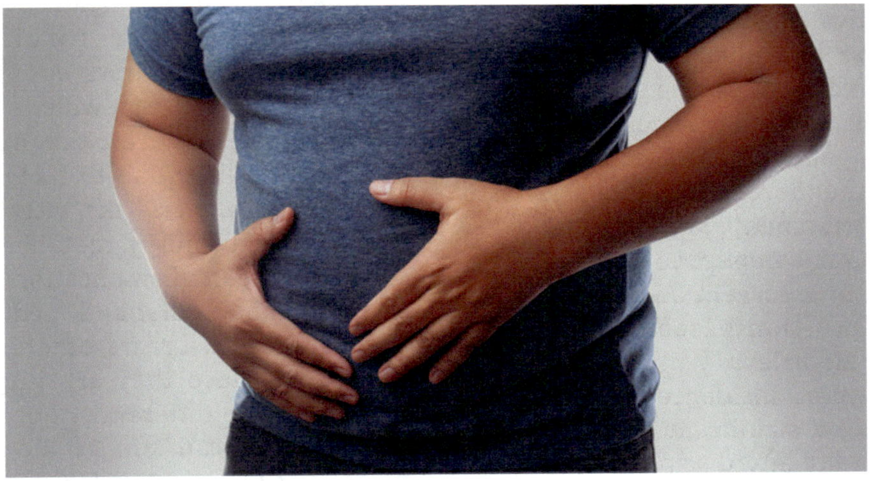

Figure 7.1. Liver disease

Source: https://www.gastroconsa.com/wp-content/uploads/2023/04/Fatty-Liver-Disease-Symptoms-870x488.jpg.

Importance of Studying Metabolic and Genetic Factors

Understanding the metabolic and genetic pathways of liver disease is valuable for several reasons that resonate throughout clinical practice and research. First, these pathways provide significant insights into the pathophysiology of diseases such as NAFLD and hemochromatosis. By examining the underlying metabolism, scientists can identify early biomarkers for diagnosis, as well as intervention targets, which can have significant implications for patient prognosis. Metabolic dysregulation that underlies these diseases indicates that research in these areas is not merely speculative but has practical implications for the development of targeted therapies. Furthermore, the linkage of genetic predispositions to metabolic disturbances can sustain the risk of liver disease, and this helps to underscore the requirement for a multidisciplinary approach to the management of these complicated diseases. Furthermore, analysis of genetic variation on metabolic pathways can inform about interconnectedness among lifestyle determinants and liver health. New research indicates that gene mutations can change an individual's response to diet, exercise, and body clocks, directly impacting the liver. For instance, understanding how specific genetic markers affect metabolism can be used to provide tailored dietary and exercise recommendations for individuals who are at risk of liver disease. This personalized approach is showcased in research focused on the relationship of sleep rhythms with metabolic well-being and suggests that scientists will need to factor in genetic and metabolic profiling in current liver disease models. Insights from such investigations have the potential to develop lifestyle interventions tailored to a person's genome, which would then result in better treatments and long-term health. The relevance of research in metabolic and genetic factors is equally applicable to public health, particularly in the prevention and intervention for liver disease. As obesity and metabolic syndrome become more prevalent, the need to intervene and address the root causes of these conditions is urgent. Research shows that how genetics and metabolism interact can inform more broad-based public health interventions aimed at reducing risk factors of liver disease. Collaboration between researchers in public health, genetics, and metabolism can make possible groundbreaking discoveries that enhance our understanding of liver pathologies as well as transferable implications for effective community health interventions. Specifically, genetic predisposition-based populations for metabolic disorders will undoubtedly contribute to lowered incidence rates for liver disease, reflecting a significant imperative for ongoing research and interdisciplinary research collaboration in this vital health science field (Arble *et al.*, 2015; Fu *et al.*, 2013).

7.1. Overview of Metabolic Liver Disorders

Grasping metabolic liver disorders is essential to see how liver diseases affect the health of the public. Because of these disorders, which involve metabolic errors, people may develop problems like fat buildup, scarring of the liver, and cirrhosis. Lipid metabolism, storing carbohydrates, and detoxification are some of the many metabolic functions of the liver. When metabolic pathways fail because of genetics or other causes, it can cause major problems with liver function. Consequently, early detection and intervention become critical, particularly in pediatric populations where many conditions manifest with subtle or atypical symptoms (Alisi *et al.*, 2015). Improvements in finding biomarkers and using imaging are helping doctors diagnose diseases early, which allows for prompt treatment. When we know more, the healthcare community can respond better to how metabolism affects the liver, which helps patients. There are many inherited metabolic liver disorders that show difficulties in both detecting and managing these conditions. Wilson's disease, which disrupts copper metabolism, and hemochromatosis, which results from too much iron, demonstrate the problems that can occur in the liver due to metabolic problems. Similarly, disorders like fatty acid oxidation defects affect energy metabolism, leading to significant health complications (Buckley *et al.*, 2011). Although diet and medication can help some of these disorders, others are still difficult to treat because they are very complex and often present differently. For instance, early interventions can still be life-saving in cases of urea cycle disorders (UCD), underlining the need for swift identification and management. The different ways these metabolic disorders present and develop highlight the need for more research to improve diagnostics and find new treatments that can improve how patients feel and their outlook. New treatments such as gene therapy may be effective in handling metabolic liver disorders that have a genetic cause. The potential of adopting approaches such as adeno-associated virus (AAV)-based vectors represents a significant leap in the field, offering hope for conditions previously deemed untreatable (Buckley *et al.*, 2011). Research on how to use gene therapy for newborns and fetuses could make it possible to correct genetic defects at an early stage, which could transform the way these disorders are handled. Even though some diseases are controlled by the use of drugs, gene therapy might offer a permanent cure. Such advances in treatments underline the role of innovation in managing metabolic problems, so the field of liver disease management could get more advanced as we learn more. Continued collaboration between geneticists, hepatologists, and researchers is essential to enhance therapeutic efficacy, paving the way for improved health outcomes in patients impacted by metabolic liver disorders (Figure 7.2).

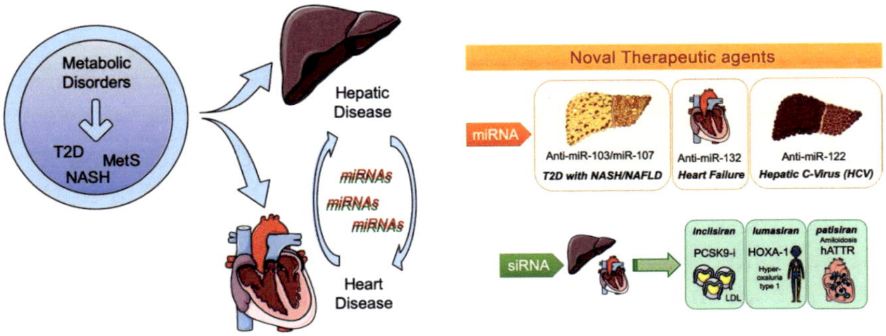

Figure 7.2. Metabolic disorders affecting the liver and heart.

Source: https://ars.els-cdn.com/content/image/1-s2.0-S1043661824000276-ga1_lrg.jpg.

7.1.1. Definition and Classification of Metabolic Disorders

Metabolic disorders constitute a broad category of diseases encompassing dysfunction in the metabolism of the body, which disrupts the normal biochemical processes necessary to achieve homeostasis. The disorders can be brought about by genetic mutations, dietary deficiencies, or environmental factors, leading to impaired cell functioning and accumulation of toxic compounds. The classification of metabolic disorders commonly has the sections of carbohydrate metabolism disorders, lipid metabolism disorders, amino acid metabolism disorders, and miscellaneous other genetic metabolic disorders. Each is distinct but interconnected, as impairment in one metabolic pathway can affect others, particularly in the complex context of metabolic networks. Identification of these categories allows healthcare practitioners to diagnose and treat these diseases effectively, especially in the case of genetic liver diseases, which primarily present as manifestations of underlying metabolic disturbances. Of the various categories, hereditary metabolic disorders, or inborn errors of metabolism (IEMs), are noteworthy due to their genetic origin. These illnesses are a result of enzyme deficiencies that disrupt normal metabolic processes, with resultant accumulation of intermediate substrates and eventual clinical presentation. These include phenylketonuria, galactosemia, and the glycogen storage diseases (GSDs), most of which are defined by liver dysfunction as a primary feature and exhibit significant growth- and development-altering effects in affected individuals. Since the liver plays such a key role in metabolic processes, it is the focus for comprehension of the consequences of these diseases. Therefore, accurate classification based on metabolic pathways not only educates disease etiology but also enhances the validity of therapeutic therapies and diet management regimens. Beyond genetic origins, environment or lifestyle-determined acquired metabolic disorders remain a crucial aspect of metabolic classification. Conditions such as type 2 diabetes mellitus (T2DM), NAFLD, and metabolic syndrome all demonstrate the manner in which lifestyle aspects can lead to significant metabolic derangements. They tend to result from an interaction between genetic susceptibility and environmental determinants such as diet and physical inactivity and are underlined by insulin resistance (IR), alterations in lipid metabolism, and increased inflammation. Clinically, the overlap of genetic and acquired metabolic disorders highlights the fact that the therapy must be holistic in nature, embracing lifestyle modification alongside drug treatment. The overlap between the two categories indicates the complexity of metabolic disorders and their far-reaching effects on liver function, necessitating further studies to define the interface of multifarious metabolic pathways in both hereditary and acquired contexts.

7.1.2. Common Types of Metabolic Liver Disorders

Metabolic liver disorders are conditions that mostly occur when the body cannot manage metabolic functions well, which causes fats, sugars, or other substances to build up in the liver. One of the most prevalent forms of these disorders is metabolic-dysfunction-associated steatotic liver disease (MASLD). Before, it was called NAFLD, and MASLD is marked by fat accumulation in the liver, even if little or no alcohol is consumed.

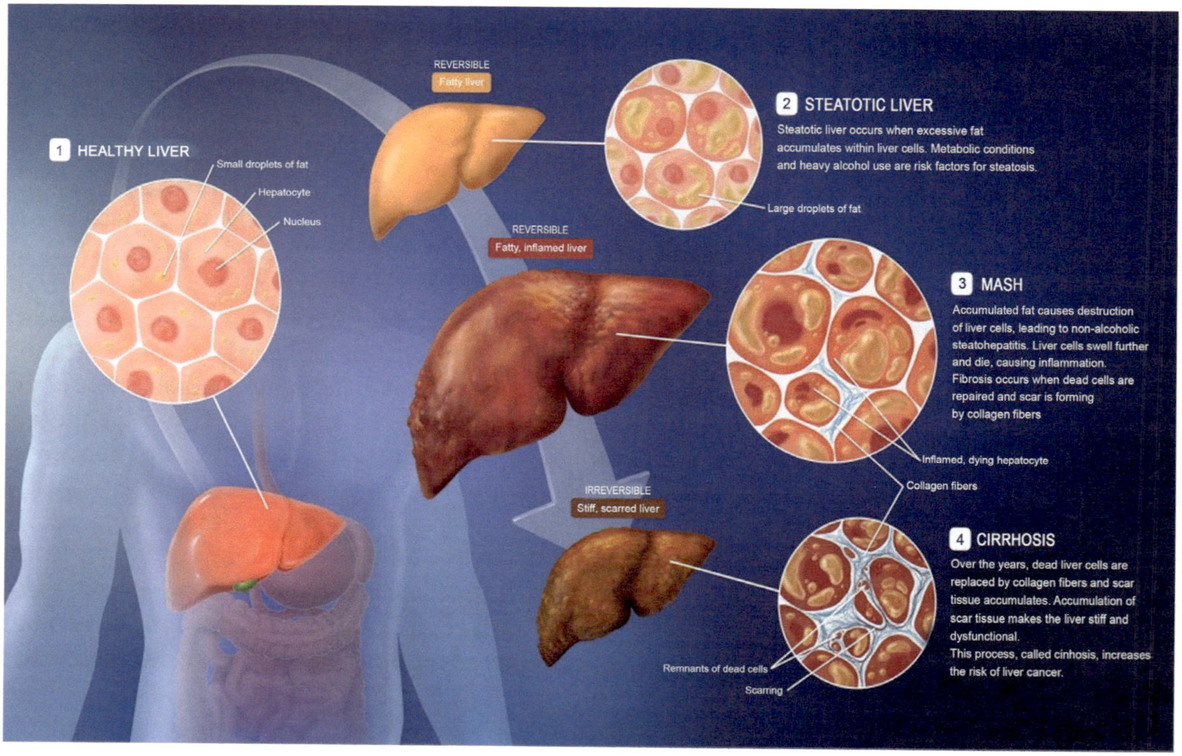

Figure 7.3. Metabolic-dysfunction-associated steatohepatitis (MASH).

Source: https://zymedi.com/wp-content/uploads/2024/01/unnamed-3-1024x666.jpg.

The presence of contributing factors such as obesity, type 2 diabetes, and dyslipidemia further complicates the condition, leading it to manifest as more severe forms like metabolic-dysfunction-associated steatohepatitis (MASH) and, in some cases, hepatic fibrosis, cirrhosis, or HCC. As obesity rates rise globally, understanding MASLD's multifactorial etiology has become crucial in mitigating its impact on public health, as highlighted by ongoing studies into genetic and epigenetic influences on disease progression (Mejía-Guzmán *et al.*, 2025). Another major metabolic liver disorder is hemochromatosis, which is passed down through families and causes too much iron to build up in the liver and other organs. Caused by genetic mutations, the most common being in the HFE gene, patients with hemochromatosis often experience a variety of symptoms, including fatigue, joint pain, and abdominal discomfort, eventually leading to complications such as liver cirrhosis (LC) and diabetes if not diagnosed and treated effectively (Figure 7.3).

The metabolic effects not only extend to liver function but also include changes in glucose metabolism and enhanced vulnerability to CVDs. Early detection via genetic testing and routine follow-up of serum ferritin levels can enable early intervention by means of phlebotomy or chelation therapy to debulk excessive iron and avoid potential liver damage. By bringing into focus genetic information, such as the heritability and metabolic pathways of hemochromatosis, researchers are better able to create more targeted treatment protocols (van der Meer *et al.*, 2024). Lastly, Wilson's disease is another fundamental metabolic disorder of liver function that results from an overaccumulation of copper due to a defect in copper transport. This autosomal recessive disorder is primarily found in children and adolescents, but in most instances may be symptom-free until later in life. Deposition of copper is the cause of hepatocellular damage, leading to liver failure and dysfunction. In addition to the hepatic manifestations, Wilson's disease is also characterized by neurological manifestations, rendering diagnosis on the basis of unpredictable clinical presentation challenging. Early intervention with the use of copper-chelating drugs such as penicillamine favors improved prognosis in patients and avoids progression to more severe forms of liver disease. Like in any other metabolic liver disease, it is advisable to know the genetic background of Wilson's disease in-depth that enables customized treatment planning and better patient care (Mejía-Guzmán *et al.*, 2025).

7.1.3. Symptoms and Diagnosis of Metabolic Disorders

It is very important to detect metabolic disorders early to reduce the damage they could cause to the liver and overall health. Often, these disorders show vague symptoms in children, which may make it difficult to diagnose them. Often, the symptoms of liver problems are not easy to spot, which can let the issue develop before it is noticed. For instance, CLD in children often does not exhibit pronounced symptoms in their initial stages, leading to delays in diagnosis and treatment (Alisi *et al.*, 2015). This leads to many undiagnosed cases, which shows that healthcare providers need to be more aware. Noticing the first signs—for example, tiredness, less appetite, or frequent abdominal pain—can be very important for quick action. Treatment is important for managing symptoms and also for improving the results of care for patients with metabolic and genetic liver diseases. A diagnosis of metabolic disorders is usually made by using clinical assessment, biochemical tests, and imaging techniques. After examining the symptoms, doctors usually perform blood tests to check liver enzyme levels, examine metabolic processes, and identify any genetic factors. When transaminases are found to be high in the blood, it may indicate that the liver is inflamed or damaged, so more tests are needed to find out the exact metabolic problem. The complexity of these disorders often necessitates a multidisciplinary approach, incorporating genetics experts and metabolic specialists, to ensure an accurate diagnosis (Bax *et al.*, 2020). Such teamwork makes it more likely to find rare illnesses that can look similar to common disorders. To treat effectively and prevent liver damage, an accurate diagnosis is essential. In addition, new technology and molecular biology have made it much easier to diagnose metabolic disorders. Techniques such as next-generation sequencing (NGS) have revolutionized the identification of genetic mutations linked to various metabolic syndromes, including liver-related issues (Bax *et al.*, 2020). With these advances, it is possible to look for genetic causes even when the symptoms are not typical or present in small amounts. For example, in disorders like mitochondrial neurogastrointestinal encephalomyopathy (MNGIE), where the clinical presentation may be diverse, genetic testing can clarify diagnosis despite initial ambiguity. Early recognition facilitated by advanced diagnostics can lead to timely therapies that modify disease progression, underscoring the importance of a proactive approach in clinical settings (Alisi *et al.*, 2015). Providing healthcare workers with the skills and tools to diagnose these conditions well can improve how patients feel and their overall health.

7.2. Genetic Factors in Liver Disorders

The genetic components of liver diseases are rendered complicated by their polyvalent presentations and the several metabolic pathways on which they manifest their impact. Out of the myriad of medical conditions affecting liver health, hereditary hemochromatosis (HH) represents a paradigm example of how genetic predisposition influences risk for disease. The disease results from mutations in the HFE gene that lead to aberrant iron accumulation in the liver and other organs. This iron overload leads to tissue damage and can induce complications like cirrhosis and HCC. The identification of the genetic etiology of such liver disease highlights the importance of personalized screening and intervention protocols.

The variation in enzyme activities, including alanine aminotransferase (ALT) and aspartate aminotransferase (AST), observed in different ethnic populations further implies that genetic backgrounds influence the liver's function and overall well-being, again proving the role of genetics in clinical assessment (Marjani *et al.*, 2016). Genetic factors significantly influence children's vulnerability to CLD, which continuously deteriorates their well-being and development. Pediatric liver diseases usually do not have early signs, which makes it difficult to arrive at an early diagnosis and results in an increased risk of serious complications like cirrhosis and HCC during adulthood. For example, Alagille syndrome, an inherited disorder involving the liver and other organ systems, exemplifies the significant role played by genes in liver architecture and function.

Genetic developments are now defining single mutations that underlie various conditions of the liver, allowing for early diagnosis and more effective management plans. Moreover, such developments are also emphasizing the need for improving our understanding of the genetic basis of liver diseases since they may provide novel therapeutic targets that could potentially make a real impact on patient outcomes (Alisi *et al.*, 2015). The interaction of environmental and genetic variables is also essential in the pathogenesis of liver diseases. For instance, people carrying some genetic defects may be asymptomatic until exposed to some environmental triggers, such as alcohol or viral infections.

This interaction presents challenges in risk prediction and requires extensive research that explores gene-environment interactions in the context of liver health. As noted in research conducted across ethnic populations, trends of variation in liver enzymes showing inherited susceptibility to liver diseases can be determined through inheritance. Introducing screening programs for targeted populations with family histories of liver diseases is thus important. Embedding genetic screens in standard clinical practice might not only enable early diagnosis but also guide tailored treatment regimens based on individual genetic profiles to maximize health benefits (Marjani *et al.*, 2016) (Figure 7.4).

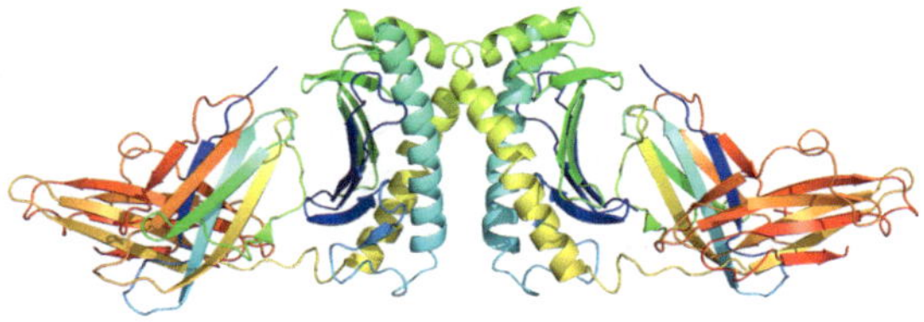

Figure 7.4. Structure of the HFE protein.

Source: https://upload.wikimedia.org/wikipedia/commons/d/d5/Protein_HFE_PDB_1a6z.png.

7.2.1. Role of Genetics in Liver Disease Susceptibility

Genetic factors play a pivotal role in determining an individual's susceptibility to various liver diseases, particularly metabolic-associated fatty liver disease (MAFLD). Several recent studies have found that PNPLA3, TM6SF2, and MBOAT7 are genetic variants that greatly increase the risk of hepatic steatosis and metabolic disorders. Diet and activity are believed to interact with these variants to make liver disease worse. For example, those with the PNPLA3 variant are more likely to have too much fat in their liver, which may harm the liver and result in steatohepatitis. Understanding the interplay between these genetic predispositions and lifestyle factors is crucial for identifying at-risk individuals and developing targeted interventions to mitigate the progression of liver diseases linked to IR and dyslipidemia, emphasizing the essential nature of genetics in liver disease susceptibility. Also, the way genetic background and metabolic stress interact demonstrates the many ways liver disease can appear. The existence of specific alleles may make people more likely to have dyslipidemia, which can then lead to and worsen MAFLD. For example, genetic factors can lead to atherogenic dyslipidemia, characterized by high triglycerides and low high-density lipoprotein (HDL) cholesterol levels, both of which are deleterious to liver health. Many times, this genetic susceptibility can only be fully seen when people are also exposed to environmental factors such as obesity or type 2 diabetes, which highlights how liver disease can have many different causes. As recent studies suggest, unraveling these relationships has significant clinical implications for prevention and treatment (Foster *et al.*, 2024). So, learning about these genetic interactions is necessary to create personalized ways to manage liver disease. Besides knowing about genetic variants, the overall effects of metabolic disorders on the liver should not be ignored. Obesity and diabetes can cause the liver to collect more iron, which makes liver-related complications worse. Because of the metabolic changes in these diseases, the body becomes more inflamed, which can harm the liver and lead to scarring. Having metabolic disorders and genetic factors can result in a variety of liver diseases, including steatosis, fibrosis, and cirrhosis. This interaction shows that a person's risk for liver diseases should be considered by examining both their genetic and metabolic factors. Consequently, leveraging genetic insights has the potential to inform clinical strategies aimed at early diagnosis and effective management of liver disorders, underscoring the critical role that genetics plays in understanding liver disease susceptibility (Foster *et al.*, 2024).

7.2.2. Inherited Liver Disorders and Their Prevalence

Inherited liver disorders comprise a diverse group of metabolic and genetic illnesses that have common pathophysiological mechanisms and clinical features. They are the outcomes of genetic mutation of enzymic activities crucial to liver metabolism, which cause the accumulation of noxious metabolites or disruption of essential metabolic pathways. For instance, conditions such as Wilson's disease and hemochromatosis illustrate how disturbance of copper and iron metabolism, respectively, can lead to extensive hepatic injury and systemic involvement. The clinical variability often causes challenges for clinicians, particularly in diagnosis in the broader context of metabolic disorders. Therefore, it is imperative to comprehend the genetic aetiology of such conditions to devise specific screening protocols and refine efficient management plans that can enormously improve patient outcomes. Inheritance of liver diseases is enormously heterogeneous across populations as well as geographical regions, depending upon several factors like genetic heterogeneity, environmental factors, and healthcare access. For example, some metabolic disorders occur more frequently in specific ethnic groups due to previous genetic drift or founder effects. While a comprehensive newborn screening policy has enhanced the detection of some metabolic liver conditions, effectiveness will be compromised if unresolved regional variations in incidence are not considered. Finally, most inherited liver disease remains underdiagnosed, particularly where less advanced metabolic screening schemes are available. It is also important to have a thorough understanding of the epidemiological patterns for these disorders so that concrete public health strategies can be made to address the identification and management of such patients in different populations. New advances in the discipline of metabolomics and genetic screening hold the potential for transforming inherited liver disorder diagnosis and the measurement of their prevalence. Techniques such as untargeted metabolomics facilitate the identification of a broader spectrum of metabolic derangements outside the limitations of traditional screening analyses that are limited to the targeting of a specific list of metabolites. These advances are instrumental in the enhancement of diagnostic accuracy and thereby facilitating earlier diagnosis and effective management of disorders that may not be overtly symptomatic until late stages. For instance, studies of disorders involving mitochondrial dysfunction, such as those for ATP synthase deficiency with specific genetic mutations, show the complexity of such diseases and the necessity for accurate, biochemically correct diagnostics (Bodamer *et al.*, 2010). More research in this field will undoubtedly yield surprises that could have a significant impact on the prevalence and understanding of inherited liver diseases, ultimately leading to better management of those affected (Fiehn *et al.*, 2019) (Figure 7.5).

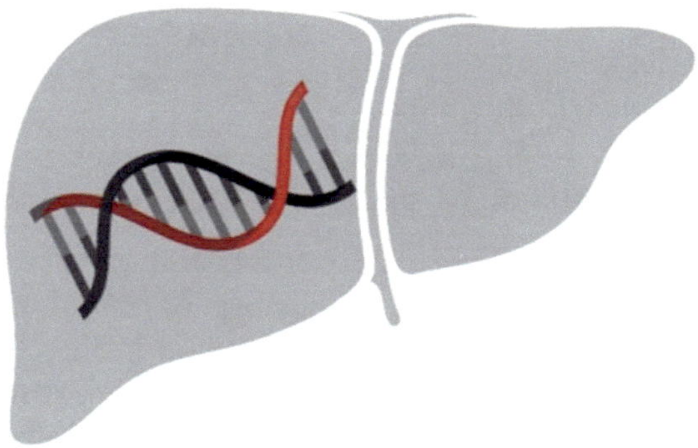

Figure 7.5. Genetics and liver disease

Source: https://med.stanford.edu/gastrohep/patient-care/liver-clinical-programs/inherited-liver-disease/_jcr_content/main/panel_builder/panel_0/panel_builder_1264095746/panel_1/image.img.full.high.jpg/H-Inherited-liver.jpg.

7.2.3. Genetic Testing and Its Implications

When genetic testing meets metabolic liver disorders, it has major effects on both medical care and patient support. Genomic technology is improving our knowledge of liver conditions, and genetic testing is very useful for diagnosing inherited metabolic disorders. For example, UCD is caused by genetic changes that make the liver unable to get rid of ammonia, which can result in serious health problems. In the case of sodium valproate-induced hyperammonemia, identifying the underlying genetic predisposition to urea cycle dysfunction can profoundly influence treatment strategies, warranting personalized approaches that mitigate risks and improve patient outcomes (Ahn *et al.*, 2018). So, using genetic tests helps doctors identify diseases correctly and provide treatments that fit the patient's genetic makeup and metabolism. As well as helping with diagnosis, genetic testing related to metabolic liver disorders can support preventive health planning. Knowing about a patient's predispositions, healthcare providers can take steps to stop the disease from getting worse. This is very important for diseases that are influenced by the environment, such as the effects of consuming high fructose on metabolic health. Research indicates that genetic variations can influence how different individuals respond to dietary inputs, highlighting the need for personalized dietary recommendations based on genetic testing outcomes (Ahn *et al.*, 2018). In addition, early identification of genetic problems using screening can give families important information about their health risks, which can help them plan for their family's health and make changes to their lifestyle to reduce the effects of genetic issues. Also, the ethical questions about genetic testing in metabolic liver disorders must be carefully considered. Matters like genetic privacy, the risk of discrimination, and effects on family members are major ethical problems. A person diagnosed with a genetic condition may experience stress, and this can also cause stress for family members who may be at risk as well. It is the job of clinicians to weigh the benefits of using genetic knowledge for treatment and prevention against the need to get informed consent and prevent misuse of genetic data. As the capabilities of genetic testing expand, developing clear guidelines and ethical frameworks will be essential to navigate the complex terrain of genetic information while maximizing its utility for managing metabolic liver disorders in a compassionate manner (Mehta *et al.*, 2018) (Figure 7.6).

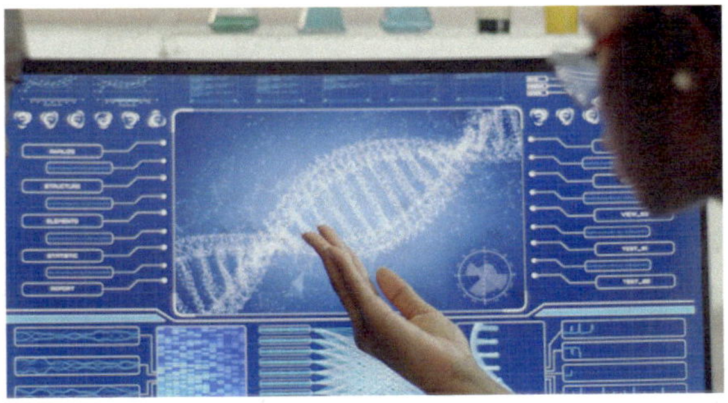

Figure 7.6. Genetic testing.

Source: https://www.cdc.gov/genomics-and-health/media/images/gen_testing.jpg.

7.3. Common Metabolic Liver Disorders

Shared metabolic liver disorders include HH, Metabolic dysfunction-associated steatotic liver disease (MASLD), and Wilson's disease. They are inherited conditions that affect the metabolism and processing of substances by the liver. Apart from NAFLD, another significant characteristic of metabolic liver disorders is metabolic dysfunction-associated steatotic liver disease (MASLD). This condition is not only prevalent in the general population but also associated with elevated risks for CVDs. Early diagnosis with timely therapeutic interventions can significantly decrease the risk of causing permanent liver damage, and consequently decrease liver-related and cardiovascular mortality rates. MASLD is often linked with overall metabolic disorders such as type 2 diabetes and extreme obesity, requiring comprehensive treatment. However, detection of the more uncommon types, such as familial partial lipodystrophy, is equally important due to their unique treatment protocols. Through the management of the nuances of various metabolic disorders, clinicians can improve the outcome of patients through the timely medical management. The management of metabolic liver diseases involves both lifestyle modifications and pharmacological treatment. Weight loss has been shown to improve liver histology in patients with steatosis; thus, nutritional counseling and training programs are a must in these patients' treatment regimens. Furthermore, pharmacotherapy may also include agents directed towards glycemic control and have a secondary effect on liver steatosis. The addition of new therapeutic strategies, such as leptin replacement therapy in some genetic diseases, has been valuable in improving outcomes of liver health. Further research into the treatment and pathophysiology of metabolic liver disease is important, particularly to establish the role of novel therapeutic agents. Thus, the region is increasingly evolving, with promising treatments and novel clinical tactics to treat the growing tide of metabolic liver diseases.

7.3.1. Metabolic Dysfunction–Associated Steatotic Liver Disease (MASLD)

Metabolic dysfunction–associated steatotic liver disease (MASLD) is a type of CLD. This condition is diagnosed when there is excessive fat build-up in the liver (hepatic steatosis), and at least one metabolic risk factor When there is also increased alcohol intake, the term MetALD, or metabolic dysfunction and alcohol associated/related liver disease is used, and differentiated from alcohol-related liver disease (ALD) where alcohol is the predominant cause of the steatotic liver disease. NAFL and NASH, now MASH, were used to show different levels of disease, and MASH indicates that the liver has additional inflammation. NAFL is less dangerous than NASH and usually does not progress to it, but this progression may eventually lead to complications, such as cirrhosis, liver cancer, liver failure, and cardiovascular disease (Figure 7.7).

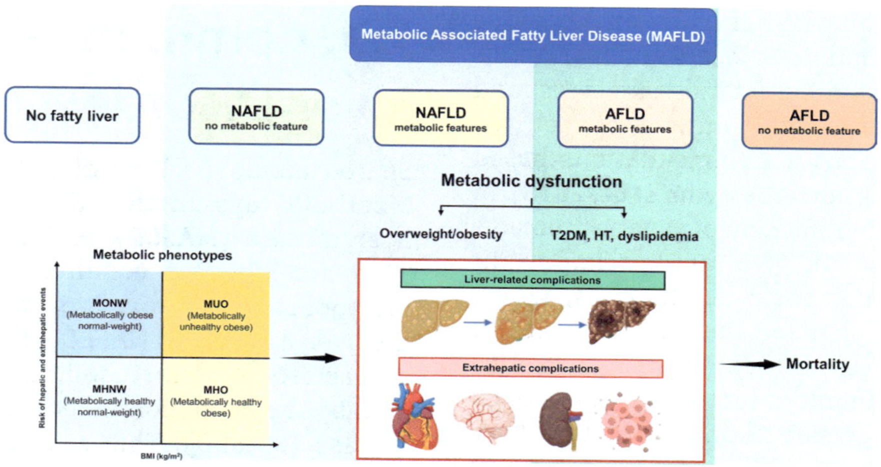

Figure 7.7. Metabolic-dysfunction-associated steatotic liver disease (MASLD).

Source: https://publinestorage.blob.core.windows.net/f2088594-c143-4702-91c0-6973e90f49c2/jcth-2022-00170s-g001.jpg.

Type 2 diabetes and obesity are important risk factors for MASLD. Overweight, metabolic syndrome (having three or more of the five conditions listed below: abdominal obesity, high blood pressure, high blood glucose, high serum triglycerides, and low serum HDL cholesterol), high-fructose diet, and older age are other risks. A liver biopsy sample after excluding other etiologies for fatty liver will confirm the diagnosis (Figure 7.8).

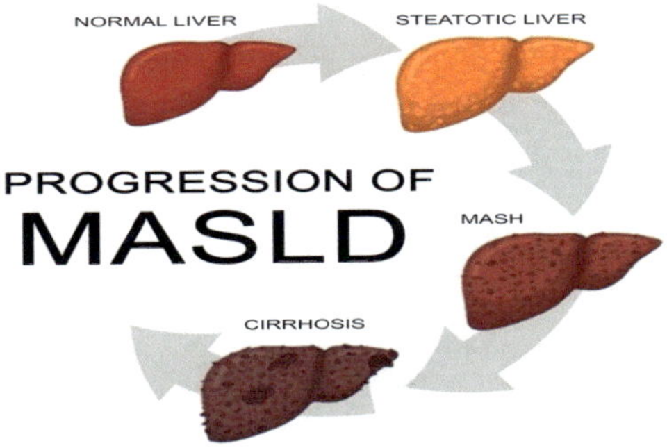

Figure 7.8. Progression of MASLD.

Source: https://www.insightsonindia.com/wp-content/uploads/2024/12/masld.jpg.

7.3.2. Hemochromatosis

Hemochromatosis, an iron overload disorder of the body, is a profound metabolic and hereditary liver disease. The most common one, HH, is an autosomal recessive disease caused by mutations in the HFE gene, specifically the p.C282Y variant. It is a result of genetic susceptibility that leads to uncontrolled dietary iron uptake, subsequently resulting in hepatic iron loading that could cause severe complications such as cirrhosis, hepatocellular carcinoma, and heart disease. Recent studies have explained the impacts of iron deposition in the varied organ systems, pointing out the neurological implications to accompany HH. An important observation demonstrates that male p.C282Y homozygotes experience increased prevalence of movement disorders, highlighting the need for early screening and intervention to avoid the intrinsic risks of iron overload and systemic consequences (Loughnan *et al.*, 2022). Furthermore, the interaction between iron deposition within the liver and other liver diseases underscores the intricacy of diagnosing and treating hemochromatosis. Most commonly, HH patients also have nonalcoholic fatty liver disease (NAFLD), adding to the complexity of the clinical presentation. This association requires close surveillance and evaluation of liver steatosis, as deranged metabolism of iron can further aggravate the underlying hepatic conditions. Imaging techniques such as multi-echo chemical-shift encoded MRI have emerged as crucial in quantifying both iron deposits in the liver and fat deposition. Such newer technologies provide physicians with the ability to accurately separate steatosis and iron deposition, allowing them to implement the correct management regimen according to each patient's requirements. The issues of hemochromatosis, therefore, must be comprehended and addressed by an interdisciplinary process involving genetic assessment, imaging, and medical management (França, 2021). In short, hemochromatosis is a significant example of how genetic and metabolic disease might cross over to impact liver functioning. From genetic mutations that target iron metabolism, the disease not only brings about pathology to the liver but also has far-reaching effects on the patient's quality of life. Identification of p.C282Y homozygosity as a causative factor underlines the significance of genetic screening in high-risk groups, facilitating early intervention by means of routine phlebotomies to control iron levels effectively. By raising awareness and knowledge about hemochromatosis and the risks associated with it, healthcare professionals can greatly enhance outcomes for those affected. Ongoing research into the pathophysiological mechanisms and treatment strategies will further enhance our capability to combat this disorder and its multifaceted implications within the area of metabolic and genetic liver disorders (Loughnan *et al.*, 2022) (Figure 7.9).

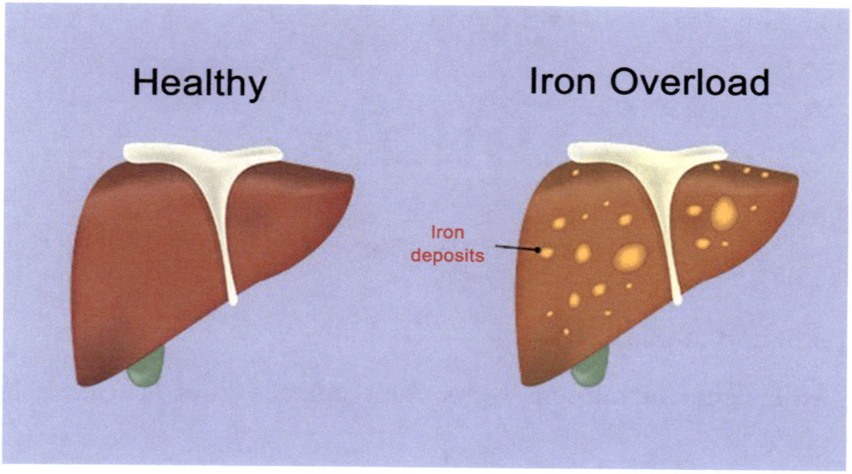

Figure 7.9. Haemochromatosis.

Source: https://images.everydayhealth.com/images/digestive-health/liver-disease/what-is-hemochromatosis-722x406.jpg?sfvrsn=a208bd22_1.

7.3.3. Wilson's Disease

Wilson's disease, which causes too much copper to build up in the body, is a major issue in metabolic and genetic liver disorders. A mutation in the ATP7B gene, which is required for copper transport, is what causes Wilson's disease. As a result, copper collects mainly in the liver, but it may also build up in the brain and other tissues, which leads to problems with the liver, brain, and mental health. Because untreated Wilson's disease can cause serious liver, brain, and health problems, early diagnosis and treatment are very important. Monitoring serum ceruloplasmin levels and liver function tests (LFTs) are essential in assessing the progression of the disorder, while specific genetic testing can confirm the diagnosis and facilitate family screening for at-risk individuals. Wilson's disease has effects on the liver as well as on other metabolic processes. Metabolic syndrome and diabetes are closely linked to the way diseases alter copper metabolism. It seems that when copper is mishandled, it may disrupt lipid metabolism and help cause fatty liver disease, as research on shared genes has shown. Wilson's disease and metabolic complications often affect the same patients, which raises the question of inflammation and oxidative stress as common risk factors for both. It has been found in research that links between liver diseases, such as Wilson's disease, and systemic metabolic dysfunction may explain how hepatic diseases can put patients at risk for cardiometabolic disorders, which calls for treating both liver and systemic health issues. Wilson's disease is managed by using both drugs and non-drug approaches to lower copper levels and stop damage to the organs. Treatment relies heavily on using chelating agents such as penicillamine, which help remove excess copper from the body through the kidneys. Also, zinc works as an important addition to treatment by reducing the uptake of copper in the gut. Still, since Wilson's disease is complex, patients need help from different specialists and should follow a special diet and regular checks for problems with the liver. As more data emerges, the interconnectedness of Wilson's disease with other metabolic disorders underscores the importance of understanding shared pathophysiological mechanisms, which may lead to innovative therapeutic targets for interventions aimed at mitigating the burden of liver-related health issues, enhancing overall patient outcomes, and highlighting the necessity of holistic patient management (Jadhav *et al.*, 2024; Wang *et al.*, 2025) (Figure 7.10).

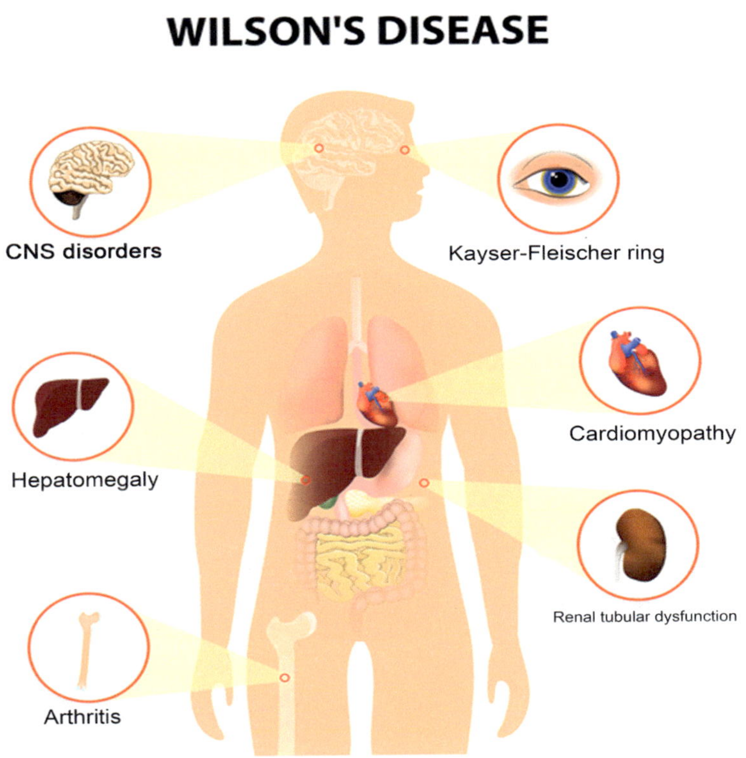

Figure 7.10. Wilson's disease.

Source: https://medlineplus.gov/images/PX0001BG_PRESENTATION.jpeg.

7.4. Genetic Liver Disorders

The intricate interaction between genetic and hepatic function has led to various genetic liver diseases, which manifest as a continuum of clinical syndromes ranging from asymptomatic elevation of enzymes to acute hepatic failure. The diseases are caused by some genetic mutations that impair the liver's metabolism of substances like fats, proteins, and carbohydrates. For instance, conditions such as Wilson's disease and hemochromatosis illustrate how the normal metabolic pathways are disrupted by genetic alterations to form toxic copper and iron deposits, respectively. Understanding these genetic underpinnings is not only crucial for early diagnosis but also crucial for tailoring treatment options to the individual patient as part of the wider drive towards personalized medicine for the treatment of liver disease. The connectivity of these genetic determinants to metabolic processes also underlines the need for further work in identifying potential biomarkers of risk determination and disease progression. The recent advances in genetic research have thrown light on the complexities of liver enzyme regulation, ascribing variations in such enzymes to more integrated metabolic and CVDs. Large genome-wide association studies (GWAS) with large biobanks, such as the UK Biobank, have revealed that numerous single-nucleotide polymorphisms (SNPs) are associated with plasma levels of liver enzymes. After replication of results with additional analyses, genetic risk for elevated liver enzyme levels has been demonstrated to be associated with increased risk for conditions such as coronary heart disease and IR. Identification of these genetic variants not only increases our understanding of liver physiology but also points to the potential application of genetic risk scores in predicting metabolic risks in humans. Further research into the molecular pathways controlled by these genetic factors may therefore offer novel therapeutic targets for the treatment of hepatic and metabolic diseases in a better manner (Alisi *et al.*, 2021). At the same time, the new field of gene therapy emerged as a promising method to treat a variety of genetic liver diseases, with promise for individuals who once had few options. The success of liver-directed gene therapy trials, particularly in hemophilia B, shows the therapeutic potential of AAV-derived vectors. Recent clinical trials have shown that one dose of these vectors can result in long-term improvement in the function of the liver as well as in the patient's general health. This achievement not only signifies the efficacy of gene replacement therapy but also sets a precedent for the treatment of other inherited metabolic disorders involving the liver. With continuous research, the phenotypes of enzymes and metabolism differentiated by unique genetic backgrounds will increasingly be held accountable for optimizing gene therapy success, paving the way for its routine use in clinical practice to treat monogenic liver diseases.

7.4.1. Alpha-1 Antitrypsin Deficiency

The significance of Alpha-1 antitrypsin deficiency (AATD) in the context of metabolic and genetic liver disorders cannot be overstated, as it exemplifies the intricate interplay between genetic mutations and organ-specific pathologies. AAT helps shield tissues from inflammation, and most of its deficiency comes from mutations in the SERPINA1 gene. Such mutations cause proteins to fold incorrectly, which collects in the liver and causes liver cell damage that may develop into cirrhosis. AATD also causes problems in the lungs, as the shortage of AAT allows enzymes to be active without control, and this often leads to emphysema. Because AATD affects both the liver and lungs, it is necessary to understand this to give affected individuals the best possible treatment and support, since it has wide-ranging effects on their health and life. Recent advancements in biotechnological methods, including the use of human induced pluripotent stem cells (iPSCs) and CRISPR-Cas9 gene editing, offer promising avenues for addressing AATD. iPSC technology makes it possible to create cells from individual patients for studying AATD in detail. They offer explanations for how the liver and lungs are damaged, which helps find new treatments. CRISPR-Cas9 gene editing allows for the correction of the genetic mutations behind AAT deficiency, which is a major step forward from simply treating the symptoms. Such innovations highlight the transformative potential of modern biotechnology to alter the landscape of treatment for genetic disorders like AATD, ultimately aiming to improve patient outcomes and alleviate the disease's burden on healthcare systems. Alternatively, there are still difficulties in managing and spotting AATD, which can cause delays or mistakes in diagnosing the condition. Lung and liver symptoms are common with AATD; nevertheless, it can also cause problems in other organs. This wider presentation highlights the need for clinicians to be more aware, because untreated AATD can cause damage to important organs that is often missed. Not paying enough attention to systemic complications can make it harder for doctors to recognize AATD, since they might mistake symptoms for something else. Thus, fostering a holistic understanding of AATD, inclusive of its effects beyond the liver and lungs, is critical for timely intervention and improved prognostic outcomes for patients suffering from this genetic disorder (Figure 7.11).

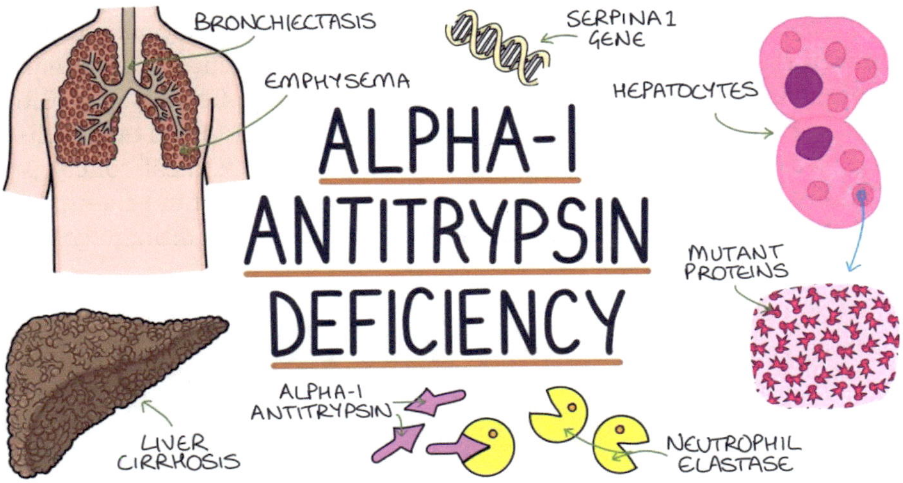

Figure 7.11. Alpha-1 antitrypsin deficiency.

Source: https://i.ytimg.com/vi/hrpNb3e869k/maxresdefault.jpg.

7.4.2. Glycogen Storage Diseases

GSDs constitute a heterogeneous group of genetic metabolic disorders with glycogen storage due to enzymatic defects in the metabolism of glycogen. The liver is predominantly involved in the disease with significant clinical manifestations such as hypoglycemia, hepatomegaly, and metabolic developmental delay. Among the various types of GSDs, Glycogen Storage Disease Type I is most unique due to its profound hypoglycemia and hypothalamic-pituitary axis abnormalities resulting in endocrine dysfunction and complicating patient management. These presentations highlight the necessity to take into account not only the metabolic manifestations of the GSDs but also the more general physiological manifestations that might follow in this patient population. There is a critical need for greater awareness and optimization in the clinical handling of GSD patients to minimize the numerous health complications experienced by such patients, as stated in earlier literature. Clinical management of GSDs entails a multimodal treatment protocol that encompasses dietary modifications, drug therapy, and regular monitoring. Diet management typically involves maintaining stable glucose levels through regular feeds with high amounts of complex carbohydrates, supplemented with cornstarch in cases where hypoglycemic attacks are to be prevented. Treatment itself, however, results in secondary complications, e.g., IR in GSDs I and III.

Thus, proper evaluation of each patient's regimen is necessary to improve their quality of life. Progress in gene-editing technologies, namely CRISPR-Cas9, presents promising avenues for contemplated treatments that could help solve the underlying genetic mutations responsible for such metabolic disorders. Such pioneering treatments need constant research and collaborative input from clinicians and biomedicine researchers to identify the pathophysiology of the conditions and refine treatment interventions to achieve the best results for patients. Rising developments in both disease modeling and therapeutic interventions are transforming the paradigm of GSDs. The capacity to develop patient-specific cellular models with human induced pluripotent stem cells (iPSCs) has the potential to allow researchers to elucidate disease mechanisms more effectively while also evaluating new pharmacological agents within a controlled environment. These developments represent a further step towards precision medicine, allowing for more targeted treatment of individuals based on their genetic makeup. Apart from the potential for fixing genetic defects, application of the CRISPR-Cas9 gene-editing technology also holds out the promise of gaining further insights into the biochemical pathways impacted by such diseases. Yet, as these new technologies mature, ethical concerns and regulatory matters must be addressed to allow for safe and effective use of potential therapy. The interface of cutting-edge research, patient management, and ethical concerns will ultimately result in improved outcomes in GSD patients (Figure 7.12).

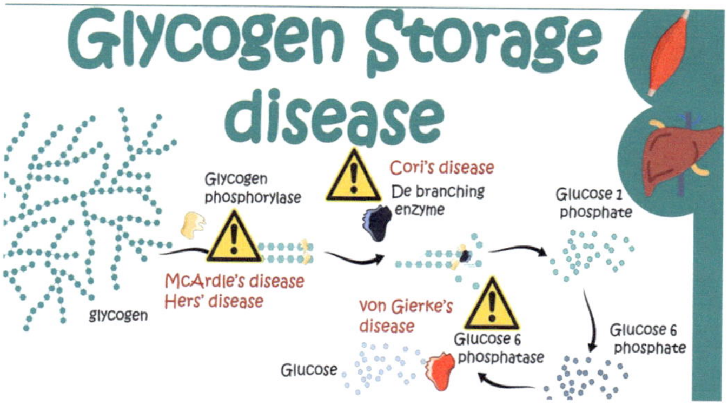

Figure 7.12. Glycogen storage diseases.

Source: https://i.ytimg.com/vi/yvaqtsSceww/maxresdefault.jpg.

7.4.3. Familial Hypercholesterolemia

The concept of familial hypercholesterolemia (FH) encompasses a genetic disorder with significant implications for lipid metabolism and cardiovascular health. Characterized by exceptionally high levels of low-density lipoprotein cholesterol (LDL-C), this condition arises from mutations in genes essential for cholesterol transport and metabolism, primarily the Low-Density Lipoprotein Receptor (LDLR), Apolipoprotein B (APOB), and Proprotein Convertase Subtilisin/Kexin Type 9 (PCSK9). Because these genes control cholesterol in the blood, any dysfunction causes LDL-C to build up, which increases the risk of atherosclerosis and heart disease. It is important to find FH early, because people with untreated high cholesterol can develop heart problems much earlier, which is why genetic screening should be done in those at risk for FH. When children have FH, the link with childhood obesity increases the dangers to their health. It has been found that obesity can worsen the genetic tendency for high cholesterol, which together increases the risk of heart disease in children. The presence of various mutations, including those in genes like Fat Mass and Obesity Associated (FTO) and Leptin Receptor (LEPR), signifies a multifaceted approach required for management (Caudle *et al.*, 2014). Since childhood obesity is increasing, especially linked to FH, it is necessary to increase awareness and use more preventive measures. Health professionals, mainly nurses, play a key role by encouraging people to adopt healthy habits in schools and communities to help reduce the lasting effects of these related diseases. Effective management of FH involves a comprehensive therapeutic approach aimed at lowering LDL-C. Statin therapy remains the primary treatment avenue; however, a notable proportion of patients may not reach target LDL-C levels or experience adverse reactions to these medications (Dayspring *et al.*, 2012). If this happens, other treatments should be considered, such as ezetimibe, which stops cholesterol from being absorbed in the intestines. It helps reduce the current lipid problems and also helps prevent the further effects of high cholesterol, such as the development of heart and blood vessel diseases. As research continues to evolve, understanding the biochemical mechanisms behind FH and promoting individualized treatment plans will be essential in enhancing patient outcomes and preserving vascular health (Figure 7.13).

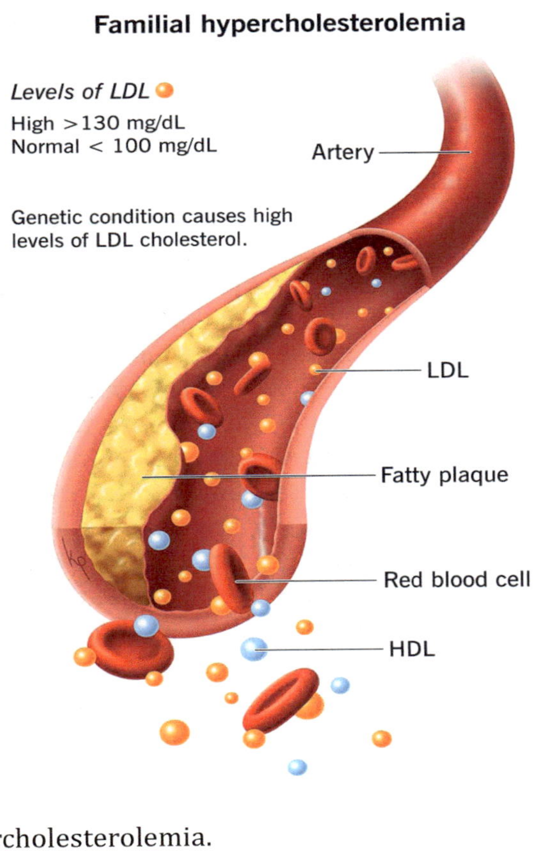

Figure 7.13. Familial hypercholesterolemia.

Source: https://my.clevelandclinic.org/-/scassets/images/org/health/articles/22067-familial-hypercholesterolemia-illustration.

7.5. Treatment and Management Strategies

Ideal management and treatment of liver diseases and metabolic and genetic conditions require an interdisciplinary therapy modality that emphasizes early diagnosis and personalized therapy. Advances in diagnosis have significantly enhanced the ability to diagnose liver diseases in their early stages, which is crucial given that most liver diseases are characterized by non-specific symptoms. For instance, understanding the pathogenesis of some conditions has led to new therapeutic opportunities. This enhancement not only positively helps to cure the present conditions but also inhibits the disease from progressing into more complicated stages, for example, cirrhosis or HCC. As such, holistic care strategies should aim for these early interventions, which may include both drug treatments and lifestyle modifications to maximize overall liver function and patient quality of life (Alisi *et al.*, 2015). Treatment of IEMs is another critical element of treatment strategies for liver disease. These genetic disorders disrupt metabolic processes and cause a wide array of disorders if not left untreated. Newborn screening currently is predominantly based on targeted assays, which can limit identification of IEMs since they are focused. To enhance diagnostic accuracy, untargeted metabolomics, in which it is possible to analyze several metabolites simultaneously, has been increasingly advised. Such all-in-one screenings may improve the potential for early diagnosis and timely treatment, ultimately averting long-term health consequences of such conditions. With metabolic screening technologies advancing in a continuous manner, such strategies will need to be optimized to tailor treatment to each patient based on their own specific metabolic profile (Fiehn *et al.*, 2019). These management strategies also need to address extended patient follow-up and education, and highlight the consequences of metabolic and genetic liver conditions throughout the life cycle. These conditions have the potential to lead to chronic health disorders, necessitating long-term management regimens involving continuous monitoring, dietary control, and educational intervention. In children, in particular, early intervention cannot be overstressed with regard to the risk of potentially developing chronic hepatopathies in the future. Integrative care, incorporating healthcare professionals, nutritionists, and genetic counselors, can offer a holistic treatment approach. By the promotion of awareness and the development of healthy lifestyle practices, the caregivers can directly impact the progression of liver conditions and improve the quality of life of such patients well into the future (Alisi *et al.*, 2015).

7.5.1. Lifestyle Modifications and Dietary Changes

Metabolic and genetic liver disorders, particularly nonalcoholic fatty liver disease (NAFLD), have garnered increased attention due to their growing prevalence and associated health complications. Making changes in your lifestyle and diet is very important for these conditions, as they can improve liver health and your metabolism. It appears that what we eat can change the way genes in the liver work, which can affect both lipid metabolism and inflammation. Accordingly, a well-designed dietary approach not only helps manage the disease but may also prevent its progression to more severe stages such as nonalcoholic steatohepatitis (NASH) and cirrhosis. Highlighting the need for better eating habits encourages people to improve their health, which supports public health efforts to reduce the increasing metabolic disorders and follow healthy lifestyle advice. Studies carried out recently have shown that some dietary changes can help reduce the risk and seriousness of NAFLD. Eating mostly fruits, vegetables, and whole grains, which is a plant-based diet, has been suggested because it provides a lot of fiber and helpful phytochemicals. Fish, nuts, and olive oil are good sources of polyunsaturated and monounsaturated fatty acids, which are recommended in this diet. At the same time, it's important to eat less processed foods, sugary foods, and salt, because these can increase liver fat and cause inflammation. These findings underscore the importance of integrating lifestyle and dietary changes into NAFLD management strategies and align with the growing recognition that nutrition plays an indispensable role in the prevention and treatment of metabolic liver disorders (Bars-cortina *et al.*, 2024). Also, nutritional genomics explains how differences in our genetic code can change our response to certain foods, which may make some people more likely to get liver diseases such as NAFLD. It looks at how what we eat can influence our genes and epigenetic factors, so that nutrition can be tailored to each person. Knowing the genetic and metabolic causes of liver problems helps healthcare professionals guide patients on dietary changes that fit their risks. With more research on diet, genetics and liver health, it becomes obvious that changing your lifestyle can help a lot. This holistic approach not only aims to manage liver disorders but also promotes sustainable health through preventive strategies that empower patients to take control of their nutritional choices and overall well-being (Rustichelli *et al.*, 2020) (Figure 7.14).

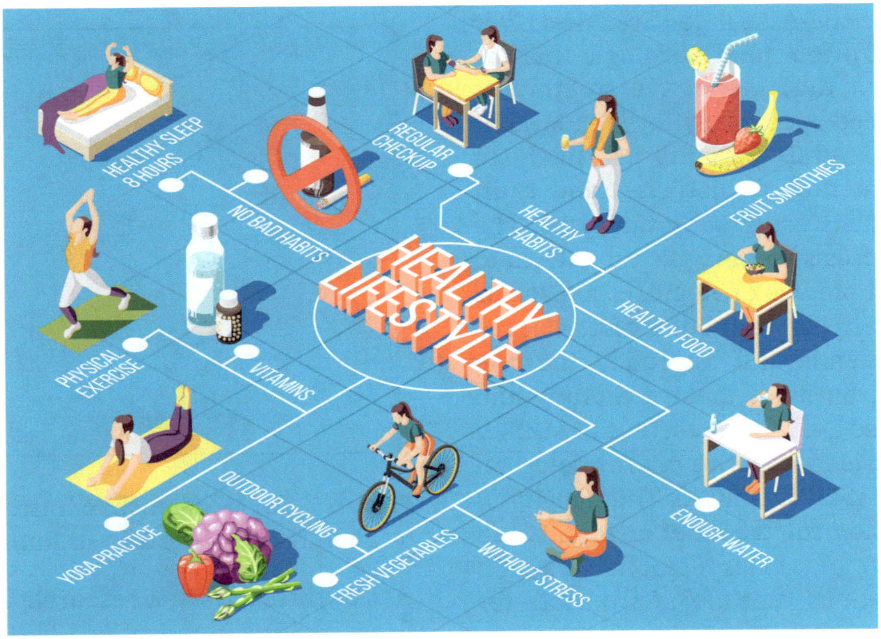
HEALTHY LIFESTYLE
HEALTHY SLEEP 8 HOURS
NO BAD HABITS
REGULAR CHECKUP
HEALTHY HABITS
FRUIT SMOOTHIES
HEALTHY FOOD
PHYSICAL EXERCISE
VITAMINS
YOGA PRACTICE
OUTDOOR CYCLING
FRESH VEGETABLES
WITHOUT STRESS
ENOUGH WATER

Figure 7.14. Healthy lifestyle.

Source: https://img.freepik.com/free-vector/healthy-lifestyle-flowchart-with-outdoor-cycling-physical-exercises-yoga-practice-regular-checkup-fresh-food-isometric-icons-illustration_1284-31-218.jpg.

7.5.2. Pharmacological Treatments

The nature of the metabolic and genetic liver diseases necessitates comprehensive pharmacological therapies that are tailor-made to address the situation of the patients. In UCD, for example, treatment is aimed at overcoming hyperammonemia, which is an instantaneous consequence of ammonia metabolism compromise due to genetic deficiencies of enzymes. Nitrogen-scavenging pharmacological agents such as benzoate and butyrate are successful in reducing serum levels of ammonia. They help prevent the neurological abnormalities brought about by ammonia accumulation and can lead to catastrophic encephalopathy if left untreated. Nutritional modifications like a eucaloric, low-protein diet supplemented with added essential amino acids are the foundation of treating these conditions and can be supplemented pharmacologically, providing a comprehensive treatment approach that is based both on metabolic homeostasis as well as the safety of the patient (Das, 2025). For Metabolic-Associated Steatotic Liver Disease (MASLD), too, pharmacologic therapy is challenging in that ineffective treatments are being designed specifically for lean MASLD patients. Lean MASLD patients are likely to have complex metabolic histories, and thus, treatment regimens are greatly impaired. The population requires strict diagnostic criteria to rule out other etiologies of steatosis, as well as addressing underlying metabolic disturbances such as dyslipidemia and IR. Today, lifestyle interventions in terms of dietary therapy and exercise regimens are of interest, but in MASLD patients who are lean, effective pharmacological treatment for MASLD is limited. The paucity of good pharmacological treatments implies an extreme necessity for further research to develop targeted medications that are appropriate for the unique physiological characteristics of these patients to ensure improved therapeutic results and quality of life (Zabotina *et al.*, 2025). Ongoing work on the pharmacologic treatment of metabolic and genetic liver disorders underscores the importance of individualized treatment, since therapeutic responses in various patients can vary significantly. For instance, in UCD patients, therapeutic strategies such as enzyme replacement therapy are poised to make major breakthroughs, holding hope for more successful treatment of these orphan genetic disorders. Simultaneously, advances in the understanding of the pathogenesis of MASLD will bring with them the potential of new drugs able to address the underlying cause and not merely control the symptoms. To make this happen, there must be intense interdisciplinary interaction among hepatologists, geneticists, and pharmacologists towards developing coordinated care pathways that maximize both established and emerging treatments. The interaction between pharmacological innovations and personalized treatment regimens is most important in managing the wide range of metabolic and genetic liver disorders in an effective manner and enhancing patient health status (Figure 7.15).

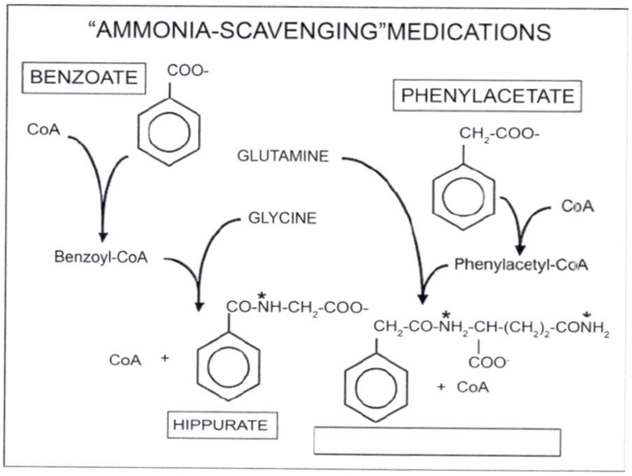

Figure 7.15. Mechanism of nitrogen scavenging by sodium benzoate and sodium phenylacetate.

Source: https://www.researchgate.net/profile/Gregory-Enns/publication/244925959/figure/fig2/AS:298490631606297@1448177120948/Mechanism-of-nitrogen-scavenging-by-sodium-benzoate-and-sodium-phenylacetate-Hippurate.png.

7.5.3. Role of Liver Transplantation

When metabolic or genetic liver problems affect the liver and overall health, liver transplantation is very important. If someone has Wilson's disease or alpha-1 antitrypsin deficiency, the liver's inability to process substances can cause cirrhosis and liver failure. As noted in studies, pediatric genetic and metabolic liver diseases are particularly significant, representing the second most common indication for liver transplantation following biliary atresia (Hassan *et al.*, 2024). The choice to do a transplant is made by looking at the liver, signs of disease outside the liver, and the likely results after surgery. So, liver transplantation is a key treatment that relieves symptoms and helps patients live much longer. As well as saving lives, liver transplantation gives families and patients hope when other treatments fail. Most metabolic liver disorders must be managed over a lifetime, and medical therapies may not be enough. Transplantation helps fix the metabolic problems that lead to a healthy liver and better metabolism throughout the body. Because early treatment matters a lot, it is especially vital for young patients. Moreover, the evolving nature of transplant methodologies, including living donor liver transplantation, has enhanced the accessibility of these life-saving procedures, expanding the donor pool and reducing wait times, thereby improving survival rates for patients with severe metabolic liver disorders (Hassan *et al.*, 2024). Also, new studies about the genetics of metabolic disorders guide the medical use of liver transplants. Genes and metabolism are closely linked, and this link can reveal special ways that diseases develop and are treated. Many studies point out that some genetic factors contribute to both metabolic disorders and psychiatric illnesses, showing that these diseases are caused by a variety of factors. Learning about these relationships shows why liver transplantation is necessary for patients with metabolic and genetic liver disorders and prepares for medicine that addresses certain genetic profiles. Besides replacing organs, liver transplantation is a key part of managing complex liver diseases and it has the ability to greatly improve the lives of many patients.

SUMMARY

The study of metabolic and genetic liver disease reveals a challenging landscape of challenge and innovation for the field. As suggested, CLD in children represents severe public health issues, with many of them underdiagnosed due to the insidious onset of early manifestations. Underdiagnosis could lead to dire outcomes, such as cirrhosis and HCC, for which early intervention is essential. The advancement that has been achieved in the elucidation of the pathogenesis of these diseases has provided avenues for identifying new targets for therapy. In the years to come, integration of this knowledge is key to further improving diagnosis and treatment protocols and eventually the patient's outcome, as well as redefining management strategies. Also, recent workshops that have emphasized the link between sleep, disruption of circadian rhythm, and metabolic health have revealed other avenues for research. The necessity of convergence and interaction between sleep researchers and metabolic experts is noted in that synergistic knowledge may further explain the physiological mechanism underlying liver diseases. Addressing the complexity of interacting factors is of great significance, considering the potential for interactions between lifestyle factors, genetic components, and metabolic function. Conducting intensive research would lead to dramatic enhancements in the prevention and therapy methods for individuals susceptible to liver diseases, encouraging an interdisciplinary treatment strategy. Lastly, the ongoing research on metabolic and genetic liver disorders represents a crucial step towards improved public health outcomes. As breakthroughs in the investigation of these complex diseases keep coming, it becomes ever more urgent to disseminate the results widely. Health care professionals must be careful to diagnose and treat these disorders, particularly in vulnerable populations such as children. The ultimate aim should be to take these findings and use them in useful applications that will not only enhance clinical practice but also foster an active strategy for liver health. By prioritizing ongoing training and collaboration, partners are paving the way toward a future where liver diseases are detected early and treated effectively, ultimately leading to healthier lives.

Metabolic and genetic liver disease analysis reveals a complex interplay between metabolic pathways and genetic polymorphisms, particularly for cardiovascular disease and diabetes. For instance, more recent genome-wide association studies (GWAS) indicate that decreased function polymorphisms in the organic cation transporter, OCT1 (SLC22A1), correlate with elevated levels of cholesterol and triglycerides and a higher risk for T2DM. This interaction is indicative of the significance of OCT1 beyond drug transport, suggesting that it also has a significant role in regulating hepatic glucose and lipid metabolism. OCT1 deficiency in models correlates with impaired thiamine-dependent pathways and is indicative of metabolic inflexibility, and this has implications for cardiometabolic disease more generally. The work remains in the full elucidation of the mechanisms responsible for linking OCT1 to such metabolic properties, noting the intricate pathways responsible for the causation of disorders related to the liver (Abad *et al.*, 2018). In terms of child health, the prevalence and diagnosis of liver disorders among children are significant public health concerns. Approximately 15,000 US children are hospitalized annually for liver disease, yet the disorder is underdiagnosed due to asymptomatic presentation in the early stages. This relative lack of visibility leads to delay in therapy and diagnosis, and adds risk for subsequent chronic diseases such as cirrhosis and HCC later in life. Recent advances have enlightened the pathogenesis of various liver diseases in children, and hence new therapeutic targets have become possible to find out. This advancement, as well as augmenting our understanding of liver diseases, has also highlighted the relevance of increased screening and early intervention strategies in children, paving the way for better health throughout life (Alisi *et al.*, 2015). The coincidence of these findings accentuates the need to connect metabolic and genetic information in the understanding of liver diseases. Scientists must look further to reveal the interaction between genetic mutations, metabolic abnormalities, and the expression of diseases, particularly in at-risk groups like children. Through the improved understanding of mechanisms like those through OCT1, a great deal can be learned in the treatment as well as prevention of both metabolic and genetic liver ailments. In addition, awareness should be raised on early detection of pediatric liver disease since early treatment has the potential to curb long-term health implications. When research is opened up, the potential for the development of improved therapy and prevention techniques that encompass the variables of liver well-being and disease management will also increase (Abad *et al.*, 2018; Alisi *et al.*, 2015).

CLOSER LOOK

INDUCED PLURIPOTENT STEM CELLS (IPSCS)

Induced pluripotent stem cells (iPSCs) are adult cells that have been genetically reprogrammed to a pluripotent state, similar to embryonic stem cells. This means they can differentiate into any cell type in the body. iPSCs are derived from somatic cells like skin or blood, making them a source of patient-specific cells for research and potential therapies (Figure 7.16).

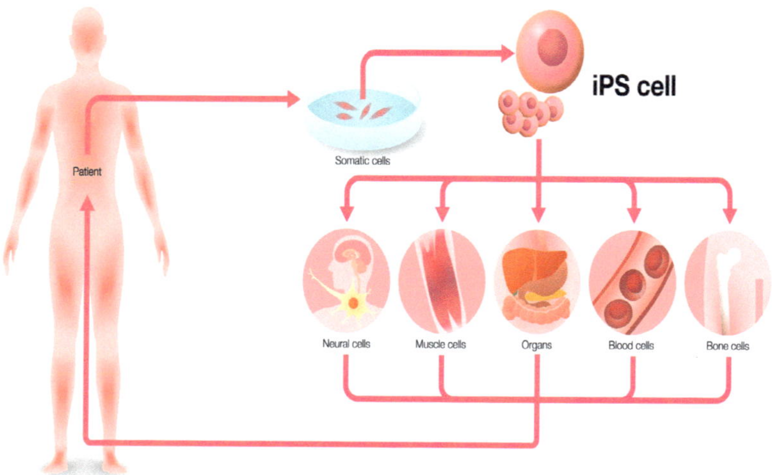

Figure 7.16. iPS Cell

Source: https://d2jx2rerrg6sh3.cloudfront.net/image-handler/picture/2019/7/By_metamorworks.jpg.

Key Aspects of iPSCs

- **Reprogramming:** iPSCs are created by introducing specific genes (Yamanaka factors: Oct4, Sox2, Klf4, and c-Myc) into adult cells, which triggers a return to a pluripotent state.
- **Pluripotency:** They can differentiate into all cell types, offering a vast potential for regenerative medicine and disease modeling.
- **Patient-specific:** iPSCs can be generated from a patient's own cells, allowing for personalized therapies and disease models.
- **Ethical Considerations:** iPSCs bypass the ethical concerns associated with using human embryonic stem cells.
- **Applications:** iPSCs are used in disease modeling, drug discovery, and regenerative medicine.

- **Disease Modeling:** iPSCs derived from patients with genetic conditions can be used to study the underlying mechanisms of the disease.
- **Regenerative Medicine:** iPSCs can be differentiated into specific cell types to repair damaged tissues or organs.
- **Drug Discovery:** iPSCs can be used to test the efficacy and safety of new drugs in a more relevant *in vitro* model.

Advantages of iPSCs

- **Unlimited Source:** iPSCs can be grown indefinitely in the lab, providing a limitless supply of cells for research and therapeutic applications.
- **No Need for Embryos:** iPSCs eliminate the ethical concerns associated with human embryonic stem cell research.
- **Patient-Specific:** iPSCs derived from a patient's own cells offer a more accurate model of disease and a potentially better match for cell-based therapies.

Challenges of iPSCs

- **Efficiency of Reprogramming:** The efficiency of converting adult cells into iPSCs can vary and is still being optimized.
- **Potential for Tumor Formation:** Some research suggests that iPSCs may have a higher risk of forming tumors compared to embryonic stem cells.
- **Integration of Reprogramming Factors:** The integration of reprogramming factors into the host cell's genome can be a concern, as it may lead to unwanted genetic changes.

References

1. Abad, J., Calvert, M. E., Chen, E. C., *et al.* (2018). *Organic Cation Transporter 1 (OCT1) Modulates Multiple Cardiometabolic Traits Through Effects on Hepatic Thiamine Content.* https://core.ac.uk/download/323063284.pdf.
2. Adeli, O. A., Toama, A., Mariam, Darvishi, M., Ramadan, F., *et al.* (2024). *A Review of The Effects of Omega-3 And Omega-6 On Alcoholic and Non-Alcoholic Fatty Liver.* https://core.ac.uk/download/599201495.pdf .
3. Ahn, I.S., Lang, J.M., Olsen, C., Ying, Z., Zhang, G., Byun, H.R., Zhao, Y., Kurt, Z., Lusis, A.J., Hsaio, E., Gomez-Pinilla, F., & Yang, X. (2018). Host Genetic Background and Gut Microbiota Contribute to Differential Metabolic Responses to High Fructose Consumption in Mice. bioRxiv. https://www.semanticscholar.org/paper/Host-Genetic-Background-and-Gut-Microbiota-to-to-in-Ahn-Lang/482173aeb51127fc5c520a0a2799e60459eae756
4. Rossi, A., Simeoli, C., Pivonello, R., Salerno, M., Rosano, C., Brunetti, B., Strisciuglio, P., Colao, A., Parenti, G., Melis, D., & Derks, T.G. (2024). Endocrine involvement in hepatic glycogen storage diseases: pathophysiology and implications for care. Reviews in Endocrine & Metabolic Disorders, 25, 707 - 725. https://www.semanticscholar.org/paper/Endocrine-involvement-in-hepatic-glycogen-storage-Rossi-Simeoli/907544680b280b3fe3aee90720c83448f0c154f9
5. Alisi, A., Alterio, A., Della Corte, C., Mosca, A., *et al.* (2015). Pediatric liver diseases: Current challenges and future perspectives. https://core.ac.uk/download/84688423.pdf (accessed on 24 May 2025).
6. Alizadeh, B. Z., Atkinson, S. R., Boezen, H. M., *et al.* (2021). Genetic analysis in European ancestry individuals identifies 517 loci associated with liver enzymes. https://core.ac.uk/download/519043164.pdf.
7. Angelís, A., Annoni, A., Biffi, A., Cantore, A., Dhawan, A., Doenecke, A., Donsante, A., *et al.* (2017). Gene therapy for monogenic liver diseases: Clinical successes, current challenges and future prospects. https://core.ac.uk/download/111014729.pdf (accessed on 24 May 2025).
8. Arble, D. M., Bass, J., Behn, C. D., Butler, M. P., *et al.* (2015). Impact of sleep and circadian disruption on energy balance and diabetes: A summary of workshop discussions. https://core.ac.uk/download/213087763.pdf (accessed on 24 May 2025).
9. Bars-Cortina, D., & Martín Barraza, J. I. (2024). Dietary pattern's role in hepatic epigenetic and dietary recommendations for the prevention of NAFLD. https://diposit.ub.edu/dspace/bitstream/2445/216596/1/nutrients-16-02956.pdf (accessed on 24 May 2025).
10. Bax, B. E. (2020). Mitochondrial neurogastrointestinal encephalomyopathy: Approaches to diagnosis and treatment. https://core.ac.uk/download/287649788.pdf (accessed on 24 May 2025).
11. Bodamer, O., Freisinger, P., Hansikova, H., Honzik, T., *et al.* (2010). Mitochondrial encephalocardio-myopathy with early neonatal onset due to *TMEM70* mutation. https://core.ac.uk/download/55758074.pdf (accessed on 24 May 2025).
12. Buckley, S. M., Chan, J. K., Howe, S. J., McKay, T. R., *et al.* (2011). Perinatal gene transfer to the liver. https://core.ac.uk/download/18302246.pdf (accessed on 24 May 2025).
13. Caudle, A. (2014). Childhood obesity and familial hypercholesterolemia: Genetic diseases that

contribute to cardiovascular disease. https://core.ac.uk/download/129590399.pdf (accessed on 24 May 2025).

14. Czekaj, O., Demianenko, Y., Kościołek, A., *et al.* (2024). Genetic implications in patients with NAFLD. https://core.ac.uk/download/597985289.pdf

15. Das, A. M. (2025). Urea cycle defects in adulthood: Clinical presentation, diagnosis and treatment in genetically encoded hepatic metabolic disorders with a potential for encephalopathy. *Metabolic Brain Disease, 40*. https://www.semanticscholar.org/paper/1f150f812b90b795860258874f20a16f51d9bffb (accessed on 24 May 2025).

16. Dayspring, T. D., Phan, B. A. P., & Toth, P. P. (2012). Ezetimibe therapy: Mechanism of action and clinical update. https://core.ac.uk/download/323069011.pdf.

17. Zabotina, Khabarova, Y. A., & Stukova, N. Y. (2025). Metabolic dysfunction-associated steatosis liver disease in lean patients: Diagnostic and treatment challenges. *Experimental and Clinical Gastroenterology.* https://www.semanticscholar.org/paper/d2c0550b79bdc8ddf3abe3b5077f49e2c024a5fa (accessed on 24 May 2025).

18. Foster, C., Gagnon, C.A., & Ashraf, A.P. (2024). Altered lipid metabolism and the development of metabolic-associated fatty liver disease. Current Opinion in Lipidology, 35, 200 - 207. https://www.semanticscholar.org/paper/Altered-lipid-metabolism-and-the-development-of-Foster-Gagnon/17b66bcc77db265c3c6de15f4592c631b2dac173

19. Fiehn, O., Ismail, I. T., & Showalter, M. R. (2019). Inborn errors of metabolism in the era of untargeted metabolomics and lipidomic. https://core.ac.uk/download/323068986.pdf.

20. França, M. (2021). Editorial for "Limits of Fat Quantification with Chemical Shift Encoded." *Journal of Magnetic Resonance Imaging, 54*. https://www.semanticscholar.org/paper/4f3c479fd374061c9e3b69c8c554c88329e0f94e (accessed on 24 May 2025).

21. François, M., Baigent, C., Catapano, A. L., Koskinas, K. C., Casula, M., Badimón, L., Chapman, M. J., *et al.* (2019). 2019 ESC/EAS guidelines for the management of dyslipidemias: Lipid modification to reduce cardiovascular risk. *European Heart Journal, 41*, 111–188. https://doi.org/10.1093/eurheartj/ehz455.

22. Frank, L. J. V., Mach, F., Smulders, Y. M., Carballo, D., Koskinas, K. C., Bäck, M., Bénétos, A., *et al.* (2021). 2021 ESC guidelines on cardiovascular disease prevention in clinical practice. *European Heart Journal, 42*, 3227–3337. https://doi.org/10.1093/eurheartj/ehab484.

23. Fu, Y. H., Hallows, W. C., & Ptáček, L. J. (2013). Solving the mystery of human sleep schedules one mutation at a time. https://core.ac.uk/download/322310898.pdf.

24. Galicia-García, U., Benito-Vicente, A., Jebari, S., Larrea-Sebal, A., Siddiqi, H., Uribe, K. B., Ostolaza, H., *et al.* (2020). Pathophysiology of type 2 diabetes mellitus. *International Journal of Molecular Sciences, 21*, 6275. https://doi.org/10.3390/ijms21176275.

25. Gul, R., Firasat, S., Schubert, M., Ullah, A., Peña, E., Thuesen, A. C. B., Hussain, M., *et al.* (2023). Identifying the genetic causes of phenotypically diagnosed Pakistani mucopolysaccharidoses patients by whole genome sequencing. *Frontiers in Genetics, 14*. https://www.semanticscholar.org/paper/50b2c34b666066558e4f6042e5b14a59378761c2 (accessed on 24 May 2025).

26. Hassan, S., Anouti, A., Tan, Q., Wangensteen, K., & Aqul, A. (2024). Liver transplantation for pediatric genetic and metabolic disorders. *Liver Transplantation: Official Publication of the American Association for the Study of Liver Diseases and the International Liver Transplantation*

Society. https://www.semanticscholar.org/paper/1d197569d85d47e820ffa06faac43cb4f231319c (accessed on 24 May 2025).

27. Jadhav, P. A., Thomas, A. B., Chopada, V. M., Bokaria, P. V., Deokate, S. B., Chougule, P. S., Chavan, P. N., *et al.* (2024). Correlation of non-alcoholic fatty liver disease and neurodegenerative disorders. *Egyptian Liver Journal*. https://www.semanticscholar.org/paper/715dfc6464a7a535c906e813012f935c0e2636a2 (accessed on 24 May 2025).

28. Kościołek, D., Urbaś, M., Kępczyk, M., Kościołek, A., Surowiecka, K., Misiak, J., Ojdana, M., *et al.* (2024). Alpha 1 antitrypsin deficiency–Etiology, symptoms in various organs, diagnosis, treatment, prognosis. *Journal of Education, Health and Sport*. https://www.semanticscholar.org/paper/100e3189ce7b60d6a69b6f95af7521dfc97f8b7a

29. Loughnan, R., Ahern, J., Tompkins, C., Palmer, C., Iversen, J., Thompson, W., Andreassen, O., *et al.* (2022). Association of genetic variant linked to hemochromatosis with brain magnetic resonance imaging measures of iron and movement disorders. *JAMA Neurology*. https://www.semanticscholar.org/paper/616bc4cb6410e0dbbd34d75169921d3da408d6e1 (accessed on 24 May 2025).

30. Marjani, A., Mehrpouya, M., & Pourhashem, Z. (2016). Serum γ-glutamyltransferase, alanine aminotransferase and aspartate aminotransferase activity in healthy blood donor of different ethnic groups in Gorgan. https://core.ac.uk/download/52205537.pdf (accessed on 24 May 2025).

31. Mehta, S., Tayabali, S., & Lachmann, R. (2018). Valproate-induced hyperammonemia—Uncovering an underlying inherited metabolic disorder: A case report. *Journal of Medical Case Reports, 12*. https://www.semanticscholar.org/paper/2601dca51ecf6add11759d34ea1e2457e997fab4 (accessed on 24 May 2025).

32. Mejía-Guzmán, J. E., Belmont-Hernández, R. A., Chávez-Tapia, N. C., Uribe, M., & Nuño-Lámbarri, N. (2025). Metabolic-dysfunction-associated steatosis liver disease: Molecular mechanisms, clinical implications, and emerging therapeutic strategies. *International Journal of Molecular Sciences, 26*. https://www.semanticscholar.org/paper/4c63d1bff27c7cfbe5c3091c5eb3445a0a04f186 (accessed on 24 May 2025).

33. Mohammadi, S., Ghaderi, S., & Fatehi, F. (2024). Iron accumulation/overload and Alzheimer's disease risk factors in the precuneus region: A comprehensive narrative review. Aging Medicine, 7, 649 - 667.https://www.semanticscholar.org/paper/Iron-accumulation-overload-and-Alzheimer's-disease-Mohammadi-Ghaderi/3a13c1f0f1e2df252674e9b856af9ad69300ad97

34. Rustichelli, M., Longo, M., Meroni, M., & Dongiovanni, P. (2020). Nutrition and genetics in NAFLD: The perfect binomium. https://core.ac.uk/download/323192564.pdf (accessed on 24 May 2025).

35. Tamimi, A., Javid, M., Sedighi-Pirsaraei, N., & Mirdamadi, A. (2024). Exosome prospects in the diagnosis and treatment of non-alcoholic fatty liver disease. *Frontiers in Medicine, 11*. https://www.semanticscholar.org/paper/2ea589f133328a9be4e8c95f4a15e372535f84cb (accessed on 24 May 2025).

36. van der Meer, D., Shadrin, A. A., Stinson, S. E., Koch, E., Rokicki, J., Rahman, Z., Bergstedt, J., *et al.* (2024). Divergent patterns of genetic overlap between severe

mental disorders and metabolic markers. https://www.semanticscholar.org/paper/f817d1b628db8e14a15483482aa9e915f3f5a051 (accessed on 24 May 2025).

37. Vorona, E., Sorkina, E., & Trebicka, J. (2024). Progressive Metabolic Dysfunction-Associated Steatotic Liver Disease (MASLD) from a Young Age Due to a Rare Genetic Disorder, Familial Partial Lipodystrophy: A Case Report and Review of the Literature. Livers.

38. Wang, X. Y., Lyu, Q., Zhang, Y. Y., Su, Y., Zhao, H., Shen, H. H., & Xie, Y. Y. (2025). Shared genetic architecture between metabolic dysfunction-associated steatosis liver disease and cardiometabolic traits comorbidities: A genome-wide pleiotropic and multi-omics study. *Metabolism and Target Organ Damage*. https://www.semanticscholar.org/paper/1b9e1ef4d6b3da8ee1389798e78f1b70ac466971 (accessed on 24 May 2025).

39. Walsh, C., & Jin, S. (2024). Induced Pluripotent Stem Cells and CRISPR-Cas9 Innovations for Treating Alpha-1 Antitrypsin Deficiency and Glycogen Storage Diseases. Cells, 13. https://www.semanticscholar.org/paper/Induced-Pluripotent-Stem-Cells-and-CRISPR-Cas9-for-Walsh-Jin/753d7151b7dc5537ee4c7d186b773b667e74251d

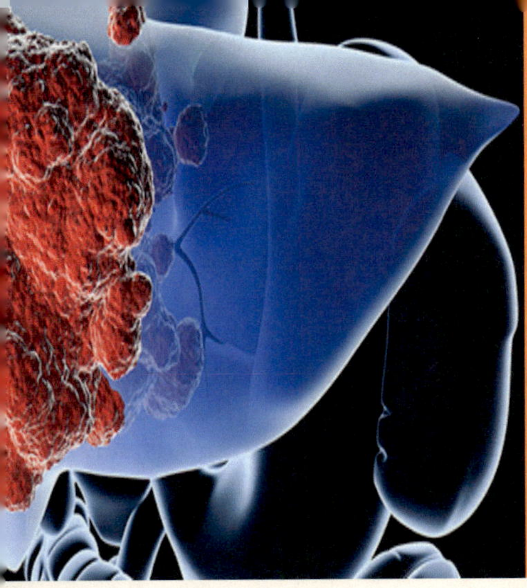

Chapter 8
LIVER TUMORS

Contents

Introduction

The study of liver tumors has been of great interest to the medical research community due to the rising global incidence of liver cancer. The most prevalent type is hepatocellular carcinoma (HCC), which has a propensity to occur in the context of chronic liver diseases (CLD) such as hepatitis B and C infection and cirrhosis. Understanding the mechanisms of cancer development is significant not only in diagnosis but also in treatment selection. Emerging evidence has demonstrated a complex pattern of genetic aberrations associated with liver tumors, which draws attention to the implementation of targeted therapy. The study of such genomic landscapes, particularly with advanced techniques such as next-generation sequencing (NGS), promises to revolutionize control of this cancer by identifying actionable targets within the tumor's molecular profiles (Janku *et al.*, 2014). The incidence of liver tumors is more than just an individual concern; it is a public health issue that touches lives all over the world. As liver cancer often progresses unnoticed, the majority of patients are symptom-free until the condition has reached late stages, thus posing early detection and treatment as challenging. The financial impact of managing advanced liver cancer is extensive; extensive resources in healthcare are used in relatively less efficient treatments due to late diagnosis. Additionally, the delay further causes poor prognosis and compromised quality of life among patients. Hence, raising awareness of risk factors and promoting early screening programs are critical components of integrated liver cancer control programs. Coupling these public health interventions with novel information obtained from genomic research is likely to offer better results through tailor-made medicine regimens according to patients' cancer profiles (Bernard Becker Medical Library Archives, 2002). In addition, the study establishes liver tumors intersect with broader concerns regarding tumorigenesis and cancer research as a whole, particularly the environmental and genetic factors affecting tumorigenesis. Recent research highlights the importance of understanding causative HCC development pathways, such as the PI3K/AKT/mTOR and Wnt signal transduction pathways. Not only are these pathways involved in tumor formation, but they are also therapeutic targets. The current gap in our knowledge of the genomic map of liver cancer underscores the necessity for an intense, active research agenda in this area. With insight into the molecular basis of liver tumors, researchers can unveil new therapeutic avenues that can provide hope to patients afflicted by this challenging disease (Janku *et al.*, 2014).

Definition of Liver Tumors

It is important to understand what liver tumors are to know their effects on health. These tumors are mainly divided into benign and malignant types, and benign ones, like hemangiomas and FNH, are not usually a major risk, but malignant tumors such as HCC and cholangiocarcinoma can be dangerous since they may behave aggressively and spread. A lot of malignant liver tumors develop in people with CLD, especially cirrhosis or hepatitis infections. The presence of liver disease and the possibility of tumors emphasize that liver cancer is not simple, and doctors must carefully consider how these tumors can change liver function and affect the patient's outcome. Because of this, a clear definition of liver tumors covers both their biological features and their effects on overall hepatobiliary health. The type of cells in and around liver tumors is very important for their development and actions. The liver, being highly vascularized and possessing a unique architecture, presents a distinct tumor microenvironment (TME) that influences tumor growth, invasion, and metastasis. 3D bioprinting technologies are improving, which shows the drive to create this complex TME. Using accurate placement of bioinks, scientists have begun to create models of liver tumors that better reflect the real disease, which helps researchers' study how cells and the surrounding matrix affect each other. These innovative approaches facilitate research not only in the context of tumor behavior but also in the exploration of treatment modalities, emphasizing the importance of personalized medicine in the management of liver tumors, particularly for hepatopancreato-biliary (HPB) cancers (Zhuang *et al.*, 2023). Correct diagnosis and treatment of liver tumors depend on accurate characterization, which is usually done using advanced imaging and examining the tissue under a microscope. Magnetic Resonance Imaging (MRI), for instance, serves as a vital tool in distinguishing various types of liver tumors by providing detailed insights into their structural and functional attributes. In addition, the difference found between *in vivo* and *ex vivo* conductivity in studies is significant for learning about tumor biology and its electromagnetic behavior. The ability to estimate conductivity *in vivo* allows for more precise modeling of tumor characteristics, contributing to diagnostics and therapeutic planning in liver cancer management (He *et al.*, 2024). Thus, a comprehensive definition of liver tumors is intertwined with advanced diagnostic modalities that not only assist in their identification but also in establishing effective treatment pathways (Figure 8.1).

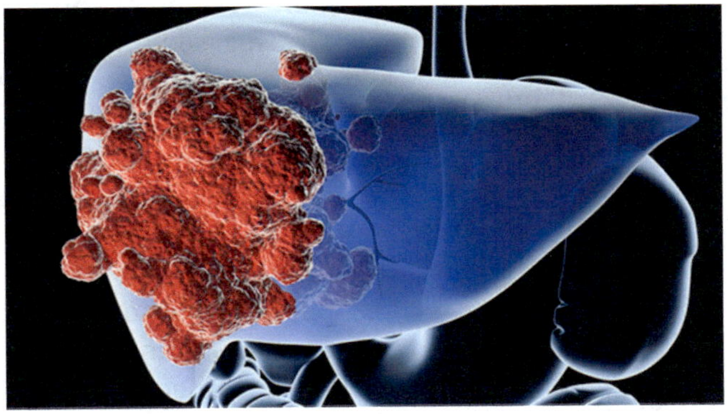

Figure 8.1. Liver tumors

Source: https://www.hopkinsmedicine.org/-/media/images/health/1_-conditions/liver-gallbladder-and-pancreas/liver-tumors-teaser-image.jpg.

Importance of Studying Liver Tumors

Investigation of liver tumors is important with increasing incidence of liver cancer worldwide, particularly in nations that have high infection rates of viruses of hepatitis and LC. The most common form of liver cancer, HCC, poses challenges to public health to a significant degree since it presents late with advanced cancer stages when treatment is minimal. Understanding the etiology, molecular biology, and methods of early detection of liver tumors will be crucial to further promote patient benefits. Also, hepatological and oncological advancements require constant investigation to discover new therapeutics that are either symptomatic or anti-cancer. Such knowledge acquired through the study of liver tumors not only assists in the creation of novel treatment strategies but also enhances screening protocols that can potentially be utilized to identify the initial onset of such tumors and have improved prognoses for the first-time offenders. The heterogeneity of liver tumors demands well-documented knowledge and comprehension of their biological composition and reaction to treatment. Liver tumors exhibit various genetic and molecular patterns that influence their virulence and drug sensitivity. For instance, ongoing research in patient-derived xenografts (PDXs) has underlined the necessity of developing model systems that mimic the natural microenvironment of the cancer. Through PDXs, researchers can screen for the efficacy of drugs and simulate tumor growth, paving the way for targeted medicine based on the unique genetic makeup of an individual's tumor (Babicky *et al.*, 2014). Thus, the study of liver tumors extends far beyond basic science; it is a component of everyday clinical practice that seeks to tailor treatment to the patient, enhancing quality of life and survival. New methodologies, including liquid biopsies, have also radically altered the study and management of liver tumors. Liquid biopsies analyze circulating tumor products, including circulating tumor cells (CTCs) and circulating tumor DNA (ctDNA), providing valuable information on tumor biology without requiring invasive procedures (Calborean *et al.*, 2018). Clinicians can monitor responses to treatments, detect recurrences, and tailor treatment strategies accordingly using these biomarkers. By bringing liquid biopsy technologies into mainstream clinical practice, medical care professionals can offer more accurate diagnosis and uniquely individualized treatment plans that are sensitive to the unique needs of patients. The worth of research on liver tumors is not only in increasing scientific knowledge, but in translating that into useful interventions that improve patient management and outcomes within a clinical setting.

8.1. Types of Liver Tumors

Liver tumors are mainly divided into benign and malignant types, which have their own traits, causes, and effects on patients. Benign liver tumors, such as hemangiomas, focal nodular hyperplasia (FNH), and hepatocellular adenomas, often remain asymptomatic and are frequently discovered incidentally during imaging studies. Most of the benign tumors in the liver are hemangiomas, which are rare and usually don't need treatment unless they cause serious symptoms or problems. Unlike the previous ones, hepatocellular adenomas are influenced by hormones, mainly oral contraceptives, and could become cancerous, which requires regular monitoring. FNH is usually symptomless and is not known to progress, so it rarely needs treatment. So, it is important to understand how benign liver tumors act to manage them well and reassure patients. Malignant liver tumors are predominantly categorized into primary and secondary (metastatic) types. Primary liver cancer is largely represented by hepatocellular carcinoma (HCC), which is often linked to chronic liver conditions such as hepatitis B or C infections, as well as cirrhosis. The prognosis for a patient with HCC depends on the stage of the tumor, the liver's functional status, and the treatment plan used. Another main type of primary tumor is intrahepatic cholangiocarcinoma, which starts in the bile ducts inside the liver. Such tumors usually act more aggressively and are found in the advanced stages, which greatly reduces the chances of recovery for patients. Also, when cancer spreads to the liver, often from breast, colon, and lung cancers, it highlights the liver's role as a frequent site for secondary tumors, so understanding their origins is very important for managing cancer. Many pathological factors play a big role in predicting how liver tumors will respond to surgical treatment. It has been shown that if the margins of the surgery are positive or lymph nodes are involved, it is more likely that the patient will not survive after hepatic resection or transplantation for cholangiocarcinoma. For instance, patients with multiple tumors or those with advanced pTNM stages demonstrate significantly poorer prognoses compared to those with solitary lesions and negative margins (Casavilla *et al.*, 1997). For this reason, the type of liver tumor determined by histology is very important for deciding how to treat them. The implications of such prognostic assessments are profound, as they inform treatment decisions and ultimately shape patient outcomes, thereby underscoring the necessity for continued research and refinement of liver cancer management strategies (Dvorchik *et al.*, 1998).

8.1.1. Benign Liver Tumors

Prevalence and nature of benign liver tumors are of significant concern in hepatology studies since they can be employed to simulate more risky conditions. The most common of the usual benign tumors are hemangiomas, hepatic adenomas, and FNH. The most frequent are hemangiomas, often asymptomatic, and typically discovered by chance on imaging for another reason. In a clinical environment, these benign lesions have to be distinguished from malignant tumors using meticulous imaging techniques as diagnostic procedures significantly influence the treatment. Techniques such as contrast-enhanced ultrasound (CEUS) and magnetic resonance imaging (MRI) have improved the ability of differentiation, allowing clinicians to make improved judgments about patient management. Research has indicated that benign liver tumors have some imaging properties that are different from malignant lesions and can lead to proper diagnoses without the need for invasive tests (Varigonda *et al.*, 2024). Hepatic adenomas, although rarer than hemangiomas, pose a specific challenge because of their hormonal dependency and malignant potential, especially among women of childbearing age. These tumors are more commonly related to the use of oral contraceptives or anabolic steroids, as this indicates the involvement of endocrine factors in the liver tumorigenesis. Hepatic adenomas are often asymptomatic clinically but develop symptoms by producing complications such as hemorrhage and abdominal pain when large or ruptured. Surgical resection is usually recommended in symptomatic adenomas and those of a particular size to an institution, reflecting an estimation of risk versus benefit during treatment planning. Moreover, characterization of the histologic subtypes of hepatic adenomas, i.e., steatotic or inflammatory types, can aid practitioners in the prediction of behavior and decisions regarding surgical therapy (Świątkowski *et al.*, 2020). Another benign liver tumor, FNH, also occurs as a well-circumscribed mass, typically in a woman. The cause is not particularly understood but is speculated to be the consequence of a vascular anomaly leading to hepatocyte hyperplastic nodules. FNH has no potential for malignant growth and is therefore distinct from other liver lesions. Diagnosis is most frequently acquired by imaging investigations, where the presence of a central scar is a typical imaging feature of FNH on MRI. Management is typically conservative, particularly in asymptomatic patients, because FNH is well tolerated in most instances. Surgical resection is, however, occasionally required to excise symptoms if they do arise or with diagnostic doubt (Świątkowski *et al.*, 2020; Varigonda *et al.*, 2024). Understanding the nature of these benign tumors is important for managing and treating patients appropriately in hepatology (Figure 8.2).

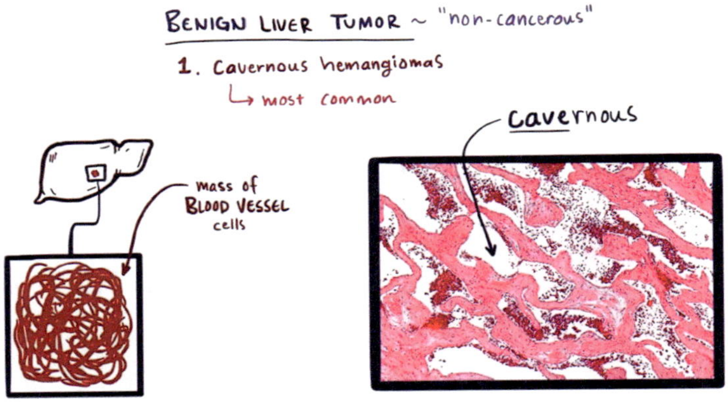

Figure 8.2. Benign liver tumors.

Source: https://d16qt3wv6xm098.cloudfront.net/KlqV95pCRUuiGi4i369g031sQs6B-XYT/_.jpg.

8.1.2. Malignant Liver Tumors

Malignant liver tumors, mainly HCC, are a major challenge in healthcare worldwide because they are very aggressive and have multiple complicated causes. Most cases of HCC happen in people with CLD, and cirrhosis greatly increases their risk. Infections with hepatitis B and hepatitis C, alcohol abuse, and nonalcoholic fatty liver disease are important factors that cause these tumors. More cases of HCC are being seen, which is linked to a rise in related liver diseases, so it is important to study the causes and processes behind HCC. In addition, new diagnostic tools, especially imaging and biomarkers, have made it easier to detect HCC early, which may improve the outcome for patients. A strong knowledge of these cancers is needed to create interventions that improve the chances of survival for people suffering from them. Treating malignant liver tumors requires surgical, radiological, and systemic methods. Removing part of the liver by partial hepatectomy or performing a liver transplant are the main ways to treat localized tumors. Because the disease is often found in the late stages and the liver is already damaged, many patients cannot have surgery. Consequently, locoregional therapies like radiofrequency ablation and transarterial chemoembolization (TACE) have gained prominence as effective palliative options. Besides, researchers are investigating systemic treatments such as targeted drugs and immunotherapies for advanced HCC. Analyzing the tumor's molecular features, such as with NGS, can help doctors decide on the best treatment and watch for variants that might predict how the patient will react to therapy or the course of the disease. There is a growing focus on liver cancer diagnosis on finding good biomarkers that can help improve accuracy and predict the outcome. Alkaline phosphatase (ALP), for instance, has been implicated in various cancers, including liver malignancies. High ALP levels might point to liver metastasis or more severe disease, which can indicate a poor outcome in certain situations. Using ALP together with aspartate aminotransferase and carbohydrate antigen 19-9 helps doctors make better decisions about treating the disease. Additionally, research into the roles of molecular markers like RB1, TP53, and TERT is shedding light on the biological complexity of malignant liver tumors and may pave the way for targeted interventions tailored to specific familial predispositions or tumor profiles (Jiang *et al.*, 2023; Ma *et al.*, 2024). This growing body of evidence reinforces the need for a multidisciplinary approach to combat these formidable tumors effectively (Figure 8.3).

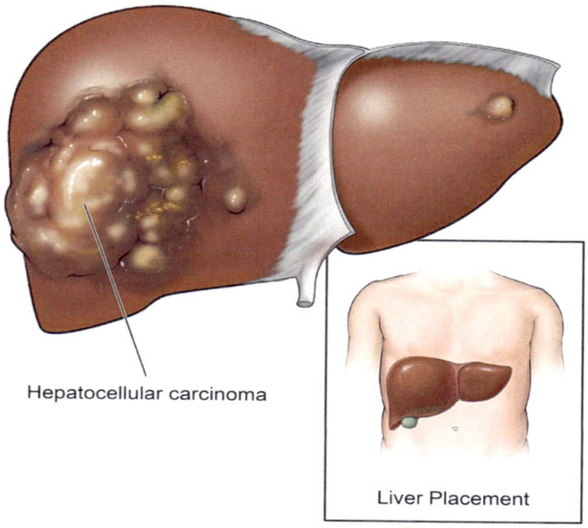

Figure 8.3. Hepatocellular carcinoma illustration.

Source: https://my.clevelandclinic.org/-/scassets/images/org/health/articles/21709-hepatocellular-carcinoma-illustration.

8.1.3. Metastatic Liver Tumors

Pathophysiology of metastatic liver cancer involves complex interactions between the hepatic microenvironment and tumor cells. Metastatic tumors typically originate from a remote site, such as the gastrointestinal tract, breast, or lungs, and metastasize to the liver, where the specific anatomical and immunological characteristics can facilitate their growth and survival. Liver metastases are then a significant prognostic factor of patient outcome in most instances. For instance, in pancreatic neuroendocrine tumors (PNET), as many as 40-93% of them present with liver metastases, highlighting the liver's key role as a secondary site for tumor development. These findings highlight the need for ongoing research into predictive markers of metastatic disease and the development of therapeutic approaches, particularly aimed at fighting hepatic metastasis, ultimately to create better survival and quality of life for those with these conditions (Aurello *et al.*, 2018). Various treatment modalities have been examined to manage metastatic liver tumors, a reflection of the need for individualized treatment. Surgical resection may be an integral treatment in appropriately chosen individuals with oligometastases. However, multiple patients are not candidates for surgery by disease extent or pre-existing liver impairment. Therefore, non-surgical treatments such as systemic therapy and regional ablative techniques like SBRT have gained popularity. In one trial assessing SBRT in patients with liver metastases, local control was much greater in tumors that received doses above certain thresholds, implying that aggressive and precise radiation may benefit this difficult patient group by improving outcomes (Feng *et al.*, 2012). This change in management practices is an indication of a shift toward maximizing the care of patients with metastatic liver tumors with the overall aim of enhancing survival, while also maximizing the efficacy of the treatment. Since the challenges posed by metastatic liver tumors are multidimensional, multidisciplinary teams of caregivers play a crucial role in the establishment of new paradigms of treatment. Hepatologists, oncologists, surgeons, and radiologists need to coordinate their efforts to come up with full treatment plans that consider the intricacies of each case. The more evidence is gathered on the efficiency of different treatments, the more crucial it is to incorporate clinical research data into practice. For instance, the application of integrated therapies that couple systemic therapy with targeted strategies, like SBRT and resection, could have synergistic effects. As well, patient selection remains critical, in that choosing the patients who will gain the most from aggressive treatment will maximize therapy outcome with minimal morbidity. The constant evolution of therapy holds hope for those afflicted with the impact of metastatic liver tumors and attests to the necessity of continued research in the matter (Figure 8.4).

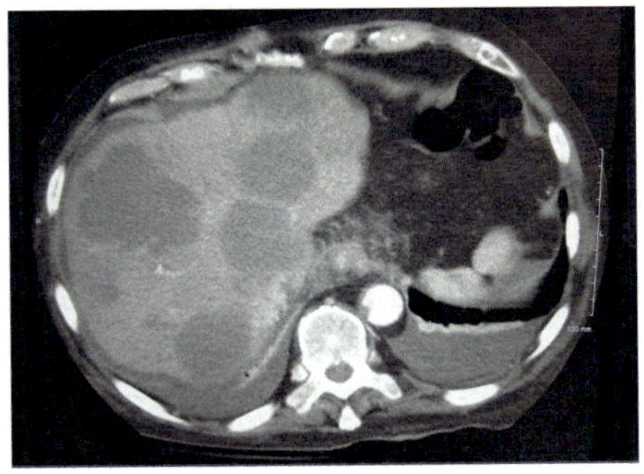

Figure 8.4. Multiple liver metastases.

Source: https://upload.wikimedia.org/wikipedia/commons/thumb/8/81/MultipleLiverMets2008.jpg/800px-MultipleLiverMets2008.jpg.

8.2. Causes and Risk Factors

Many different reasons and risk factors work together to cause liver tumors to develop. Liver cancer cases are increasing mainly because of infections with the hepatitis B and C viruses. When these viruses infect the liver for a long time, they cause constant inflammation and damage liver cells, which can result in LC and, in some people, cancer. Chronic drinking is also critical; it worsens liver damage and encourages the disease to progress. At the same time, both hepatitis and drinking too much alcohol harm the liver, which significantly increases the risk of tumors. Also, being exposed to a wide range of toxic materials is a major risk factor. Aflatoxins, which are often present in contaminated crops, have been linked to liver cancer because they can change cells in the liver and cause tumors. Consuming such toxins over a long period can make people more likely to get HCC, mainly in areas where food safety is not well controlled. Genetic factors also contribute greatly to why some people are more likely to get liver cancer. Certain genetic mutations can predispose individuals to liver tumors, especially in cases of hereditary hemochromatosis (HH) and other metabolic disorders that affect iron accumulation in the liver. Also, living with obesity or diabetes can make liver cancer more likely. The global rise in obesity rates correlates strongly with an increase in nonalcoholic fatty liver disease (NAFLD), a condition associated with a heightened risk of cirrhosis and liver tumors. IR, which is common in people with diabetes, leads to more inflammation and stress in the liver. Liver tumors can develop in a complex way because of the influence of metabolic conditions, alcohol, and viruses. In particular, the synergistic relationship between hepatitis C virus (HCV) and alcohol has been documented, where alcohol exacerbates hepatitis progression, leading to a higher incidence of tumorigenesis in affected individuals (Asahina *et al.*, 2009). For this reason, dealing with these different risk factors is important for successful liver tumor prevention and treatment.

8.2.1. Viral Hepatitis and Liver Cancer

The link between viral hepatitis and liver cancer, which includes HCC, is a global health problem. HBV and HCV are the most significant viral pathogens that lead to HCC causation. The chronic infection of viruses normally leads to chronic inflammation of the liver, cirrhosis, and ultimately, to malignancy. Chronic inflammation and fibrosis of the liver form the immunobiologic liver milieu that plays a significant role in oncogenic transformation of hepatocytes. In this regard, the fact that the liver's unique immune microenvironment is not only capable of promoting tumorigenesis but also influencing the efficacy of therapeutic interventions needs to be mentioned. The complexity of HCC arises from the fact that it is multicausal in its etiology, and it is viral infections that complement environmental and genetic factors to promote cancer growth, requiring exhaustive prevention as well as treatment strategies. Recent studies have elucidated the mechanisms of chronic viral hepatitis-caused liver cancer, with evidence of a continuum of pathophysiologic processes that are activated. Of note of concern is HCV's association with increased risk of developing liver tumors as a consequence of its interaction with other risk factors, such as alcohol consumption. Alcohol synergistically enhances liver disease progression and risk of liver cancer from HCV, suggesting the presence of a complex interaction between agents. Induction of Toll-like receptor 4 (TLR4) by the nonstructural protein NS5A of HCVs is of particular interest, as this pathway mediates liver injury and tumorigenesis. Furthermore, TLR4 activation has also been demonstrated to upregulate expression of Nanog, a marker of stem cells, with potential significance for a novel mechanism in HCV-induced liver tumorigenesis. Understanding of these mechanisms would be critical to the generation of targeted therapies. Clinical relevance of viral hepatitis-induced liver cancer should not be exaggerated, considering that the incidence of HCC remains on the rise in the majority of the world. Because the majority of HCCs arise against a backdrop of CLD due to hepatitis virus infections, early screening and treatment are essential. Advanced HCC is managed with systemic treatments such as multikinase inhibitors, but ICI use is demonstrating potential in select patient populations. Of specific interest is the special immunologic status of the liver, regulated by cirrhosis and chronic inflammation, which may complicate the response to these therapies. Therefore, the exploration of the liver's immunobiology can offer insight into the optimal treatment of liver tumors secondary to viral hepatitis. With the progression in disease microenvironment understanding, personalized medicine emerges as central to the control of liver cancer, paving the way for improved patient outcome in this high-risk population (Figure 8.5).

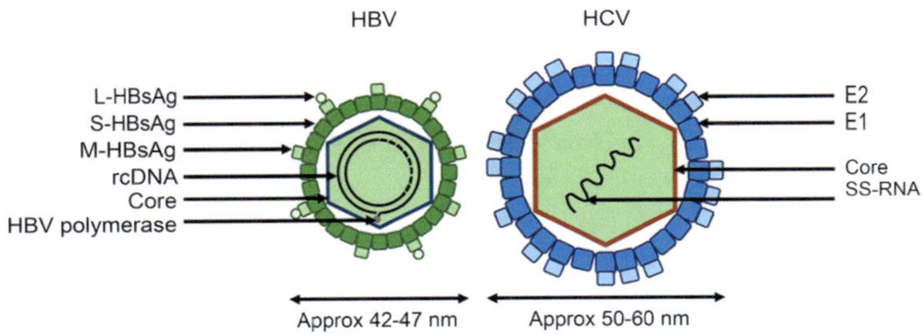

Figure 8.5. Hepatitis B virus (HBV) and hepatitis C virus (HCV) viral structures.

https://www.researchgate.net/publication/347635456/figure/fig1/AS:11431281212159424@1702560495631/Comparison-of-hepatitis-B-virus-HBV-and-hepatitis-C-virus-HCV-viral-structures-The.tif.

8.2.2. Alcohol Consumption and Liver Damage

Alcohol consumption is a significant factor influencing liver damage, with chronic intake leading to a spectrum of liver diseases, including alcoholic liver disease (ALD) and HCC. The liver breaks down alcohol mainly by using alcohol dehydrogenase and aldehyde dehydrogenase. If a person drinks too much alcohol, the body produces harmful substances, including acetaldehyde, which leads to damage in cells through oxidative stress and inflammation. Continued drinking can make the liver's antioxidant system less effective, which makes hepatocytes more likely to be damaged. If the damage to the liver builds up, its ability to heal may not keep up, which might cause fibrosis and cirrhosis, both known to be early stages of liver tumors. There is an additional complication when thinking about viral hepatitis infections, especially HCV, in the link between alcohol and liver damage. Studies have found that alcohol makes liver disease caused by HCV worse, which increases the risk of liver tumors. HCV nonstructural proteins in hepatocytes can cause TLR4 to be expressed, which increases the inflammatory response. TLR4 activation also appears to increase the expression of Nanog, a stem cell marker that could influence the formation of liver cancer. So, we must recognize that drinking alcohol when the liver is already damaged greatly increases the risk of cancer through different molecular pathways, which helps us better understand liver tumor causes. As well as the traditional ways alcohol can harm the liver, it also increases the risk of liver tumors through its effects on metabolism. Some research shows that drinking ethanol can change the way metabolic processes work, which could be linked to cancer development. As a result of oxidizing alcohol, reactive oxygen species are formed, and the amount of antioxidants such as glutathione is reduced. As a result of oxidative stress, liver cells may experience mutations, and the usual cell signaling may be disrupted, which can create conditions that help tumors to develop. Also, alcohol's effect on hormones can cause high estrogen, which is linked to cancer and adds to the challenges of alcohol-related liver damage and oncology. Collectively, these findings underscore the multifaceted relationship between alcohol consumption and liver pathology, illuminating pathways that may converge on liver tumor development (Figure 8.6).

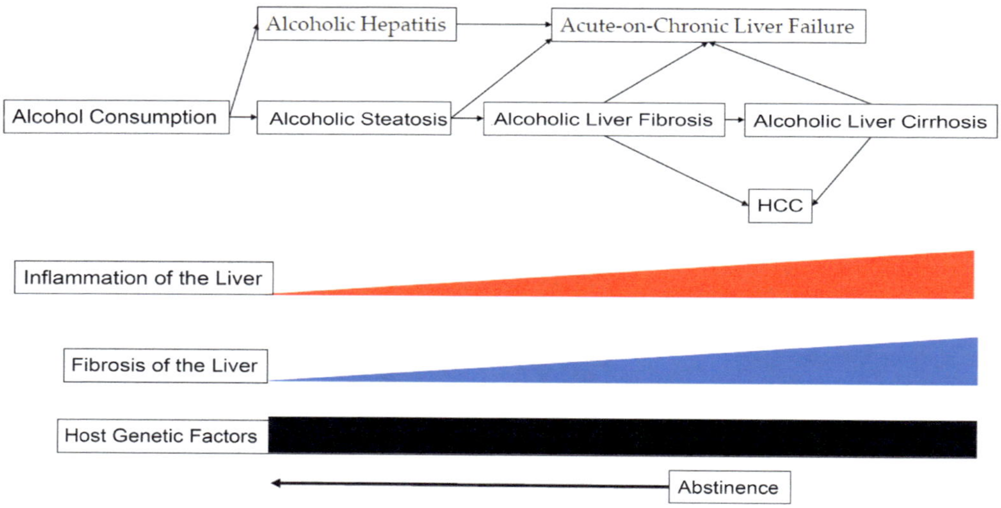

Figure 8.6. Molecular mechanisms: the connections between alcohol consumption and hepatocellular carcinoma.

Source: https://www.mdpi.com/ijms/ijms-23-09679/article_deploy/html/images/ijms-23-09679-g002.png.

8.2.3. Genetic Predispositions

The concept of genetic predispositions is highly significant in liver tumor pathogenesis. Genetic predisposition refers to a condition in which an individual is likely to develop a certain disease due to inherited genetic disorders. For hepatocellular carcinomas, some genetic syndromes or mutations may significantly increase the risk of a person. For instance, HH and alpha-1 antitrypsin deficiency are inherited conditions that have been linked to the frequency of liver tumors. Such genetic tendencies are likely to result in pathological changes that lead to HCC or other related tumors in the affected individuals, hence underlining the importance of genetic analysis in high-risk populations. Moreover, identification of hereditary syndromes for liver tumors has broad implications in screening for and preventing cancer. Genetic testing has allowed for the identification of individuals who would benefit from proactive surveillance and treatment early in their lives. For example, those with a history of cancer in their families or specific genetic markers can be tested to be regularly checked. As identified by research at The University of Texas M.D. Anderson Cancer Center, identification of patients' genetic background can enhance assessment of their cancer risk profile, paving the way for more targeted and effective management strategies, including genetic counseling and lifestyle modifications to mitigate risk factors for liver tumors (Clifford *et al.*, 2017). Moreover, the dynamic interaction between genetic susceptibility and the environment should not be overlooked when conducting research on liver tumors. Genotypic exposure to dietary habits, alcohol consumption, and certain toxins may affect tumor development by interacting with the individual's genetic profile. The retrospective epidemiologic evidence suggests that while genetic factors give insights into the susceptibility of an individual to liver cancer, environmental agents may have key roles as modifiers of risk. For instance, increased body mass index (BMI) and certain dietary habits may amplify the impact of genetic factors. Understanding such interaction is significant for the development of overall prevention programs that account for both genetic and environmental contributions to liver tumor causation (White *et al.*, 2016).

8.3. Symptoms and Diagnosis

Liver tumors usually cause symptoms that are not easy to notice, which makes it hard to detect them early. At first, liver tumors may not cause any symptoms, which means that regular screening is essential for people with CLD or hepatitis. As the tumor gets worse, common symptoms might be abdominal pain, weight loss that cannot be explained, jaundice, and a change in appetite. Because these symptoms can resemble other mild conditions, people might not get diagnosed quickly. So, because the symptoms are not always apparent, healthcare professionals should be vigilant to catch liver tumor cases early. Better imaging methods have greatly changed how liver tumors are diagnosed. Tools such as ultrasound, computed tomography (CT), and magnetic resonance imaging (MRI) provide detailed visualization, enhancing the ability to detect hepatic lesions. Because of these techniques, more hepatic tumors are now found, causing surgeons to often examine and suggest treatments for benign lesions that could cause symptoms. It is still difficult to make a correct diagnosis, because benign tumors can sometimes cause serious problems that resemble those of cancer. Although imaging can accurately identify common benign lesions, such as hemangiomas and liver cysts, it may struggle to distinguish between benign hepatic adenomas and malignant tumors, emphasizing the need for further diagnostic evaluations in ambiguous cases (Iwatsuki *et al.*, 1990). If the images do not give a clear diagnosis, more tests might be needed. Biopsy procedures, such as fine-needle aspiration (FNA), can supply histological confirmation and guide treatment protocols. Besides classifying tumors, accurate diagnosis is important because it guides the choice of treatment, which can vary from close monitoring for benign tumors to surgical removal or use of drugs for malignant tumors. For instance, studies indicate that patients presenting with metastatic pancreatic neuroendocrine tumors (PNETs) often experience liver metastases at diagnosis, which significantly influences their prognosis (Aurello *et al.*, 2018). For this reason, it is very important to understand the signs and use effective methods to diagnose liver tumors, as this helps choose the best and possibly life-saving treatment options.

8.3.1. Common Symptoms of Liver Tumors

The presentation of liver tumors is usually insidious in nature and hence delays early diagnosis. Classic symptoms that appear are significant weight loss, anorexia, and persistent abdominal pain, particularly in the right upper quadrant. These are not necessarily suggestive of malignancy and therefore result in misdiagnosis or delay in treatment. Patients usually report fullness after little food intake, which might be due to the physical presence of the tumors inside the abdominal cavity. Jaundice, with signs of yellow skin and eyes, also appears in most cases as liver impairment occurs after tumor growth. Such a constellation of symptoms, both localized and systemic, can confuse medical practitioners unless proper examination is conducted. Physicians should have a very high index of suspicion when such symptoms occur, particularly in patients with a history of liver disease. Obstruction and inflammation of the bile ducts also worsen the clinical syndrome in liver tumor patients. These mechanisms have a tendency to create pruritus or intense itching because bile salts pool within the bloodstream when drainage is blocked. In addition, patients may have ascites, or fluid in the abdominal cavity, causing abdominal swelling and pain. This is indicative of a bad disease and must be treated immediately. Liver tumors tend to be related to liver enlargement or hepatomegaly, which is also palpable on physical examination. All in all, these symptoms embody the multi-component impact that liver tumors have on liver function and overall health and quality of life. The onset of these symptoms makes early detection and treatment especially paramount. In the case of individual tumor types, the presentation of symptoms may vary. As an example, pancreatic neuroendocrine tumors (PNETs) will metastasize to the liver, and from evidence it can be seen that 40-93% of these are presented with liver metastasis, once more highlighting the liver's role as a common site of metastasis (Aurello *et al.*, 2018). Symptoms in metastatic patients can also include those already mentioned, along with potential hepatic compromise as the tumor devastates normal liver architecture. Moreover, hepatic hemangiomas—liver vascular neoplasms—can also present differently, sometimes asymptomatic and incidentally detected by imaging. Nevertheless, when symptomatic, they can also produce pain or discomfort depending on size and location, also illustrating the diverse symptomatology of various liver tumor presentations (Fennell *et al.*, 1980). Awareness of these symptoms not only aids clinical diagnosis but also informs prognosis and treatment planning in affected patients (Figure 8.7).

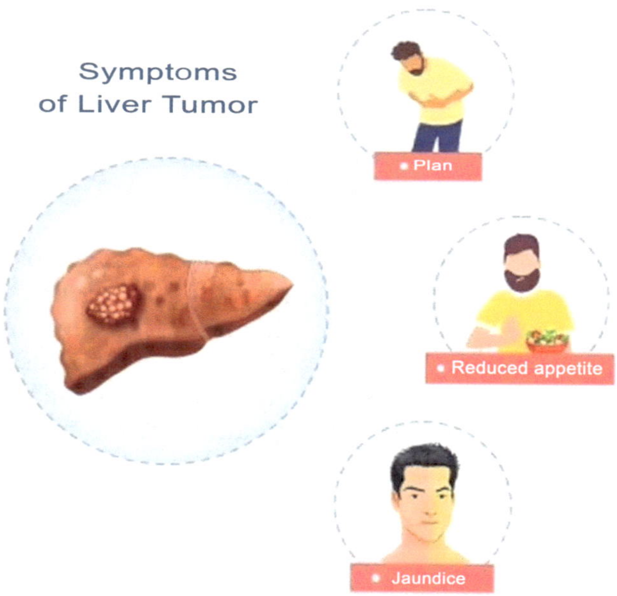

Figure 8.7. Symptoms of liver tumor.

Source: https://www.gastroclinix.com/wp-content/uploads/elementor/thumbs/Symptoms-of-liver-cancer-q6xbyobpgghr2l5vuooj1uh996hof2a94ab3zrmvqk.webp.

8.3.2. Diagnostic Imaging Techniques

The evaluation and control of liver tumors rely heavily on diagnostic imaging, which uses several techniques to improve the accuracy of diagnosis. Among these methods, magnetic resonance imaging (MRI) stands out for its ability to provide detailed visualization of liver anatomy and pathology. Recent advancements in MRI, particularly the application of machine learning (ML) algorithms, have significantly improved the classification of liver tumors. Studies have shown that using shape and texture features in these algorithms improves their performance, and the Extra Trees model is especially effective at classification. This development not only enhances diagnostic precision but also supports clinicians in making informed treatment decisions, underscoring the importance of innovation in medical imaging techniques in the context of liver tumors (Kandoriya *et al.*, 2024). Another important way to diagnose liver lesions is with ultrasound, which is accessible and can provide real-time images. Recent trials using advanced ultrasound systems, such as the Resona A20 Series, focus on multifrequency convex probes that incorporate cutting-edge techniques, including high-frame-rate contrast-enhanced ultrasound (HiFR CEUS) and shear wave elastography (SWE). These innovations allow for detailed visualization and characterization of liver lesions, facilitating accurate diagnoses of conditions like HCC and cholangiocellular carcinoma (CCC). Preliminary findings suggest the ability of these ultrasound techniques to characterize tumors based on elasticity and fat content, demonstrating efficacy in over 90% of cases evaluated (Jung *et al.*, 2024). The development of technology is making it more straightforward that ultrasound is becoming a main method for diagnosing liver problems. Liver tumor management has improved a lot thanks to the use of different diagnostic imaging methods, which help doctors diagnose and track tumors more accurately. Every imaging technique is useful, and MRI is best for seeing small details in soft tissue, whereas ultrasound can be used in real time and is widely available. Furthermore, the integration of artificial intelligence (AI) and ML into MRI analysis shows promise for enhanced prediction and categorization of tumor types, enabling more tailored therapeutic strategies. Overall, the collaborative application of MRI, ultrasound, and emerging technologies fosters a multidimensional understanding of liver tumors, ultimately contributing to improved patient outcomes and more effective clinical pathways in the management of this complex disease (Figure 8.8).

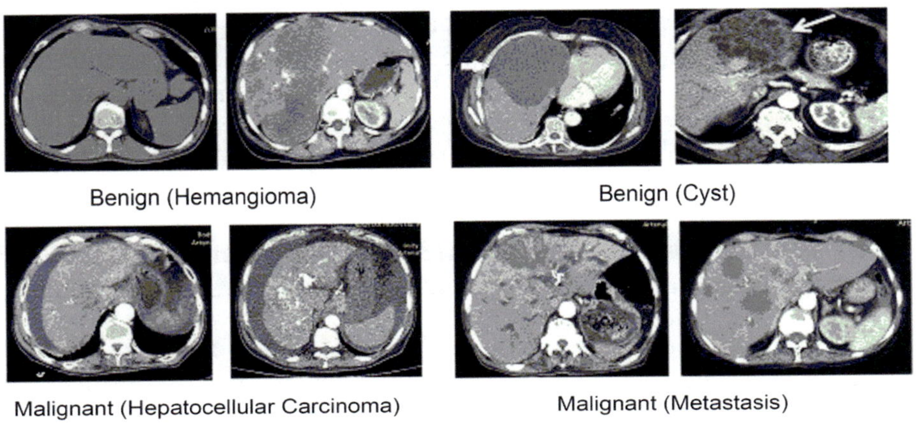

Figure 8.8. Liver tumor CT dataset images.

Source: https://www.researchgate.net/publication/359725187/figure/fig1/AS:11431281256808408@1719571374823/Liver-tumor-CT-Dataset-images.jpg.

8.3.3. Biopsy and Histological Examination

The test protocol for liver neoplasms typically calls for biopsy and histological examination, as both procedures provide significant information about the character and behavior of the neoplasms. A biopsy involves removing an inconsequential sample of liver tissue to be analyzed for cell abnormalities. This is particularly important for the differentiation of malignant from benign lesions and the diagnosis of some forms of liver tumors, such as HCC. Histological assessment allows pathologists to analyze the cellular architecture, morphology, and presence or absence of necrosis or inflammation. This, with the use of these guidelines, will allow clinicians to inform treatment decisions and make prognostic judgments, directing the way to individualized patient management regimens.

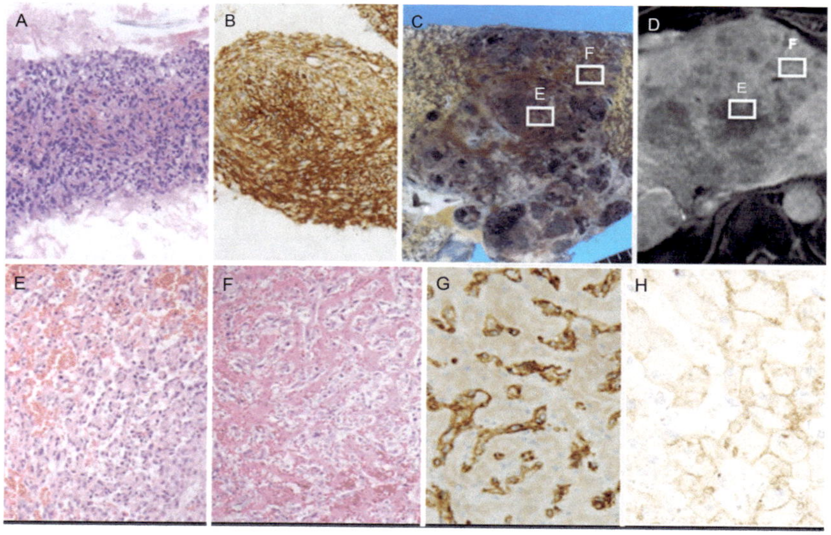

Figure 8.9. Histological findings from a liver tumor biopsy revealed the solid proliferation of spindle cells. A: Hematoxylin and eosin (HE); C: Macroscopically, a large tumor and many satellite nodules were observed in the liver; D: A hepatobiliary phase image obtained using gadolinium-ethoxybenzyl-diethylenetriamine-enhanced magnetic resonance imaging, depict almost the same plane of C; E: The proliferation of atypical spindle cells and hemorrhage were seen; F: Tumor cells had spread to the sinusoids in most of the liver, although normal hepatic cells remained; G: Tumor cells were positive for CD34; H: Tumor cells were negative for OATP1B3, and hepatic cells were positive for OATP1B3.

Source: https://www.researchgate.net/publication/322745427/figure/fig2/AS:587459402416128@1517072644812/Histological-findings-from-a-liver-tumor-biopsy-revealed-the-solid-proliferation-of.png.

The types of biopsy procedures used are not standardized, and the options can be FNA, core biopsies, or even open surgical biopsies in a few cases. All have their sets of pros and cons. For instance, FNA is less invasive but may not provide sufficient material for a definitive diagnosis, while core biopsies will provide larger samples and more reliable information about tissue composition. As noted, advances in imaging modalities enhance these techniques' sensitivity, allowing for more precise lesion targeting. At the histologic level, the examination can discern typical patterns by tumor type, i.e., hepatocellular-injury-type liver injury necrosis, underscoring the importance of correlating imaging findings and biopsy within diagnostic protocols (Kawano *et al.*, 2024). The correlation between histology and clinical findings is equally crucial. For instance, histologic characteristics such as grade of malignancy, inflammatory infiltrates, and necrosis may affect treatment and prognosis. The histologic context of liver tumors not only aids in diagnosis but can also guide therapeutic decisions, particularly in advanced disease. The histologic examination provides a basis for successful treatment planning tailored to the patient's disease status, as well as overall health. Also, the longer methods improve, the accuracy and worth of biopsy and histological examination reinforce their role as the "golden standard" in cancer diagnosis, just like with any other tumor forms (Saprykina *et al.*, 2024) (Figure 8.9).

8.4. Treatment Options

The treatment of liver tumors, mainly HCC, is not simple and usually requires using various approaches that match the patient's needs. Liver tumors found early are usually treated with surgery, which can result in a cure. However, the choice for surgery is limited by how big the tumor is, where it is found, and how well the liver functions, which can make it less effective. People who do not qualify for resection may be offered radiofrequency ablation and TACE as alternatives. They are designed to treat the tumor without harming much of the healthy liver tissue. Nonetheless, the prognosis for patients with advanced HCC remains poor, especially in light of the tumor's complex biology and resistance to standard interventions, prompting ongoing research into innovative treatments and combinations of existing modalities (Kim *et al.*, 2024). Recently, immunotherapy has changed the way cancer is treated in many types of cancer, including liver tumors. The immune response is often suppressed in the tumor microenvironment (TME) of liver cancer, making the application of immunotherapy particularly challenging yet critical. ICI has demonstrated good results, helping the body to spot and eliminate cancer cells. Still, their usefulness for HCC is not always the same, due to the liver's special immunosuppressive environment and the many types of HCC. Researchers are still exploring the immune system in liver tumors to find biomarkers that can show if immunotherapy will be effective. By tailoring treatment plans based on individual immune profiles, researchers hope to overcome existing barriers and optimize therapeutic outcomes for patients facing liver cancer (Nittayacharn *et al.*, 2023). New ways of delivering medicine are being studied to help improve how well drugs affect liver tumors. Using microbubbles filled with lipids for ultrasound-guided drug delivery has attracted interest because it may increase the accuracy of therapy. Initial research indicates that nanobubbles loaded with Doxorubicin can improve how the drug gets to liver tumors when used with ultrasound, helping to increase the drug inside the tumor and lower the risk of side effects elsewhere. This way of treatment greatly improves the therapeutic index, which is important for diseases that have few treatments and can be very toxic. As such, integrating innovative delivery systems with established treatments forms a promising avenue of research aimed at refining the therapeutic arsenal against liver tumors, ultimately paving the way for more tailored, effective interventions that enhance patient outcomes (Nittayacharn *et al.*, 2023).

8.4.1. Surgical Interventions

Management of liver tumors frequently requires surgical procedures, which are paramount to enhancing patient outcomes. Surgical interventions may vary from the resection of part of the liver to orthotopic liver transplantation (OLT), based on the tumor's characteristics, size, location, and the patient's general health. Resection is commonly done for local lesions that are considered to be resectable, where the goal is the attainment of clear margins to reduce the risk of recurrence. The challenge is that liver anatomy is so delicate, requiring an expert operating team to cut through vascular associations without harming the healthy liver. Resection, furthermore, is occasionally secondarily augmented by liver transplantation in highly select individuals with terminal liver cancer. This intervention does more than merely resect the lesion; it excises the underlying liver disease, providing a curative solution in select instances. Recent advancements have enhanced the efficacy and feasibility of surgical treatment of liver tumors. The 35-year-old woman with metastatic mixed acinar-endocrine carcinoma, for instance, is a case study that shows the complexity of curing liver tumors that have neuroendocrine features. Despite early misdiagnosis and prolonged non-surgical therapy with sunitinib and peptide receptor radionuclide therapy, a decision for liver transplantation was finally made due to tumor progression and symptomatic obstructive jaundice. Such an experience once again highlights the worth of personal treatment plans and the role of surgery in the control of long-term disease, especially if there is complex tumor involvement. The evolving understanding of tumor behavior and biology is most important in making decisions on surgery to ensure that patients get appropriate and potentially curative treatment (Both D *et al.*, 2017). Moreover, the multi-disciplinary approach is key to optimizing surgical outcomes for liver tumors. Inter-disciplinary collaboration between hepatologists, oncologists, radiologists, and surgeons facilitates careful patient assessment and management planning. Preoperative imaging studies, including advanced modalities like magnetic resonance imaging (MRI) and positron emission tomography (PET), provide important information on tumor staging and vascular extension. These modalities help define the surgical plan and determine respectability of the tumor. Furthermore, technical improvement in surgery, e.g., laparoscopic procedures, reduces morbidity and recovery times. Providing regular follow-up after surgical interventions is also crucial, as this allows for easy detection of recurrence or complications. Overall, these are the factors representing the highly variable landscape of surgical options for liver tumors, separating the optimal paths toward managing the patient (Figure 8.10).

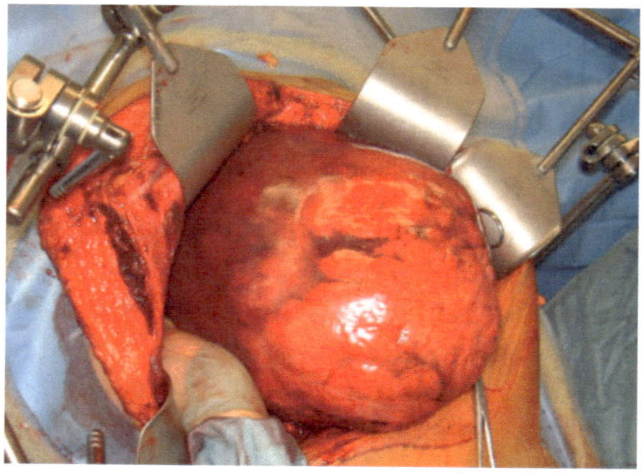

Figure 8.10. The massive liver tumor was at an early stage of the challenging operation.

Source: https://www.researchgate.net/profile/Hanan-El-Mahallawi/publication/6807838/figure/fig4/AS:202831505170436@1425370207064/The-massive-liver-tumor-at-an-early-stage-of-the-challenging-operation.png.

8.4.2. Chemotherapy and Targeted Therapy

Because of chemotherapy and targeted therapy, patients with tumors that cannot be removed by surgery now have more options for treatment. Chemotherapy, which is usually effective against fast-dividing cells, has had problems treating liver tumors because of their particular microenvironment and resistance. Even so, gemcitabine and cisplatin are commonly used chemotherapy drugs for advanced biliary cancers. Chemotherapy may not greatly increase long-term survival, but it is still important in palliative care to relieve symptoms and improve how patients feel when surgery is not possible. Targeted therapies are now being used as a promising way to treat liver tumors, mainly when the tumors have certain genetic mutations. Targeted treatments have made a huge difference in oncology by working to stop cancer growth by targeting the unique problems inside cancer cells. For biliary cancer, targeted approaches focusing on mutations such as those in the fibroblast growth factor receptor (FGFR) or isocitrate dehydrogenase (IDH) genes exemplify a shift towards personalized medicine. They may greatly enhance the results and give hope when chemotherapy has not worked well. As research continues to illuminate the genetic landscape of liver tumors, targeted therapies will likely play a more central role in treatment protocols, improving both survival rates and the quality of care for affected patients (Proskuriakova *et al.*, 2022). In addition, HCC, which is the most common type of liver cancer, creates unique problems and chances for treatment. For advanced HCC, treatment options like TACE and hepatic arterial infusion chemotherapy (HAIC) are increasingly utilized alongside targeted therapies to create a multimodal treatment strategy. It has been found that using chemotherapy and targeted drugs together can help the treatment work more effectively by using both types of drugs at once. For instance, recent advancements in systemic therapies targeting pathways like the vascular endothelial growth factor (VEGF) have shown potential when used in conjunction with traditional chemotherapy regimens. As targeted therapy continues to evolve, it is essential to integrate these innovative treatments into existing paradigms to better address the complexities of liver tumors and enhance patient outcomes (Guo *et al.*, 2022) (Figure 8.11).

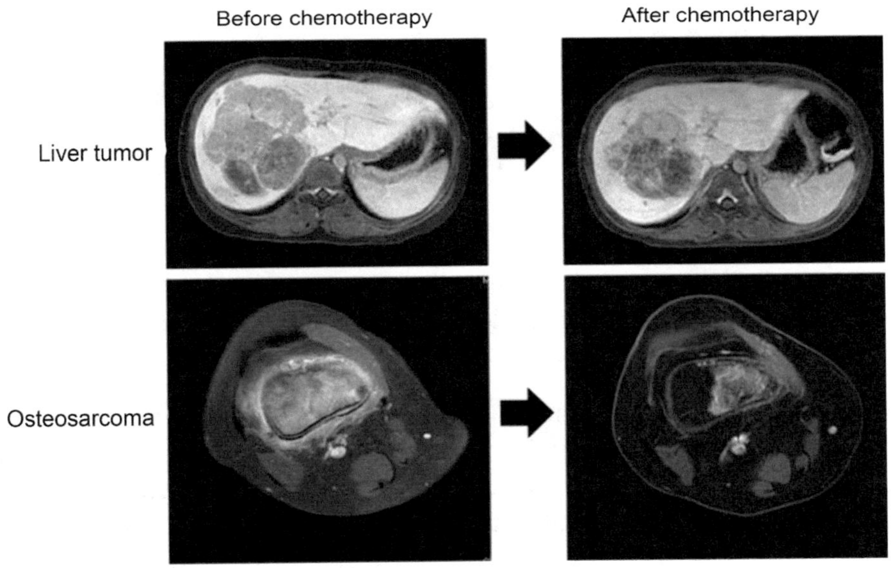

Figure 8.11. Reduced tumor masses in the liver and bone after chemotherapy.

Source: https://www.researchgate.net/profile/Yasushi-Fuchimoto-2/publication/231861263/figure/fig1/AS:214315983478788@1428108320373/Reduced-tumor-masses-in-the-liver-and-bone-after-chemotherapy-Magnetic-resonance-imaging.png.

8.4.3. Radiation Therapy

Radiotherapy has emerged as a principal component in the treatment of liver tumors, primarily as a palliative measure or in unresectable patients. It is a surgery-free method employing high-energy particles or waves to destroy cancer cells. For liver tumor conditions, the precision of radiotherapy is particularly useful because of the intricate organ anatomy and proximity to significant structures. Traditional external beam radiation is hampered in that it harms adjacent healthy tissue; however, more modern technologies, such as SBRT, permit sharp accuracy in targeting higher doses with a smaller impact on adjacent organs.

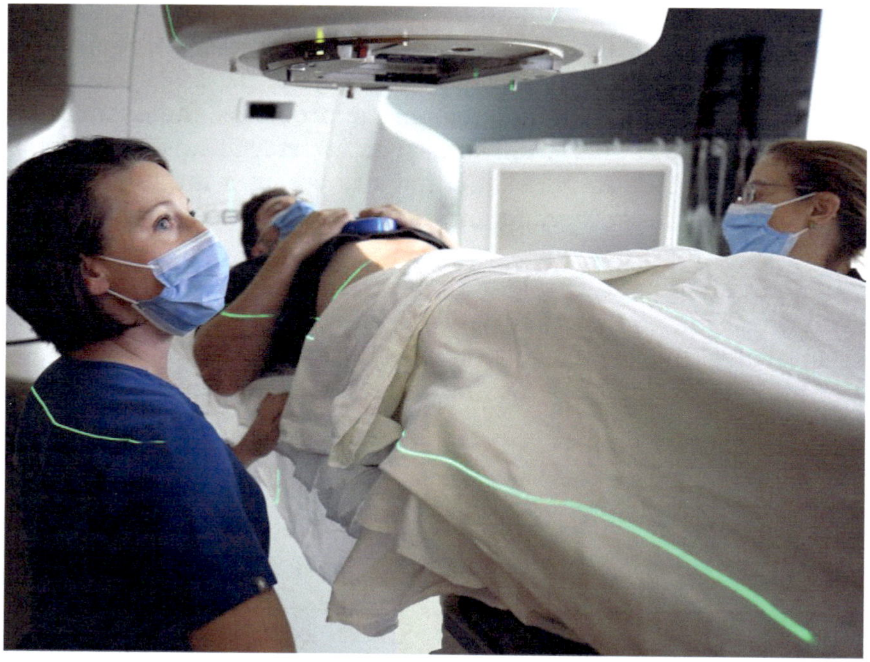

Figure 8.12. Radiation therapy.

Source: https://www.massgeneralbrigham.org/content/mgb-global/global/en/patient-care/international/treatments-and-specialties/cancer-care/liver-cancer/_jcr_content/root/container_924996778/hero_banner.coreimg.jpeg/1724688336118/liver-cancer-1428x1110.jpeg.

The patients subsequently experience a remission of symptoms and, in some cases, actual shrinkage of the tumor, paving the way for subsequent surgery or enhanced overall quality of life. Selective internal radiation therapy (SIRT) has also been marketed as a specialized form of radiation therapy for liver cancer patients, especially with inoperable tumors or metastatic disease. By injecting Yttrium-90 resin microspheres directly into the blood supply of the liver, this treatment confines radiation effects to the tumor and avoids the healthy liver. Specifically, SIRT has worked well in hard-to-treat diseases, such as metastatic tumors derived from solitary fibrous tumors (SFTs), which are highly resistant to standard therapies. As one can observe in studies that document the application of SIRTs in SFTs, patients have experienced a significant reduction of tumor and relief of symptoms following therapy. The success of such interventions reflects the need for further investigation of SIRT as a mode of treatment, with optimism in the patient population with limited alternatives (Badran *et al.*, 2024). Furthermore, while radiation treatment offers great promise, obstacles still exist in optimizing its application to liver tumors. The success of radiation can be influenced by tumor type, size, and location. The heterogeneity of liver cancers calls for treatment strategies tailored to patient-specific profiles. Furthermore, the tolerance to cumulative dose by the liver due to its radiosensitivity continues to be a persistent concern. New evidence now indicates that the association with immunotherapy provides an improved tumor control without the risks associated with radiation. This evolving landscape of liver cancer treatment calls for continued research and clinical trials to improve the understanding of long-term benefits and limitations of radiation therapy so that patients receive the optimum and most specific treatment (Liang, 2024) (Figure 8.12).

8.5. Prognosis and Survival Rates

The outlook for people with liver tumors, mainly HCC, depends on many things, such as the health of their liver and the tumor's features. HCC is known to be the second most common cause of cancer deaths worldwide, which makes it a difficult condition for doctors to treat. The results of treatment are very different depending on how advanced the disease is when it is found, and patients with small tumors and healthy livers tend to live much longer.

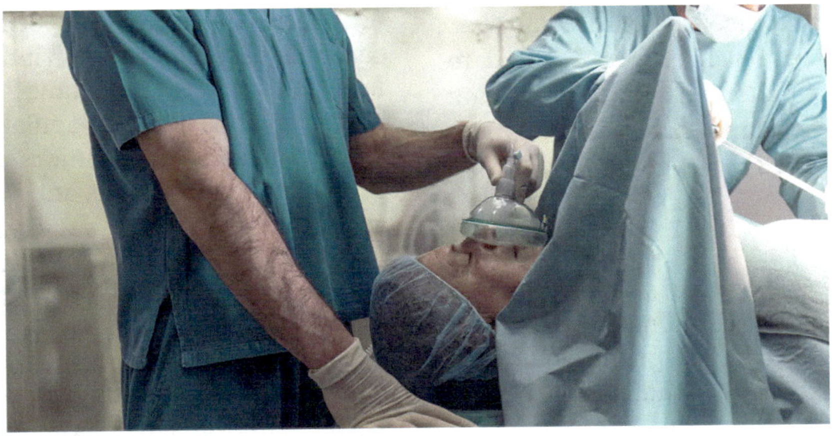

Figure 8.13. Prognosis and Survival Rates

Source: https://media.post.rvohealth.io/wp-content/uploads/2021/01/middleaged-man-put-under-anesthesia-1200x628-facebook-1200x628.jpg.

Most HCC cases are discovered at an advanced stage, so only around 20%-30% can benefit from interventions that might cure the disease, such as liver transplantation or anatomical targeting. Consequently, the five-year survival rate in the United States for HCC patients lags at approximately 16%, indicating the urgent need for improved diagnostic and therapeutic strategies (Busuttil *et al.*, 2015). Following patients with cholangiocarcinoma, especially those who have OLT, helps to discover what affects their survival from liver tumors. In a study of 54 patients, the researchers found that the extent of tumor removal and the surgical margins played a major role in patient survival. If the tumor was removed completely, one-year survival was 64%, but this dropped to

26% after five years. It was found that having multiple tumors, lymph node involvement, and positive surgical margins were major predictors of poor results. Excluding patients with these predictors revealed significantly improved survival rates, underscoring the importance of precise surgical strategies in enhancing prognosis (Casavilla *et al.*, 1997). Adding novel diagnostic and prognostic biomarkers to the management of liver tumors can help improve the outcomes of patients. With new research, targeted therapies and customized treatment plans are now more possible for people with liver cancer. Using immunotherapy along with standard treatments gives patients with advanced liver tumors a better chance of fighting the disease. Creating and confirming prognostic biomarkers is very important, as they help doctors determine the risk level of patients and what treatment to use to increase survival. As such, ongoing research efforts devoted to refining prognostic tools and strategies remain pivotal in the evolving landscape of liver cancer treatment (Figure 8.13).

8.5.1. Factors Influencing Prognosis

The prognosis of liver tumors is established based on a multivariable combination of clinical and pathological variables. Of primary concern is metastatic disease status. Studies have shown that the character of the primary tumor has a significant impact on liver tumor prognosis; for example, in patients undergoing hepatic resection for metastatic colorectal neoplasm, positivity of surgical margins and extension of tumor beyond the liver anticipate poor outcomes (Bonham *et al.*, 1999). In addition, tumor burden, as indicated by the number of lesions and their pattern in the liver, is also of significant concern. Tumors with bilateral or multifocal involvement will generally indicate a worse prognosis, therefore underscoring early complete assessment and planning for management. Lastly, awareness of these prognosticators can make therapy and patient care so targeted that results are optimized and risks associated with advanced liver cancer are reduced. Besides tumor characteristics, patient-specific variables have a strong prognostic influence. Age, baseline liver function, and general functional status are significant in survival evaluation in patients with liver cancer. Patients with previous liver disease, for instance, cirrhosis, will have deficient hepatic function, which adversely affects their ability to tolerate aggressive treatment such as surgical resection or TACE. In this case, the Child-Pugh score is a methodical way to assess liver function, directing clinical treatment and therapeutic decisions (Abdelaziz *et al.*, 2011). Furthermore, the time interval between the first treatment of the primary tumor and recurrence of liver metastasis is of essential importance to prognosis, with shorter intervals tending towards an unfavorable prognosis. These patient-specific factors must be carefully assessed to offer individually tailored interventions that optimize survival in this heterogeneous patient population. The modality of treatment for liver tumors carries significant prognostic significance, and various modalities are associated with varying outcomes. For example, TACE is now a palliative intervention for unresectable HCC. The efficacy of TACE can be inconsistent based on some variables, including the presence of PVT and arterioportal shunts, which have been shown to significantly impact local tumor response (Abdelaziz *et al.*, 2011). This validates the necessity for precise imaging and clinical evaluation prior to treatment initiation. Additionally, as treatments evolve, the use of additional therapies or combined regimens has been reported to enhance efficacy and patient outcomes. Optimal understanding of the interaction between treatment modalities and factors related to patients will ultimately enable individualized planning for treatment that maximizes survival and quality of life in patients with liver tumors.

8.5.2. Survival Rates for Different Types of Liver Tumors

Survival rates of various forms of liver tumors can vary considerably with tumor origin, stage at presentation, and treatment modalities. HCC, which is the most common primary liver malignancy, generally has worse prognostic outcomes, especially at advanced stages. The five-year survival for localized HCC is approximately 30%, declining dramatically to about 3% with metastasis. In contrast, when liver tumors are of a neuroendocrine nature, i.e., pancreatic neuroendocrine tumors (PNETs), survival is much improved. PNETs may initially bear liver metastasis but, if treated by resection of the tumor, can offer a median overall survival of 128 months and an 83% survival at five years for well-differentiated tumors, pointing to the impact of tumor biology and treatment on survival. Surgical advances and adjuvant therapy have further modified survival in the treatment of liver tumors. Research has shown that complete resection of liver tumors, such as colorectal cancer metastases, can significantly increase overall survival. In a clinical trial of patients with initially unresectable colorectal liver metastases (CRLM), survival figures indicated overall median survival in patients treated with FOLFOX/FOLFIRI-bevacizumab at 39.9 months, as opposed to 18.3 months in those with tumors remaining unresectable. This contrast highlights the importance of early treatment and the potential of systemic therapies, including FOLFOX, to improve patient survival. Of interest, adjuvant treatment following liver surgery can enhance relapse-free survival rates, reflecting a broad trend in cancer therapy that seeks to optimize patient survival. Understanding the complexity of survival rates in liver tumors involves consideration of tumor differentiation and position. For example, the latter group of patients with well-differentiated tumors has significantly improved prognoses compared to those who are diagnosed with poorly differentiated subtypes, which incidentally normally indicate a more aggressive clinical course and poor prognosis. The grade of the tumor remains a significant prognostic factor; while overall survival for G1 PNETs is about 128 months, this significantly decreases in the case of G3 tumors, with a median survival of only 49.7 months. These variations stress the significant role played by tumor features in survival projection and highlight the need for personalized therapeutic measures. Accordingly, further investigation into the biological and molecular features of liver tumors is important to improve the rate of survival and provide insight into future clinical practice in managing these cancers (Figure 8.14).

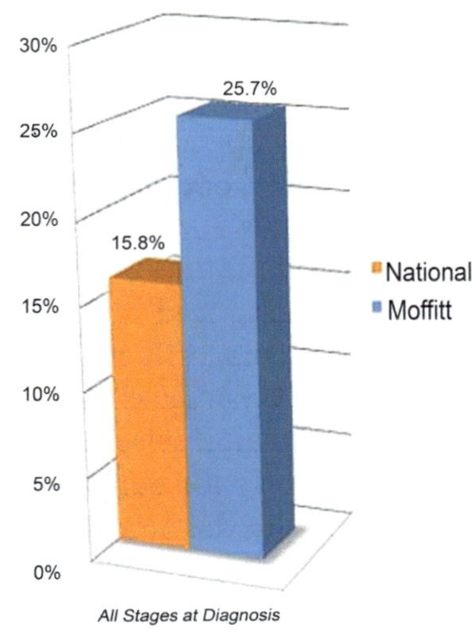

Figure 8.14. Survival rates for liver cancer patients.

Source: https://iytmed.com/wp-content/uploads/2015/12/5_liver-chart.jpg.

8.5.3. Importance of Early Detection

The significance of early diagnosis of liver tumors, particularly HCC, cannot be overestimated. A slow-growing malignant liver illness with few symptoms, early detection becomes essential to improve the prognosis of patients. The asymptomatic character of the early stage of HCC results in a high number of patients being diagnosed in the advanced stage, when few therapeutic options are available. The establishment of a diagnosis prior to the onset of severe symptoms significantly enhances the possibilities for curative therapies. Global guidelines stipulate that surveillance at fixed intervals should be performed among populations with a high risk; however, existing methods of diagnosis fall short in sensitivity for identifying tumors at the earliest phase, rendering early detection unlikely (Cox *et al.*, 2016). These limitations underscore the pressing need for innovative screening technologies capable of identifying HCC at its earliest, most developing stages. The recent advances in biomarker studies and metabolic profiling also hold great potential for enhancing the earlier detection of liver tumors. Metabolic studies have been successful in detecting specific metabolites that dramatically differentiate between HCC and other liver conditions like CLD. For example, the sugar alcohols level has been found to be elevated in patients with HCC compared to patients with CLD and healthy controls, reflecting a potential early tumorigenesis marker (El-Said *et al.*, 2020). The distinct metabolic alterations of HCC could bring crucial biomarkers for early detection. In addition to accentuating the biological intricacy of HCC, these findings indicate that harnessing metabolomic and proteomic platforms will be crucial in designing simple, non-invasive assays to diagnose liver tumors at their early stages, particularly where the elevated prevalence of HCC is seen in resource-limited areas (El-Said *et al.*, 2020). Embracing enhanced early detection strategies can have significant implications for public health and patient prognosis. Detection of liver tumors in an early stage enables medical systems to intervene early, which reduces the risk of death among patients. Early detection guarantees a decrease in the health burden imposed by HCC, which is among the leading causes of cancer-related mortality globally (Cox *et al.*, 2016). Hence, it is crucial to give priority to clinical and research validation of emerging biomarkers and diagnostic tests. With the insight into liver tumorigenesis deepening, there is the potential to reformulate early detection rates at their very foundation, which would ultimately lead to improved clinical outcomes as well as reduced mortality from liver tumors (El-Said *et al.*, 2020). Such a refinement of diagnostic capability will not just enhance patient care but reduce the economic load involved in curing advanced-stage liver cancer (Figure 8.15).

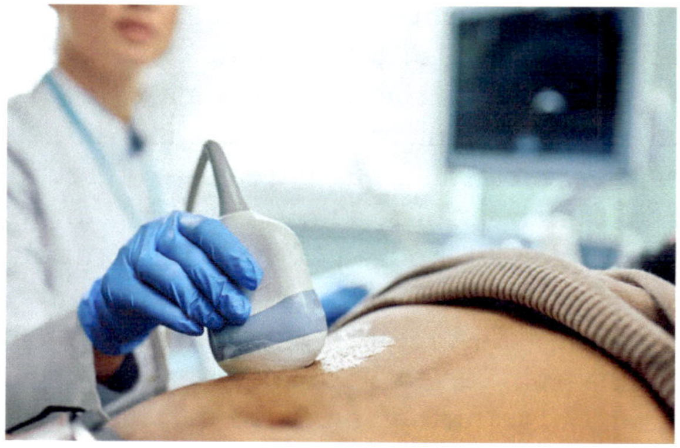

Figure 8.15. Detecting liver tumors.

Source: Vhttps://v.wpimg.pl/MzUxN2Q0Yhs0GjgBfktvDndCbFs4EmFYIFp0EH4Bf0JlAGFUOFwoCDAIIRw2QjgKNA8-HCFcYhslEWFEYB8pEyYIIlMoHygXNx0qHWJVKU1gTHoLfAJ7QjdVegM3B2BCM0t2HzIFfUlgSXlWZQF6T3cF.

8.6. Research and Advances

Lately, there has been a surge of research on liver tumors, which has provided important information about their diagnosis and treatment. The use of MRI and CT scans has made it easier to find liver tumors sooner, which helps patients get better treatment and outcomes. New studies point out that using different specialties together helps design personalized treatment plans for patients with liver tumors. For instance, Caplin *et al.* (2017) underscore the necessity of having specialized protocols and coordinated care networks to optimally manage these neoplasms. With these frameworks, both the diagnosis and the choice of therapy are made easier, and patients receive treatment that matches their tumor and condition. There have been important improvements in treating liver tumors, mainly for HCC and metastatic conditions. Because of targeted therapies and immunotherapies, treatment options have improved for cases that were previously hard to treat. It has been found that using systemic therapies with ablation and TACE can give patients with liver tumors better outcomes. Furthermore, Bronsther *et al.* (1992) highlight the promising results of using liver transplantation in cases of extensive hepatic cell proliferation, illustrating how innovative surgical interventions can effectively manage complicated cases of adenomatous lesions. This shows a wider move towards personalized medicine, where people's treatment is guided by their genetic and molecular information. With more research, the outlook for treating liver tumors is getting better. New medicines and improved therapies are created through ongoing clinical trials. Looking into different ways to combine treatments and provide drugs could greatly improve the effectiveness of what is used now. Improved genetic sequencing techniques are helping researchers learn more about tumor biology, which might result in finding new biomarkers for early detection and predicting outcomes. Researchers and clinicians need to join forces so that new discoveries are used in medical practice. The integrative approach highlighted by *et al.*Caplin *et al.* (2017) not only addresses the complexities of liver tumors but also sets the foundation for improved outcomes in patients facing these challenging conditions. With further progress, these developments are expected to change the way liver tumors are handled, managed, and defeated.

8.6.1. Current Research Trends in Liver Tumor Treatment

The therapeutic setting for liver tumours has dramatically evolved, particularly with regard to unraveling the TME and its impact on therapy. Recent directions of research are tilting more towards unraveling the complexity of the TME, specifically metastatic processes. For instance, peritoneal metastasis of colorectal cancer research emphasizes the significance of the TME in enabling metastatic activity and points to a need for novel therapeutic strategies against this microenvironment. By identifying the structural components and functional characteristics of the TME, researchers anticipate that it is possible to design interventions capable of re-engineering the stroma to inhibit the formation of metastasis and improve patient outcomes. This line of inquiry not only suggests a trend toward more directed approaches but also toward a better understanding of the biologic interactions that define tumor behavior in liver tumors (Ceelen *et al.*, 2020). At the same time, new therapeutic modalities are being explored to augment traditional methods of liver tumor management. Radioembolization and chemoembolization are two such modalities that have been considered. Current comparative studies demonstrate that both methods yield similar disease control rates and toxicities when applied to unresectable intrahepatic cholangiocarcinoma. The research shows that even though the two procedures have an equivalent therapeutic window, their varying mechanisms under some clinical situations have different advantages. This ongoing research into interventional radiology underscores the importance of treatment planning on a patient-specific basis, creating an era where the preferred technique can be maximized based on patient profiles in terms of history, tumor burden, and overall condition (Akinwande *et al.*, 2017). With continuous advancement in the discipline, the addition of systemic treatment to the local interventions is the current vogue in the investigation of liver tumors. Directed therapies based on the body's immune system, complemented by molecular profiling technologies, are spearheading the move toward more personalized treatments.

Current research is trying to identify the best molecular characteristics that predict response to therapy and thereby enable clinicians to select the optimal multimodality therapy for liver tumors. While these research trends are being felt, the promise is moving away from one-size-fits-all to a more nuanced one that takes into account the heterogeneity of liver tumors. The hopes of greater prognostic accuracy and therapeutic efficacy by means of such targeted methods offer a hopeful horizon in the unrelenting fight against liver cancers, ultimately attempting to enhance survival and quality of life for patients (Akinwande *et al.*, 2017; Ceelen *et al.*, 2020) (Figure 8.16).

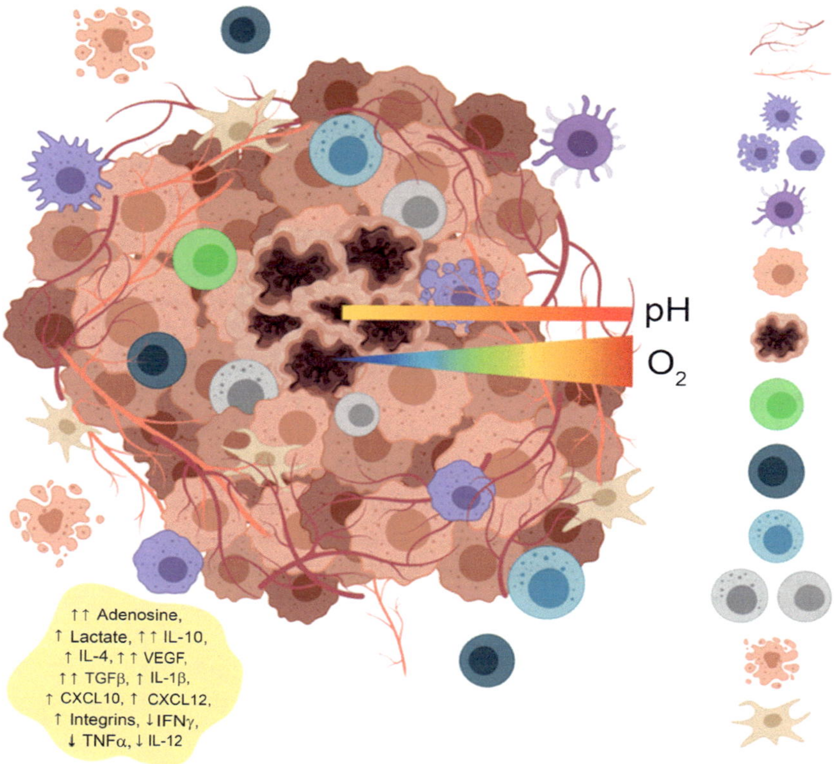

Figure 8.16. Component of the tumor microenvironment (TME).

Source: https://upload.wikimedia.org/wikipedia/commons/thumb/4/4c/Components-of-the-tumor-microenvironment.png/800px-Components-of-the-tumor-microenvironment.png.

8.6.2. Innovations in Diagnostic Techniques

There have been many improvements in liver oncology, especially in how liver elastography has made it possible to diagnose liver problems without invasive procedures. With this method, doctors can check the stiffness of tissue to distinguish malignant liver tumors from benign ones. The basic idea is that cancers often have more cells, which causes them to be stiffer than benign tumors. Liver elastography uses the differences in tissue stiffness to help diagnose liver diseases, which reduces the need for liver biopsies. Besides, better ultrasound equipment and AI help make HCC diagnoses more accurate and allow doctors to determine the risk for each patient. With ongoing research underscoring the utility of elastography in predicting HCC progression and evaluating treatment responses, these innovations mark a significant leap toward improving patient management in liver oncology (Cerban *et al.*, 2025). It is critical to use precise diagnostic methods in liver tumors, as they help decide on the best treatment plan, especially for liver transplantation. Innovations in perfusion technology have emerged as particularly promising, especially for utilization in cases involving donation after circulatory death (DCD). Using machine perfusion helps to keep organs alive during transplantation, which lowers the risk of ischemia–reperfusion injury. Using these techniques, which involve both warming and cooling the liver, may revolutionize how liver grafts are managed in transplant oncology. Although there is no proof yet that machine perfusion lowers tumor recurrence, many are hopeful that it can enhance the function and outcomes of the transplanted organ. Continued exploration into the applications of machine perfusion in transplant settings suggests significant potential for future breakthroughs in the management of liver tumors (Finotti *et al.*, 2024). Using modern imaging methods has improved the ability to find liver tumors. MRI and CT scans today use new imaging methods and contrast agents to better see both the shape of tumors and their blood vessels. Because of these advancements, liver tumors can be better staged, and doctors can design more suitable treatment plans for each patient. Better imaging can find smaller tumors sooner, which may help patients live longer. Also, using imaging along with liquid biopsies can provide more information about tumor changes and how patients respond to treatment. As these innovations continue to evolve, they will play an increasingly critical role in the early detection and characterization of liver tumors, ultimately contributing to improved prognostic outcomes for patients (Cerban *et al.*, 2025).

8.6.3. Future Directions in Liver Cancer Research

With ongoing liver tumor research, the future of liver cancer research remains centered on non-invasive diagnostic techniques with a concentration towards improving early detection and HCC characterization. Current diagnosis largely depends on invasive procedures, such as needle biopsies, which are dangerous for patients. New techniques with next-generation imaging technologies are being developed to scan ultrasound images with special regard to the textural features of liver tissue. Employing higher-order Grey Level Cooccurrence Matrices (GLCM) together with accurate textural models, researchers are working towards establishing a reliable, computerized HCC diagnosis. This paradigm has the promise to provide timely information to clinicians, enabling proactive treatments and ultimately enhancing patient prognosis without the complications that occur in standard biopsy protocols and thus representing a promising horizon for liver cancer research (Badea *et al.*, 2012). The research on immunotherapy is also ostensibly a focal area of interest in the war against liver cancer, especially in the instance of HCC. Accumulating evidence identifies the significant hindrances caused by immunosuppression and immune dysfunction in patients, especially those who are suffering from CLD. Advances in the knowledge of mechanisms underlying T-cell-mediated immunosuppression suggest that therapies designed to restore immune vigilance could significantly improve patient prognosis. Clinical trials have also begun to uncover that approximately 20% of advanced HCC patients may benefit from treatment methods targeting the restoration of antitumor immunity. Future research must then aim at establishing the mechanisms of immune impairment in the remaining population of patients to develop more targeted therapies capable of enhancing immunity to HCC, and look forward to an increase in survival in this patient population (Karin *et al.*, 2018). In the end, the systematic approach integrating new diagnostic approaches and immunotherapeutic protocols has the promise of revolutionizing the treatment of liver cancer. To optimize the use of such advances, interdisciplinarity involving many specialties—molecular biology, pharmacology, and medical imaging, among others—will be required. The principles of translational research should be adhered to by researchers, with findings from the laboratory translated successfully into the clinic. Along with this, patient-centered studies that consider the diverse needs of liver cancer-stricken patients also hold importance. With the formulation of an innovation, learning, and collaborative culture, the future of liver cancer studies can offer more effective treatments, better detection methods, and ultimately, a better quality of life for liver tumor patients (Badea *et al.*, 2012; Karin *et al.*, 2018) (Figure 8.17).

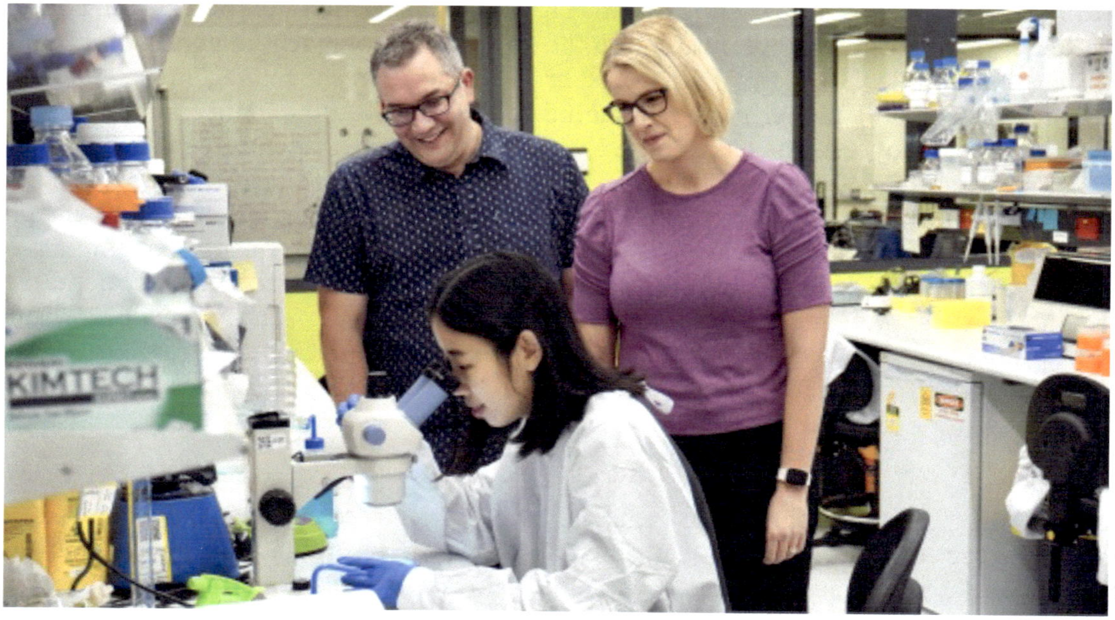

Figure 8.17. Future investigations

Source: https://www.petermac.org/images/news/DSC05650.jpg.

SUMMARY

The liver's fundamental role in detoxification and metabolism makes it particularly vulnerable to a range of malignancies, the primary among them being HCC, the most common. As highlighted, the rising incidence of primary liver cancer, with approximately 30,000 new cases each year being reported in the United States, paints a picture of an urgent demand for effective diagnostic and therapeutic interventions. Awareness of the risk factors, such as cirrhosis and chronic hepatitis infection, is important for earlier treatment and improved outcomes. Last but not least, awareness about liver tumors is important for both patients and physicians, so that diagnosis can be done at the right time. Moreover, advances in medical imaging technology are vital in the treatment of liver tumors. Techniques such as CT and Magnetic Resonance Imaging (MRI) facilitate detailed studies of tumor characteristics for more accurate diagnosis and personalized therapy. As affirmed by existing clinical studies, imaging techniques facilitate the delineation of tumor size and vascularity of HCC tumors, which are crucial for treatment planning. For instance, measurement of tumor volume within contrast-enhanced CT imaging provides essential information that can be applied in the direction of treatment intervention, e.g., TACE. Ongoing research must continue to further these imaging modalities in terms of maximizing patient care as well as maximizing the accuracy of liver tumor evaluations, since this is at the core of optimizing patient outcomes. Ultimately, the issue of liver tumors, specifically HCC, highlights the need for a multifaceted solution that addresses prevention, early detection, and potent treatment regimens. The presence of PVT and arterioportal shunts significantly affects treatment responses, underlining the importance of understanding tumor biology and patient individuality. This need dictates an interdisciplinarity in management approach, encompassing surgery, medicine, and supportive care to address the disease and the patient's individual needs. As development in the discipline advances, collaboration and interdisciplinary investigation will be central in the management of the increasing liver tumor burden and quality of life in those affected. Outcomes from current research provide a firm foundation upon which to base future developments in the treatment of liver cancer, presenting the ongoing work necessary to address this important health issue.

The complex arena of liver neoplasms has a spectrum of tumors with varied biological characteristics and clinical implications. Traditionally, liver tumor classification has given significance to cellular origins and morphological patterns, but recent advancements have underscored a paradigm shift towards consideration of the physiological activities of the tumors. For instance, differentiation between malignant and benign hepatocellular neoplasms may be enhanced by attention to the liver-restricted metabolic pathways, such as albumin and bile acid production and glucose regulation. This novel paradigm not only improves understanding of tumor biology but also builds a critical connection between metabolic dysregulation and tumorigenesis, in particular HCCs that are metabolically heterogeneous (Aoki *et al.*, 2024). Such observations highlight the imperative need to include metabolic profiling in liver tumor assessment and management. Furthermore, the identification of intrinsic molecular pathways has profound implications for the classification of liver tumors. Existing research focuses on the signaling pathways of normal hepatobiliary differentiation processes, with homology to the majority of tumors. Those critical pathways, such as Wnt/β-catenin, RAS, NOTCH, and TGF-β, are important in determining tumor features and also in influencing prognosis. Most significantly, lost essential metabolic processes in tumors can lead to dedifferentiation and neomorphosis toward biliary cells or show elevated glycolytic metabolism. This transformation can lead to vast changes in tumor behavior and complicate diagnosis and therapy even further (Aoki *et al.*, 2024). This dynamic knowledge base forms the groundwork for the future study of stratifying liver tumors based on their metabolic signatures and corresponding signal transduction pathways. Finally, a focus on physiological liver tumor classifications opens rich soil to devise targeted therapy regimens. Through an understanding of the mechanisms driving metabolic alterations in liver neoplasms, researchers can hopefully delineate novel biomarkers that could be implemented in early detection and tailored treatment regimens. Translation of studying metabolic function tests into the clinical environment might not only refine prognostic estimates, but also revolutionize the therapeutic environment for liver tumor patients. Further research on the intersection between liver metabolism and oncogenesis provides a promising potential to transform treatment approaches that directly address the unique metabolic demands of liver tumors (Aoki *et al.*, 2024). With regard to this, the union of sophisticated molecular diagnostics with traditional histopathological assessments will set the liver cancer management agenda for the future, holding promise for improved patient outcomes.

CLOSER LOOK

TRANSARTERIAL CHEMOEMBOLIZATION (TACE)

TACE is a minimally invasive procedure used to treat cancer, particularly liver cancer, by combining the delivery of chemotherapy drugs with the blockage of blood flow to the tumor. It works by infusing chemotherapy directly into the blood vessels feeding the tumor, then using an embolic agent to block those vessels, trapping the chemotherapy and reducing its systemic effects. TACE is often used for unresectable HCC (Figure 8.18).

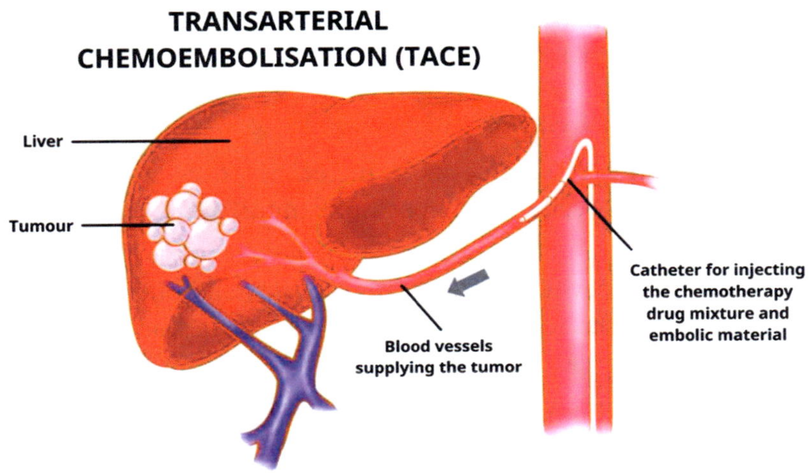

Figure 8.18. Transarterial chemoembolization (TACE).

Source: https://www.fvhospital.com/wp-content/uploads/2024/10/tace-202404.jpg.

How TACE Works

- **Chemotherapy Delivery:** Chemotherapy drugs are infused directly into the arteries supplying the tumor through a catheter inserted into a major artery, typically the femoral artery. This delivers a higher concentration of chemotherapy to the tumor than systemic treatment, reducing the need for higher systemic doses and minimizing side effects.
- **Embolization:** Following chemotherapy delivery, embolic agents are used to block the tumor-feeding blood vessels. This can be achieved with materials like Lipiodol, Gelfoam, or microparticles.
- **Synergistic Effect:** The combination of chemotherapy and embolization aims to achieve a synergistic effect, enhancing the treatment's effectiveness. The embolization reduces blood flow to the tumor, which can increase the effectiveness of the chemotherapy by allowing it to linger longer in the tumor.

- **Minimally Invasive:** TACE is a minimally invasive procedure, performed using imaging guidance (like fluoroscopy) and a catheter. This reduces the need for major surgery and associated risks.

Benefits of TACE

- **Targeted Treatment:** TACE allows for targeted delivery of chemotherapy to the tumor, potentially sparing healthy tissue.
- **Reduced Systemic Toxicity:** By delivering chemotherapy directly to the tumor, TACE minimizes the amount of drug circulating in the bloodstream, reducing systemic side effects.
- **Effective for Unresectable HCC:** TACE is a standard treatment option for unresectable HCC, particularly in patients with cirrhosis.

Considerations and Potential Risks

- **Side Effects:** TACE can cause side effects, including post-embolization syndrome (fever, pain, nausea, fatigue), as well as other complications like allergic reactions to the embolic agent.
- **Individualization:** The specific chemotherapy drugs, embolic agents, and technique used in TACE may vary based on the patient's condition and the characteristics of the tumor.
- **Repeated Sessions:** In some cases, multiple TACE sessions may be needed to achieve the desired treatment effect.

References

1. Abdelaziz, O., Ackermann, H., Emad-Eldin, S., Mohammed, A., *et al.* (2011). *Portal Vein Thrombosis and Arterioportal Shunts: Effects on Tumor Response After Chemoembolization of Hepatocellular Carcinoma.* https://core.ac.uk/download/14530356.pdf (accessed on 24 May 2025).

2. Addeo, P., Cusumano, C., Goichot, B., Guerra, M., Faitot, F., Imperiale, A., & Bachellier, P. (2022). Simultaneous Resection of Pancreatic Neuroendocrine Tumors with Synchronous Liver Metastases: Safety and Oncological Efficacy. Cancers, 14. https://www.semanticscholar.org/paper/Simultaneous-Resection-of-Pancreatic-Neuroendocrine-Addeo-Cusumano/1a3fcde941d566f1951dfc876914a31f6a1eff50

3. Aisaborhale, E. E. (2016). *Relationship Between Primary Liver Hepatocellular Carcinoma Volumes on Portal-Venous Phase CT Imaging* [Master's thesis, Boston University]. https://open.bu.edu/bitstream/2144/15388/1/Aisaborhale_bu_0017N_10836.pdf

4. Akinwande, O., Foltz, G., Mills, A., Noda, C., *et al.* (2017). *Chemoembolization Versus Radioembolization for The Treatment of Unresectable Intrahepatic Cholangiocarcinoma in A Single Institution: Image-Based Efficacy and Comparative Toxicity.* https://core.ac.uk/download/286537351.pdf (accessed on 24 May 2025).

5. Aoki, T., Nishida, N., Minami, Y., & Kudo, M. (2024). The impact of normal hepatobiliary cell zonation programs on the phenotypes and functions of primary liver tumors. *Liver Cancer, 14*, 92–103. https://www.semanticscholar.org/paper/82cd58aa5d022842f6a4867f858fca879326ab0f (accessed on 24 May 2025).

6. Asahina, K., Deshaies, R., Duan, L., Dynnyk, A., *et al.* (2009). *Toll-Like Receptor 4 Mediates Synergism Between Alcohol and HCV in Hepatic Oncogenesis Involving Stem Cell Marker Nanog.* https://core.ac.uk/download/4880714.pdf.

7. Aurello, P., Crovetto, A., Debs, T., Mangogna, A., *et al.* (2018). *Treatment Options for PNET Liver Metastases: A Systematic Review.* https://core.ac.uk/download/159636090.pdf (accessed on 24 May 2025).

8. Babicky, M. L., French, R. P., Hoh, C. K., Jaquish, A., *et al.* (2014). *Generation of Orthotopic Patient-Derived Xenografts from Gastrointestinal Stromal Tumor.* https://core.ac.uk/download/323066735.pdf.

9. Badea, R., Mitrea, D., Nedevschi, S., Socaciu, C., *et al.* (2012). *The Role of The Superior Order GLCM in The Characterization and Recognition of The Liver Tumors from Ultrasound Images.* https://core.ac.uk/download/30311780.pdf.

10. Badran, O., Dereza, S., Mireb, L., Neeman, Z., & Bar-Sela, G. (2024). Case report: Successful treatment of solitary fibrous tumor with selective internal radiation therapy (SIRT). *Diseases, 12.* https://www.semanticscholar.org/paper/f327451ff378993dc3dfbecf1f8056aae4b8733f (accessed on 24 May 2025).

11. Bernard Becker Medical Library Archives. (2002). *Focal Spot, Summer 2002.* Washington University School of Medicine. https://core.ac.uk/download/129069324.pdf (accessed on 24 May 2025).

12. Bond, M., Bolhuis, K., Loosveld, O. J. L., de Groot, J. D., Droogendijk, H., Helgason, H., Hendriks, M., *et al.* (2024). First-line systemic treatment for initially unresectable colorectal liver

metastases: Post hoc analysis of the CAIRO5 randomized clinical trial. *JAMA Oncology*. https://www.semanticscholar.org/paper/fb7952fee090506568bdd6b00577bf88560170be

13. Bonham, A. C., Dodson, F., Dvorchik, I., Fung, J. J., *et al.* (1999). *Hepatic Resection for Metastatic Colorectal Adenocarcinoma: A Proposal of a Prognostic Scoring System*. https://core.ac.uk/download/12205499.pdf (accessed on 24 May 2025).
14. Bronsther, O., Iwatsuki, S., Marino, I. R., Scantlebury, V., *et al.* (1992). *Total Hepatectomy and Liver Transplant for Hepatocellular Adenomatosis and Focal Nodular Hyperplasia*. https://core.ac.uk/download/12204786.pdf (accessed on 24 May 2025).
15. Busuttil, R. W., Faltermeier, C., & Zarrinpar, A. (2015). *A Surgical Perspective on Targeted Therapy of Hepatocellular Carcinoma*. https://core.ac.uk/download/323077917.pdf.
16. Calborean, V., Miscoci, A., Pirvu, C. D., Pădureanu, V., *et al.* (2018). *The Importance of Circulating Tumor Products As "Liquid Biopsies" In Colorectal Cancer*. https://core.ac.uk/download/216808108.pdf (accessed on 24 May 2025).
17. Caplin, M., Falconi, M., Fusai, G. K., Lykoudis, P., *et al.* (2017). *Treatment Challenges in And Outside a Specialist Network Setting: Pancreatic Neuroendocrine Tumors*. https://core.ac.uk/download/168403284.pdf (accessed on 24 May 2025).
18. Casavilla, F. A., Dvorchik, I., Fung, J. J., Iwatsuki, S., *et al.* (1997). *Hepatic Resection and Transplantation for Peripheral Cholangiocarcinoma*. https://core.ac.uk/download/12205423.pdf (accessed on 24 May 2025).
19. Castro, G. D., & Castro, J. A. (2014). *Alcohol Drinking and Mammary Cancer: Pathogenesis and Potential Dietary Preventive Alternatives*. https://core.ac.uk/download/159292661.pdf
20. Ceelen, W., De Wever, O., Heriot, A. G., & Narasimhan, V. (2020). *Targeting the Tumor Microenvironment in Colorectal Peritoneal Metastases*.
21. Cerban, R., Iacob, S., Ester, C., Ghioca, M., Chitul, M., Iacob, R., & Gheorghe, L. (2025). Liver elastography methods for diagnosis of de novo and recurrent hepatocellular carcinoma. *Diagnostics*. https://www.semanticscholar.org/paper/6b41cbb3c471c74b15c1ed52db957706563981e8 (accessed on 24 May 2025).
22. Clifford, M. (2017). *Clinical Applicability of Proposed Algorithm for Identifying Individuals at Risk for Hereditary Hematologic Malignancies* [Doctoral dissertation, Boston University]. https://core.ac.uk/download/130044936.pdf (accessed on 24 May 2025).
23. Cox, I. J., Crossey, M. M., Fye, H. K., Gomez-Romero, M., *et al.* (2016). *Hepatocellular Carcinoma: Review of Disease and Tumor Biomarkers*. https://core.ac.uk/download/77011285.pdf (accessed on 24 May 2025).
24. De Both, A., De Man, M., Geboes, K., Hoorens, A., *et al.* (2017). *Treatment of a Mixed Acinar-Endocrine Carcinoma with Uptake On 68gallium-Dotatoc Positron Emission Tomography-Computed Tomography: A Case Report*. https://core.ac.uk/download/84594808.pdf (accessed on 24 May 2025).
25. Dvorchik, I., Fung, J. J., Iwatsuki, S., Lee, R. G., Marsh, J. W., Madariaga, J. R., & Starzl, T. E. (1998). Treatment of hilar cholangiocarcinoma (Klatskin tumors) with hepatic resection or transplantation. https://core.ac.uk/download/12205465.pdf (accessed on 24 May 2025).
26. El-Said, H., Elfert, A., Fiehn, O., & Helal, M. (2020). Sugar alcohols have a key role in pathogenesis of chronic liver disease and hepatocellular carcinoma in whole blood and liver tissues. https://core.ac.uk/download/323071553.pdf.

27. Feng, J., Lamond, J., Yang, J., Brady, L., Good, M., & Lanciano, R. (2012). Stereotactic body radiation therapy for patients with heavily pretreated liver metastases and liver tumors. https://core.ac.uk/download/pdf/8729451.pdf.

28. Fennell, R. H., Iwatsuki, S., Johnson, M. L., Kano, T., Shaw, B. W., & Starzl, T. E. (1980). Excisional treatment of cavernous hemangioma of the liver. https://core.ac.uk/download/12203859.pdf (accessed on 24 May 2025).

29. Finotti, M., Romano, M., Grossi, U., Dalla Bona, E., Pelizzo, P., Piccino, M., & Scopelliti, M., *et al.* (2024). Innovations in liver preservation techniques for transplants from donors after circulatory death: A special focus on transplant oncology. *Journal of Clinical Medicine, 13*. https://www.semanticscholar.org/paper/0acdb8afdebab7dc69ed324eda09688a79863acd (accessed on 24 May 2025).

30. Fong, L., Keenan, B. P., & Kelley, R. K. (2019). Immunotherapy in hepatocellular carcinoma: The complex interface between inflammation, fibrosis, and the immune response. https://core.ac.uk/download/323074225.pdf.

31. Guo, Y., & Liu, Z. (2022). Progress in the treatment of hepatocellular carcinoma based on hepatic arterial infusion chemotherapy. *Advances in Clinical Medicine*. https://www.semanticscholar.org/paper/75ac4aac7d3cce8423fe6a93e8bf501cded7089a (accessed on 24 May 2025).

32. He, Z., Soullié, P., Lefebvre, P. M., Ambarki, K., Felblinger, J., & Odille, F. (2024). Changes of *in vivo* electrical conductivity in the brain and torso related to age, fat fraction and sex using MRI. *Scientific Reports, 14*. https://www.semanticscholar.org/paper/5203956b52ad87bb42591c44bea8cb220047e3d9 (accessed on 24 May 2025).

33. Iwatsuki, S., Starzl, T. E., & Todo, S. (1990). Excisional therapy for benign hepatic lesions. https://core.ac.uk/download/12204545.pdf (accessed on 24 May 2025).

34. Janku, F., Kaseb, A. O., Kurzrock, R., & Tsimberidou, A. M. (2014). Identification of novel therapeutic targets in the PI3K/AKT/mTOR pathway in hepatocellular carcinoma using targeted next generation sequencing. https://core.ac.uk/download/323066908.pdf.

35. Jiang, T., Zeng, Q., & He, J. (2023). Do alkaline phosphatases have great potential in the diagnosis, prognosis, and treatment of tumors? *Translational Cancer Research, 12*, 2932–2945. https://www.semanticscholar.org/paper/971b780d4fdc8937b3c0a2f5b817143e16b0aa69 (accessed on 24 May 2025).

36. Jung, E., Kaiser, U., Herr, W., Stroszczynski, C., & Jung, F. (2024). Novel high-resolution contrast agent ultrasound techniques HiFR CEUS and SR CEUS in combination with shear wave elastography, fat assessment and viscosity of liver parenchymal changes and tumors. *Clinical Hemorheology and Microcirculation*. https://www.semanticscholar.org/paper/3fd645d9b410f09a0467e6d683fb0fdd6251dda6 (accessed on 24 May 2025).

37. Kandoriya, J., & Degadwala, S. (2024). Advanced machine learning techniques for liver tumor classification in MRI imaging. *International Journal of Scientific Research in Computer Science, Engineering and Information Technology*. https://www.semanticscholar.org/paper/4cff158d3983d4c456cf27ed34096f4b5cde4af0 (accessed on 24 May 2025).

38. Karin, M. (2018). New insights into the pathogenesis and treatment of non-viral hepatocellular carcinoma: A balancing act between immunosuppression and immunosurveillance. https://core.ac.uk/download/323065762.pdf.

39. Kawano, M., Yano, Y., Yamamoto, A., Yasutomi, E., Inoue, Y., Kitadai, J., Yoshida, R., *et al.* (2024). Risk factors for immune checkpoint inhibitor-induced liver injury and the significance of liver biopsy. *Diagnostics, 14*. https://www.semanticscholar.org/paper/eb03365a0b34bfec3cecbd851a7dcea7b9880ce4 (accessed on 24 May 2025).

40. Kim, J., & Seki, E. (2024). Inflammation and immunity in liver neoplasms: Implications for future therapeutic strategies. *Molecular Cancer Therapeutics*. https://www.semanticscholar.org/paper/c79968189bde8350dffc47358e1af053fbc7ed01 (accessed on 24 May 2025).

41. Liang, Y. (2024). Role of CAR-T-based immunotherapy in the treatment of hepatocellular carcinoma. *Highlights in Science, Engineering and Technology*. https://www.semanticscholar.org/paper/4328c0493bf310eb5db795db46d2683cf122acc4 (accessed on 24 May 2025).

42. Ma, M., Shang, K., Wang, J., Teng, X., Li, P., & Wang, J. (2024). A patient with multiple primary malignant neoplasms with high variant allele frequencies of RB1, TP53, and TERT. *Biomarker Research, 12*. https://www.semanticscholar.org/paper/f906f003347c9aea997675048111dfff5ec8d7e0 (accessed on 24 May 2025).

43. Nittayacharn, P., Abenojar, E., Cooley, M. B., Berg, F., Counil, C., Jafari Sojahrood, A., Khan, M. S., *et al.* (2023). Efficient ultrasound-mediated drug delivery to orthotopic liver tumors–Direct comparison of doxorubicin-loaded nanobubbles and microbubbles. *bioRxiv*. https://www.semanticscholar.org/paper/582e86e9eaa8bf9e1cf1d77462967e1e3737ec7d (accessed on 24 May 2025).

44. Park, Y.W., Vollmuth, P., Foltyn-Dumitru, M., Sahm, F., Ahn, S.S., Chang, J., & Kim, S.H. (2023). The 2021 WHO Classification for Gliomas and Implications on Imaging Diagnosis: Part 1—Key Points of the Fifth Edition and Summary of Imaging Findings on Adult-Type Diffuse Gliomas. Journal of Magnetic Resonance Imaging, 58.

45. Proskuriakova, E., & Khedr, A. (2022). Current targeted therapy options in the treatment of cholangiocarcinoma: A literature review. *Cureus, 14*. https://www.semanticscholar.org/paper/a0de6c83d10888931b770f04b7fe5be33cab372d (accessed on 24 May 2025).

46. Saprykina, E. A., Teplyakov, V. V., Shaposhnikov, A., Lazukin, A. V., Ukhvarkin, A. P., & Dobrosotsky, S. V. (2024). Diagnostic efficacy of trephine biopsy and core biopsy of bone and soft tissue tumors. *Bone and Soft Tissue Sarcomas, Tumors of the Skin*. https://www.semanticscholar.org/paper/05f4bc6ec3127d1bfaf39ad1d3091d4df935dbb9 (accessed on 24 May 2025).

47. Świątkowski, F., Zielińska, D., Tański, W., Gajdzis, P., & Chabowski, M. (2020). Liver angiomyolipoma. *Srpski Arhiv za Celokupno Lekarstvo*. https://www.semanticscholar.org/paper/1bf0c7829e97455615cdaa5daa77046183a09e63 (accessed on 24 May 2025).

48. Varigonda, M., Yarlagadda, J., Naga Sai, T. C., Patnaik, S., Bhrugumalla, S., & Gunturi, S. R. V. (2024). The role of diffusion-weighted MRI in correlation with contrast-enhanced MRI and histopathology in the evaluation of focal liver lesions. *Cureus, 16*. https://www.semanticscholar.org/paper/84657d1553247de920c57bb9bba85a15d349ad23 (accessed on 24 May 2025).

49. White, R. E. (2016). *Risk Factors for Developing Inflammatory Breast Cancer: An Epidemiological Study of a Single Patient Population* [Master's thesis, Boston University]. Boston University OpenBU. https://open.bu.edu/bitstream/2144/14382/9/White_bu_0017N_10446.pdf (accessed on 24 May 2025).

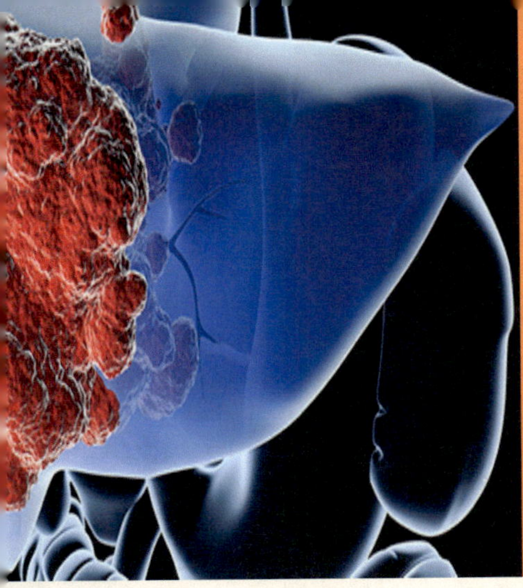

Chapter 9

VASCULAR DISORDERS OF THE LIVER

Contents

Introduction

The liver is one of the key organs in the human body and plays a wide range of physiological functions, including detoxification, metabolism, and the production of proteins essential in the body. Among these wide-ranging functions, vascular integrity plays a critical role in maintaining normal blood circulation and liver function. Vascular liver diseases like portal hypertension, hepatic venous occlusive disease, and liver cirrhosis (LC) disrupt this delicate balance. Their effect on the liver extends beyond the organ itself to generate systemic effects and significantly affect the patient's quality of life. An understanding of the subtleties of these vascular diseases is necessary for the identification of individualized therapeutic strategies and effective management protocols. The pathophysiology of vascular liver diseases often involves complex interactions between hemodynamic changes and the accompanying liver parenchymal illnesses. For instance, portal hypertension is usually caused by increased resistance to portal blood flow, typically secondary to hepatic cirrhosis or fibrosis. Increasing portal vein pressure contributes to the formation of esophageal varices and splenomegaly that may cause major complications if not properly treated. Besides, some etiologic agents, such as alcohol consumption and viral hepatitis, can increase liver damage, which further pollutes the vascular environment of the organ. Understanding these risk factors allows physicians to tailor patient care based on patient-level risk profiles, maximizing treatment efficacy and outcomes. There is an ever-growing amount of evidence that places greater emphasis on the global burden of liver vascular disease, with a shocking pattern of morbidity and mortality from these diseases. Different studies contributed that the prevalence of liver diseases due to environmental vascular malfunction keeps on increasing, and with it comes economic and health burdens for target populations. For instance, among communities with scarce healthcare facilities, lack of access to efficacious treatments adds to the public health problem caused by environmental vascular disorders, contributing to liver diseases. Therefore, the promotion of better diagnostic methods and treatments is essential to help overcome such challenges. Efforts must also be made towards enhancing awareness, along with training medical professionals in the effective identification and management of signs and symptoms of liver vascular disorders. Recognition of the broader burden of diseases emphasizes the importance of joint prevention, research, and therapy.

Definition of Vascular Disorders

Vascular disorders refer to many conditions that mainly impact the vascular system, mainly the blood vessels that supply organs. The result of these disorders might be either a blockage or an irregular flow of blood, which can lead to insufficient tissue perfusion or the development of thrombosis. In the liver, vascular disorders refer to illnesses of the hepatic arteries, portal veins, and hepatic veins, which are key for the liver's function and balance in the body. The liver, because it is highly vascularized, is more likely to experience changes in its blood vessels, which may result in severe conditions such as portal hypertension and liver fibrosis. It is important to understand how vascular health affects the liver to explain the causes of many liver diseases. Vascular liver disorders (VLDs) can significantly disrupt normal physiological processes, presenting both diagnostic and therapeutic challenges. Such conditions usually happen when there is an increased tendency to clot in the blood vessels, which causes clots to form in the hepatic veins and the portal circulation. Recent research suggests that VLDs might be partly explained by Virchow's triad (hypercoagulability, blood stasis, and damage to the endothelium). However, their exact mechanisms are not fully understood because they are rare and few animal models are available. Because of this gap, there is a strong need for more studies on the molecular details of VLDs. The rise of complications such as liver fibrosis as a consequence of these disorders necessitates an urgent exploration of therapeutic interventions, highlighting their relevance in clinical settings (Giuli *et al.*, 2023). The link between liver function and vascular health is very clear in patients with cirrhosis, since both bleeding and thrombosis are major issues. It has been found that the balance of blood clotting is disturbed in cirrhosis, which raises the risk of both bleeding and blood clots. Knowing about these risks justifies doing systematic assessments ahead of invasive procedures, which could lower the risk of complications in vascular liver disorders. Also, well-known risk factors for blood clots in the portal and hepatic venous systems should be carefully considered when caring for patients. The identification of thrombophilia and the application of targeted therapies could pave the way for improved outcomes in patients suffering from VLDs, reinforcing the importance of vascular evaluations in this context (Northup *et al.*, 2020) (Figure 9.1).

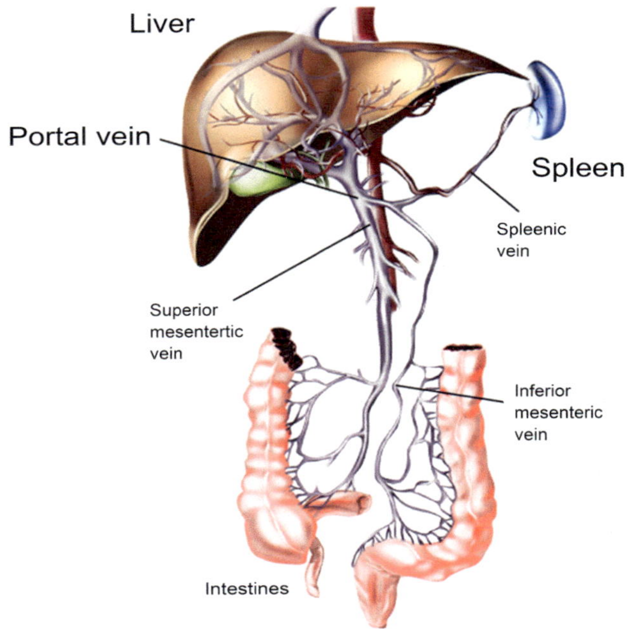

Figure 9.1. Vascular liver diseases.

Source: https://www.valdig.eu/wp-content/uploads/2022/05/img_portal_vein.jpg.

Importance of Liver Health

The liver is a central element of general well-being, functioning as an essential metabolic detoxification and storage organ. Its intricate system of blood vessels is tasked with regulating the flow of blood, providing a specialized pathway for nutrient-rich blood to be cleansed. Maintaining liver function is particularly important considering its role in many biochemical processes, such as digestion and immune activity. Liver diseases, particularly those involving vascular integrity, may lead to severe complications such as portal hypertension, which results from increased pressure within the portal venous circulation. It typically precedes severe liver disease and highlights the interdependent relationship between liver function and vascular disease. Taking care of liver health first, both via diet and lifestyle choices, individuals can lower the risk of having such life-threatening illnesses. Recognition of the significance of liver health also comes with embracing the effects of liver diseases on global public health. Studies have shown that non-communicable diseases, which include liver illnesses, contribute significantly to global mortality and warrant a call for prevention and effective therapies. Particularly, diseases such as cirrhosis and vascular complications of cirrhosis can lead to a high death rate, emphasizing the importance of increasing public awareness and early diagnosis. The Global Burden of Diseases, Injuries, and Risk Factors Study has provided very important data presenting the rising incidence and mortality of liver diseases, again underlining the importance of comprehensive public health interventions towards promoting liver health. In the face of such disconcerting trends, the management of liver health not only favors the individual but also mitigates global public health concerns (Roth *et al.*, 2018). Promoting liver health thus demands multi-modal management that includes both medical management as well as lifestyle modification and public education. Regular screening of liver function as well as vascular complications can enable prompt detection and intervention, with timely interventions where warranted. In addition, health education campaigns among populations to educate them on the risks of poor liver health, such as unsafe consumption of alcohol and viral hepatitis, can promote better lifestyles. It is also essential for health care providers to be multi-layered in their consideration of each patient's case while adhering to established guidelines (Mach *et al.*, 2019). By encouraging coordination of public health strategy and individual health management, the incidence of liver vascular disorders can be restricted to a large extent, leading to improved health outcomes and augmenting the quality of life of diseased patients (Figure 9.2).

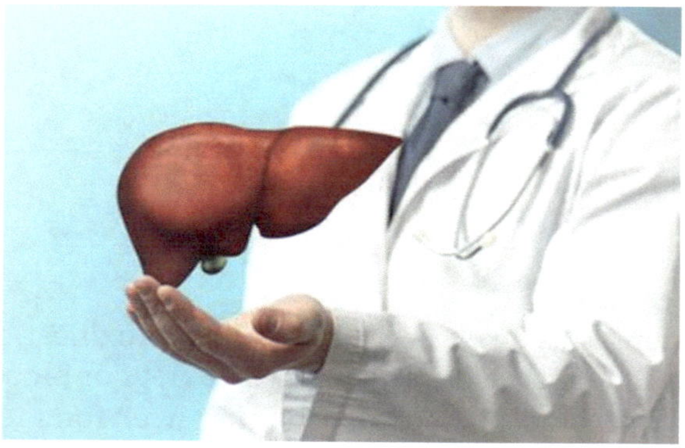

Figure 9.2. Liver Health

Source: https://smb.ibsrv.net/imageresizer/image/article_manager/1200x1200/2036/1147300/heroimage0.513549001713388482.jpg.

9.1. Types of Vascular Disorders

It is very important to be aware of different vascular disorders of the liver to help with their diagnosis and treatment. One prominent category is portal vein thrombosis (PVT), which occurs when a blood clot obstructs the portal vein, leading to compromised blood flow to the liver. Risk factors for this condition are cirrhosis, malignancies, and certain surgical procedures. PVT may not show any symptoms, or it might cause abdominal pain, fluid in the abdomen, and problems with liver function. Because of improved diagnostic imaging, PVT can be found earlier and treated more quickly. The type of treatment is chosen based on the severity and causes of the thrombosis, which shows how important it is to identify and address these issues in patients with hepatic vascular complications. Another significant vascular disorder is hepatic vein thrombosis (HVT), also known as Budd-Chiari syndrome (BCS), characterized by the obstruction of hepatic veins due to thrombosis. This condition can result from hypercoagulable states, liver cirrhosis (LC), or malignancies impacting venous drainage from the liver. Symptoms of BCS in the clinic may be abdominal pain, swelling of the liver, and jaundice, and if not treated, it can rapidly lead to liver failure. It is important to tell this syndrome apart from other liver diseases, because it needs different treatment methods. Anticoagulation therapy, angioplasty, or surgical procedures like shunt creation may be used to help the liver drain blood properly. A thorough understanding of the pathophysiology, clinical presentation, and management of HVT is vital for practitioners involved in caring for patients with liver-related vascular disorders (Murray *et al.*, 2022; Northup *et al.*, 2020). Other than the mentioned conditions, changes in liver hemostasis can lead to both blood clots and bleeding problems. Patients with chronic liver disease (CLD) often exhibit complex hemostatic changes characterized by a combination of thrombocytopenia and dysregulation of clotting factors, ultimately leading to a fragile state where both bleeding and thrombosis may coexist. Because of their blood-clotting issues, patients with hemostatic dysfunctions are more likely to have complications from procedures like liver biopsies and endoscopies. Being aware of the risk of thrombosis in PVT and also the risk of bleeding helps doctors design better treatment plans. This is very important for improving patient outcomes, especially in those dealing with problems caused by advanced liver disease. Ultimately, recognition and appropriate management of these diverse vascular disorders are critical in providing holistic care for liver patients, confirming the intricate relationship between liver function and vascular health (Murray *et al.*, 2022; Northup *et al.*, 2020).

9.1.1. Portal Hypertension

Portal hypertension pathophysiology is intrinsically linked with CLD, the most common etiology being cirrhosis. In cirrhosis, fibrosis and regenerative nodules is resulting from distortion of the architecture of the liver, leading to increased resistance to portal blood flow. The resistance leads to elevated portal venous pressure, and this may result in a cascade of complications, including esophageal varices formation, splenomegaly, and ascites. The complex interaction between increasing portal pressure and impaired hemostatic mechanisms creates significant challenges in clinical management.

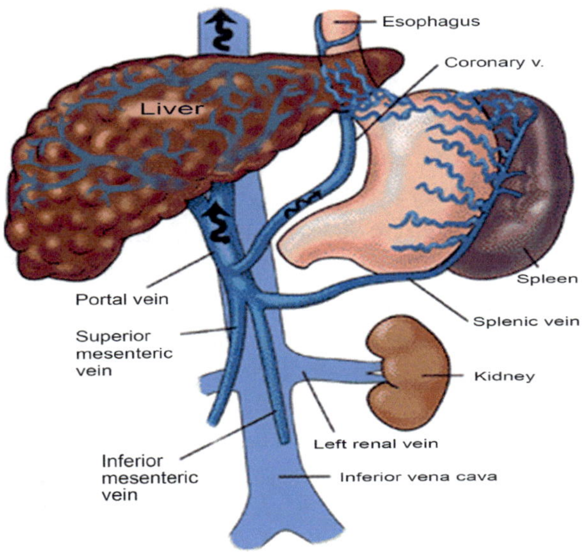

Figure 9.3. Portal hypertension.

Source: https://gastrointestinalcancersurgerydelhigurgaon.com/wp-content/uploads/2020/03/3338075_orig.jpg.

The patients present with hemostatic abnormalities in the form of thrombocytopenia, which also makes procedure-based intervention challenging, as there is an increased risk of bleeding during invasive interventions. Furthermore, the evaluation of risk for bleeding in this population is now more nuanced and demands a more intricate appreciation of hemostatic balance, particularly in the context of portal hypertension (Northup *et al.*, 2020). Portal hypertension has a deep impact on clinical outcomes, particularly when its implications are viewed in the context of intervention and surgery. As patients with severe liver disease often have multiple comorbidities, establishing the risk of bleeding is a challenging process. The traditional laboratory assessments, such as prothrombin time and platelet count, are often not indicative of the patient's actual hemostatic state and lead to underestimation of the risk of bleeding (Northup *et al.*, 2020). Therefore, the development of global hemostatic testing and viscoelastic testing has provided a window to better appreciate coagulation profiles of such patients. These newer methods, although useful, remain limited, in particular, to predicting individual bleeding events. Thus, detailed risk assessment involving portal pressure measurements, indices of liver function, together with individual patient factors, is required to maximize surgical risks in portal hypertensive patients. Therapeutically, portal hypertension treatment involves both surgical and nonsurgical interventions with the aim of reducing portal pressure as well as preventing the consequences of its complications. Pharmacological intervention, such as using non-selective beta-blockers, is employed in reducing portal hypertension through the reduction of heart rate and cardiac output, thereby preventing variceal hemorrhage. In addition, endoscopic therapy, such as variceal ligation, is central to the prevention of hemorrhage related to esophageal varices. Where medical and endoscopic management are unsuccessful, interventional surgery options like the placement of a transjugular intrahepatic portosystemic shunt (TIPS) or liver transplantation might be considered. Each of these treatments possesses its specific risks and advantages, and it takes a multidisciplinary group of hepatology, surgery, and interventional radiology to ensure that patients receive the most effective and best-suited treatment for their respective diseases complicated by portal hypertension (Figure 9.3).

9.1.2. Budd-Chiari Syndrome

BCS is a major problem affecting the liver's blood vessels, where hepatic veins become blocked, which leads to portal hypertension and congestion of the liver. The classification of this condition depends on the main reasons behind it, which are called primary or secondary. Primary BCS is often related to myeloproliferative neoplasms (MPNs), where genetic mutations cause increased blood viscosity and thrombosis within the hepatic venous system. In Morocco, a study looking back at cases found that 29 patients with BCS had a strong connection to MPNs, and 10% of these cases were related to a genetic predisposition. The prominence of clinical manifestations such as decompensated portal hypertension highlights the critical need for early diagnosis and intervention in managing BCS effectively (Jebari *et al.*, 2024). The use of new imaging and diagnostic techniques has improved the ability to find BCS. Imaging techniques, including Doppler ultrasound, CT scans, and magnetic resonance imaging (MRI), facilitate the assessment of hepatic vein patency and the presence of thrombosis. The methods are used to diagnose BCS by showing the typical signs of hepatic vein blockage and other vascular problems. In the context of clinical evaluation, patients often present with symptoms ranging from abdominal pain and ascites to more severe manifestations like acute liver failure (ALF). Importantly, differential diagnosis between BCS and other hepatic vascular disorders, such as sinusoidal obstruction syndrome (SOS), is essential. While both conditions can lead to similar complications, they exhibit distinct pathological features, risk factors, and management strategies (Lu *et al.*, 2023). Because BCS is complex, care must be personalized to fit the needs of each patient. Anticoagulation therapy is sometimes given to break up any current clots and prevent further venous occlusions. Sometimes, angioplasty or stenting is done to clear blocked veins. Furthermore, dealing with the underlying causes, especially in patients with MPNs, is very important for better patient outcomes. Despite the range of treatments, a large number of patients still had complications from portal hypertension, which highlights the severity of BCS. An integrated approach that combines both medical and surgical interventions is vital to mitigate the risks and enhance the quality of life for patients afflicted with this complex disorder (Jebari *et al.*, 2024) (Figure 9.4).

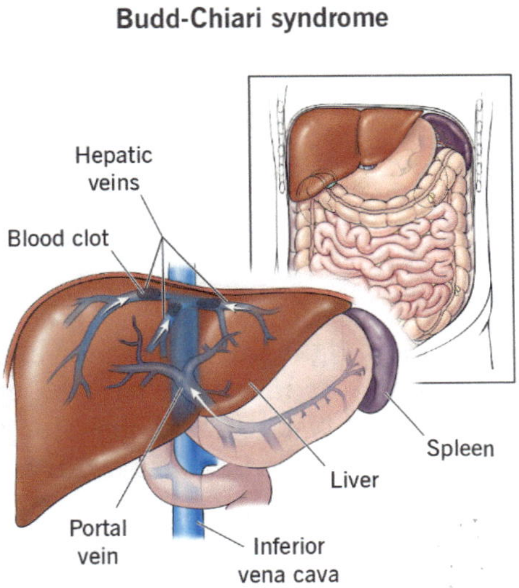

Figure 9.4. Budd-chiari syndrome.

Source: https://my.clevelandclinic.org/-/scassets/images/org/health/articles/21097-budd-chiari-syndrome.jpg.

9.1.3. Hepatic Artery Thrombosis

Hepatic artery thrombosis is an emergent hepatic vascular illness that refers to the obstruction of blood supply through the hepatic artery. Hepatic artery thrombosis can occur in various clinical contexts, such as following liver transplantation, where it leads to severe complications such as graft loss and liver failure. The pathophysiologic mechanism of hepatic artery thrombosis is multicausal and often involves reasons like surgical intervention, vascular anatomy-related complexities, and patient-related factors like coagulopathy. The variably reported incidence rate of hepatic artery thrombosis, 5% to 25% in the post-transplant setting, also highlights the importance of remaining vigilant on the part of healthcare providers since early detection and intervention are critical toward avoiding detrimental consequences affecting liver function as well as overall patient survival (Zhang, 2021). The clinical presentation of hepatic artery thrombosis varies from asymptomatic to severe liver dysfunction, necessitating a high index of suspicion in high-risk populations. Abdominal pain, hepatomegaly, and jaundice are noted as presenting symptoms; however, other patients have no symptoms until there is extensive liver damage. Imaging studies constitute the bulk of diagnostic testing, with Doppler ultrasonography being the first line employed for assessment of blood flow and diagnosis of thrombosis of the hepatic artery. If the initial imaging does not prove definitive, CT or magnetic resonance imaging (MRI) can be used to produce a wider survey of hepatic vascular structures. Treatment strategies tend to focus on the reestablishment of adequate blood flow and can involve the use of anticoagulation therapy and, in the more severe instances, surgery designed to address the thrombotic episode (Gimson, 2020). Understanding hepatic artery thrombosis in the setting of global vascular liver disorders underscores the interrelatedness of vascular health and liver function. Complications of hepatic artery thrombosis, moreover, can snowball into more severe presentations, such as ischemic hepatopathy, which will highlight the necessity of total management beyond the fact of the initial thrombosis. Practitioners must employ a multidisciplinary approach that will address not only the thrombotic event but also possibly its resultant complications. By interdisciplinary collaboration, healthcare professionals can optimize patient outcomes, providing integrative care that may include monitoring, nutritional support, and liver transplantation modalities where the damage is permanent. An emphasis on preventive interventions and early intervention can ultimately optimize the prognosis of patients affected with hepatic artery thrombosis and other vascular liver diseases (Zhang, 2021) (Figure 9.5).

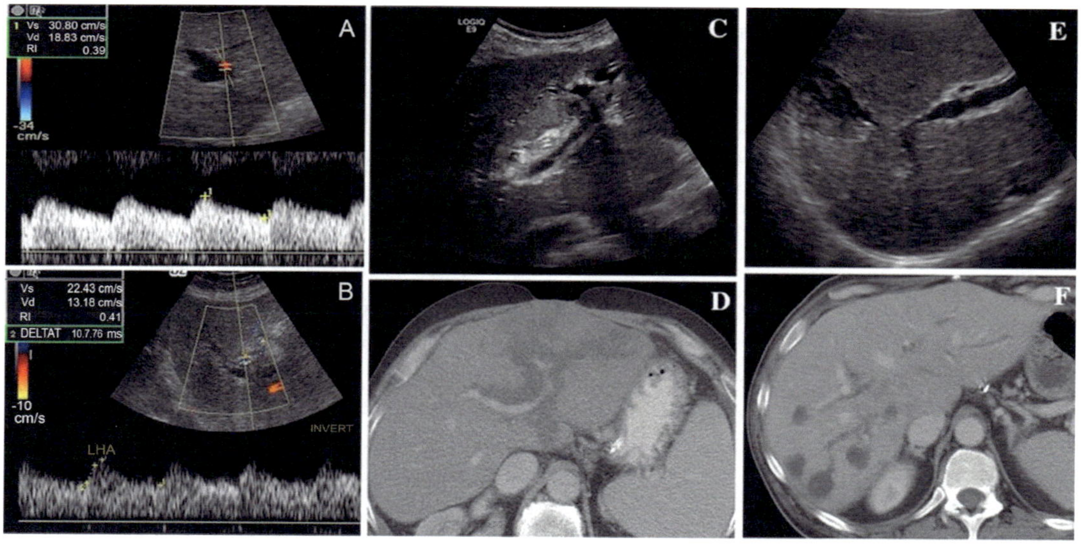

Figure 9.5. Hepatic artery thrombosis. a, b Doppler Ultrasound through right and left hepatic arteries demonstrates a tardus-parvus pattern of intrahepatic flow. No flow was identified at the hepatic hilum. c Gray scale ultrasound shows increased periportal echogenicity due to biliary sloughing and sludge, confirmed on CT, d as low attenuation casts in the biliary tree. e Gray scale ultrasound shows cystic collections in keeping with bilomas in the liver parenchyma. f Corresponding CT scan shows multiple bilomas. Extent of biliary injury at times maybe underestimated on ultrasound.

Source: https://www.researchgate.net/publication/344667220/figure/fig13/AS:946825792077843@1602752268472/Hepatic-artery-thrombosis-a-b-Doppler-Ultrasound-through-right-and-left-hepatic.jpg.

9.2. Causes of Vascular Disorders

Vascular disorders affecting the liver may have a complicated cause, often involving genetics, the environment, and personal habits. A major reason for hepatic vascular problems is cirrhosis of the liver, which makes the portal blood flow more difficult and leads to significant portal hypertension. Resistance occurs because cirrhosis causes fibrosis, which reduces blood flow to the liver and results in the creation of varices and ascites. Moreover, conditions such as alcoholic liver disease (ALD) can exacerbate this process, highlighting the interplay between chronic alcohol consumption and vascular impairments in liver function. Because cirrhosis and vascular disorders are so connected, it is important to treat both liver health and blood vessel health at the same time. Thrombosis, which is a blood clot, is another important reason for vascular disorders in the liver, especially in the hepatic veins or portal vein. Several possible causes for BCS, which blocks hepatic venous outflow, include hypercoagulable states, cancers, and inflammatory diseases. Because of the inflammation and vascular damage from liver disease, individuals are more likely to have blood clots, which can worsen liver function. It is important to know the causes of venous thrombosis, since early recognition and treatment can prevent liver failure. For this reason, understanding the causes of thrombosis in liver disorders is still very important for creating better treatments and helping patients. Infections and inflammation are important reasons why vascular problems occur in the liver. When pathogens cause inflammation in the blood vessels, it may result in hepatic SOS, which causes the liver's blood flow to be disrupted and its function to be affected. The immune system's response to infections, for example, by viruses like hepatitis, can also cause more inflammation and damage in the blood vessels. This points out that taking care of liver and blood vessel health is important, and this can be done by vaccinating and regularly screening for viral infections. In addition, how systemic inflammation contributes to liver vascular problems is a major research topic, highlighting how different parts of the body can affect each other. Because there are many causes, a complete approach to diagnosis and treatment is needed for people with liver disease, considering both the liver and the blood vessels.

9.2.1. Genetic Predispositions

Genetic susceptibility plays a key part in the pathogenesis of most liver vascular diseases, dictating susceptibility to disease to a large degree. Environmental stress may interact with genetic susceptibility to enhance liver endothelial dysfunction and fibrosis, processes of critical significance in vascular diseases. For example, genetic mutations in lipid metabolism genes can intensify fat accumulation in the liver, evolving into NAFLD, which is a major risk factor for liver vascular complications. It should be understood that the genetic nature of such disorders is crucial because it not only guides diagnosis but also treatment strategies, allowing for a more personalized approach toward the management of liver vascular disorders. The interaction between environment and genetics requires in-depth investigation, as patients with inherited diseases may require tailored therapies that factor in both their genetic makeup and the environmental inputs they experience. Genetic vulnerabilities in pediatric hepatology are increasingly recognized as causal agents in infantile vascular liver disease. Pediatric genetic and metabolic liver diseases often necessitate liver transplantation, indicating the severity and complexity of these diseases. Most of these disorders are caused by genetic metabolic defects that can lead to massive hepatic involvement as well as extra-hepatic manifestations complicating the clinical management. For instance, certain genetic diseases impair the liver's ability to metabolize toxins or produce essential proteins, resulting in vascular complications that can ultimately need surgical repair. These findings of genetic predispositions highlight the importance of early genetic screening for risk populations to possibly have improved outcomes by means of early management and intervention strategies that are tailored for patients' own genetic background (Hassan *et al.*, 2024).

Current studies increasingly correlate genetic predispositions with vascular dysfunction in NAFLD patients and neurodegenerative diseases and produce a complex interaction that is yet to be explored. Both conditions share common risk factors such as metabolic syndrome and chronic inflammation, which are governed by genetic variability. For instance, some genetic profiles may predispose an individual to heightened inflammatory outcomes, both impairing liver and neurological function. The interconnections between NAFLD and vascular impairment show shared pathophysiological mechanisms that overlap, giving credence to the fact that genetic predisposition may be a point of convergence linking these conditions. An effective understanding of such mechanisms may usher in new therapeutic approaches addressing the root causes of such interrelated disorders. Thus, a holistic approach combining genetic testing with traditional clinical analysis is mandatory for effective diagnosis and treatment (Jadhav *et al.*, 2024) (Figure 9.6).

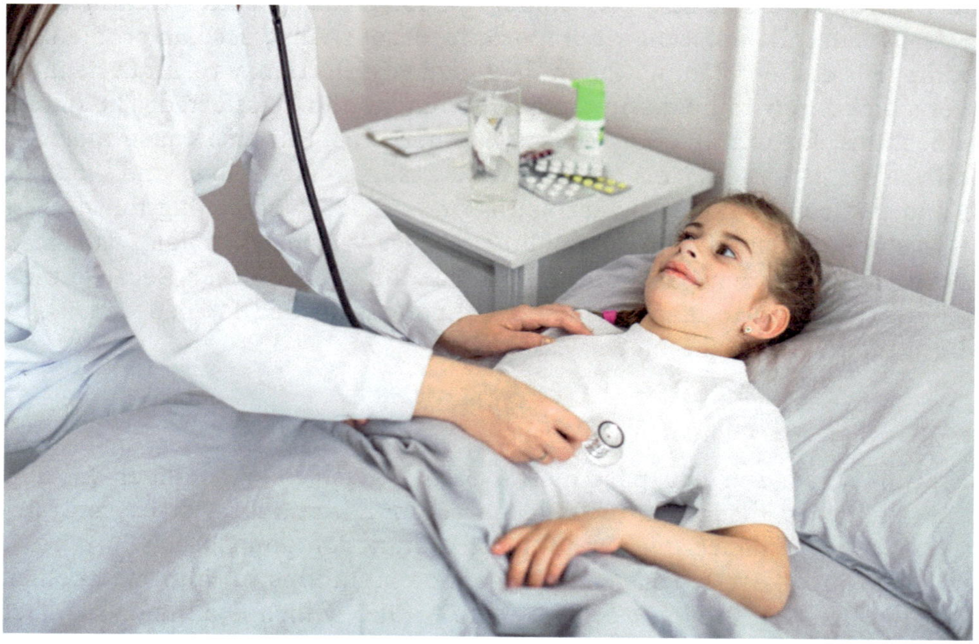

Figure 9.6. Genetic Predispositions

Source: https://www.ankurahospitals.com/wp-content/uploads/2024/11/Pediatric-Liver-Disease.jpg.

9.2.2. Lifestyle Factors

Lifestyle choices are very important in the development and worsening of liver vascular disorders. The liver is damaged greatly by not moving enough, eating unhealthy foods, and drinking too much alcohol. A lack of physical activity makes people more likely to become obese, have hypertension, and develop IR, which all negatively affect the liver. The accumulation of fat in the liver is what causes NAFLD, which is often triggered by extra weight. It has been found that remaining inactive makes these conditions worse and increases metabolic problems. Eating lots of refined sugars and saturated fats can greatly harm the body, because it causes inflammation and oxidative stress, which can result in more serious problems in the blood vessels and liver. Lifestyle factors and how they influence a person's emotions should be considered in liver vascular disorders. Long-term stress and depression may cause metabolic problems, and IR is one of them, which is linked to many chronic diseases involving liver dysfunction, such as type 2 diabetes and heart problems. Since mental health and physical health are linked, it is important to support both by giving diet and exercise advice together with emotional support. It has been found that those who feel a lot of psychological distress tend to eat too much and exercise less, which can make liver problems worse. To that end, addressing both mental and physical lifestyle factors may prove essential for improving health-related quality of life and mitigating the risk of developing vascular disorders of the liver (Deana *et al.*, 2023). Besides, making healthy changes in lifestyle, such as eating well and exercising regularly, can help prevent liver vascular disorders. It appears that programs designed to improve diet and exercise can help people manage their weight, improve insulin sensitivity, and reduce liver fat, which may prevent liver disease. More physical activity is associated with healthier endothelial cells, which helps the vascular system function more efficiently. The role of nitric oxide (NO) in vascular health, for instance, is closely tied to the body's ability to regulate its response to insulin; as insulin sensitivity improves, so does the endothelial response, leading to better vascular function (Kearney, 2013). For this reason, making sure people are physically active, eat a healthy diet, and manage their mental health is essential for liver health and to reduce the number of vascular disorders.

9.2.3. Underlying Liver Diseases

It is necessary to understand the interaction of underlying liver pathology with vascular diseases in managing hepatic diseases. CLD, hepatitis, and cirrhosis fundamentally modify the hepatic vascular bed to form severe complications, one being portal hypertension. This elevated pressure in the portal vein system can be due to increased resistance from fibrosis and vascular abnormalities. The pathophysiologic changes that accompany liver disease will evoke a prothrombotic state, which exacerbates vascular complications and proper blood flow.

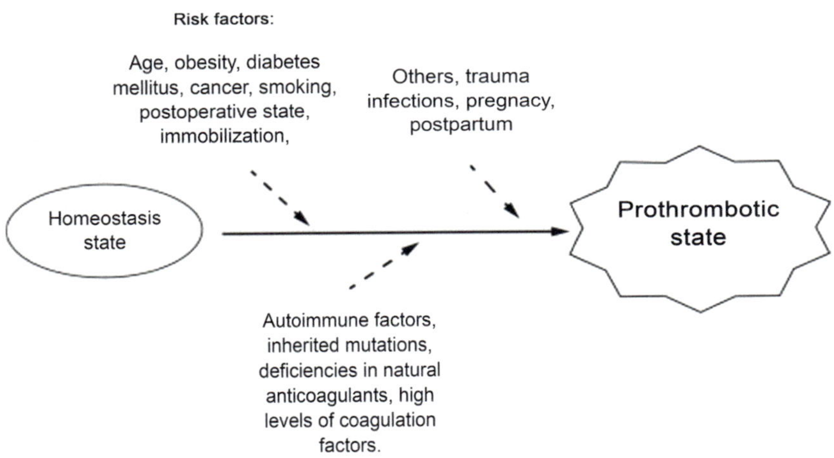

Figure 9.7. Prothrombotic state.

Source: https://ars.els-cdn.com/content/image/1-s2.0-S0065242321000275-f05-01-9780128246276.jpg.

The event sequence establishes the way liver function is inherently linked to vascular control, and how concerted approaches in diagnosis and therapy are essential. The intrahepatic mechanisms of vascular liver diseases are often founded on alterations to normal hepatic hemodynamics, which are further augmented by chronic liver injury. For instance, ALD and NAFLD are able to initiate inflammation and fibrosis to induce vascular remodeling. This remodeling is able to interfere with the delicate balance of the hepatic sinusoids and impair endothelial function. The resultant damage compromises not just the architecture's structure of the livers architecture but also its regulatory function for blood flow. Patients then present with an increased risk of hepatic decompensation and thrombosis. These findings reveal the urgent need for the development of targeted therapies that will aim to correct both the liver's underlying disease and its vascular complications, which could open the door for improving patient outcomes. Quite recently, research has put into perspective the potential contribution of new therapies in alleviating the vascular complications of liver diseases. The development of new drug delivery systems, such as vitamin A-modified micelles and biomimetic nanoclusters, has shown potential therapeutic efficiency in targeting hepatic vascular diseases. The preclinical experiments mark their potential to curb fibrosis significantly and improve hemodynamic indexes in models of liver pathology, thereby emphasizing the requirement for tailored treatment modalities. In addition, the study of anticoagulation therapy offers a complementary strategy in the management of the prothrombotic picture encountered in vascular liver disease. In targeting the molecular pathways for vascular dysfunction in liver disease, these drugs not only decrease such complications as portal hypertension but can also enhance overall liver function, underscoring the interrelatedness of hepatic and vascular treatment options (Giuli *et al.*, 2023; Wang *et al.*, 2025) (Figure 9.7).

9.3. Symptoms and Diagnosis

Vascular disorders of the liver often cause symptoms that are not specific, which can make it difficult to diagnose. Liver hematomas, which might happen during pregnancy, usually have vague symptoms, so early detection is hard. Some patients can have abdominal pain, nausea, or discomfort, but not the main signs of liver failure. Because this condition can progress rapidly, it is important to diagnose it as soon as possible to avoid serious complications like hepatic rupture. Evaluating liver problems and seeing hematomas is best done using ultrasonography and CT imaging. Given that symptoms may not present until the condition has advanced, a high index of suspicion among clinicians is necessary to ensure appropriate imaging and supportive care are implemented promptly, thus enhancing patient outcomes during this critical period of management (Saad *et al.*, 2025). In the context of extrahepatic portal vein obstruction (EHPVO), symptomatology also plays a pivotal role in diagnosis. At the start, people often do not experience any symptoms, which makes it hard to detect the condition early. With the progression of the disorder, patients may start to show concerning symptoms like vomiting blood, spleen enlargement, or other problems in the digestive tract. Because EHPVO is a chronic condition, it can cause serious problems, and healthcare workers should be aware of the possible symptoms. Using Doppler ultrasound, MRI, and CT scans helps confirm the presence of obstruction in the portal vein and also evaluates the alternate routes for blood flow. These imaging modalities not only enhance diagnostic accuracy but also assist in guiding therapeutic interventions that are critical in managing the complications associated with EHPVO effectively (Babu *et al.*, 2024). Vascular disorders of the liver are best diagnosed by using both a full medical examination and advanced imaging methods. Unclear symptoms may cause a delay in finding out what is wrong, which is why a full patient history and physical exam are necessary. Healthcare providers should watch out for unusual symptoms, mainly in groups that are more likely to develop complications, for example, pregnant women or those with existing health problems. Looking for signs early through regular screening can help prevent serious complications in those who are not yet showing symptoms. It is also important to have multidisciplinary care, since managing these cases well often requires hepatologists, radiologists, and surgeons to collaborate. By employing a systematic approach to diagnosis, healthcare professionals can enhance the detection and treatment of liver vascular disorders, optimizing patient outcomes and reducing the associated morbidity and mortality (Babu *et al.*, 2024; Saad *et al.*, 2025).

9.3.1. Common Symptoms of Vascular Disorders

Liver vascular disorders can have many various symptoms, some of which coincide with other conditions of the liver. Their most prominent symptom is HE, a form of mental deterioration that occurs when the liver is unable to purge toxins from the bloodstream. With the accumulation of toxins, patients become confused, disoriented, and even comatose in severe cases. Development of HE typically prompts a thorough evaluation for potential liver vascular anomalies. IPSVS are particularly significant in this context because they can potentially lead to bypass of the portal venous system, worsening the symptoms of HE in patients without a history of liver disease. Hence, the identification of vascular disorders is imperative for effective treatment and management of such complex symptoms (Villegas *et al.*, 2025). Another common symptom associated with vascular liver disease is abdominal pain, which is highly variable in nature and intensity. The pain results from increased pressure within the portal venous system, leading to a condition known as portal hypertension. The pain will also be described as aching and stabbing or simply sharp and may be localized or diffuse in the abdomen. The symptom is also frequently coupled with other presentations, such as ascites, where there is an accumulation of excess fluid within the abdominal cavity, making the clinical presentation even more complicated. The presence of abdominal pain also suggests potential vascular complications such as splenic or HVT and thus needs to be monitored closely to prevent severe consequences such as hemorrhage resulting from varices caused by portal hypertension (Xie *et al.*, 2021). Cutaneous changes such as spider angiomata and palmar erythema may also reflect underlying vascular diseases that compromise liver function. Spider angiomata are small vascular lesions with a central focus and radiating capillaries, which occur commonly in patients with chronic liver disease. Palmar erythema, or reddening of the palms, is yet another symptom of a vascular nature that occurs in liver diseases. Both symptoms often occur with high estrogen levels resulting from liver failure and are signs of advanced disease progression. Vascular symptom identification is of primary importance, as they are of great diagnostic significance, requiring further study of vascular structures in relation to liver status. Elucidation of relationships between vascular symptoms and liver function is the key to clinicians developing comprehensive treatment plans and optimizing patient outcomes.

9.3.2. Diagnostic Imaging Techniques

Assessing and managing liver vascular disorders depends greatly on diagnostic imaging, as the hepatic blood vessels are very complex. Non-invasive methods such as ultrasound (US), CT, and magnetic resonance imaging (MRI) have evolved significantly, providing clinicians with enhanced visualization of vascular abnormalities. Doppler imaging with ultrasound helps detect blood flow problems in major vessels, which can lead to the discovery of PVT and hepatic vein obstruction. Its main strengths are its immediate results, no use of ionizing radiation, and accessibility in hospitals and clinics. Nevertheless, some patient conditions, such as obesity or a lot of gas in the bowel, can make it hard to see the vascular structures properly. CT also plays a key role in vascular liver disorders by giving clear cross-sectional images that can clearly show the structure and problems of the blood vessels. CT angiography is very helpful for examining the blood vessels of the liver and detecting problems such as hepatic artery stenosis or pseudoaneurysms, which are important for transplantation and TIPS procedures. A contrast agent makes it easier to see blood vessels during an angiogram. On the other hand, the dangers of using iodinated contrast in patients with kidney problems, which are common in cirrhosis, mean that special care should be taken when planning the procedure. Magnetic resonance imaging (MRI) stands out for its superior soft tissue contrast and lack of ionizing radiation, making it particularly beneficial for patients requiring multiple imaging assessments. MRI allows doctors to observe the liver's blood flow and structure, which can help diagnose SOS and hepatic fibrosis. Besides, both diffusion-weighted MRI and MR angiography can find liver perfusion and vascular problems more accurately than common methods. FDG-PET/CT is being used more often in vascular disorders and appears to help detect malignant changes in vascular lesions early on. As the field of diagnostic imaging continues to progress, the integration of these modalities will enhance the diagnostic accuracy and management strategies for vascular disorders of the liver, ultimately improving patient outcomes (Figure 9.8).

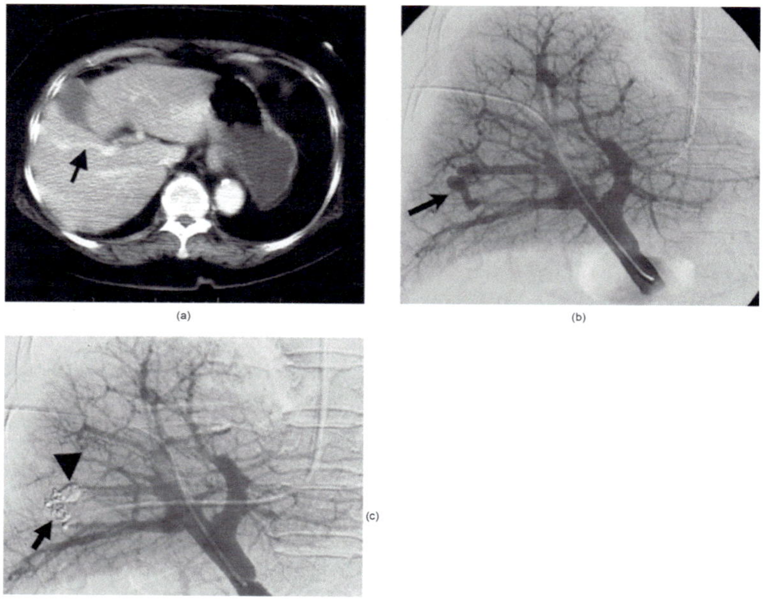

Figure 9.8. An 82-year-old woman with an intrahepatic portosystemic venous shunt (IPSVS) in the right hepatic lobe. (a) Contrastenhanced abdominal CT shows an abnormal vessel running through the right hepatic lobe (arrow). (b) Direct portography shows only one shunt between the right hepatic vein and the right portal vein (arrow). (c) Direct portogram taken after the embolisation procedure shows the complete obliteration of the IPSVS.

Source: https://www.researchgate.net/profile/Hiroyuki-Morishita-2/publication/6731414/figure/fig1/AS:362558600040455@1463452114827/An-82-year-old-woman-with-an-intrahepatic-portosystemic-venous-shunt-IPSVS-in-the-right.png.

9.3.3. Laboratory Tests and Liver Function Assessments

In assessing liver function, particularly in vascular liver conditions, laboratory tests play an extremely significant role. The tests mostly consist of a measurement of biochemical markers such as alanine aminotransferase (ALT), aspartate aminotransferase (AST), alkaline phosphatase

(ALP), and bilirubin. All these enzymes provide critical information regarding hepatic function and injury. However, routine coagulation tests like prothrombin time (PT) and international normalized ratio (INR) are often unable to predict cirrhotic patients' risk of bleeding because they do not adequately reflect the intricacy of hemostatic process alterations caused by liver disease. These shortcomings necessitate more comprehensive methods that incorporate aspects of coagulation as well as liver function. With the evolution in our knowledge of the hemostatic system in CLD, incorporating newer laboratory tests that reflect this complexity becomes increasingly pertinent in making clinical judgments and the management of vascular-related complications (Northup *et al.*, 2020). Furthermore, new diagnostic tests expand our capacity to evaluate liver function and its associated vascular disease. Global hemostasis assays, such as the thrombin generation assay and viscoelastic studies such as thromboelastography (TEG) and rotational thromboelastometry (ROTEM), provide a more nuanced view of coagulopathy in liver disease.

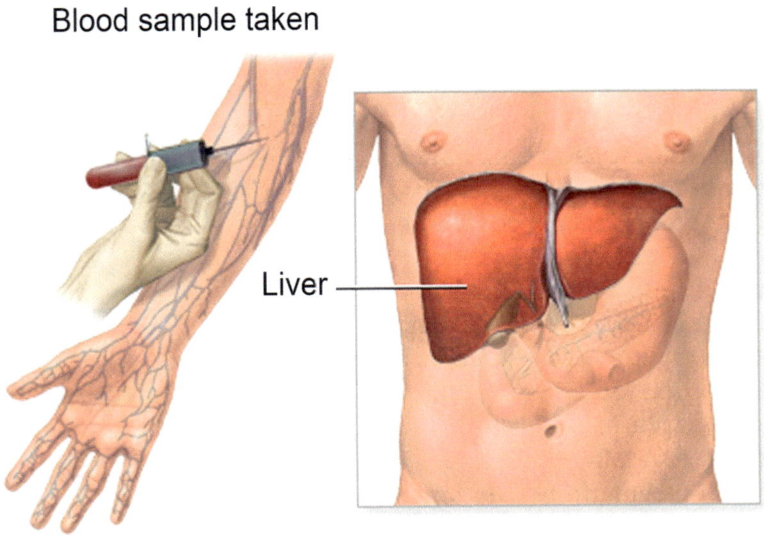

Figure 9.9. Liver function tests.

Source: https://ufhealth.org/assets/adam/9533.jpg.

These assays are able to demonstrate a normal or enhanced thrombin-generating capacity even with a bleeding disorder by conventional tests. This divergence validates the application of certain laboratory tests, as the predictive value of the standard tests is most often false in the context of cirrhosis. For this reason, clinicians must be mindful and keep in mind the inherent biases of standard markers when they arrange invasive procedures for patients with vascular liver disease. Continuing research and advancements in these hemostatic tests also demonstrate the dynamic cross-talk between liver function and vascular health (Finn *et al.*, 2020). Utilization of these advanced tests is also becoming progressively more applicable in the clinical environment for patients undergoing liver vascular disease procedures. Grasping how hemostatic changes influence bleeding risk necessitates a shift in paradigm towards algorithms of individualized patient management. While traditional measurements reflect an increasing risk of bleeding, a more comprehensive assessment in international tests may signify a less risk profile and help with more specific therapeutic interventions. Individualized approaches may lead to better outcomes by ensuring a balance between bleeding risk and procedural safety. Lastly, the incorporation of advanced laboratory testing into liver function tests offers a high-tech model for managing patients with vascular liver disease, emphasizing the need for continuous evolution of clinical guidance in accordance with evolving evidence in this complex field (Northup *et al.*, 2020) (Figure 9.9).

9.4. Treatment Options

Treatment for liver vascular disorders is chosen based on the condition and what caused it. As an example, BCS is a major issue in hepatic vascular disorders when the hepatic veins are blocked. Treatment modalities include both pharmacological and interventional approaches. Anticoagulation therapy is usually used to stop thrombus formation and help reopen blocked vessels. If the liver is severely damaged or there are serious issues, doctors may need to do percutaneous balloon angioplasty or TIPS. Ultimately, the choice of treatment is heavily influenced by the patient's overall clinical status and the severity of the vascular obstruction, illustrating the need for individualized care in managing such complex liver disorders (Gamanagatti *et al.*, 2021). In addition to BCS, gastric antral vascular ectasia (GAVE) presents a unique challenge in the realm of hepatic vascular conditions. In GAVE, there is an excessive growth of blood vessels in the gastric antrum, which usually causes gastrointestinal bleeding. Because medical care has often failed, surgery is generally only used when everything else has been tried, because it can be risky and lead to serious problems. Recent progress has introduced new ways to treat, such as endoscopic treatments that include laser therapy and argon plasma coagulation. These new techniques are as effective as surgery but cause less risk of serious problems. Consequently, these approaches emphasize a shift toward safer, less invasive treatment options in managing GAVE, ultimately enhancing patient outcomes (Patel *et al.*, 2017). The effectiveness of treatment for liver vascular disorders depends on the interventions used and on regularly checking and adjusting the patient's therapy. Improving and developing new solutions depends on progress in research and technology. Regular check-ups with imaging and lab work help determine if treatments are working, which can lead to changes if needed. Therapies like gene therapy and targeted treatments using molecules are expected to play a big role in managing liver vascular disorders. Thus, a comprehensive treatment strategy that incorporates both established and novel approaches will likely enhance the management of hepatic vascular diseases, ultimately striving for improved patient quality of life and survival (Gamanagatti *et al.*, 2021; Patel *et al.*, 2017) (Figure 9.10).

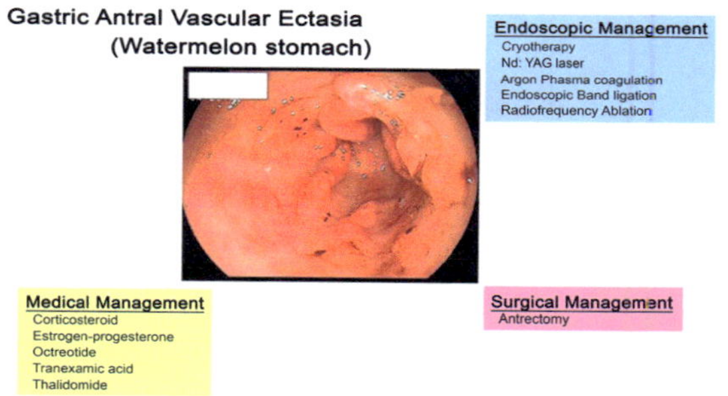

Figure 9.10. Management of gastric antral vascular ectasia. Nd: YAG, neodymium-yttrium-aluminum garnet laser.

Source: https://www.researchgate.net/publication/322709056/figure/fig1/AS:11431281145342345@1681405027075/Management-of-gastric-antral-vascular-ectasia-Nd-YAG-neodymium-yttrium-aluminum-garnet.tif.

9.4.1. Medical Management

Effective medical treatment of liver vascular disorders depends on the explicit understanding of the pathophysiologic mechanisms and complications. Subtlety to this therapeutic method is the attainment of the proper diagnosis, which typically occurs via a multidisciplinary evaluation process consisting of imaging tests like Doppler sonography, CT scans, or MRI scans. The imaging tests enable clinicians to visualize vascular malformations, quantify blood flow, and identify potential thrombotic events. Early diagnosis is also essential since delay can lead to dire consequences such as hepatic ischemia or ALF. Treatment of the disorders also often involves diligent observation of liver function tests and early intervention in order to avoid complications, thus enhancing the patient's prognosis. Application of this integrative model allows doctors to formulate individualized treatment plans that adequately address the unique challenges of vascular diseases of the liver. Vascular disease patients with liver involvement typically present with ascites or abdominal discomfort based on the extent and location of the disease, which needs specific therapeutic intervention.

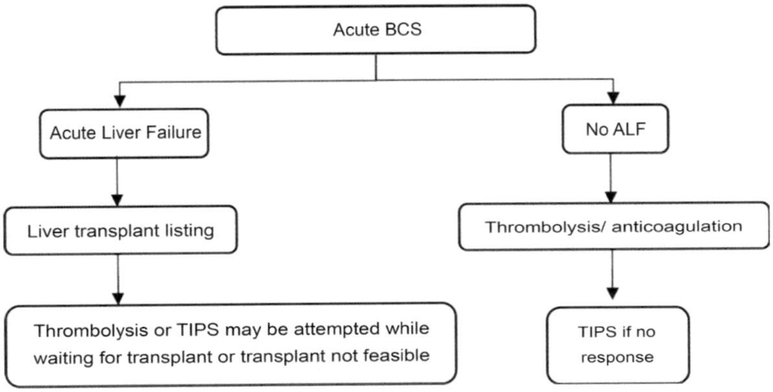

Figure 9.11. Approach to management of acute budd-chiari syndrome.

Source: https://www.researchgate.net/profile/Suprabhat-Giri/publication/353113620/figure/fig5/AS:11431281079582195@1660750933416/Approach-to-management-of-acute-Budd-Chiari-syndrome.png.

The management may involve pharmacological interventions, e.g., anticoagulation therapy, in conditions such as BCS to avert thrombosis. Evaluation of the risk of thrombosis is particularly relevant in patients suffering from vascular diseases of the liver, especially when combined with other conditions such as COVID-19, which has been reported to exacerbate thrombotic complications (Thromboprophylaxis Working Group, 2023). Therefore, proper observation of the patient's risk for thromboembolism allows physicians to prescribe appropriate anticoagulants, based on the severity of the liver illness and the patient's background. The application of evidence-based guidelines for anticoagulant use also contributes to the efficacy of treatment and patient safety, towards the aim of optimizing outcomes and decreasing morbidity and mortality risk among vulnerable populations. In addition to pharmacological treatment, medical management also involves supportive care interventions that significantly influence patient recovery. Nutritional support is also an important part of the management of liver disease, since nutrition is essential in preserving liver function and general health. Specific diets could be necessary for the patient based on their individual needs, supplementing any deficiencies that could exacerbate the disease. Lastly, follow-up on an outpatient basis guarantees continued monitoring and maintenance of any developing complications. Existing specialist opinion about the treatment of aldehyde metabolism disorders emphasizes the role of structured treatment regimens in emergency and critical care that can be extended to manage acute vascular events of liver diseases effectively (Emergency *et al.*, 2024). The structured management strategies ultimately target the preservation of liver function, enhancing the quality of life, and improving survival in patients with vascular liver complications (Figure 9.11).

9.4.2. Surgical Interventions

Surgical interventions for vascular disorders of the liver are characterized by their complexity and the necessity for a tailored approach, particularly in patients with anatomical variations such as situs inversus totalis (SIT). It is very important to plan surgery carefully in advance; advanced imaging is key to seeing the special blood vessels involved in SIT cases.

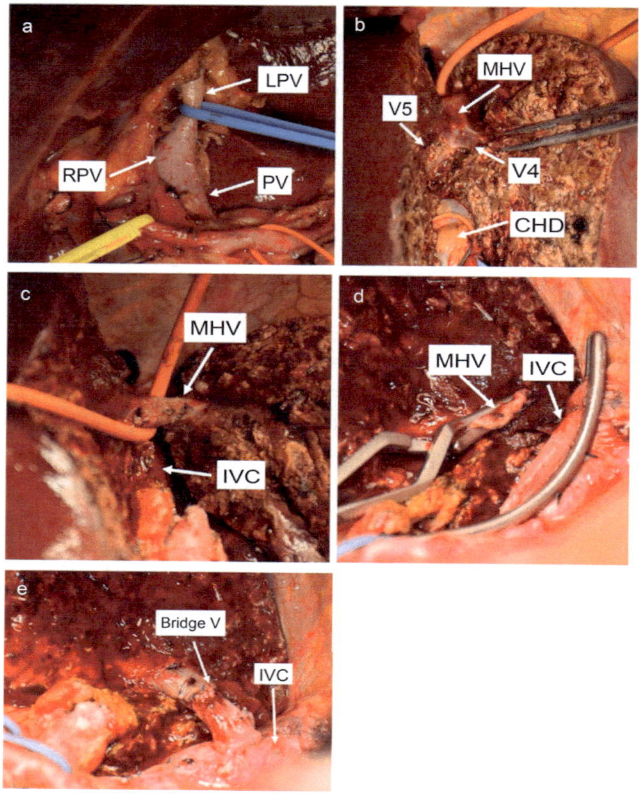

Figure 9.12. Intraoperative vascular operation: (a) dissected the first hepatic hilum, showing the left and right branches of the portal vein; (b) the trunk of middle hepatic vein and its branches; (c) cut off the branch of the segment 4 originating from the middle hepatic vein; (d) the middle hepatic vein and the left hepatic vein were cut off from the root. The left liver lobe and the Spiegel lobe were removed to expose the inferior vena cava; (e) using the left main branch of the portal vein as a vein graft to reconstruct the middle hepatic vein.

Source: https://www.researchgate.net/publication/346507776/figure/fig2/AS:983477734342659@1611490772985/ntraoperative-vascular-operation-a-dissected-the-first-hepatic-hilum-showing-the-left.png.

It is important to understand these variations since traditional surgery may have problems with patients who have their organs flipped. As many surgeons are right-handed, the left-handed dexterity required during procedures in such patients often poses an additional challenge, necessitating innovative surgical strategies that can adapt to these anatomical distinctions (Eitler *et al.*, 2022).

Because of this, these patients might need surgeons to use different surgical methods and tools to fit their unique body structures. Doctors also use surgery to manage PVT and HVT, which are types of hepatic vascular disorders. Earlier, hepatic vascular surgery targeted large vessel thrombosis, but now it is also influenced by new ideas about hemostasis in patients with CLD. TIPS procedures are often used to manage PVT. TIPS not only alleviates portal hypertension symptoms but also serves as a conduit for increased intrahepatic blood flow, thereby addressing the risk of further thrombotic events (Northup *et al.*, 2020). New surgical methods are being developed to avoid complications in vascular diseases, so safer and more effective procedures can be used for these patients. Also, because patients with liver vascular disorders can easily bleed during surgery, it is essential to understand the challenges they have with blood clotting. Usual tests for coagulation, including prothrombin time and platelet counts, may not accurately show how well patients with cirrhosis can clot their blood, which is why better tests are needed to assess bleeding risk. Surgical teams must navigate the dualities of prohemostatic and antihemostatic pathways that exist within this population, often complicating the decision-making process surrounding interventions (Northup *et al.*, 2020). Thus, progress in viscoelastic testing has given surgeons more information for personalized treatment, which has made procedures safer for patients with liver vascular conditions. Such tailored approaches are vital for not only enhancing surgical outcomes but also promoting patient safety in this challenging clinical landscape (Figure 9.12).

9.4.3. Lifestyle Modifications

Lifestyle modifications are now a key component of treatment and prevention strategies in the treatment of vascular liver diseases. The modifications consist of several habits, including diet, exercise, and avoidance of harmful substances, that, when integrated, aim to enhance the functioning of the liver and overall well-being. Convergent evidence suggests that a proper diet rich in fruit, vegetables, whole grains, and lean protein may significantly reduce the risk of liver damage secondary to many vascular diseases. In addition, the incorporation of regular exercise can improve metabolic health, with secondary effects including the enhancement of hepatic arterial blood flow and the reduction of liver disorder complications. By considering these lifestyle choices, patientscan participate actively in their care, and it will result in improved clinical outcomes as well as quality of life. Moreover, alcohol consumption has been a long-standing cause of liver disease, and alcohol reduction or abstinence is important in the context of lifestyle modification. The liver does not have good regenerative capacity, and hence, diminished alcohol use is essential to prevent further vascular damage. Medical authorities uniformly advise moderation, based on evidence from studies correlating heavy drinking with increased fibrosis and cirrhosis, frequently aggravated in pre-existing vascular liver disease. Abstinence not only eliminates undue strain on the liver but also facilitates better compliance with therapeutic regimens. Support groups or counselling are also recommended to enhance the support for sobriety activities since the collective experiences form a good foundation for behavioural modification. A customized effort towards lifestyle adjustment, particularly about alcohol consumption, is therefore necessary for effective control of liver disease. Finally, the influence of sex and gender in deciding the efficacy of lifestyle modifications in the management of vascular liver diseases should receive special attention. Evidence indicates that these differences may impact disease pathology, progression, and sensitivity to treatment and hence imply the need for adjustment of lifestyle intervention accordingly. Men and women may react differently to dietary modification and exercise due to differences in metabolic rate, endocrine impact, and psychosocial factors. For example, women will most likely derive more benefits from some forms of exercise or from dietary restriction compared to men. With clinicians attempting to implement personalized care, they must consider these sex and gender variables to ensure that they optimize patient outcomes. By incorporating such personalized lifestyle adjustments into models of treatment, medical practitioners can significantly improve the quality of care delivered to patients with liver vascular disease (F-Jarvis *et al.*, 2020; Visseren *et al.*, 2021).

9.5. Complications of Vascular Disorders

Problems in the liver's blood vessels can seriously affect how the liver works, which can lead to many health complications. One critical condition concomitant with liver vascular disorders is the development of nonalcoholic fatty liver disease (NAFLD), often exacerbated by IR and type 2 diabetes. Having these metabolic disorders is worrying since they increase the seriousness of liver diseases. Having elevated fasting glycemia and glucose intolerance is typical of pre-diabetes, which leads to diabetes and can also bring on vascular complications such as atherosclerotic cardiovascular disease and fatty liver. Consequently, diagnosing and managing these diseases effectively is vital for preventing the advancement of hepatic vascular disorders, as proper intervention can mitigate the associated risks and improve patient outcomes in this vulnerable population (Tć-Živković, 2022). Also, there is a strong link between liver vascular disorders and renal complications. When the liver is not working properly, there is a greater chance for patients to develop chronic kidney disease, especially if they are obese and have IR. Different subtypes of pre-diabetes are linked to different risks, especially when obesity and fatty liver are present, which increases the risk of cardiovascular and renal diseases. Because NAFLD and type 2 diabetes have similar causes, taking care of the vascular system is very important. Unfortunately, failure to address these intertwined conditions may lead to more severe health complications, including progression to hepatocellular carcinoma (HCC), a dire consequence of chronic hepatic stress associated with vascular dysfunction (Saki *et al.*, 2021).

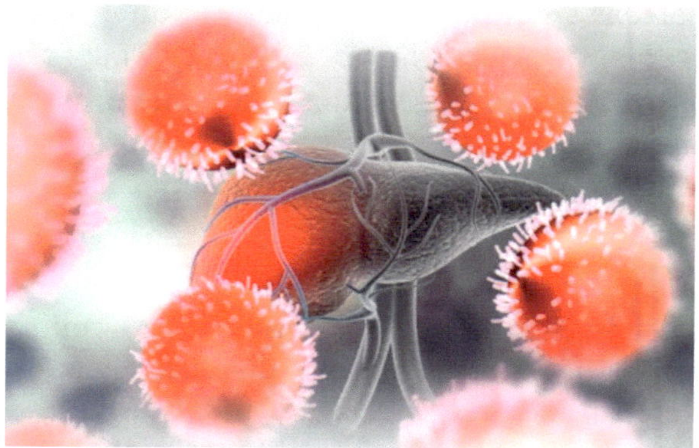

Figure 9.13. Hepatic vascular disorders

Source: https://www.webconsultas.com/sites/default/files/styles/wc_adaptive_noticia__small/public/media/2022/02/14/enfermedades_vaculares_hepaticas_riesgo_covid.jpg.webp

So, it is important to understand these relationships when planning management strategies. These vascular complications can cause problems in the liver and kidneys and may also affect the general health of people. Liver vascular disorders tend to cause patients to deal with several issues, such as a higher risk of heart-related illnesses and death. Understanding the different types of pre-diabetes helps people manage their risks better and stresses the importance of strong screening and prevention. Changing your diet and being more active helps a lot in managing these vascular complications and stopping them from getting worse. Sometimes, using specific medications may be required to manage comorbid conditions, mainly in people with severe IR and liver problems. Therefore, a proactive and integrated approach toward the cardiovascular and metabolic health of patients suffering from vascular disorders of the liver is crucial to improving overall health outcomes (Tć-Živković, 2022) (Figure 9.13).

9.5.1. Risk of Liver Failure

The risk of liver failure, particularly in vascular liver disorders, cannot be overstated, as it is a serious complication of acute and chronic pathological processes. Such disorders as PVT greatly modify hepatic circulation, leading to extreme ischemia and thus compromised hepatocyte function. The compromised hepatic perfusion may trigger a sequence of hepatic damage that progressively aggravates liver pathology, leading to cirrhosis. CLD patients, especially those with cirrhosis, are generally in a delicate balance between bleeding disorders and hypercoagulability due to alterations in hemostatic factors related to liver disease, and their procedural risk profiles become more complicated. The intricacy of such conditions necessitates a graduated approach to managing bleeding risks with particular focus on patient hemostatic system stability while receiving treatment (Northup *et al.*, 2020). In addition, pathogenic mechanisms of liver-related vascular diseases can predict a heightened vulnerability to liver failure in subjects with telomere biology disorders (TBDs). Clinical manifestations that involve TBDs, i.e., dyskeratosis congenita, have serious implications, including susceptibility to HCC and other vascular lesions. These multi-complex system illnesses reveal an intrinsic risk of both liver failure and dysfunction, caused by a combination of vascular and hematological pathology. As has been described throughout the literature, convergence of condition results in a cumulative risk profile, particularly where compromised hepatic vasculature insults ongoing liver pathology. These considerations highlight the necessity of longitudinal monitoring and intervention strategies targeting these cross-cutting health problems, especially among patients showing clinically relevant telomere-related impairment (Niewisch *et al.*, 2019).

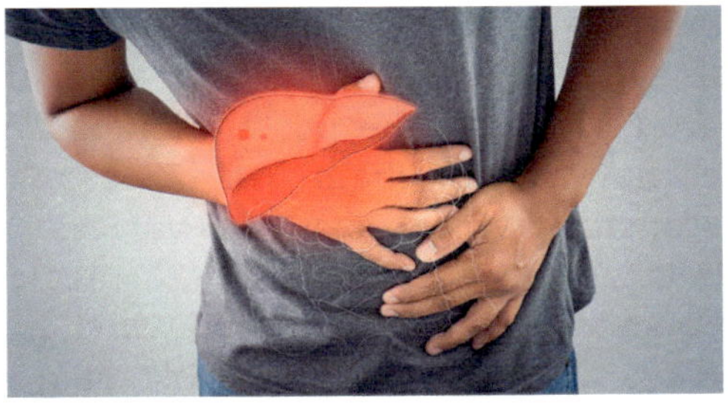

Figure 9.14. Risk of liver failure

Source: https://www.webconsultas.com/sites/default/files/styles/wch_image_schema/public/media/0d/temas/insuficiencia_hepatica.jpg

Finally, procedural interventions among those with pre-existing vascular and hepatic defects heighten the likelihood of liver failure, presenting a critical clinical conundrum. Interests such as paracentesis, endoscopy, or liver biopsy (LBx), despite their diagnostic and managerial necessity, carry the risks of complications in the form of bleeding and infection that could precipitate ALF. General guidelines emphasize individualized risk assessment, especially considering the complex relationship between liver function and hemostatic status. Individuals with advanced portal hypertension or decompensated liver disease are in a very precarious balance, where low-risk procedures can be harmful if appropriate measures are not taken. Therefore, clinicians ought to adopt an equitable, proactive approach by the application of advanced hemostatic tests and clinical experience to minimize risk and optimize care in patients with vascular diseases of the liver in order to finally prevent liver failure development (Northup *et al.*, 2020) (Figure 9.14).

9.5.2. Development of Varices

Liver disease patients are at risk of varices, especially in the esophagus, mainly because of portal hypertension, which is a frequent result of CLD. When blood flow to the liver is blocked by cirrhosis, which causes the liver's structure to change and fibrosis to occur, portal hypertension results. Because of the increased pressure, the portal venous system creates new routes, mainly in the esophagus and stomach, which result in varices. They are enlarged veins that usually do not cause symptoms at first, but can burst, which is very dangerous and may cause severe bleeding in the gastrointestinal tract. CLD, especially fibrosis and cirrhosis from viral hepatitis or ALD, is the main reason for varices to develop, which calls for close observation and early treatment in affected people. Variceal management depends on treating the liver disease and preventing the complications that can happen with variceal bleeding. The usual methods are drugs such as beta-blockers, which successfully lower portal pressure and the chances of varices bleeding. As well, endoscopic techniques may be used to treat varices that are present, using either band ligation or sclerotherapy to destroy the variceal tissue. Sometimes, when patients have recurrent variceal bleeding, invasive treatment such as TIPS could be considered. The procedure decompresses the portal system, but it can bring about its own risks and lasting problems. As emphasized in current guidelines, integrating a multidisciplinary approach involving hepatologists and gastroenterologists is crucial in optimizing management strategies for patients at risk for variceal development and related complications, thus improving overall patient care outcomes (Sarkar *et al.*, 2020). Liver disease can also play a role in variceal development that impacts reproductive health, which should be recognized and managed differently. It seems that the combination of portal hypertension and hormone changes during pregnancy can raise the risk of varices developing and rupturing. In women who already have liver disease and are pregnant, the increased blood volume and changes in blood flow can greatly raise the risk of variceal bleeding. It is important that hepatologists and maternal-fetal medicine doctors work together to address the difficulties of managing liver disease and varices in pregnant patients. Such collaboration is essential not only for safeguarding maternal health but also for ensuring fetal well-being, particularly given the multifaceted challenges posed by vascular disorders of the liver in this vulnerable population (Finn *et al.*, 2020) (Figure 9.15).

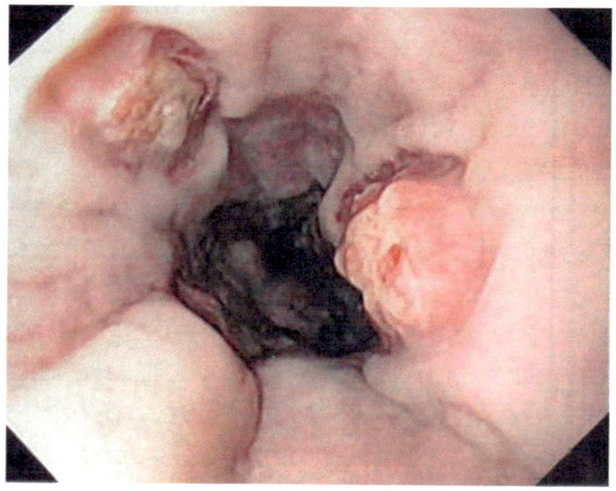

Figure 9.15. Esophageal varices seven days after banding, showing ulceration at the site of banding.

Source: https://upload.wikimedia.org/wikipedia/commons/0/09/Esophageal_varices_-_post_banding.jpg.

9.5.3. Impact on Overall Health

The connection between liver vascular disease and overall body health is immense, as this disease is bound to initiate a spate of systemic complications. Liver vascular diseases such as portal hypertension and HVT have a direct impact on the organs' capacity to digest nutrients and cleanse blood, with a rippling effect on metabolic equilibrium across the body. When circulation of the blood is blocked, it may lead to pathologies like ascites, where there is an accumulation of fluid in the cavity of the peritoneum, leading to abdominal discomfort and immobility. These complications not only decrease the quality of life but also present serious challenges to the healthcare system, as patients may have to undergo lengthy and recurrent medical interventions. Hence, the long-term effects of hepatic vascular diseases extend beyond regional issues, and it is significant to understand their general health implications and early detection as well as treatment methodologies. Moreover, hepatic vascular diseases have a direct correlation with other varieties of health issues beyond liver function, like cardiovascular disease and diabetes. The liver is also a crucial organ for cholesterol homeostasis and insulin sensitivity, and impairment of its vascular system can lead to metabolic dysregulation. For instance, elevated portal pressure can result in the release of pro-inflammatory cytokines, worsening systemic inflammation, which has been implicated as an etiological factor in cardiovascular and metabolic diseases. Thus, patients with liver vascular diseases are more susceptible to subsequent chronicity that will seriously impair overall health and life expectancy. As can be testified by many investigations, including antimicrobial resistance investigations, the cost of subsequent health complications warrants vigilant observation and multidisciplinary care of patients (Murray *et al.*, 2022; Visseren *et al.*, 2021). Lastly, psychosocial impacts of vascular disease on liver health are an important concern in their overall health effect. Patients may become seriously distressed by ongoing symptoms, frequent physician visits, and the threat of serious disease complications. This distress and uncertainty tend to trigger depression and anxiety, which in turn exacerbate physical deterioration through mechanisms such as inflammation and immunosuppression secondary to stress. Moreover, the psychological stigma of liver ailments discourages patients from seeking medical help on time, and thus, managing becomes even tougher. Therefore, addressing the multifaceted mental and physical implications of hepatic vascular disorders is not only about having a narrow understanding of the physiological effects but also about using supportive mental health frameworks that aid in navigation. Having an interdepartmental response that deals with both physical and mental implications would dramatically decrease the burden on such life-altering patients.

SUMMARY

Vascular liver disease is a significant diagnostic and therapeutic challenge, underlining the sophistication of the liver's interaction with the cardiovascular system. Evidence of cardiac involvement in CLD patients suggests an intimate relationship in which alterations in vascular dynamics potentiate hepatic dysfunction. For instance, LC patients have important changes such as higher resting heart rates and left ventricular mass, which indicate the necessity for comprehensive cardiovascular assessment in these patients. These findings demonstrate that cardiovascular structural and functional alterations are not secondary events but may be significant indicators of liver disease severity and prognosis (Cozzolino *et al.*, 2025). Recognition of this interrelatedness facilitates a profound understanding of patient management and care, and a more holistic understanding of treating vascular presentations in liver disease. Additionally, genetics, through examples such as GSDs, elucidates critical pathways between metabolic defect and vascular complication in the context of the liver. The case of glycogen storage disease type I, with its complicated inflammatory hepatic adenomas, highlights the relationship between metabolic and vascular dysregulation. These patients are typically presented with hepatomegaly as well as systemic symptoms, and thus, monitoring for vascular complications is necessary with caution, including hemorrhagic events due to hepatic adenomas. The correlation of such vascular complications with liver function is of critical significance, and gene sequencing provides useful information about the pathophysiology behind this (Wang *et al.*, 2024). Thus, the application of genetic diagnostics together with traditional assessments has promise for improving the quality of treatment of vascular liver disease, particularly in children. Lastly, knowledge of the presentation of vascular diseases in liver disease not only enhances practice but also offers opportunities for further research. Investigation of the complex interrelationships between hepatic dysfunction, vascular integrity, and patient outcomes could lead to the generation of synergistic treatments addressing liver and cardiovascular disease simultaneously. Such a synergistic treatment may ensure that cardiologists and hepatologists collaborate, facilitating interdisciplinary care for the patient. With the recognition of the complexity of vascular interactions in liver disease, healthcare providers can attempt to achieve better prognosis and quality of life of these patients. This holistic approach can usher in a revolution in treatment paradigms, addressing symptoms of liver dysfunction as well as circulatory disturbances that have far-reaching implications for patient care.

The complex interplay between vascular liver diseases involves a range of conditions that necessitate cautious assessment in the clinical environment. Among these is the congenital portosystemic shunts (CPSS), rare vascular anomalies that form abnormal communications between the portal and systemic venous systems. Portosystemic shunts can variably present as multi-system disorders with a plethora of manifestations that can masquerade as other common childhood disorders, such as hyperinsulinemia or raised aminotransferases. Diagnosis typically necessitates advanced imaging modalities, e.g., Doppler ultrasound or angio-CT scans, which have been instrumental in the identification of these vascular malformations. Early detection is significant since it can significantly influence management strategies and patient outcomes, making the specificity of a diagnostic approach in cases of unexplained endocrine or liver disease crucial (Bahadori *et al.*, 2022). Furthermore, when vascular liver disease occurs, the distinction between acquired and congenital malformations needs to be highlighted. For instance, diabetic complications such as diabetic peripheral angiopathy are dominated by extreme endothelial dysfunction and vascular injury, and most frequently lead to critical conditions that influence liver function. A systematic approach to treatment, identified in recent studies, includes new treatments, including magnetic-laser therapy, with the goal of enhancing vascular activity and microcirculation in various tissues, including the liver. It not only addresses localized vascular impairments but also tries to mitigate systemic diabetic complications, ensuring overall well-being in patients with underlying liver pathologies (Zabulonov *et al.*, 2015). In conclusion, the study of liver vascular disease discloses a multifaceted setting that brings together congenital defects, acquired disease, and new forms of treatment. Knowledge of the subtleties of CPSS and diabetic vascular deficiencies is paramount for clinicians tasked with providing comprehensive care. Multidisciplinary patterns of diagnosis and treatment are more likely to guarantee successful outcomes and improve the quality of life in patients. This combined perspective not only solidifies the central insight into liver vascular pathology but also promotes the necessity of early intervention and ongoing research in this field (Bahadori *et al.*, 2022; Zabulonov *et al.*, 2015).

CLOSER LOOK

ESOPHAGEAL VARICES

Esophageal varices are enlarged, weakened veins in the esophagus that can bleed severely. They are often a consequence of portal hypertension, a condition where blood pressure in the portal vein (which carries blood from the intestines, pancreas, and spleen to the liver) becomes elevated. This increased pressure forces blood into smaller vessels in the esophagus, leading to the varices (Figure 9.16).

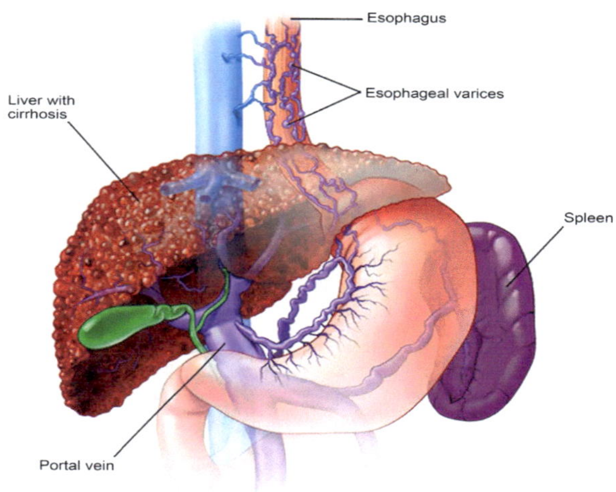

Figure 9.16. Esophageal Varices

Source: https://www.mayoclinic.org/-/media/kcms/gbs/patient-consumer/images/2013/11/15/17/39/an00758_-ds00676_-ds00785_-ds00820_im02167_ans7_esphogeal_varicesthu_jpg.jpg.

Causes and Risk Factors

- **Portal Hypertension:** The most common cause is portal hypertension, often due to liver diseases like cirrhosis.
- **Cirrhosis:** Scarring of the liver (cirrhosis) impedes blood flow, leading to portal hypertension.
- **Other Conditions:** Conditions like schistosomiasis can also contribute to portal hypertension and varices.

Symptoms

- **Usually Asymptomatic:** Esophageal varices themselves don't usually cause symptoms until they bleed.

- **Bleeding:** If varices rupture, they can cause severe upper gastrointestinal bleeding, which can be life-threatening.
- **Other Signs of Liver Disease:** Jaundice (yellowing of the skin), ascites (abdominal fluid buildup), edema (swelling), and upper abdominal pain can be signs of underlying liver disease.

Diagnosis

- **Endoscopy:** A procedure where a flexible tube with a camera is inserted into the esophagus to visualize the veins.
- **CT Scan:** A computerized tomographic scan can also be used to visualize the esophagus and identify varices.

Treatment

- **Managing Portal Hypertension:** Treating the underlying cause of portal hypertension is crucial.
- **Medications:** Beta-blockers can help reduce blood pressure in the portal vein and lower the risk of bleeding.
- **Endoscopic Band Ligation:** A procedure where elastic bands are used to tie off the varices, preventing them from bleeding.
- **Other Procedures:** TIPS can be used to reduce portal pressure.

References

1. Babu, D., Priya, A., & Yadav, K. A. C. (2024). A rare case of esophageal variceal bleeding from portal hypertension due to extrahepatic portal vein obstruction in a two-year-old. *International Journal of Basic & Clinical Pharmacology*. https://www.semanticscholar.org/paper/e05f51b349862f7a756fd87285a572fed72c13cc (accessed on 24 May 2025).
2. Bahadori, A., Kuhlmann, B., Debray, D., Franchi-Abella, S., Wacker, J., Beghetti, M., Wildhaber, B., *et al.* (2022). Presentation of congenital portosystemic shunts in children. *Children, 9*. https://www.semanticscholar.org/paper/40b7b588a6cf0d91a76c817dff504da3c27ded09 (accessed on 24 May 2025).
3. Balali-Mood, M., Naseri, K., Tahergorabi, Z., Khazdair, M. R., & Sadeghi, M. (2021). Toxic mechanisms of five heavy metals: Mercury, lead, chromium, cadmium, and arsenic. *Frontiers in Pharmacology, 12*, Article 643972. https://doi.org/10.3389/fphar.2021.643972.
4. Živković Beljić, T. (2022). Prediabetes: From diagnosis to prognosis. *Galenika Medical Journal*. https://www.semanticscholar.org/paper/8c59d05dc6179927a367f0c2425d2213ad2e96ad (accessed on 24 May 2025).
5. Cozzolino, D., Nevola, R., Ruggiero, A., Romano, C., Umano, G. R., Aitella, E., Sardu, C., *et al.* (2025). The cross-talk between the heart and the liver: The involvement of the mitral valve as a novel actor upon the ancient scene of liver cirrhosis. *Journal of Cardiovascular Development and Disease, 12*. https://www.semanticscholar.org/paper/999c9fdeac5d4b763f7275d5b43591dc6cfcdaf2 (accessed on 24 May 2025).
6. Deana, C., Vetrugno, L., Cortegiani, A., Mongodi, S., Salve, G., Mangiagalli, M., Boscolo, A., *et al.* (2023). Quality of life in COVID-related ARDS patients one year after intensive care discharge (Odissea study): A multicenter observational study. *Journal of Clinical Medicine, 12*. https://www.semanticscholar.org/paper/6cf8ce186af524698be547e7670a190e297fff77 (accessed on 24 May 2025).
7. Eitler, K., Bibok, A., & Telkes, G. (2022). Situs inversus totalis: A clinical review. *International Journal of General Medicine, 15*, 2437–2449. https://doi.org/10.2147/ijgm.s295444.
8. Finn, R. S., Qin, S., Ikeda, M., Galle, P. R., Ducreux, M., Kim, T. Y., Kudo, M., *et al.* (2020). Atezolizumab plus bevacizumab in unresectable hepatocellular carcinoma. *New England Journal of Medicine, 382*(20), 1894–1905. https://doi.org/10.1056/nejmoa1915745.
9. Gamanagatti, S., & Hemachandran, N. (2021). Hepatic venous outflow tract obstruction: Causes, natural history, and treatment. *Clinical Liver Disease, 18*. https://www.semanticscholar.org/paper/35eada962f166371aad6a17be8a5d8cb8ffa6c74 (accessed on 24 May 2025).
10. Gimson, A. (2020). Vascular disorders of the liver. In *Oxford Textbook of Medicine*. https://www.semanticscholar.org/paper/11e7432ca5b07857465b2a8dc123123b99f850b32 (accessed on 24 May 2025).
11. Giuli, L., Pallozzi, M., Venturini, G., Gasbarrini, A., Ponziani, F., & Santopaolo, F. (2023). Molecular mechanisms underlying vascular liver diseases: Focus on thrombosis. *International Journal of Molecular Sciences, 24*, Article 799404. https://www.semanticscholar.org/paper/799404eb6841cde5ba11eb909f425163c102afe2 (accessed on 24 May 2025).
12. Hassan, S., Anouti, A., Tan, Q., Wangensteen, K., & Aqul, A. (2024). Liver transplantation for pediatric genetic and metabolic disorders. *Liver Transplantation: Official Publication of the*

American Association for the Study of Liver Diseases and the International Liver Transplantation Society. https://www.semanticscholar.org/paper/1d197569d85d47e820ffa06faac43cb4f231319c (accessed on 24 May 2025).

13. Jadhav, P. A., Thomas, A. B., Chopada, V. M., Bokaria, P. V., Deokate, S. B., Chougule, P. S., & Chavan, P. N. (2024). Correlation of non-alcoholic fatty liver disease and neurodegenerative disorders. *Egyptian Liver Journal*. https://www.semanticscholar.org/paper/715dfc6464a7a535c906e813012f935c0e2636a2 (accessed on 24 May 2025).

14. Jebari, Y., Kadiri, M., Chabib, F., Lagdali, N., Borahma, M., & Ajana, F. (2024). Budd Chiari syndrome (BCS) and Myeloproliferative Neoplasms (MPN): A Moroccan experience center. *Saudi Journal of Medical and Pharmaceutical Sciences*. https://www.semanticscholar.org/paper/039ac5c811381484e9580ba84c379812b0461a52 (accessed on 24 May 2025).

15. Kearney, M. (2013). Changing the way, we think about endothelial cell insulin sensitivity, nitric oxide, and the pathophysiology of type 2 diabetes. *Diabetes, 62*(4), 1386–1388. https://www.semanticscholar.org/paper/acc5999175742bf3c48d7617fc1cfd42ae084539 (accessed on 24 May 2025).

16. Lu, F., Jia, S., Lu, H., Zhao, H., Li, Z., Zhuge, Y., Romeiro, F., *et al.* (2023). Primary Budd-Chiari syndrome versus sinusoidal obstruction syndrome: A review. *Current Medical Research and Opinion, 40*, 303–313. https://www.semanticscholar.org/paper/9553cfe7c1fedb15a224a03c4978bdd548624390 (accessed on 24 May 2025).

17. Mach, F., Baigent, C., Catapano, A. L., Koskinas, K. C., Casula, M., Badimón, L., Chapman, M. J., *et al.* (2019). 2019 ESC/EAS guidelines for the management of dyslipidemias: Lipid modification to reduce cardiovascular risk. *European Heart Journal, 41*, 111–188. https://doi.org/10.1093/eurheartj/ehz455.

18. Jarvis Mauvais-, F., Bairey Merz, C. N., Barnes, P. J., Díaz Brinton, R., Carrero, J. J., DeMeo, D. L., De Vries, G. J., *et al.* (2020). Sex and gender: Modifiers of health, disease, and medicine. *The Lancet, 396*, 565–582. https://doi.org/10.1016/s0140-6736(20)31561-0.

19. Medicine Chinese Society of Emergency, Care Chest Pain Branch of China International Exchange, Association Multidisciplinary Joint Committee on Cardiopulmonary, Workgroup of the Chinese Experts Consensus on Alde. (2024). [Chinese experts' consensus on aldehyde metabolism disorder guided the early management of emergency and critical care medicine (2023)]. *Zhonghua Wei Zhong Bing Ji Jiu Yi Xue, 36*(1), 6–15. https://www.semanticscholar.org/paper/4770ac93d955166111b4d8c243bf7452506d5974 (accessed on 24 May 2025).

20. Murray, C. J. L., Ikuta, K. S., Sharara, F., Swetschinski, L. R., Robles Aguilar, G., Gray, A. P., Han, C., *et al.* (2022). Global burden of bacterial antimicrobial resistance in 2019: A systematic analysis. *The Lancet, 399*, 629–655. https://doi.org/10.1016/s0140-6736(21)02724-0.

21. Niewisch, M. R., & Savage, S. A. (2019). An update on the biology and management of dyskeratosis congenita and related telomere biology disorders. *Expert Review of Hematology, 12*(12), 1037–1052. https://doi.org/10.1080/17474086.2019.1662720.

22. Northup, P., García-Pagán, J., Garcia-Tsao, G., Intagliata, N., Superina, R., Roberts, L., Lisman, T., *et al.* (2020). Vascular liver disorders, portal vein thrombosis, and procedural bleeding in patients with liver disease: 2020 practice guidance by the American Association for the Study of Liver Diseases. *Hepatology, 73*(1), 366–413. https://doi.org/10.1002/hep.31646.

23. Patel, A. J., Patel, S., Wickremesinghe, P., & Vadada, D. (2017). Radiofrequency ablation using Barrx® for the endoscopic treatment of gastric antral vascular ectasia: A series of three cases and a review of the literature on treatment options. *Clinical and Experimental Gastroenterology, 10*, 113–120. https://www.semanticscholar.org/paper/dc684f1f5bdf5a20e88d23e2e53025db0f122c5f (accessed on 24 May 2025).

24. Roth, G. A., Abate, D., Abate, K. H., Abay, S. M., Abbafati, C., Abbasi, N., Abbastabar, H., *et al.* (2018). Global, regional, and national age-sex-specific mortality for 282 causes of death in 195 countries and territories, 1980–2017: A systematic analysis for the Global Burden of Disease Study 2017. *The Lancet, 392*(10159), 1736–1788. https://doi.org/10.1016/s0140-6736(18)32203-7.

25. Saad, A. F., Chahine, K. M., Saade, G., & Sibai, B. (2025). Liver hematoma in pregnancy: Challenges, management strategies, and outcomes. *O&G Open*. https://www.semanticscholar.org/paper/19173dba546847ddb64711fc8a14682f569b1fcc (accessed on 24 May 2025).

26. Saki, K., Mansouri, V., Abdi, S., Fathi, M., Razzaghi, Z., & Haghazali, M. (2021). Assessment of common and differentially expressed proteins between diabetes mellitus and fatty liver disease: A network analysis. *Gastroenterology and Hepatology from Bed to Bench, 14*(Suppl), S94–S101. https://www.semanticscholar.org/paper/30721ad0de745a4e4274e8a4b602c1a457f70510 (accessed on 24 May 2025).

27. Sarkar, M., Brady, C. W., Fleckenstein, J., Forde, K. A., Khungar, V., Molleston, J. P., Afshar, Y., *et al.* (2020). Reproductive health and liver disease: Practice guidance by the American Association for the Study of Liver Diseases. *Hepatology, 73*(1), 318–365. https://doi.org/10.1002/hep.31559.

28. Thromboprophylaxis Working Group on Guidelines for COVID Management of Anticoagulation in Hospitalized Patients, Embolism Pulmonary, Society Pulmonary Vascular Diseases Group of the Chinese Thoracic Society, Physicians Pulmonary Vascular Disease Working Committee of Chinese Medical Association, Prevention National Cooperation Group on Embolism Treatment of Pulmonary, *et al.* (2023). Practice guidelines of thromboprophylaxis and management of anticoagulation in hospitalized patients with COVID-19. *Zhonghua Yi Xue Za Zhi, 103*, 1–23. https://www.semanticscholar.org/paper/c8b4d7d12ee9930831851047b062a49d13bcba35 (accessed on 24 May 2025).

29. Villegas, D., Levy, J., Moreno, M., & Rimer, R. (2025). Successful embolization of symptomatic intrahepatic portosystemic venous shunts through trans-splenic access–A case report. *American Journal of Interventional Radiology*. https://www.semanticscholar.org/paper/788014084965f5b1bfb66403493fa28d4dbea77e (accessed on 24 May 2025).

30. Visseren, F. L. J., Mach, F., Smulders, Y. M., Carballo, D., Koskinas, K. C., Bäck, M., Bénétos, A., *et al.* (2021). 2021 ESC guidelines on cardiovascular disease prevention in clinical practice. *European Heart Journal, 42*, 3227–3337. https://doi.org/10.1093/eurheartj/ehab484.

31. Wang, A., Wu, J., Yuan, X., Liu, J., & Lu, C. (2024). A case study of a liver transplant-treated patient with glycogen storage disease type Ia presenting with multiple inflammatory hepatic adenomas: An analysis of clinicopathologic and genetic data. *BMC Medical Genomics, 17*. https://www.semanticscholar.org/paper/39fec190d601b825d2a888e6cbf2ea81511b764f (accessed on 24 May 2025).

32. Wang, Y., Wang, L., Wen, Y., Wu, X., & Cai, H. (2025). Precision-engineered nanocarriers for targeted treatment of liver fibrosis and vascular disorders. *World Journal of Innovation and Modern Technology*. https://www.semanticscholar.org/paper/f071460303104a0ae96342e07c6e2d0fc4422590 (accessed on 24 May 2025).

33. Wichmann D, Sperhake JP, Lütgehetmann M, Steurer S, Edler C, Heinemann A, Heinrich F, Mushumba H, Kniep I, Schröder AS, Burdelski C, de Heer G, Nierhaus A, Frings D, Pfefferle S, Becker H, Bredereke-Wiedling H, de Weerth A, Paschen HR, Sheikhzadeh-Eggers S, Stang A, Schmiedel S, Bokemeyer C, Addo MM, Aepfelbacher M, Püschel K, Kluge S. Autopsy Findings and Venous Thromboembolism in Patients With COVID-19: A Prospective Cohort Study. Ann Intern Med. 2020 Aug 18;173(4):268-277. doi: 10.7326/M20-2003. Epub 2020 May 6. PMID: 32374815; PMCID: PMC7240772.

34. Xie, F., Wang, J., & Yang, Q. (2021). Recurrent pyogenic liver abscess after pancreatoduodenectomy caused by common hepatic artery injury: A case report. *World Journal of Clinical Cases, 9*, 9198–9204. https://www.semanticscholar.org/paper/9df59237695a694c166c57d43c1e3259b697a900 (accessed on 24 May 2025).

35. Zabulonov, Y., Chukhraiyeva, O., Vladimirov, A., Chukhraiyev, M., & Zukow, W. (2015). Diabetic peripheral angiopathy treatment using a multi-laser therapy device. *Journal of Education, Health and Sport, 5*. https://www.semanticscholar.org/paper/328e24e2350496cd98e8ec5541bf5b2bdce2a842 (accessed on 24 May 2025).

36. Zhang, S. (2021). Expert consensus on perioperative vascular complications for liver transplantation (2021). *Zhonghua Wai Ke Za Zhi [Chinese Journal of Surgery], 59*(8), 641–645. https://www.semanticscholar.org/paper/cb4d1bdeff794478ca203778ecece4c69ed701ee (accessed on 24 May 2025).

37. Zhang, Y., Yan, Y., & Song, B. (2019). Noninvasive imaging diagnosis of sinusoidal obstruction syndrome: A pictorial review. *Insights into Imaging, 10*. https://doi.org/10.1186/s13244-019-0791-x.

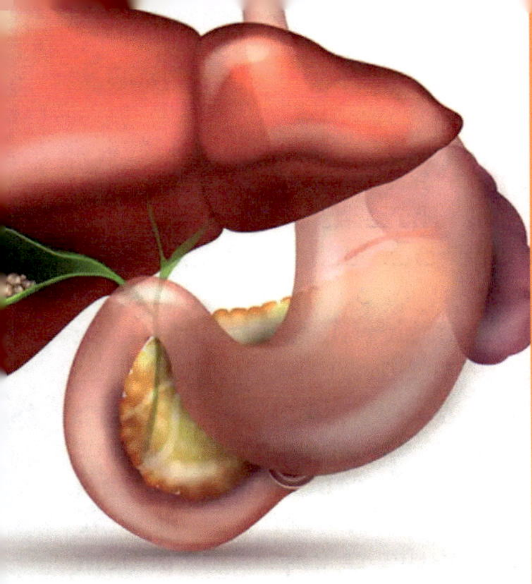

Chapter 10
BILIARY TRACT DISEASES

Contents

Introduction

Diseases of the biliary tract encompass a broad spectrum of disorders of the biliary apparatus, i.e., the gallbladder, bile ducts, and associated structures. These diseases can lead to significant morbidity and are typically accompanied by various presentations such as pain, jaundice, and gastrointestinal abnormalities. The pathogenesis of biliary tract diseases is multifactorial, with some of the factors being inflammation, obstruction, and infection. The significance of these conditions is underlined by their risk of causing acute and chronic complications, including cholecystitis, cholangitis, and even cancers of the biliary system. It is necessary to appreciate the epidemiology and clinical presentation of these conditions so that they can be managed and treated, especially since they overlap very commonly with other systemic diseases. The prevalence of biliary tract disease might markedly vary depending on geographic, cultural, and socioeconomic factors. Particularly, nations with diverse patterns of diet and access to healthcare should be expected to exhibit increased rates of some biliary conditions. For instance, the prevalence of liver fluke infection is much higher in poor nations where particular environmental and agricultural factors predispose to infection. Infection hazards are considerable in as much as liver flukes have been proven to be biological carcinogens, leading to increased morbidity as well as chronic liver disease. The epidemiologic foundation of biliary tract diseases emphasizes the necessity for public health interventions that will diminish risk factors for these diseases in diverse populations. Care of biliary tract diseases is a unique challenge for clinicians due to the variety of underlying causes and the severity of complications. For example, DILI with long-term drug therapy with drugs like linezolid illustrates how certain drugs can cause biliary issues such as lactic acidosis and hepatotoxicity. Doctors are thus increasingly being compelled to remain vigilant to toxic drug effects and interactions with underlying biliary disease. Through this, ongoing research into the etiology and treatment of biliary tract disease is imperative to improving patient outcomes and guiding clinical practice. With the continuous evolution in diagnostic strategies and therapeutic options, the hope is to gain better insights into these diseases and develop effective strategies to reverse their impact on public health (Figure 10.1).

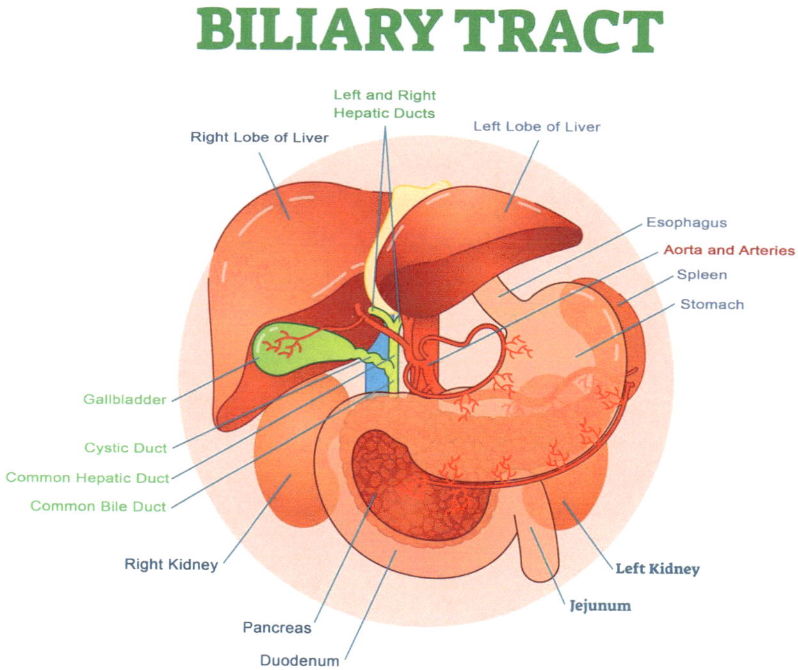

Figure 10.1. Biliary tract.

Source: https://www.verywellhealth.com/thmb/fiHWPHtgHC1BfewDlPHoekUeNhQ=/1500x0/filters:no_upscale():max_bytes(150000):strip_icc()/GettyImages-930064116-83edb075ecfc48e0919dbd03b1235c63.jpg.

Definition of Biliary Tract Diseases

The biliary tract includes the gallbladder, bile ducts, and related structures, and diseases in this area are called biliary tract diseases. Diseases of this type are usually classified into obstructive and inflammatory categories. Obstructive diseases, for example, choledocholithiasis, cause gallstones or tumors to block bile flow, which may result in cholangitis or pancreatitis. In contrast, inflammatory disorders include conditions like cholecystitis and primary sclerosing cholangitis (PSC). Because these diseases can seriously harm a patient, they need to be found and managed as soon as possible. Both the structure and function of the biliary system must be considered since disturbances can cause symptoms such as jaundice and abdominal pain. So, any complete definition of biliary tract diseases should cover their causes, their mechanisms, and the symptoms they cause. Imaging tests and laboratory examinations are usually used to diagnose diseases of the biliary tract. The biliary tree can be seen, and any abnormalities detected with the help of ultrasound, MRCP, and CT scans. They give important details about whether there are blockages, swelling, or possible cancer changes in the biliary system.

Laboratory tests that look at liver enzymes and bilirubin are necessary to determine how well the liver is working and the degree of biliary blockage. When imaging and biochemical reports are combined, it is easier to make the correct diagnosis and decide on the right treatment. Reliance on various diagnostic techniques points to how difficult and important it is to correctly identify and understand diseases of the biliary tract in clinical care. How biliary tract diseases are managed depends a lot on the particular condition involved. An example is that acute cholecystitis frequently calls for surgical treatment, which is often done by laparoscopic cholecystectomy. Sometimes, obstructive disorders are treated by using endoscopic or percutaneous techniques to open the bile duct and restore its normal function. In addition, some diseases of the biliary tract, for example, PSC, might need ongoing care, since they can develop complications such as cholangiocarcinoma, which is linked to chronic cholangitis. The relationship between biliary tract diseases and secondary malignancies is noteworthy; research has shown that hepatobiliary cancers can be associated with higher risks of second primary cancers, emphasizing the need for vigilant surveillance in affected populations (Chen *et al.*, 2021). Because of these challenges in management and the relationships between biliary conditions, it is important to keep researching and educating in the field of biliary tract diseases.

Importance of the Biliary System in Digestion

The biliary tract is crucial to the process of digestion, facilitating the emulsification and absorption of dietary fat. The system consists of the liver, gallbladder, and bile ducts that collaborate in bile secretion and storage, a compound that is crucial for fat digestion. Bile acids (BAs), the primary bile constituents, are bile detergents that emulsify gross fat globules to smaller micelles that increase the surface area for lipase enzymes to further hydrolyze fats into absorbing units. The complex interplay between bile secretion and production is crucial to promote metabolic homeostasis, with special emphasis on the requirement of a well-working biliary apparatus for effective digestion. Interference with bile secretion or transport, most commonly resulting from gallstones or obstructive biliary illness, can result in malabsorption and other dysfunctions that presage underlying biliary tree disease, emphasizing the importance of comprehending this system in the context of gastrointestinal health. Dysbiosis of the biliary system can occur in numerous forms, with significant repercussions on the efficiency and health of digestion. For instance, cholestasis or gallbladder disease may influence bile secretion and lead to jaundice and malabsorption of fat. The relationship between the biliary system and metabolic disease has been an increasingly prominent target of interest in the last few years. Research has revealed that BAs are not only digestive enzymes, but they also perform critical functions within glucose and lipid metabolism, influencing energy homeostasis and potentially serving as therapeutic targets for chronic liver diseases (CLD). Investigating the complexity of bile acid signaling pathways and their regulation can shed light on conditions such as NAFLD and PSC, which are increasing in prevalence in modern society (Alpini *et al.*, 2020). Thus, an understanding of the numerous roles played by bile in digestion can become a basic premise in the management of biliary tract diseases. Additionally, the significance of the biliary system's influence can be appreciated through its anatomical and physiological contribution to gastrointestinal health. The gallbladder, as a major organ of the system, holds bile and pumps it into the duodenum during the consumption of dietary fat. Changes in gallbladder function, at times indicated by the formation of gallstones, have severe health consequences, including cholecystitis and pancreatitis. Dysfunction of the gallbladder is associated with excessive bile storage and secretion, further affecting digestion and nutrient absorption. The incidence of gallstone disease and complications underscores the significance of gallbladder physiology in digestive efficiency (Ahmad *et al.*, 2024). This exchange highlights the necessity of learning about the pathophysiology of gallbladder conditions and their relevance to patient health in order to make sure that advances in treatment strategies are aligned with the fundamentals of digestion.

10.1. Anatomy of the Biliary Tract

The gallbladder and bile ducts, which make up the biliary tract, help digest and absorb fats by moving bile from the liver to the small intestine. The biliary system consists of structures within the liver (intrahepatic) and outside the liver (extrahepatic). The bile ducts in the liver join together to make the common hepatic duct, which leaves the liver. The extrahepatic part consists of the common bile duct, which goes through the pancreas and then enters the duodenum. The gallbladder, which is below the liver, holds and concentrates bile until it is needed for digestion. Since the biliary tract is very complex, understanding it is essential for diagnosing and treating diseases of the biliary tract, as problems such as cholangitis or choledocholithiasis are often caused by this anatomy. Understanding how anatomical structures relate to different diseases in the biliary tract is very important. As an example, choledochal malformations, which are congenital defects, may require surgery because of the serious complications they can cause. As demonstrated by an international Delphi survey, consensus exists about the importance of removing the entire extrahepatic biliary tract in cases of congenital choledochal malformation (CCM), with reconstruction performed via Roux-en-Y hepaticojejunostomy (Bruggink *et al.*, 2022).

The structure of the bile ducts helps explain why biliary intraepithelial neoplasms, which may develop into cholangiocarcinoma, are common. Since the biliary tract and pancreas are formed from the same embryological source, their diseases are often similar, which stresses the value of knowing the biliary tract anatomy in these cases. The anatomy of the biliary tract affects the appearance of biliary tract lesions, which makes it difficult for clinicians to distinguish between different pathologies. Both intraepithelial neoplasms in the biliary tract and the pancreas exhibit comparable characteristics, such as shared immunohistochemical phenotypes indicative of a common carcinogenic process (Alvaro *et al.*, 2019). Both systems having intraductal papillary neoplasms show how important it is to understand anatomy when checking for signs of cancer. With this knowledge, healthcare professionals can take early steps and improve patient outcomes. Moreover, the anatomical proximity of biliary and pancreatic structures provides insight into the mechanism of diseases affecting these regions, emphasizing the interconnectedness of anatomy and pathology in the biliary tract (Figure 10.2).

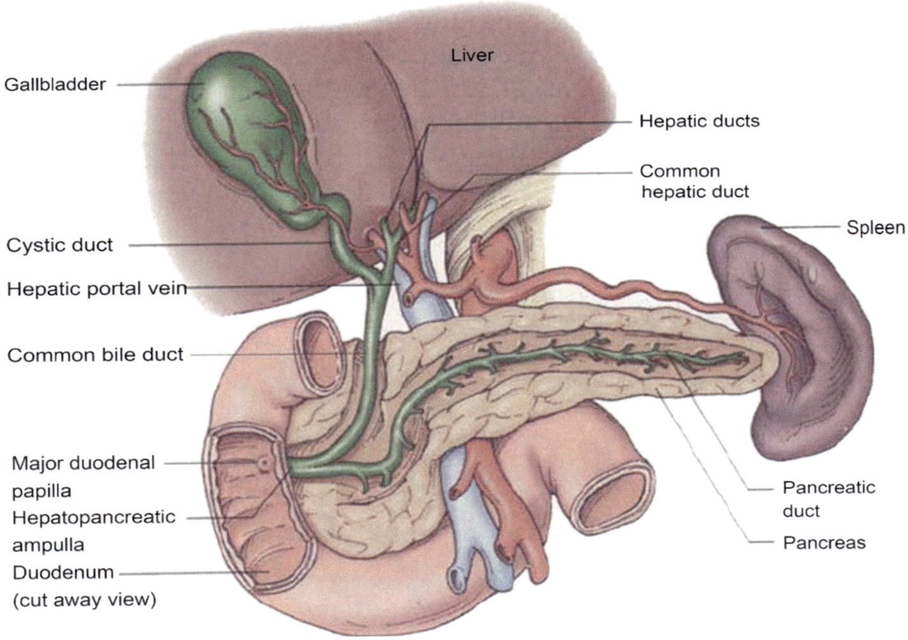

Figure 10.2. Anatomical details of a human biliary system.

Source: https://www.researchgate.net/profile/Mushtak-Al-Atabi/publication/258405778/figure/fig1/AS:297498032787460@1447940466483/Anatomical-details-of-a-human-biliary-system.png.

10.1.1. Components of the Biliary System

The biliary system plays a significant role in digestion by facilitating the transport, storage, and secretion of bile, which is a fluid employed for the emulsification of fats. The primary organs of the system are the liver, gallbladder, and ductal system of bile. The liver secretes bile in association with bile salts, cholesterol, and waste, which is conveyed to the gallbladder and there stored in a concentrated state. When fat moves to the small intestine, hormonal stimuli provoke the gallbladder to contract and release bile into the common bile duct so that it can proceed to the duodenum. The harmonious working of these structures not only aids in digestion but also indicates the intricate relationship between the various structures of the biliary system, which are susceptible to changes in various biliary tract diseases. Compounding the complexity of the biliary system's functioning are conditions related to it that can interrupt its normal processes. Biliary tract diseases can manifest in cholestasis, biliary atresia, and cholangitis types, impacting the system's structures in varying ways. Cholangitis, for example, often caused by BI, can lead to inflammation and bile duct obstruction, which significantly impacts bile flow. Epidemiologic data show that bacterial infection in bile samples is a risk factor for various biliary diseases, with significant associations between particular bacteria like *Escherichia coli* and gallstone development (Alebouyeh *et al.*, 2016). This interaction highlights the significance of thorough examination and management of biliary system health, especially in symptomatic patients with biliary tract disease. Apart from obstructions and infections, the anatomy of the biliary system also results in a chain of complications following surgery or operations such as liver transplantation. Biliary complication occurrence following transplant, for instance, occurs at a significant rate and affects the quality of the graft and donor health (Barr *et al.*, 2009). Complications are often meant to denote the biliary duct's function and can include strictures, leaks, and infections. Understanding the complex anatomy and susceptibility to post-operative complications emphasizes the importance of establishing the functioning of the biliary apparatus prior to and following surgery. As such, further research on the parts of the biliary apparatus and associated diseases is essential in minimizing surgical complications and patient prognosis in biliary apparatus diseases (Figure 10.3).

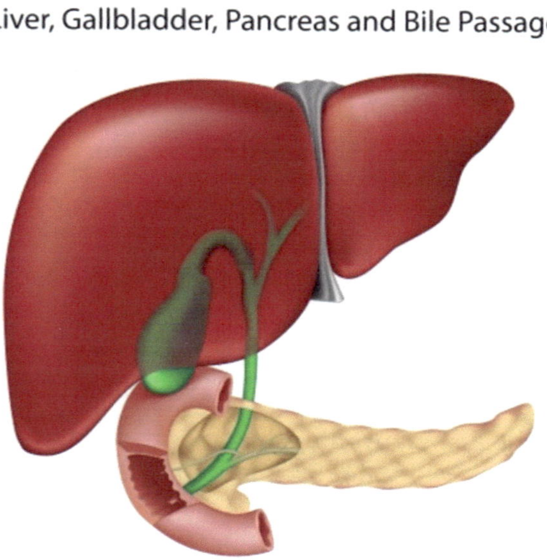

Figure 10.3. Liver, gallbladder, and bile passage.

10.1.2. Functions of the Gallbladder and Bile Ducts

The gallbladder is important in the biliary system because it stores bile, which is made by the liver. After eating a meal, especially one high in fats, the gallbladder squeezes and bile is pushed into the duodenum through the bile ducts. It is necessary for lipids to be emulsified and absorbed, which this release helps with. It also helps to make bile more concentrated than the liver can do alone, and it adds BAs, bilirubin, and cholesterol to the bile. Concentrating bile allows it to break down fats in food, which helps the body absorb needed nutrients. If the gallbladder is not working properly, the body might not absorb nutrients well, which can lead to GI symptoms and nutrient shortages. The bile ducts, which consist of both intrahepatic and extrahepatic parts, help move bile from the liver to the gallbladder and then to the intestine. Cholangiocytes, which are specialized epithelial cells, line the ducts and are responsible for regulating bile production and secretion. Scientific research points out that cholangiocytes play many roles, such as responding to different stimuli and being involved in inflammation. Their immunological features are especially important in biliary tract diseases since problems with them can lead to cholangiopathies, which mainly affect these cells. For this reason, cholangiocytes are involved in both normal bile flow and in the development of liver diseases that block bile transport, which shows how important they are for liver health. The way the gallbladder works is closely linked to the health of the bile ducts, which can have a big effect on the biliary tract. Cholestatic liver diseases, which involve a blockage of bile flow, explain the connection; they demonstrate that issues in the bile ducts can result in gallbladder problems such as inflammation, stones, or even cancer. These structures are closely related, because they both use the same mechanisms for their normal operation and when they become diseased. So, being aware of the gallbladder and bile duct functions helps with the diagnosis and treatment of diseases in the biliary tract. A comprehensive approach that considers gallbladder disorders within the broader context of liver and biliary network function will enhance therapeutic strategies for managing these complex conditions (Alpini *et al.*, 2023) (Figure 10.4).

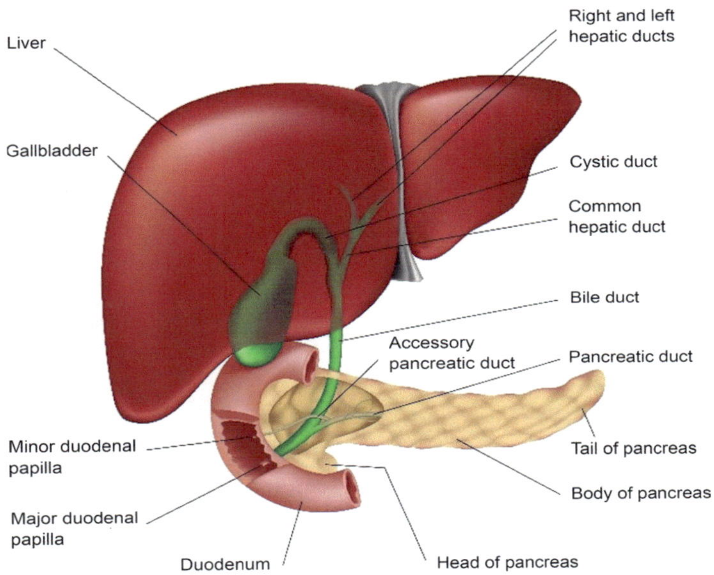

Figure 10.4. The function of the gallbladder.

Source: https://graphdiagram.com/chart/2015/01/the-function-of-the-gallbladder.jpg.

10.1.3. Relationship with the Liver and Pancreas

Liver and pancreas share a significant relationship when it comes to biliary tract disease, as they both play central roles in metabolism and digestion. The liver is primarily responsible for the production of bile, which is vitally important for fat emulsification and absorption in the intestine. The pancreas secretes digestive enzymes and hormones that also contribute to nutrient digestion and the control of glucose. Such interdependence is best exemplified under the milieu of disease, such as pancreatitis or LC, that could interrupt bile flow and play a role in the primary liver disease. Here, therefore, the malfunctioning of one organ can have damaging consequences on the other, highlighting the fine and sophisticated balance required to attain gastrointestinal health. Further illustrating the synergy between the liver and pancreas, the relationship has been observed to be synergistic in cholestatic disorders, where bile flow is compromised. In such a scenario, cholestasis may cause an increase in biliary tree pressure, with secondary inflammation in both the pancreas and the liver as a consequence. The impact is particularly important in hepatobiliary conditions such as primary sclerosing cholangitis, where pancreatic complications are more likely. These interactions are mediated by the molecular mechanisms that are complex and involve inflammatory mediators that are able to cause fibrosis or changes in cellular structure in the two organs. Knowledge of these associations is, as such, critical to the treatment and management of diseases of the biliary tract, which might necessitate a multidisciplinary approach involving both the health of the pancreas and liver. The new advances in molecular pathology have brought to light the importance of assessing the interaction between the liver and pancreas when making a diagnosis and treatment plan for biliary tract disease. For instance, the World Health Organization classification of tumors of the digestive system now gives greater emphasis to the role of molecular markers in distinguishing among various tumors involving both organs. Because chronic bile duct obstruction is a common cause of secondary tumors of the pancreas, their recognition and awareness play an important role in the management of patients and therapeutic strategy. With increasing evidence revealing the complex molecular mechanisms connecting the liver and pancreas, the picture becomes clearer as to how alterations in one organ can cascade into disease in the other, thereby emphasizing the necessity for an integrated approach in clinical care for diseases of the biliary tract (Nagtegaal *et al.*, 2019; Zheng *et al.*, 2020) (Figure 10.5).

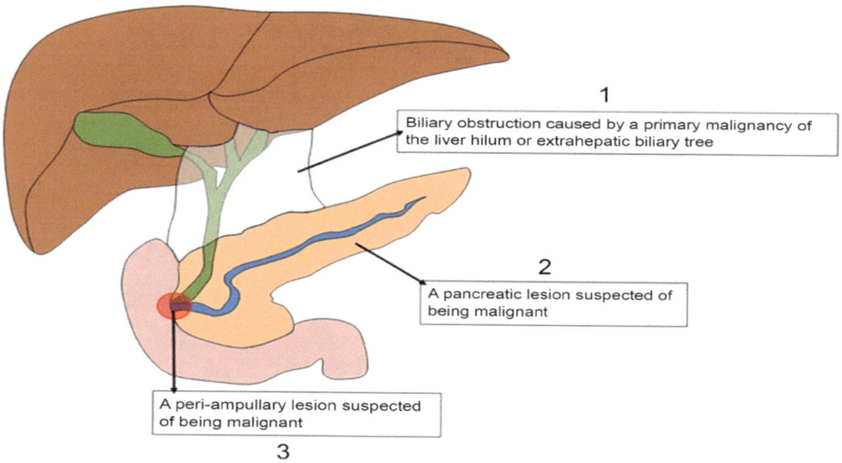

Figure 10.5. Schematic of the liver and pancreas showing the inclusion criteria. To be included, patients must have one of the three indicated inclusion criteria.

10.2. Common Biliary Tract Diseases

Diseases of the biliary tract, which include the gallbladder and bile ducts, can have a major effect on gastrointestinal health. The most common of these problems is cholelithiasis or the development of gallstones, which affects millions worldwide. If gallstones block the bile ducts, people may experience severe abdominal pain, jaundice, and acute cholangitis. The main reason gallstones form is usually an unbalance in bile, which leads to cholesterol crystals or pigment stones. Knowing the reasons behind cholelithiasis is important, since it helps people choose better ways to prevent and treat the condition, such as making lifestyle changes and undergoing cholecystectomy when needed. Cholangitis, which is another important biliary tract disease, is caused by inflammation of the bile ducts due to bacteria that enter the ducts when they are blocked. The condition may develop fast and can lead to serious body symptoms like fever, chills, and jaundice, which are signs of sepsis and can be deadly if not treated. Timely diagnosis and treatment are paramount. According to recent studies, the identification of Gram-negative bacteria, such as *Escherichia coli* and Klebsiella pneumoniae, plays a critical role in guiding antimicrobial therapy for cholangitis patients (Liu *et al.*, 2024). So, knowing the types of pathogens and their antibiotic resistance can greatly affect patient outcomes during treatment, which highlights the need for targeted therapy in managing biliary tract infections. Along with gallstones and cholangitis, the biliary tract can be involved in malignant conditions such as cholangiocarcinoma and rhabdomyosarcoma, which mostly affect children. Cholangiocarcinoma is difficult cancer that develops in the epithelial cells of the bile ducts and its common symptoms are not specific, which can make it harder to detect and manage. Conversely, rhabdomyosarcoma of the biliary tract, while rare, poses unique challenges due to its presentation, typically presenting as obstructive jaundice in children (Święszkowska *et al.*, 2024). Treating cancers of the biliary tract is not simple and usually involves several specialists, chemotherapy, and surgery. It is important to be aware of these diseases so that treatment can begin early and more patients can survive, which means research and careful monitoring should continue.

10.2.1. Cholecystitis

Cholecystitis, an inflammation of the gallbladder, is a significant condition in the category of biliary tract diseases. It typically arises due to obstruction of the cystic duct, most often due to gallstones, leading to increased intraluminal pressure and resultant inflammation of the gallbladder wall. The acute inflammation can subsequently progress to more severe complications such as necrosis and perforation, thereby requiring early diagnosis and treatment. Interestingly, the prevalence of gallbladder illness due to cholecystitis appears to be much higher in industrialized nations, where aspects of lifestyle such as diet and obesity significantly contribute to gallstone formation. Studies reveal that an understanding of the multifactorial pathophysiology of cholecystitis, including its etiologic determinants and presentations, is crucial in the development of effective treatment plans, particularly in those who are at risk of developing such a condition (Ambrosi *et al.*, 2017). Cholecystitis treatment is usually a mix of medication and surgery, where the acute inflammation is suppressed and recurrence prevented. Laparoscopic cholecystectomy remains the standard against which acute cholecystitis should be treated and is favoured due to its minimal invasiveness and shorter convalescence. However, conservative management should be utilized in certain conditions, especially in patients with serious comorbidities that can jeopardize surgery. Furthermore, the simplicity of cholecystitis may necessitate an overall appreciation for how it correlates with other biliary tract diseases. Cholestatic liver diseases, for instance, can disrupt bile flow and complicate gallbladder disease, thus highlighting the worldwide approach required in cholecystitis management (Alpini *et al.*, 2023). Understanding of these associations is paramount in comprehensive patient care as well as the development of effective therapeutic strategies. In addition, chronic cholecystitis can be a unique array of challenges in biliary tract diseases. Unlike its acute counterpart, chronic cholecystitis often presents insidiously, with patients experiencing recurrent episodes of abdominal pain and gastrointestinal upset. Over time, chronic inflammation can lead to gallbladder fibrosis and abnormalities in gallbladder function and may predispose patients to more severe complications, including risk for gallbladder cancer. Thus, an aggressive diagnostic approach is required, often relying on imaging techniques that can identify both gallstones and inflammation. It is essential to know the relationship of cholecystitis to broader biliary illness in planning long-term management for those affected. Owing to a growing prevalence of chronic gallbladder disease, ongoing research into better diagnostic criteria and intervention remains crucial (Alpini *et al.*, 2023; Ambrosi *et al.*, 2017) (Figure 10.6).

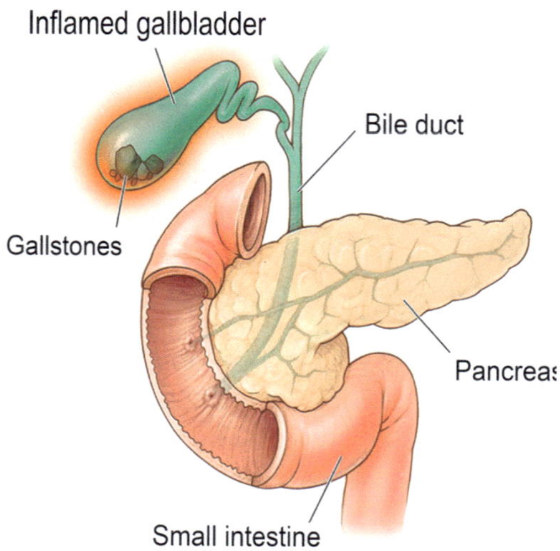

Figure 10.6. Cholecystitis.

Source: https://my.clevelandclinic.org/-/scassets/images/org/health/articles/15265-cholecystitis-gallbladder-inflammation.

10.2.2. Choledocholithiasis

The fact that choledocholithiasis or stones in the common bile duct is complex makes it an important condition among biliary tract diseases. This situation may cause symptoms as simple as mild abdominal pain or as severe as acute cholangitis, which is a dangerous infection of the bile ducts. Some patients show symptoms that are not specific to a disease, which can make it hard to diagnose them. Abdominal ultrasound and CT scans are necessary to find the stones and also to detect any problems, like the bile ducts becoming swollen. Detecting these stones early is crucial, as delayed treatment can result in exacerbation of the disease and can increase the risk of septicemia and other serious infections, thus underscoring the urgent need for effective diagnostic approaches (Abdullah *et al.*, 2004). Because of new medical technology, there are now several ways to treat choledocholithiasis. ERCP is a major approach for removing stones from the biliary system because it allows physicians to access and extract the stones easily. Other techniques, such as laparoscopic common bile duct exploration (CBDE) and percutaneous approaches, have gained traction, particularly in complex cases or those unresponsive to initial therapies. Treatment should be personalized for each patient, taking into account whether there is biliary disease, the patient's health, and the possible risks of each method. Such consideration is critical to optimizing patient outcomes and minimizing complications (Abdullah *et al.*, 2004). In pregnant patients, choledocholithiasis management must be done with extra care because it can harm both the mother and the fetus. In the past, doctors treated acute biliary diseases in pregnant women conservatively, but now, because of minimally invasive procedures, treatment is safer and more effective. Observational studies suggested that when choledocholithiasis occurs in pregnancy, surgeons can use cholecystostomy or laparoscopic cholecystectomy, depending on the trimester. These approaches not only provide relief from symptoms but also significantly reduce the risk of complications, validating that minimally invasive strategies can be effectively employed in managing biliary tract diseases in pregnant women without substantial maternal or fetal morbidity (Figure 10.7).

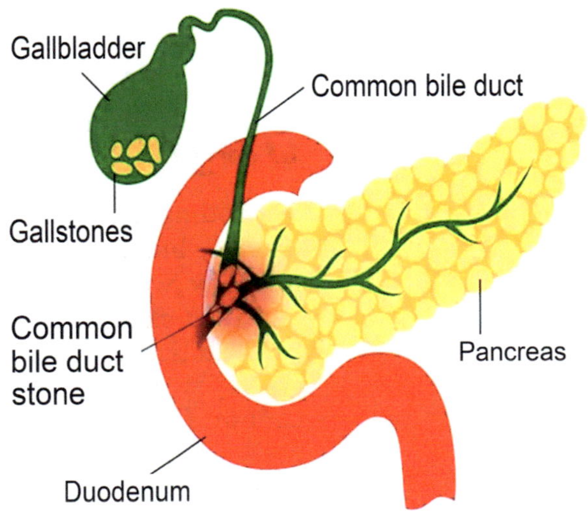

Figure 10.7. Choledocholithiasis.

Source: https://lirp.cdn-website.com/69c0b277/dms3rep/multi/opt/CBD+stone-640w.jpg.

10.2.3. Cholelithiasis

Cholelithiasis, or gallstones within the gallbladder, is a prevalent condition that significantly influences biliary tract disease. Gallstones are traditionally classified into two types: cholesterol stones and pigment stones, of which cholesterol stones are responsible for the majority. Pathophysiology of cholelithiasis involves derangement of constituents of the bile, resulting in crystallization of cholesterol. This condition is related to several risk factors, including obesity, diabetes, and certain diet-related factors responsible for supersaturation of cholesterol in the bile and stasis of the bile. The presentation can range from asymptomatic gallstones to biliary colic or acute cholecystitis, where gallstones obstruct the cystic duct to produce inflammation and pain. Early symptom recognition and early intervention are essential in order to prevent complications of untreated cholelithiasis. Knowing the microbiological underpinning of cholelithiasis could make our approach to the control of biliary tract disease more potent. Recent studies have shown that changes in the bile microbiota are indeed associated with the outcome in the patient. For instance, the presence of some bacteria, such as *E. coli* and *K. pneumoniae* havebeen associated with higher mortality in patients with a range of complications of cholelithiasis. The interaction between gallstones, bile content, and microbial invasion exists within a multifaceted environment wherein pathogenic microbes can worsen conditions in the biliary tract with a possible role in chronic inflammation and carcinogenesis. Characterization of these correlations not only promotes the understanding of the disease process but also helps to identify the necessity of targeted therapy aimed at both gallstone disease and predisposed microbial infection in an attempt to improve clinical outcomes in patients presenting with biliary tract disease, such as cholelithiasis (Agrusa *et al.*, 2019).

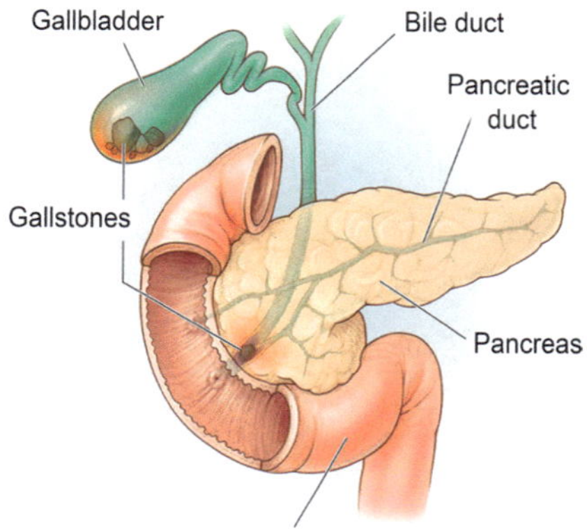

Figure 10.8. Gallstones.

Source: https://my.clevelandclinic.org/-/scassets/images/org/health/articles/7313-gallstones.jpg.

Complications arising from cholelithiasis are generally best addressed through multidimensional diagnosis. Patients can have diverse clinical presentations, usually warranting a thorough investigation to determine underlying biliary tract disease. Clinical evaluation usually encompasses meticulous history-taking and biochemical investigations to measure liver function and identify any biliary obstruction, usually reflected by raised enzyme markers like alkaline phosphatase (ALP) and 5-nucleotidase (5NT). Research has established that although increased AST and ALT levels are reflective of hepatic cell damage, 5NT is very specifically indicative of bile duct blockage and cholestasis. Biochemical markers assist the clinician in determining the severity of the condition and in choosing effective therapies, such as surgical interventions. Delayed treatment of the proper therapy may progress the disease, leading to complications such as acute cholecystitis or even malignant transformation related to chronic inflammation of the gallbladder and biliary system (Batta *et al.*, 2011) (Figure 10.8).

10.3. Symptoms and Diagnosis

Depending on the kind and severity of the disease, biliary tract symptoms can show up in many ways. Usually, jaundice, abdominal pain, and changes in bowel habits are common presentations. Jaundice, which makes the skin and eyes yellow, usually happens when bile cannot flow properly. When a patient has acute cholecystitis, they usually feel intense pain in the right upper abdomen and may also have fever and nausea. COVID-19 and similar severe illnesses can cause the immune system to weaken, which may result in fewer local symptoms. This creates a unique challenge in diagnosis, necessitating heightened vigilance among healthcare providers during patient evaluations, particularly in critically ill patients, as described in Kaverina *et al.* (2024). Being aware of the various symptoms of biliary tract diseases is important for prompt diagnosis and effective treatment. When diagnosing biliary tract diseases, healthcare workers depend on physical examination, imaging, and laboratory tests. At the beginning, doctors examine the patient, then run tests in the lab to measure liver function by checking enzyme levels and bilirubin. Ultrasound is very important for seeing abnormalities in the biliary system. In the most serious cases of COVID-19, the usual symptoms may be hidden because the local response is reduced by systemic problems. Thus, dynamic ultrasound examination emerges as a vital diagnostic tool, enabling the identification of complications like acute cholecystitis even when local signs are subdued (Kaverina *et al.*, 2024). Because of the urgency in acute cases, the use of imaging techniques is even more important, which adds to the difficulty of diagnosing biliary tract diseases when the patient has other health problems. There is also a link between biliary system diseases and acute illnesses, especially acute pancreatitis, which adds to the difficulty of diagnosis. When acute pancreatitis and biliary problems are present together, the symptoms of the former can hide the signs of the latter, which can make diagnosis difficult. Acalculous cholecystitis, which happens in both biliary disease and pancreatitis, is a good example of this problem since it can cause serious organ failure if it is not treated right away. Inflammation throughout the body because of acute pancreatitis may result in biliary stricture, which can eventually cause the liver to become impaired. So, spotting the signs of biliary tract diseases in acute pancreatitis is very important for proper treatment and involves careful observation and advanced imaging.

10.3.1. Common Symptoms Associated with Biliary Tract Diseases

Diseases of the biliary tract typically have a broad range of symptoms that play an important role in a patient's quality of life and may be reflective of underlying disease. Abdominal pain is the most frequent presenting symptom and often involves the right upper quadrant and is either acute or chronic in nature. It can vary from a mildly annoying sensation to excruciating attacks, typically induced by fat-rich meals, and is indicative of gallbladder disease. Vomiting and nausea can also be developed by patients, contributing to the discomfort of bile duct anomalies. The development of these symptoms requires investigation since they may represent complications like inflammation and obstruction of the biliary tract. Early detection and management of these symptoms are significant because they can be the precursor to conditions like acute cholecystitis or biliary colic, with dangerous risks that may need surgical intervention. Another frequent symptom of biliary tract diseases is jaundice, which results from the blood build-up of bilirubin due to obstruction or dysfunction of bile flow. Jaundice can manifest in terms of yellow discoloration of the skin and sclera, and generally is associated with other symptoms such as dark-coloured urine and pale-colored stools. The etiologies of jaundice in these circumstances can range from gallstones obstructing the bile ducts to more severe diseases like cholangitis or biliary cirrhosis. Also, concomitant evidence of fever and chills may suggest an infection that needs prompt assessment. In particular, the development and duration of jaundice can provide a good clue to the severity of the biliary pathology and guide clinical judgment and treatment planning, particularly when managing the potential complications related to biliary pathologies. Fever is also an important symptom reported in patients with biliary tract pathologies, usually in conjunction with jaundice and abdominal pain.

This symptom can be a sign of systemic response to infection or inflammation, particularly in acute cholangitis—a severe infection of the bile duct. Incidence of cholangitis is high according to recent studies, striking a large number of patients with biliary tract infections. Studies reveal that 20.6% of patients present with cholangitis when they present with symptoms of the biliary system (Gupta *et al.*, 2023). Other signs of the system, such as fatigue and malaise, may present along with the fever, indicating a more widespread inflammatory process. These have to be closely observed as the outcomes of the patients depend greatly on an early diagnosis and treatment, particularly in managing complications associated with acute pancreatitis-inducing biliary diseases (Li *et al.*, 2024b) (Figure 10.9).

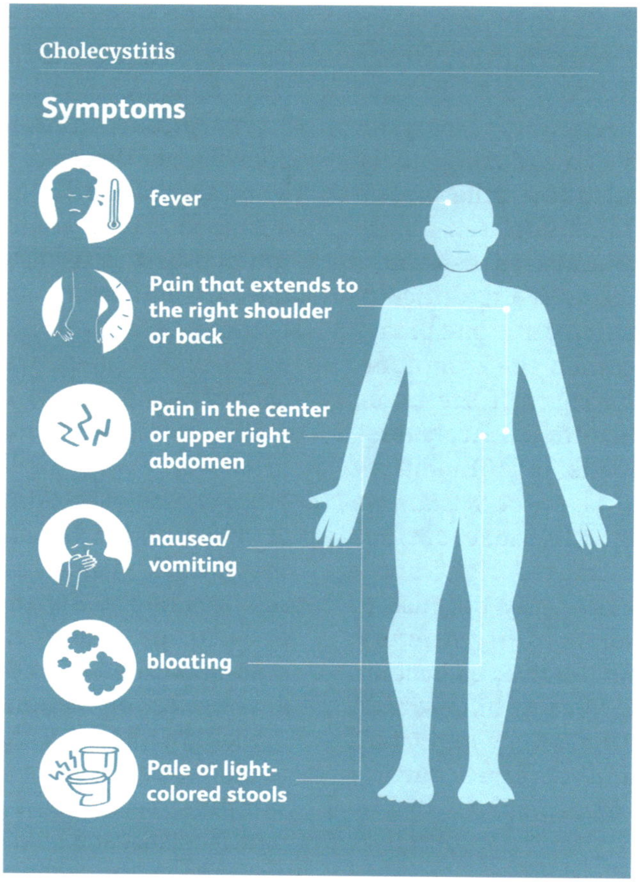

Figure 10.9. Cholecystitis symptoms.

Source: https://www.verywellhealth.com/thmb/dRfEii8rxCG6gEW0iSJ07gX91No=/1500x0/filters:no_upscale():max_bytes(150000):strip_icc()/cholecystitis-overview-4588159_final-207595402f314785 9fbb224f5b0520a4.png.

10.3.2. Diagnostic Imaging Techniques

In the management of biliary tract diseases, advanced imaging techniques are essential for correctly diagnosing different conditions of the bile ducts. Techniques such as ultrasound, CT, and magnetic resonance imaging (MRI) are commonly utilized to visualize the biliary anatomy and detect abnormalities. Because it is accessible and can detect obstruction or dilation in the bile ducts, ultrasound is usually the first test done, but it cannot see the intrahepatic bile ducts clearly. CT images the biliary system in cross-section, which helps detect tumors and other abnormalities, making it helpful for diagnosing biliary cancers. MRCP is a non-invasive way to examine the biliary tree on an MRI scan, without using contrast agents, which helps doctors understand the anatomy and any problems. It is very important to distinguish between benign and malignant lesions when assessing biliary tract diseases. Combining imaging results with findings from clinical exams is necessary for correct characterization. For instance, cholangiocarcinoma (CCA) presents unique imaging features that can aid in its differentiation from other biliary tract diseases. Using dynamic contrast-enhanced MRI and appropriate imaging techniques helps show the special patterns of these lesions, which improves how accurately they can be diagnosed. Additionally, detecting both intrahepatic cholangiocarcinoma (iCCA) and other subtypes is crucial, as their origins influence treatment decisions and prognostic outcomes. Consequently, the evolution of imaging techniques continues to significantly impact the understanding of biliary tract pathology, as evidenced by the growing body of research on the complexities of iCCA and similar entities within the biliary system, highlighting their pathophysiology and imaging characteristics (Alvaro *et al.*, 2018). Because of new imaging technology, it is now easier to accurately assess biliary tract diseases. Techniques such as ERCP and percutaneous transhepatic cholangiography (PTC) are integral for both diagnosis and therapeutic interventions, such as stone extraction or stent placement. Making imaging biomarkers is relevant since they can give information about how neoplastic lesions behave, which helps doctors decide on treatment. Research suggests that similarities exist between biliary and pancreatic neoplastic lesions regarding molecular and histological features, an aspect that is increasingly relevant in imaging studies (Alvaro *et al.*, 2019). These similarities allow for new ideas in diagnosis and new treatments. Thus, ongoing exploration of these imaging techniques will likely enhance prognosis and treatment strategies for patients suffering from biliary tract diseases, improving overall outcomes in this challenging area of medicine (Figure 10.10).

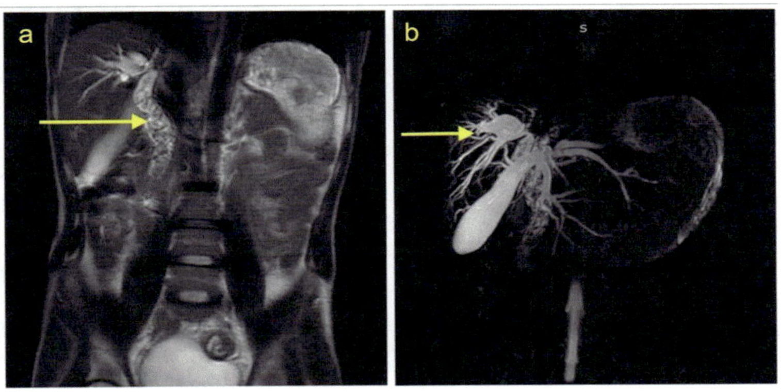

Figure 10.10. MRI (a) demonstrating extensively dilated common bile duct filled with hydatid cyst material seen as hypointense lesions (indicated by the yellow arrow). and MRCP (b) demonstrating dilated intrahepatic bile ducts (indicated by the yellow arrow).

Source: https://www.researchgate.net/publication/343220116/figure/fig1/AS:917552645558272@1595773006293/MRI-a-demonstrating-extensively-dilated-common-bile-duct-filled-with-hydatid-cyst.jpg.

10.3.3. Laboratory Tests and Their Significance

Laboratory tests are most crucial to the diagnosis and treatment of biliary tract disorders, including a broad spectrum of conditions affecting the bile ducts, gallbladder, and liver. Laboratory tests provide valuable information regarding the underlying pathophysiologic processes and enable clinicians to devise an appropriate therapeutic approach. For example, liver function tests, including serum bilirubin, ALP, and transaminases, are utilized in the diagnosis of cholestasis or hepatobiliary inflammation, which may present with conditions like cholangitis or cholestasis. Abnormal tumor markers, including carcinoembryonic antigen (CEA), are employed to identify malignant biliary tract illnesses and lead to further diagnostic workups and treatment. Clinical presentation of biliary tract illness has shifted, as laboratory tests serve not only a diagnostic but also a prognostic function, and the result of treatment. Laboratory tests have a more critical function than merely in the diagnosis; they belong to monitoring disease development and response to treatment in patients with biliary tract illnesses. For instance, measurement of inflammatory markers such as the neutrophil/lymphocyte ratio has been found to be a marker of outcomes in advanced biliary tract cancer (BTC). From studies, it has been established that increased subcutaneous adipose tissue radiodensity (SATr) is predictive of adverse outcomes in patients with such disorders as a prognostic indicator and that it can be employed to guide therapeutic interventions. Moreover, awareness of pathogen susceptibility from bile cultures, particularly regarding BI complicating biliary infections, is important to tailor antibiotic therapy. This interdisciplinarity emphasizes the necessity of laboratory tests not just for diagnosis but also for the handling of the complexity of biliary tract disease (Liu *et al.*, 2024; Sugiura *et al.*, 2025). In short, laboratory investigations are a very important component of the diagnostic and treatment protocol of biliary tract disease. They provide an immense amount of information that helps clinicians to recognize underlying disease, formulate a treatment protocol, and track patient improvement. Enhanced understanding of the correlation between laboratory findings and clinical results can significantly improve management of these diseases, given the rising prevalence of biliary tract diseases and their related complications, including sepsis. With continued study showing correlations between markers in the lab and outcome of disease, adding these tests to practice will provide more assured decision-making and ultimately improved patient outcome for biliary tract diseases (Liu *et al.*, 2024; Sugiura *et al.*, 2025) (Figure 10.11).

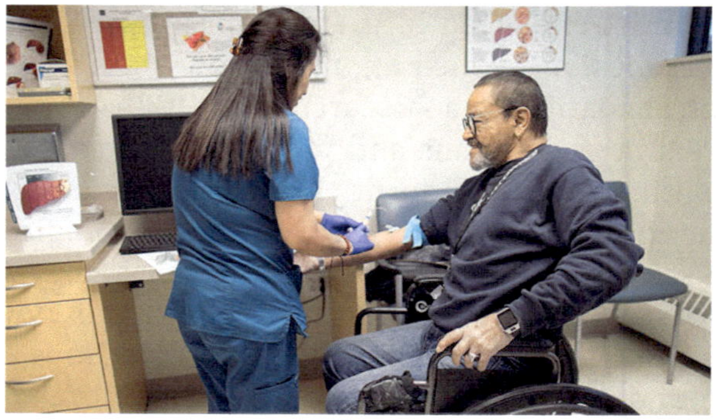

Figure 10.11. Laboratory tests

Source: https://www.mountsinai.org/files/MSHealth/Assets/HS/Care/Liver-Diseases/MSHS-Liver-BileDuct-2col-770x420.jpg.

10.4. Treatment Options

There are many ways to treat biliary tract diseases, and the approach usually depends on the condition and how severe it is. When someone has cholelithiasis, often dietary changes and medicines are enough to manage the symptoms. If issues like cholangitis or acute pancreatitis happen because of stones, more invasive treatments may be necessary. ERCP is crucial for these conditions, since it helps in diagnosis, stone removal, and placing stents when required. In addition, recent improvements in interventional radiology, such as percutaneous biliary drainage, indicate a strong focus on improving patient results with minimally invasive interventions. If the disease is advanced, such as cholangiocarcinoma or gallbladder carcinoma, the treatment options can be more complicated. At present, doctors use surgery, chemotherapy, and new targeted therapies. Surgical removal is the main way to potentially cure cancer, but a lot of patients have cancer that cannot be removed by surgery. In these scenarios, clinical trials exploring novel therapies, such as targeted agents and locoregional treatments, are essential, as supported by findings indicating that patients with advanced cholangiocarcinoma and gallbladder carcinoma have limited options, yet some experience stable disease or partial responses to advanced therapies like hepatic arterial infusion protocols (Falchook *et al.*, 2013). It shows that we need to keep studying to find the most effective treatments. Another critical consideration is the role of the bile microbiota in influencing treatment outcomes and survival for patients with pancreatic and biliary tract diseases (Agrusa *et al.*, 2019). Studies have shown that microbes in bile can change the course of diseases, which is why a new approach is needed to understand biliary problems. It means overseeing immediate symptoms and complications, and also analyzing each patient's profile, paying attention to microbiological aspects. Integrative strategies may guide care plans to improve therapy, making sure patients receive support from different specialists using traditional and innovative research on microbes. This evolving field underscores the potential for improved strategies in managing biliary diseases, paving the way for enhanced survival and quality of life among affected patients (Figure 10.12).

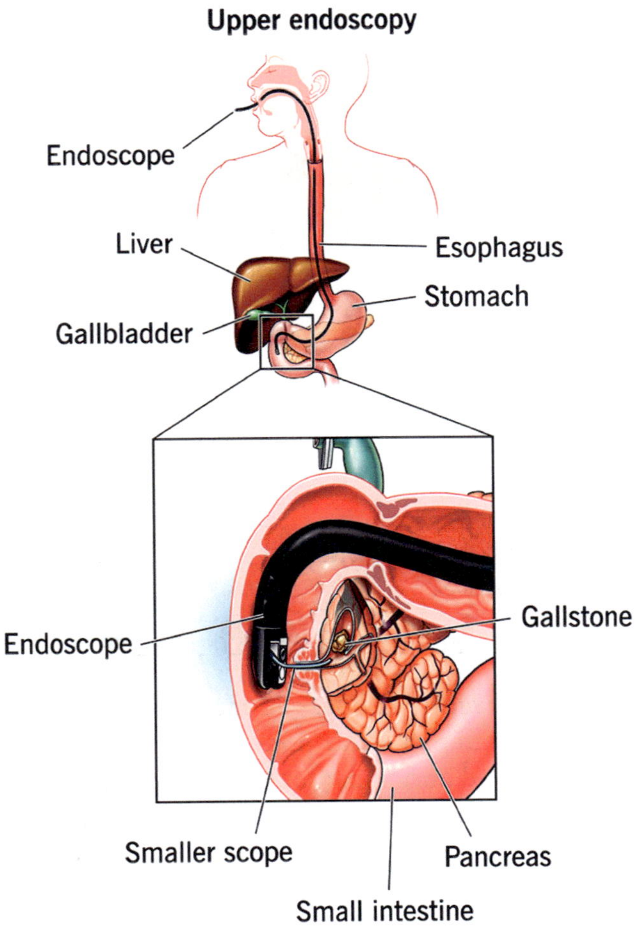

Figure 10.12. Endoscopic retrograde cholangiopancreatography (ERCP).

Source: https://my.clevelandclinic.org/-/scassets/images/org/health/articles/4951-ercp.

10.4.1. Medical Management and Lifestyle Changes

Successful medical management of biliary tract pathologies is not a monolithic, monotonous process but a complex multidisciplinary procedure with personalized management of each patient. The therapeutic treatment most frequently includes pharmacological therapy to decompress symptoms and address the causative pathophysiology, such as obstruction of bile drainage or cholestasis. Ursodeoxycholic acid is a frequently used medication to decrease bile secretion and reduce cholestatic manifestations, particularly in patients with cholestatic liver disease. The management plan may also involve regular follow-up with imaging techniques like ultrasound to monitor alterations in biliary anatomy or the development of gallstones. Further, the highly interrelated nature of liver function and gallbladder disease calls for synergistic therapeutic strategies to overcome intrahepatic and extrahepatic complications, necessitating further research into their interrelationship, as hinted at by recent research (Alpini *et al.*, 2023).

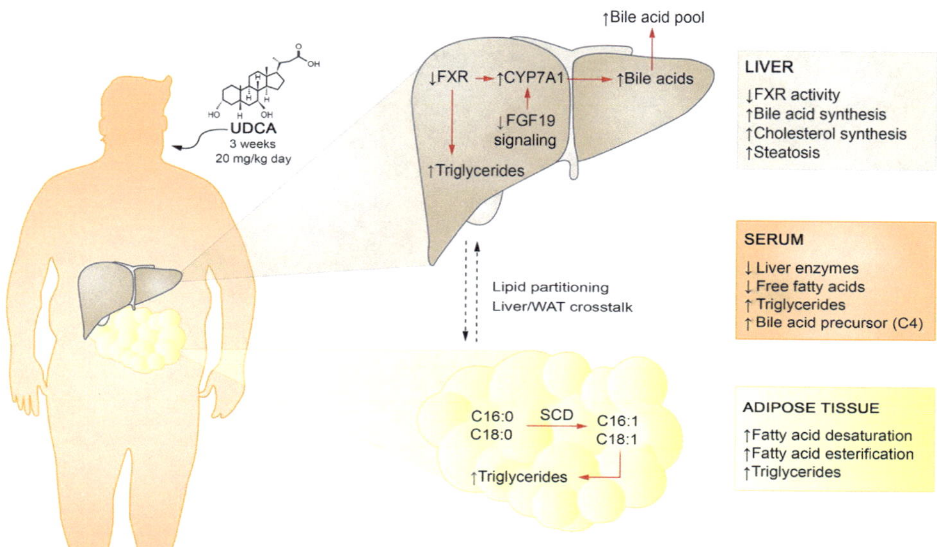

Figure 10.13. Ursodeoxycholic acid exerts farnesoid X receptor-antagonistic effects on bile acid and lipid metabolism in morbid obesity.

Source: https://ars.els-cdn.com/content/image/1-s2.0-S0168827815000100-fx1_lrg.jpg.

Aside from pharmacologic interventions, lifestyle modifications play an important role in the management of biliary tract disease. Of particular note is diet, for which patients can employ a low-fat, well-balanced diet rich in fibre and antioxidants that can potentially reduce gallstone formation and overall preservation of biliary function. Maintenance of a healthy weight is also of primary concern; obesity is a significant risk factor for gallstones and hence for biliary disease. Regular physical activity is also recommended to aid metabolic health and optimal gallbladder function. Also, attention to and control of underlying disease conditions such as diabetes or hyperlipidemia, which can speed biliary disease, are components of an overall lifestyle intervention program. This multifaceted approach is essential in the mitigation of disease risk and maintaining optimal health (Binda *et al.*, 2022). Furthermore, understanding the role of gut microbiota in biliary health has also been a matter of increased focus in relatively newer studies. Imbalance of microflora can potentially be an essential element in the etiology of biliary disease, opening new avenues for both lifestyle and medical interventions. The eubiosis paradigm of dysbiosis for biliary function predicts that a healthy gut microbiota will prevent complications of biliary disease. Since our understanding of the correlation continues to grow, treatment can be constructed to modulate dysbiotic states and, potentially, improve patient clinical outcomes. Therefore, the integration of microbiota-based strategies with natural therapy and lifestyle changes would enhance the effectiveness of therapy and is an area of fascinating future clinical study in the case of biliary tract disease (Binda *et al.*, 2022) (Figure 10.13).

10.4.2. Surgical Interventions

When medical treatments for biliary tract diseases are not enough or when anatomical changes are needed, surgery is very important. Liver resection is considered a useful treatment for different diseases such as HCC and tumors in the bile duct. With new techniques, the operation is safer and more effective, especially through improved control of bleeding and bile. Still, after surgery, patients may experience liver insufficiency or biliary leaks, which show that these procedures are not without risk. Given these risks, it is vital to have skilled surgeons with specialized experience in hepatic surgery to optimize patient outcomes and promote long-term survival, illustrating the critical intersection of surgical expertise and patient management in biliary tract diseases (Grazi *et al.*, 2007). When advanced biliary tract diseases may harm the liver, transplantation is often an important option for treatment.

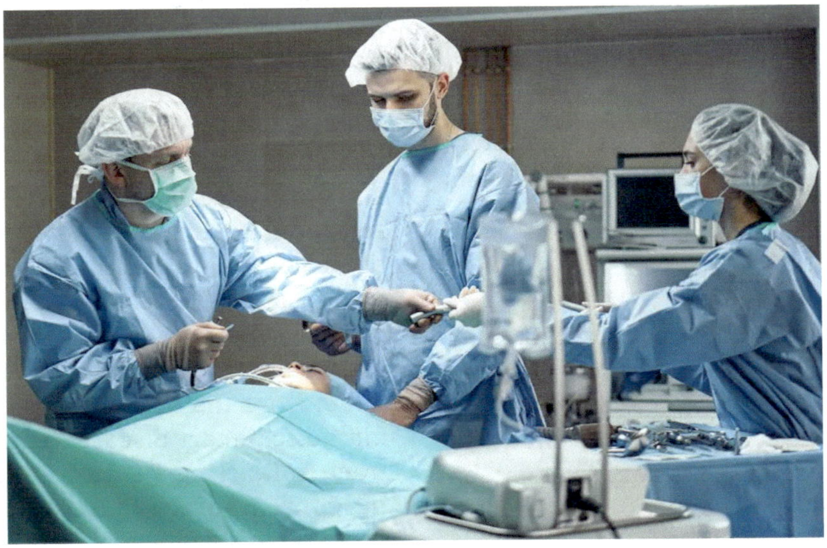

Figure 10.14. Surgical interventions

Source: https://choledochalcysts.com/wp-content/uploads/2024/10/image-2.webp.

The practice of right lobar living donor liver transplantation (LDLT) has gained traction, particularly in cases of severe liver dysfunction where traditional grafts are not viable options. It is important because it can save lives and also provide a solution for those who need a liver transplant. But, this way of transplantation can be controversial because it has led to different issues for both the donor and the recipient. It has been found that many patients experience major health problems and these affect their bile ducts and overall life expectancy. Careful preoperative assessment and donor education play critical roles in minimizing risks and ensuring that the benefits of transplantation outweigh the potential harms (Barr *et al.*, 2009). The success of surgery for biliary tract diseases depends largely on knowing the patient's condition well and making a well-planned surgical plan. Liver resection and transplantation are best done with a team of hepatologists, surgeons, and other medical staff to make sure patients receive the best care both before and after surgery. The purpose is to prevent complications and give the patient the best outcome. Improvements in surgical techniques and management are made by ongoing research, which helps to lower the risk of complications and increase the chances of survival. As the field of hepatobiliary surgery evolves, the integration of innovative surgical practices and robust patient management strategies remains pivotal to advancing the treatment of biliary tract diseases, ultimately enhancing patient quality of life and prognosis (Figure 10.14).

10.4.3. Endoscopic Procedures

Endoscopic procedures have revolutionized the treatment of biliary tract conditions, offering less aggressive alternatives to conventional surgery. Such interventions include methods such as ERCP, whereby the biliary system can be visualized and intervened upon directly. With ERCP, medical professionals are able to diagnose and manage biliary pathology, including choledocholithiasis, cholangitis, and strictures effectively. With the help of specialized equipment, physicians can remove stones in the bile ducts that are obstructed, place stents to straddle the obstruction, and sample bile for microbiological analysis to plan additional treatment (Cook *et al.*, 1999). Adding these procedures to practice has greatly improved the patient outcome and reduced the need for more aggressive surgical interventions, limiting hospitalization and associated complications. The significance of endoscopic treatment extends beyond the alleviation of acute symptoms; it is in the prolonged influence on disease management and survival in patients. Current research has acknowledged the ability of the bile microbiota to influence the outcomes of patients with biliary tract disease (PBD). For instance, the presence of specific pathogenic bacteria, such as *E. coli*, has been correlated with higher morbidity and mortality in these patients (Agrusa *et al.*, 2019). By collecting samples of bile endoscopically during procedures, physicians can identify the presence of bacteria and administer antibiotic therapy accordingly. This not only attacks existing infections but also minimizes the risk of post-operative complications, setting the stage for better biliary condition management. Weighing its role even further, technological progress has enhanced its effectiveness and safety. High-resolution imaging and the development of sophisticated endoscopic equipment have enabled improved visualization of the biliary anatomy, thus allowing more directed interventions. Patient-selection criteria also have evolved such that endoscopic intervention can now be offered to a greater number of patients with comorbid disease who would otherwise be excluded as good surgical candidates. These developments underscore the key stage role of endoscopy in multidisciplinary disease treatment of the biliary tract, solidifying its position as a cornerstone in contemporary gastrointestinal practice (Cook *et al.*, 1999). With ongoing progress in clinical practices through enhanced research and development of new technologies, the potential of endoscopic treatment for managing complex biliary disorders continues to generate significant interest within the profession (Figure 10.15).

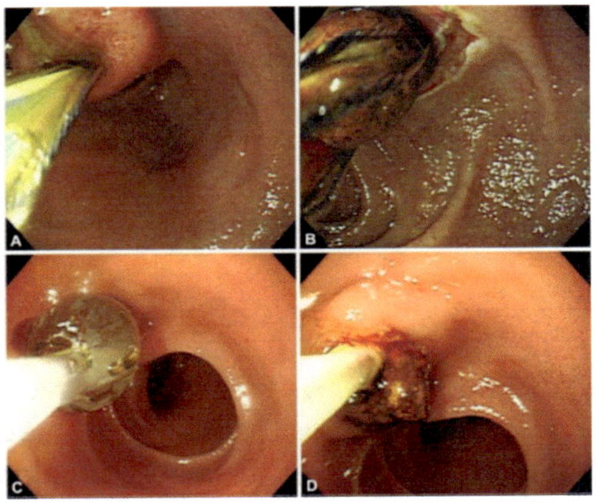

Figure 10.15. Endoscopic views of common bile duct (CBD) stone removal by using only endoscopic sphincterotomy (EST) or endoscopic papillary balloon dilatation (EPBD) in a patient with Billroth II gastrectomy. (A, B) After only EST of the major papilla was performed, a CBD stone was removed with a stone basket catheter. (C, D) After EPBD followed by EST, relatively large stones were easily extracted out of the bile duct with a balloon catheter.

Source: https://www.researchgate.net/profile/Soon-Baik/publication/233950526/figure/fig2/AS:202897112473604@1425385849406/Endoscopic-views-of-common-bile-duct-CBD-stone-removal-by-using-only-endoscopic.png.

10.5. Complications of Biliary Tract Diseases

The serious issues caused by biliary tract diseases increase the risk of illness and death in patients, which calls for careful management. A significant difficulty is when bile leaks out after surgery, which is common after obstruction from stones or cancer. Patients who have biliary leakage may feel more abdominal pain, become febrile, and show signs of infection, which makes it necessary to watch them closely. Management may require surgery to fix the leak or procedures using an endoscope to handle the biliary obstruction that often leads to these problems. Since the biliary tree is very complex, there is a high risk of leakage that can make it difficult for surgeons to avoid complications after surgery, mainly because of the possible consequences of prolonged drainage or damage to nearby structures. Biliary tract diseases may also cause liver insufficiency, which happens when there is cholestasis or severe liver damage from ongoing biliary obstruction. For people with pre-existing liver problems, this condition can become very dangerous because it can result in liver failure. It is very important to identify liver insufficiency early, which highlights the need for routine monitoring of liver function in patients with biliary diseases. Healthcare professionals need to know the pathophysiology of liver dysfunction, as these patients may sometimes need specialized care such as biliary diversion or liver transplantation, which highlights the challenges and interactions between biliary diseases and liver health. Also, there is a risk of infection after surgery in the biliary tract, especially for those who have had transplants. Studies have noted a concerning incidence of bacteremia and fungemia in recipients of liver transplants, often exceeding 70% (Hansbrough *et al.*, 1976). Many of these infections happen when pathogens enter through the grafts, often because biliary drainage is not working well. So, it is important to use active measures to detect mechanical complications and to take steps to avoid graft contamination in the postoperative period. Because of these challenges, surgeons and postoperative caregivers must be skilled, since how biliary complications are handled can determine the outcome and life expectancy of a patient. Being aware of these dangers is very important for better patient results in biliary tract diseases.

10.5.1. Potential for Infection

The risk of infection of biliary tract disease is further enhanced by diseases such as choledocholithiasis and cholangitis, which create a setting for the growth of bacteria.

When there are obstructions due to gallstones or malignant tumors, the unimpeded movement of bile is disrupted. Bile becomes stagnant and is a suitable medium for bacterial growth, and thus creates infections such as cholangitis. This condition is characterized as a triad of jaundice, fever, and right upper quadrant pain, requiring immediate medical intervention to prevent systemic complications. The prevalence of infection in biliary tract diseases emphasizes the necessity of early diagnosis and intervention, as untreated infection can escalate to life-threatening sepsis or septic shock, sharply increasing morbidity and mortality rates. Antimicrobial resistance (AMR) also complicates the condition of biliary tract disease-related infections. The infections in this condition are not only common but also increasingly challenging to treat due to new resistant strains of bacteria, potentially leading to longer hospital stays and higher health costs. Studies place the number of fatalities due to AMR at millions globally, with some of these pathogens, such as *Escherichia coli* and Staphylococcus aureus, having very high rates of occurrence in biliary infections. The effects of AMR are particularly felt in poor-resource settings where access to effective antibiotics is limited. Therefore, understanding the dynamics of AMR is crucial in the development of effective treatment approaches and policies aimed at preventing the spread of infection in patients with biliary tract infection (Murray *et al.*, 2022). Besides BI, cholangiocarcinoma is another challenge in the scope for infection within the biliary system. This extremely virulent form of cancer, which is highly prevalent in endemic regions for liver fluke infection, shares a common etiology of chronic biliary inflammation and poses a high secondary infection risk. The tumor microenvironment also can modulate the immune system and leave the patients immunocompromised, so infections can take place during treatment regimens like chemotherapy and surgery. Without adequate management of underlying diseases like PSC or choledocholithiasis, nosocomial infection risk remains high. Thus, an extensive understanding of the connection between cholangiocarcinoma and infection susceptibility is not only essential for patient management but also for the optimization of therapeutic approaches against this dual burden (Brindley *et al.*, 2021).

10.5.2. Risk of Pancreatitis

Biliary tract diseases often cause pancreatitis, which is a major challenge for medical professionals. Pancreatitis usually happens when gallstones block the bile ducts, which causes the pancreas to become inflamed and pressurized. Acute pancreatitis can occur quickly and become very serious, which can seriously affect both the patient's life and their quality of life. The most prevalent etiology of severe acute pancreatitis (SAP) is closely associated with biliary tract diseases, which account for approximately 69.75% of cases. This statistic underscores the importance of early detection and management of biliary obstruction to mitigate the possible progression to pancreatitis, as delayed treatment can lead to complications such as organ failure and sepsis, thereby increasing morbidity and mortality rates in affected individuals (Li *et al.*, 2024a). Clinical results for people with SAP also indicate that many patients die, which demonstrates the serious consequences of late treatment. A study looking back at cases found that 13.58% of SAP patients died within 90 days, mainly because of problems caused by inflammation in the pancreas. Among these patients, common complications such as acute kidney injury (AKI), abdominal bleeding, and organ failure were prevalent and significantly influenced survival rates. It appears that proactive actions, which may involve monitoring and surgery for people with major biliary obstructions, are necessary. Identifying high-risk patients through clinical assessment and biochemical markers can guide more effective treatment strategies and ultimately reduce the mortality associated with this serious condition (Li *et al.*, 2024a). Choledocholithiasis, which is gallstones in the bile duct, is important to mention in biliary tract diseases because it can cause pancreatitis. A blocked bile duct causes pancreatic enzymes to become active, which can result in acute pancreatitis. Elevated serum ALP and aminotransferases were the key indicators in a recent study that showed the common occurrence of choledocholithiasis. Also, a large number of people demonstrated signs of pancreatitis, which supports the link between choledocholithiasis and the risk of pancreatitis. These findings emphasize the importance of utilizing diagnostic criteria, such as those established by the American Society for Gastrointestinal Endoscopy (ASGE), to enhance early detection and facilitate timely intervention, therefore reducing the risk of pancreatitis related to biliary tract diseases (Figure 10.16).

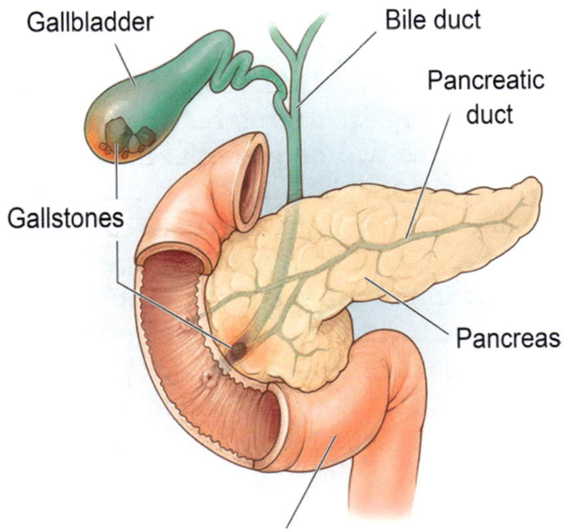

Figure 10.16. Pancreatitis illustration.

Source: https://my.clevelandclinic.org/-/scassets/images/org/health/articles/8103-pancreatitis-illustration.

10.5.3. Long-Term Effects on Liver Function

The long-term effect on liver function in biliary tract disease offers great insight into the pathophysiology of chronic cholestasis. The research shows that disturbance of bile acid levels is a critical factor in causing liver damage, inflammation, and fibrosis, all contributing to impairing liver function in the long term. Toxic BAs at high levels can induce cellular injury and trigger inflammatory responses that promote further tissue damage. This cumulative effect underscores the importance of addressing bile acid metabolism in patients with cholestatic liver disease. Available evidence has only now begun to point to potential therapeutic targets, like bile acid receptors, as these play an extremely significant role in regulating bile acid production and output. Hence, modulation of these pathways presents a potential intervention and treatment strategy that can hinder the long-term harmful effects on liver function associated with chronic biliary tract disease (Alpini *et al.*, 2020). Long-term liver function is generally compromised by surgical procedures for the treatment of biliary tract diseases. Liver resection is now a highly effective mode of treatment for diseases such as HCC and bile duct tumors. Advances in surgical techniques, particularly meticulous hemostasis and biliostasis maneuvers, have enhanced patient outcomes and reduced postoperative complications such as liver insufficiency and biliary leakage. However, these complications significantly impact long-term liver function and survival. In particular, a disease necessitating liver resection may result in compensatory mechanisms of the remnant liver tissue with possible alteration in its functional capacity over time. Maintenance of the skill of the operating staff is necessary since skilled surgeons can better minimize complications and thus more effectively preserve liver function in the long term (Grazi *et al.*, 2007). Moreover, gut health as an interaction in liver function is a matter of major concern while establishing long-term outcomes in patients with biliary tract diseases. The gut-liver axis has been referred to as a priority research field, as altered gut microbiota composition and increased intestinal permeability can hasten the progression of liver disease. Chronicity-induced liver injury can lead to alterations in bile acid composition, which then influence gut health and inflammatory responses. Therapies of the gut-liver axis, such as bile acid receptor modulators, have the potential to decrease symptoms and enhance liver function in patients with chronic cholestatic disease. This dual strategy of treating both the liver function and the gut is a multi-pronged, holistic strategy to enhance long-term effect on the liver, which emphasizes the multi-factorial nature of biliary tract disease and therapy (Alpini *et al.*, 2020).

10.6. Prevention and Risk Factors

Understanding and managing the risk factors for biliary tract diseases is very important in their prevention. Among the most common risk factors is obesity, which is linked to a higher risk of gallbladder disease and biliary cancers. Data suggests that as the socioeconomic development index (SDI) increases, the age-standardized mortality rate attributable to high body mass index (BMI) escalates, particularly in females. Because of this link, it is important to have public health measures that help manage weight and prevent obesity, especially in groups more likely to get gallbladder diseases. Consequently, developing preventive strategies that address these demographic trends could significantly reduce the burden of biliary tract diseases and improve outcomes for affected individuals (Qiu *et al.*, 2025). Besides obesity, other risk factors for biliary tract diseases are age and gender. It is clear from statistics that gallbladder and BTC are more common as people age, and women are more likely to have these conditions than men. Such a difference may be caused by hormones and reproductive factors, so it needs further study. Also, quick identification and care of BI in biliary disorders is crucial for avoiding disease progression, since patients with benign biliary conditions may develop severe complications such as sepsis. Therefore, integrating age and gender-specific health initiatives into preventive frameworks will be essential in addressing the increasing prevalence of biliary tract diseases among diverse populations (Liu *et al.*, 2024). In addition, knowing the types of microbes and their susceptibility in biliary tract infections can improve ways to prevent them. Cultures from patients with biliary disorders often contain *Escherichia coli* and Klebsiella pneumoniae, gram-negative bacteria, shows the importance of proper antibiotic use. Because of antimicrobial resistance, it is important to keep monitoring and quickly identify factors that add risk, such as comorbidities, which can make treatment more challenging for people with the infection. By recognizing the patterns of bacterial infection and their associated risk factors, healthcare professionals can develop more effective interventions, tailored to the unique clinical profiles of biliary disease patients, ultimately reducing complications and improving overall health outcomes (Liu *et al.*, 2024).

10.6.1. Dietary Influences on Biliary Health

The relationship between dietary factors and biliary health has been a focus of research in the etiology of biliary tract disease, particularly cancer risk. Increased consumption of fruits and fish in recent studies has been found to be inversely correlated with the risk of biliary cancer, suggesting that these dietary patterns may confer protective effects. Of note was a prospective study of over 638,000 participants, which revealed that the participants with the highest tertile of fruit intake experienced significantly reduced incidence of biliary cancer compared with those in the lowest tertile, and had a hazard ratio of 0.65. Similarly, high fish intake also demonstrated a protective effect, further validating the hypothesis that dietary intake has a significant bearing on biliary health and the prevention of biliary disease. As researchers explore these connections further, it becomes increasingly evident that nutrition can be a key component in reducing the risk of biliary cancers (Gunchick *et al.*, 2023). In addition to the direct influence of single food items, the role of overall patterns of diet and lifestyle factors cannot be discounted in the case of biliary well-being. Obesity, as characterized by elevated BMI, has proven to be a critical risk factor for biliary tract diseases, with BTC in particular. The meta-analysis of cohorts revealed a positive and significant association between obesity and the risk of biliary cancer with a hazard ratio of 1.66. This further signifies that proper diet control and exercise are important for maintaining a healthy weight and preventing the risk of biliary disease. Through the encouragement of eating habits that support balanced weight, health workers can prevent chronic disease in the biliary system and enhance general wellness (Gunchick *et al.*, 2023). Moreover, current research supports the prospect that the gut microbiome can influence biliary health. The balance among the populations of microbes within the gastrointestinal tract—eubiosis—is important to bile metabolism and may impact the pathogenesis of biliary disease. Research suggests that dysbiosis, or microbial imbalance, might be associated with increased risks for such diseases as biliary lithiasis and cholestatic disease. With integration of dietary influences with an understanding of microbiota dynamics, clinicians can better identify the causes of biliary health issues. This emerging field of investigation can provide novel avenues for therapeutic approaches to promote biliary health and decrease the rising disease burden of biliary diseases in the population (Figure 10.17).

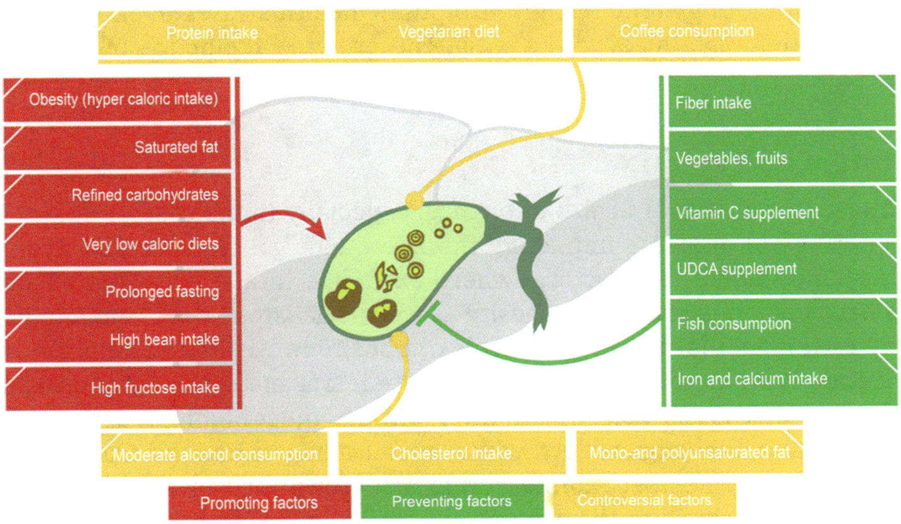

Figure 10.17. Effects of major dietary factors (promoting-, preventing-and controversial factors) on gallstone formation.

Source: https://www.researchgate.net/publication/373971916/figure/fig1/AS:11431281189040049@1694872717471/Effects-of-major-dietary-factors-promoting-preventing-and-controversial-factors-on.ppm.

10.6.2. Genetic Predispositions

Knowing about genetic predispositions gives important clues about the epidemiology of biliary tract diseases. These conditions, such as gallbladder and BTCs, demonstrate that family history can play a role in their development. Some genetic changes are found more often in particular groups, which could point to a genetic link. Noticing these differences helps us understand diseases better, catch them early, and provide the right treatment. Because genetics plays a role, it is important to recognize family history in both medical care and public health programs. With these methods, we can develop better ways to screen high-risk groups, which may allow us to manage diseases earlier and with better outcomes. Certain dog breeds are more likely to develop biliary problems, which shows that genetics can greatly affect a disease's onset. It is known that some breeds are more likely to get congenital portosystemic shunts and gallbladder mucocele, which suggests both genetics and environment play a role in these diseases. It supports veterinary care and can also reveal useful ideas for human medicine about the effects of genetics on the biliary tract. By being aware of breed-related illnesses, veterinarians can better diagnose them and find suitable ways to manage or treat them, which reflects the wider impact of genetics in medical research. Some of the worldwide health problems related to the gallbladder and the BTC can be linked to genetic factors. Studies in epidemiology reveal that certain populations are more likely to get these cancers, and this is often connected to their hereditary background and ethnicity, which is very important to know. In recent years, the number of gallbladder and BTC cases has gone up a lot. However, there are still clear differences in the rates between regions, which are likely affected by both genetic and socio-economic factors. Placing importance on the link between genes and disease outcomes, healthcare stakeholders can focus more on prevention and treatment for individuals at higher risk of disease. The integration of genetic insight into public health strategies may ultimately guide the development of more effective measures against the growing incidence of biliary tract diseases (Su *et al.*, 2024; Watson *et al.*, 2017).

10.6.3. Lifestyle Choices and Their Impact

Lifestyle is a major determinant of health outcomes, especially in the case of biliary tract disorders that encompass a range of ailments impacting the bile ducts, gallbladder, and liver. Dietary habits are one of the key modifiable risk factors, where excessive intake of saturated fats, sugars, and processed foods has been associated with obesity as well as gallstone development. United European Gastroenterology estimates that increasing levels of obesity in various nations are associated with increasing prevalence of biliary disease, indicating that dietary management is crucial in minimizing the incidence of biliary diseases. Public health interventions must highlight assistance to individuals with healthy low-fat and low-sugar diets while encouraging intake of fruits and vegetables to enhance overall well-being. Socioeconomic status also continues to affect food choice, thereby necessitating support programs at the community level in order to enhance access to healthy foods, particularly in poorer communities where poor diets are most prevalent (Rose *et al.*, 2022). Another lifestyle factor that affects biliary tract disease is alcohol consumption. Excessive alcohol use is a recognized risk factor for liver disease and encompasses biliary disease, like cholangitis and pancreatitis. The relationship between alcohol and the burden of gastrointestinal disease highlights the urgent need for alcohol reduction focused interventions. Recent evidence illustrates that certain groups understandably expect worsening biliary health with rising alcohol burden, and therefore, public health campaigns need to react to this issue (Rose *et al.*, 2022). Moreover, individuals need education regarding moderation and how alcohol can produce long-term effects on their health. Establishing environments that deter excessive consumption, along with adequate support mechanisms for alcohol dependency, can greatly minimize the risk of biliary tract disease and improve public health in general. Physical exercise is another critical component of a healthy lifestyle that influences the risk of biliary tract disease. Regular physical activity will assist with achieving a healthy weight, lowering cholesterol levels, and enhancing metabolic function, all of which are beneficial for preventing gallstone formation and other biliary diseases. Research shows that those with regular exercise have a much lower risk of developing gallbladder disease than their sedentary peers. Furthermore, the interplay between lifestyle and work environment again underscores the need for organizational policy that promotes active living, for example, the provision of exercise facilities and promotion of work-life balance. Integration of physical activity in everyday life is essential not only for individual health but also as a public health intervention to prevent the rising incidence of biliary tract disease. Thus, policymaking against physical inactivity and communal activities is necessary to assist in enhancing the health of the population and reducing the incidence of these disorders.

Summary

In conclusion, the management of biliary tract diseases (BTDs) involves an interdisciplinary approach that incorporates both diagnostic and therapeutic manoeuvres targeting the unique characteristics of the presented conditions. The molecular advancement, in particular focusing on miRNA methylation analysis, offers promising directions towards the differentiation between malignancies like BTC and benign conditions. Most importantly, the marked increase in the methylation level of miR-1247 in BTC patients is of significant diagnostic value, facilitating earlier treatment and improved prognosis. This attests to the critical role of genetic studies in our improvement in understanding and control measures of BTDs that are often complex and multifactorial in nature (Ohtsubo *et al.*, 2022). Furthermore, the association between underlying conditions, particularly diabetes, and biliary tract disease is central when deciding the prognosis of a patient and treatment strategies. Research shows that diabetic individuals with PLA have very divergent clinical presentations, hence advocating for individualized treatment strategies in consideration of comorbidities. The correlation of underlying biliary disease with the rates of infection suggests that medical practitioners must be vigilant in the follow-up of such patients in an effort to prevent complications. The observation that Klebsiella pneumoniae is the dominant major pathogen in such a scenario necessitates the application of specific antibiotic therapy that is essential in preventing recurrence and ensuring patient safety (Song *et al.*, 2020). Finally, management of biliary tract disorders transcends the immediate moment of clinical attention; it is one to be kept in mind for early diagnosis, control of risk factors, and investigation into new therapy. As technology in diagnostics evolves, with the potential even of applying plasma miRNA measurement, the healthcare system could enhance the quality of care delivered to the affected population as well. The interplay between disease mechanism and patient variables underscores the need for ongoing research and coordination among gastroenterologists, surgeons, and oncologists to advance an integrated concept of biliary tract disease. By placing a priority on a worldwide understanding, we are better able to counter the problems presented by these often complex conditions and seek improved patient outcomes in the years to come.

In the consideration of the diseases of the biliary tract, understanding the pathophysiology and potential therapy is crucial. Recent research has shown that low-grade inflammation is a unifying concept in regulating functional gastrointestinal disease, particularly of the biliary tract. This form of inflammation is likely to manifest as an increase in activated eosinophils and neutrophils in the gastrointestinal tract mucosa, highlighting the intimate interaction between immune mechanisms and gastrointestinal function. These interactions can be a causative agent in visceral hypersensitivity, often a presenting symptom in patients who have biliary disease. Knowledge of these mechanisms gives a foundation for how treatments that reverse symptoms and modify the impact of gastrointestinal illness on health outcomes can be developed (Ivashkin *et al.*, 2024). Pharmacologic treatment of biliary tract disease can be significantly increased by multitarget therapy strategies, particularly through the use of agents like trimebutine. This medication is intended to regulate a number of gastrointestinal functions, thus normalizing motility and reducing visceral hypersensitivity. The effectiveness of Trimebutine is complemented by its ability to modulate enterohormone production and by its action in reducing proinflammatory cytokine levels, implicated in the pathogenesis of functional gastrointestinal disorders. With the treatment of both the symptomatology and the underlying inflammation of biliary tract diseases, trimebutine is a major therapeutic advance in modalities, adding strength to its potential to serve as a cornerstone of therapy in such disorders (Ivashkin *et al.*, 2024). In BTC, new treatments are being discovered, particularly for those with HER2 amplification. The investigational agent zanidatamab was shown to be effective in early clinical trials, targeting HER2-overexpressing cancer cells. The results indicated high efficacy in a high proportion of patients with HER2-positive tumors to achieve a notable reduction in tumors, showing therapeutic promise in advanced disease. While recent side effects of the investigational treatments were reported, predominantly mild to moderate, the results support the need for ongoing investigation to verify and confirm the therapeutic applications of zanidatamab in treating BTC. The ever-changing nature of treatment highlights the importance of up-to-date research to maximize patient outcomes in biliary tract disease.

CLOSER LOOK

MAGNETIC RESONANCE CHOLANGIOPANCREATOGRAPHY (MRCP)

MRCP is a non-invasive imaging technique that uses MRI to visualize the bile ducts and pancreatic ducts. It is a valuable tool for diagnosing and evaluating conditions affecting the biliary and pancreatic systems, such as gallstones, pancreatitis, and tumors. MRCP offers detailed images without the risks associated with more invasive procedures like ERCP (Figure 10.18).

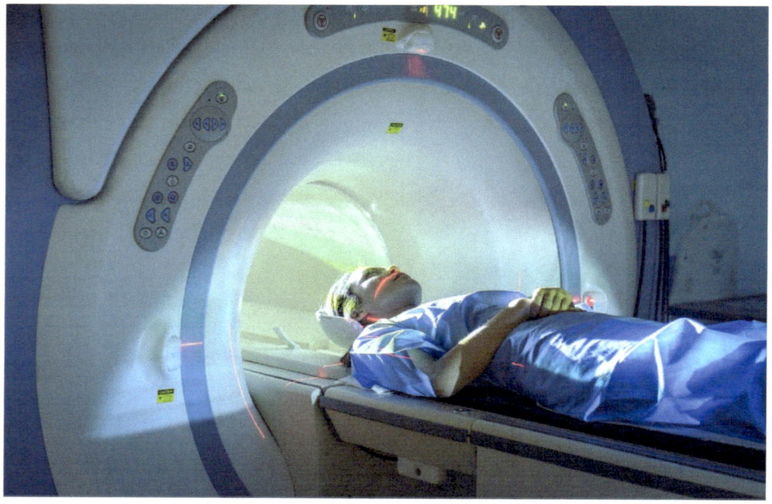

Figure 10.18. Magnetic Resonance Cholangiopancreatography (MRCP)

Source: https://www.verywellhealth.com/thmb/NCjSSjNgZ7cGK7lx0801u0PRfQI=/1500x0/filters:no_upscale():max_bytes(150000):strip_icc()/GettyImages-548557055-c18df2b5b8c64952a67d713fb7e9787e.jpg.

How It Works:

- MRCP uses strong magnetic fields and radio waves to create detailed images of the biliary and pancreatic ducts.
- A contrast agent (dye) may be used to further enhance the images, particularly for visualizing small details.
- The process is non-invasive, meaning it doesn't involve any incisions or insertion of tools into the body.
- MRCP does not use radiation, making it a safe alternative to other imaging techniques like CT scans.

Why It Is Used:

- **Diagnosing Conditions:** MRCP can help diagnose various conditions affecting the bile ducts and pancreas, such as gallstones, blockages, pancreatitis, and tumors.
- **Evaluating Symptoms:** It is often used to investigate symptoms like jaundice, abdominal pain, or unexplained weight loss.
- **Planning Treatment:** The detailed images provided by MRCP help healthcare providers plan treatment strategies.
- **Avoiding Invasive Procedures:** In some cases, MRCP can replace or reduce the need for more invasive procedures like ERCP.

Procedure:

- Patients typically lie on a scanner table during the MRCP procedure.
- The procedure may involve a contrast agent injection.
- The scan typically takes around 15-45 minutes, depending on whether other MRI scans are also being performed.
- After the scan, patients can usually resume their normal activities.

Benefits:

- **Non-Invasive:** No incisions or tools are inserted into the body.
- **Radiation-Free:** No exposure to harmful radiation.
- **Detailed Images:** Provides high-resolution images of the biliary and pancreatic system.
- **Accurate:** Can accurately detect abnormalities in the bile ducts and pancreas.
- **Useful for Diagnosis and Treatment:** Helps in diagnosing conditions and planning treatment.

Limitations:

- **Cannot Be Used in Everyone:** Individuals with certain metal implants or claustrophobia may not be suitable for MRCP.
- **May Not Be as Effective as ERCP in Some Cases:** MRCP may not be as effective as ERCP in certain situations, especially when specific areas need to be targeted.

References

1. Abdullah, A. A., Gianawati, I., Lalisang, T. J., & Lesmana, T. (2004). Diagnostic approach and treatment of choledocholithiasis. https://media.neliti.com/media/publications/70564-EN-diagnostic-approach-and-treatment-of-cho.pdf (accessed on 24 May 2025).
2. Agrusa, A., D'arpa, F., Di Carlo, P., Fasciana, T., Giammanco, A., Gulotta, G., Rodolico, V., *et al.* (2019). The microbiota of the bilio-pancreatic system: A cohort, STROBE-compliant study. https://core.ac.uk/download/224993662.pdf (accessed on 24 May 2025).
3. Aguirre-Sanchez, R.C., Herrera-Sanchez, A.H., Perez-Osorio, C.E., & Cardenas-Marrufo, M.F. (2024). ASGE Predictors for the Diagnosis of Choledocholithiasis: Validation in a Public Hospital of Merida, Yucatan, México. The International Journal of Gastroenterology and Hepatology Diseases. https://www.semanticscholar.org/paper/ASGE-Predictors-for-the-Diagnosis-of-Validation-in-Aguirre-Sanchez-Herrera-Sanchez/1295321972d220140339c2dd095b359b65fd6a97
4. Ahmad, M., Bansal, T., Dhingra, V., Fatima, M., *et al.* (2024). Establishing normal gallbladder volume: A comparative study of dual energy computed tomography and ultrasound measurements in a North Indian population. https://core.ac.uk/download/620836641.pdf (accessed on 24 May 2025).
5. Alebouyeh, M., Alizadeh, A. H. M., Majidi, M. R. S., Sherafat, A., *et al.* (2016). Association of diverse bacterial communities in human bile samples with biliary tract disorders: A survey using culture and polymerase chain reaction-denaturing gradient gel electrophoresis methods. https://core.ac.uk/download/52205553.pdf (accessed on 24 May 2025).
6. Alpini, G., Baiocchi, L., Ceci, L., Francis, H., Gaudio, E., Han, Y., Kennedy, L., *et al.* (2023). Gallstone and gallbladder disease: Biliary tract and cholangiopathies. https://core.ac.uk/download/599513205.pdf (accessed on 24 May 2025).
7. Alpini, G., Francis, H., Kennedy, L., Kundu, D., *et al.* (2020). Bile acid receptor therapeutics effects on chronic liver diseases. https://core.ac.uk/download/299809078.pdf (accessed on 24 May 2025). (accessed on 24 May 2025).
8. Alvarez Rodríguez, J., Canullán, C. M., Chiappetta Porras, L. T., Nápoli, A., *et al.* (2009). Minimally invasive management of acute biliary tract disease during pregnancy. https://core.ac.uk/download/pdf/8305846.pdf .
9. Alvaro, D., Arcidiacono, P. G., Capurso, G., Cardinale, V., *et al.* (2019). Common features between neoplastic and preneoplastic lesions of the biliary tract and the pancreas. https://core.ac.uk/download/231748248.pdf (accessed on 24 May 2025).
10. Ambrosi, A., Capuzzolo, S., Cianci, P., Fersini, A., *et al.* (2017). Acute cholecystitis: Diagnostic pitfall and timing of treatment. https://core.ac.uk/download/322430088.pdf (accessed on 24 May 2025).
11. Barr, M. L., Bogin, V., Broelsch, C. E., Bronsther, O., Campsen, J., Chan, S. C., *et al.* (2009). Complications of right lobe living donor liver transplantation. https://core.ac.uk/download/12205665.pdf (accessed on 24 May 2025).
12. Batta, A. (2011). Cholecystitis & an enzyme study. *International Journal of Current Biomedical and Pharmaceutical Research*. https://core.ac.uk/download/pdf/14665.pdf (accessed on 24 May 2025).

13. Benoit, D., De Bus, L., Depuydt, P., Libbrecht, L., *et al.* (2010). Severe drug-induced liver injury associated with prolonged use of Linezolid. https://core.ac.uk/download/55761329.pdf

14. Binda, C., Capurso, G., Coluccio, C., Cucchetti, A., Dajti, E., Ercolani, G., Fabbri, C., *et al.* (2022). Biliary diseases from the microbiome perspective: How microorganisms could change the approach to benign and malignant diseases. https://core.ac.uk/download/523413605.pdf (accessed on 24 May 2025).

15. Binda, C., Gibiino, G., Coluccio, C., Sbrancia, M., Dajti, E., Sinagra, E., Capurso, G., *et al.* (2022). Biliary diseases from the microbiome perspective: How microorganisms could change the approach to benign and malignant diseases. *Microorganisms, 10.* https://www.semanticscholar.org/paper/069393dd5f9c3579f784e382a2755681ba9ff9e9 (accessed on 24 May 2025).

16. Boru, E. C., Guida, A., Iossa, A., Rengo, G., *et al.* (2017). 25th International Congress of the European Association for Endoscopic Surgery (EAES), Frankfurt, Germany, 14–17 June 2017: Oral presentations. https://core.ac.uk/download/141696623.pdf.

17. Brindley, P. J., Bachini, M., Ilyas, S. I., Khan, S. A., Loukas, A., Sirica, A. E., Teh, B. T., *et al.* (2021). Cholangiocarcinoma. *Nature Reviews Disease Primers, 7.* https://doi.org/10.1038/s41572-021-00300-2.

18. Bruggink, J. M., Davenport, M., Hulscher, J. B. F., Kuebler, J., *et al.* (2022). Controversies in choledochal malformation in children: An international survey among pediatric hepatobiliary surgeons and gastroenterologists. https://core.ac.uk/download/518437209.pdf (accessed on 24 May 2025).

19. Carpino, G., *et al.* (2018). Intrahepatic cholangiocarcinoma: Review and update. https://core.ac.uk/download/159269704.pdf.

20. Chen, T., Forsti, A., Hemminki, A., Hemminki, K., *et al.* (2021). Second primary cancers after liver, gallbladder and bile duct cancers, and these cancers as second primary cancers. https://core.ac.uk/download/479169366.pdf (accessed on 24 May 2025).

21. Cook, A., Jenkins, L. M., & Plant, P. (1999). *A Casemix Analysis of Hospital Admissions in Six Specialties for Barking & Havering Health Authority.* https://core.ac.uk/download/10631591.pdf (accessed on 24 May 2025).

22. Falchook, G. S., Fu, S., Hess, K. R., Hong, D., *et al.* (2013). *Targeted Therapy of Advanced Gallbladder Cancer and Cholangiocarcinoma with Aggressive Biology: Eliciting Early Response Signals from Phase 1 Trials.* https://core.ac.uk/download/323067036.pdf.

23. Grazi, G. L. (2007). *Liver Resections: Complications and Survival Outcome.* https://core.ac.uk/download/11162431.pdf (accessed on 24 May 2025).

24. Gunchick, V., & Zheng, W. (2023). Abstract 3026: Dietary intakes and biliary tract cancer risk: Results from cohort studies including 638,860 Chinese and European adults. *Cancer Research.* https://www.semanticscholar.org/paper/b59e5bbaca34e32e19c8b5371a177215c97ce1cd (accessed on 24 May 2025).

25. Gupta, V., Gupta, R., Aggarwal, M., Singh, S., Kaur, H., Chaudhary, J., Gupta, M., *et al.* (2023). Bacteriological and antimicrobial susceptibility profile in biliary tract infections: A retrospective study. *Journal of Gastrointestinal Infections.* https://www.semanticscholar.org/paper/18b00024ce501fbc2cac1bfbf19826de6a6476e5 (accessed on 24 May 2025).

26. Hansbrough, J. F., Hoelscher, M., Porter, K. A., Putnam, C. W., *et al.* (1976). *Infections Complicating*

Orthotopic Liver Transplantation: A Study Emphasizing Graft-Related Septicemia. https://core.ac.uk/download/12203778.pdf (accessed on 24 May 2025).

27. Harding, J.J., Fan, J., Oh, D.Y., Choi, H.J., Kim, J.W., Chang, H., Bao, L., Sun, H., Macarulla, T., Xie, F., Metges, J.P., Ying, J., Bridgewater, J., Lee, M., Tejani, M.A., Chen, E.Y., Kim, D.U., Wasan, H.S., Ducreux, M., Bao, Y., Lindsey, S., Bachini, M., Morement, H., Boyken, L., Ma, J., Garfin, P.M., & Pant, S. (2024). A plain language summary of the results from the phase 2b HERIZON-BTC-01 study of zanidatamab in participants with HER2-amplified biliary tract cancer. Future Oncology, 20, 2319 - 2329.
28. Harrington, D., Lamberton, P. H. L., & McGregor, A. (2017). *Human Liver Flukes*. https://core.ac.uk/download/96882191.pdf.
29. Ivashkin, V. T., Bordin, D., Lapina, T., Livzan, M., Okhlobystin, A. V., Poluektova, E., Trukhmanov, A., *et al.* (2024). Role of inflammation and motility disorders in the development, course and consequences of functional gastrointestinal and biliary tract diseases (Literature review and expert panel resolution). *Russian Journal of Gastroenterology, Hepatology, Coloproctology*. https://www.semanticscholar.org/paper/aec419b55b88e07c9088eeb31e43dcdcd3600fac (accessed on 24 May 2025).
30. Kaverina, A. A., Wawrinchuk, S. A., Kosenko, P., Boyarintsev, N., & Shcherbakov, G. E. (2024). Diagnosis and treatment of biliary tract diseases in patients with COVID-19. *Yakut Medical Journal*. https://www.semanticscholar.org/paper/54459067849cbf544926c342906fa08d778f5ee9 (accessed on 24 May 2025).
31. Li, J., Gao, J., Huang, M., Fu, X., & Fu, B. (2024a). Risk factors for death in patients with severe acute pancreatitis in Guizhou Province, China. *Gastroenterology Research and Practice, 2024*. https://www.semanticscholar.org/paper/98fc4c0f7a58c64b93f2a53a5d59b974783ac670 (accessed on 24 May 2025).
32. Li, Q. Y., Luo, Y., & Sun, B. (2024b). Progress in the diagnosis and treatment of acute pancreatitis complicated by biliary tract diseases. *Zhonghua Wai Ke Za Zhi [Chinese Journal of Surgery], 63*(1), 76–80. https://www.semanticscholar.org/paper/acab8bff35e0dd8dc5f818f2bbb7f7b28976cdf0 (accessed on 24 May 2025).
33. Liu, T., Li, M., Tang, L., Wang, B., Li, T., Huang, Y., Xu, Y., *et al.* (2024). Epidemiological, clinical and microbiological characteristics of patients with biliary tract diseases with positive bile culture in a tertiary hospital. *BMC Infectious Diseases, 24*. https://www.semanticscholar.org/paper/4548d605166b46e00e1a31dbc5c0c68b0879beff (accessed on 24 May 2025).
34. Łukasiewicz, S., Czeczelewski, M., Forma, A., Baj, J., Sitarz, R., & Stanisławek, A. (2021). Breast cancer—Epidemiology, risk factors, classification, prognostic markers, and current treatment strategies—An updated review. *Cancers, 13*, 4287. https://doi.org/10.3390/cancers13174287.
35. Murray, C. J. L., Ikuta, K. S., Sharara, F., Swetschinski, L. R., Robles Aguilar, G., Gray, A. P., Han, C., *et al.* (2022). Global burden of bacterial antimicrobial resistance in 2019: A systematic analysis. *The Lancet, 399*, 629–655. https://doi.org/10.1016/S0140-6736(21)02724-0.
36. Nagtegaal, I. D., Odze, R. D., Klimstra, D. S., Paradis, V., Rugge, M., Schirmacher, P., Washington, K., *et al.* (2019). The 2019 WHO classification of tumors of the digestive system. *Histopathology, 76*, 182–188. https://doi.org/10.1111/his.13975.
37. Ohtsubo, K., Miyake, K., Arai, S., Fukuda, K., Suzuki, C., Kotani, H., Tanimoto, A., *et al.* (2022). Methylation of tumor suppressive miRNAs in plasma from patients with pancreaticobiliary

diseases. *Cancer Diagnosis & Prognosis, 2*(3), 378–383. https://www.semanticscholar.org/paper/234d836d7f6b6f09ab4ff5c6992612d72eaebe19 (accessed on 24 May 2025).

38. Oneda, E., Astore, S., Gandolfi, L., Melocchi, L., & Zaniboni, A. (2024). Which therapy in biliary tract cancer? Review of main concerns in diagnosis and choice of therapy in advanced setting, current standard, and new options. Expert Opinion on Pharmacotherapy, 25, 1807 - 1823.

39. Qiu, S., Zeng, W., Zhang, J., Xie, J., & Chen, X. (2025). The global and regional burden of gallbladder and biliary tract cancer and attributable risk factors: Trends and predictions. *Liver International, 45*(4), e70025. https://www.semanticscholar.org/paper/4c8b3c10b7855aa6703034f295ceb64c730cc0b7.

40. Rose, T. C., Pennington, A., Kypridemos, C., Chen, T., Subhani, M. M., Hanefeld, J., Ricciardiello, L., *et al.* (2022). Analysis of the burden and economic impact of digestive diseases and investigation of research gaps and priorities in the field of digestive health in the European Region—White Book 2: Executive summary. *United European Gastroenterology Journal, 10*, 657–662. https://doi.org/10.1002/ueg2.12298.

41. Song, H. M., Wang, X., Lian, Y., & Wan, T. (2020). Analysis of the clinical characteristics of 202 patients with liver abscess associated with diabetes mellitus and biliary tract disease. *The Journal of International Medical Research, 48*. https://www.semanticscholar.org/paper/cd88845f477c46e96fbacc0ae2ca900a914cc4d2 (accessed on 24 May 2025).

42. Su, J., He, X., & Liang, Y. (2024). *Global, Regional, and National Burden and Trends Analysis of Gallbladder and Biliary Tract Cancer From 1990 to 2019 and Predictions to 2030: A Systematic Analysis for the Global Burden of Disease Study 2019*. https://core.ac.uk/download/614658454.pdf (accessed on 24 May 2025).

43. Sugiura, R., Kawamoto, Y., Kuwatani, M., Kawakubo, K., Harada, K., Ohara, M., Yonemura, H., *et al.* (2025). Subcutaneous adipose tissue radiodensity as a predictor of poor prognosis in advanced biliary tract cancer. *Journal of Hepato-Biliary-Pancreatic Sciences*. https://www.semanticscholar.org/paper/04eb7ccf36bcdb62f5e9b2e320a1c00e09f7a52a (accessed on 24 May 2025).

44. Święszkowska, E., Broniszczak, D., Kaliciński, P., Szymczak, M., Stefanowicz, M., Grajkowska, W., & Dembowska-Bagińska, B. (2024). Rhabdomyosarcoma of the biliary tract in children: Analysis of single center experience. *Cancers, 16*. https://www.semanticscholar.org/paper/69a854851323388960f1c831db892ae69ab4bf15 (accessed on 24 May 2025).

45. Watson, P. (2017). *Canine Breed-Specific Hepatopathies*. https://core.ac.uk/download/83938995.pdf (accessed on 24 May 2025).

46. Xie, X., Kong, S., & Cao, W. (2023). Targeting protein glycosylation to regulate inflammation in the respiratory tract: novel diagnostic and therapeutic candidates for chronic respiratory diseases. Frontiers in Immunology, 14. https://www.semanticscholar.org/paper/Targeting-protein-glycosylation-to-regulate-in-the-Xie-Kong/6fea526e50df00a8b8d73e9a56459ee295183aae

47. Zheng, D., Liwinski, T., & Elinav, E. (2020). Interaction between microbiota and immunity in health and disease. *Cell Research, 30*, 492–506. https://doi.org/10.1038/s41422-020-0332-7.

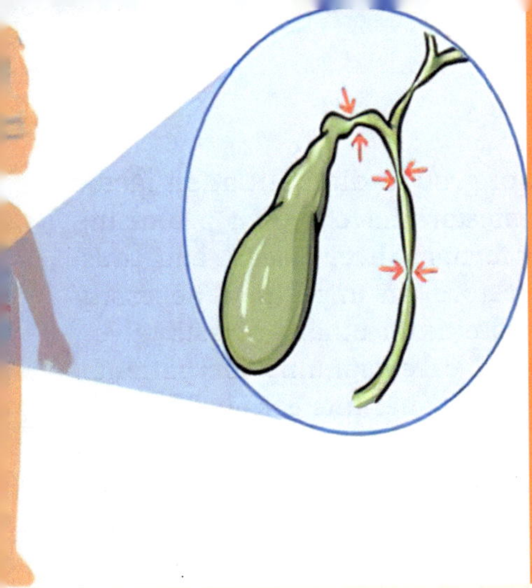

Chapter 11

BILIARY ATRESIA AND PEDIATRIC LIVER DISEASES

Contents

Introduction

The pathology of biliary atresia (BA) and pediatric liver disease represents a crucial part of pediatric medicine due to the severe impact of these diseases on a child's development and health status in the future. Biliary atresia, an obstruction of the bile ducts at birth, is the most frequent indication for liver transplant in children. Its etiology can be. mostly idiopathic, representing. significant challenges to early diagnosis and treatment. Effective management is based on a clear understanding and knowledge of the pathophysiology of the disease, with the Kasai procedure being a safe and common surgical intervention aimed at restoring biliary drainage. Its success is, however, unpredictable, and a majority of patients will eventually proceed to develop liver failure; hence, continued research into alternative therapy and the role of new surgical techniques in prolonging native liver survival. One of the more significant challenges of the treatment of biliary atresia is finding biomarkers that would potentially diagnose biliary atresia separately from other liver ailments in children. Numerous new studies have appeared concerning the diagnostic biomarker roles of growth differentiation factor 15 (GDF15) and fibroblast growth factor 21 (FGF21). These biomarkers have shown promising potential for differentiating mitochondrial hepatopathies from other forms of liver disease and, thus, enhancing diagnostic accuracy and informing treatment. It is, therefore, an imperative necessity from here on to carry out further studies on the role of these proteins in biliary atresia, given their potential to have a significant impact on clinical outcome and care planning for patients. Awareness of the interaction of these biomarkers with liver disease not only permits earlier diagnosis but also potentially better prognostication. Moreover, inadequacies of current interventions and requirements for new therapeutic approaches identify the place of multidisciplinary collaboration in pediatric hepatology. Substantial progress has been made in defining the outcome of salvage operations following Kasai, offering evidence on optimal practice in preservation of native liver function. Recent literature reports a series of interventions, such as redo-Kasai procedures and radiologic interventions, to address the complications arising after the initial operation. As liver transplantation remains the most definitive management for the majority of children with BA, the identification of effective salvage strategies is the greatest challenge. Interdisciplinary dialogue among multidisciplinary teams of pediatric surgeons, hepatologists, and transplant experts is vital to share innovative solutions and optimize long-term survival rates in children with biliary atresia and other liver diseases.

Definition of Biliary Atresia

Biliary atresia is a rare but severe disease in children characterized by a congenital absence or obstruction of the bile ducts, which hampers the normal bile flow from the intestine to the liver. The obstruction leads to bile accumulation in the liver and causes cholestasis and eventually liver injury. Infants with biliary atresia typically present in the initial weeks of life with jaundice, pale stools, and dark urine. With the continuation of the disease, chronic injury may take place, which leads to fibrosis, cirrhosis, and ultimately liver failure if left untreated (Kerola *et al.*, 2019). Biliary atresia affects approximately 1 out of 20,000 live births and is the most frequent indication for infant and childhood liver transplantation (Kerola *et al.*, 2019). Early diagnosis and surgical intervention, in the shape of the Kasai portoenterostomy, are key to favorable outcomes. However, the majority of children end up requiring liver transplantation as the disease advances. The pathophysiology of biliary atresia is poorly understood, with difficulty in treating it effectively. Even following successful portoenterostomy, restoration of bile flow does not always coincide with long-term liver health, as most patients continue to experience progressive liver fibrosis. Current research has elucidated some key molecular pathways to this fibrogenesis, with the involvement of several fibrogenic growth factors such as transforming growth factor-beta (TGF-β) and matrix metalloproteinases (MMPs) remaining persistently elevated despite surgery (Kerola *et al.*, 2019). Importantly, MMP-7 has exhibited distinctive upregulation in biliary atresia patients when compared to both fibrotic and non-fibrotic controls. Unraveling these mechanisms at the molecular level is essential for the design of targeted therapies that can potentially improve prognosis and augment native liver survival rates. Additional biomarker research on biliary atresia is essential to intervene early and treat hepatic fibrosis. Recent evidence suggests that some biomarkers, such as endoglin, IL-8, and MMP-7, are directly related to liver stiffness measurements and are likely to significantly enhance the prediction of progression of liver disease among affected children. These results highlight the need for incorporating analyses of biomarkers into clinical care for improved monitoring and treatment. With our increasing understanding of biliary atresia, the search for disease-specific interventions will be crucial in optimizing interventions that target both the mechanical and physiological bases of the disease. This kind of strategy will not only improve patient outcomes but also pave the way for upcoming technologies in the treatment of pediatric liver diseases (Figure 11.1).

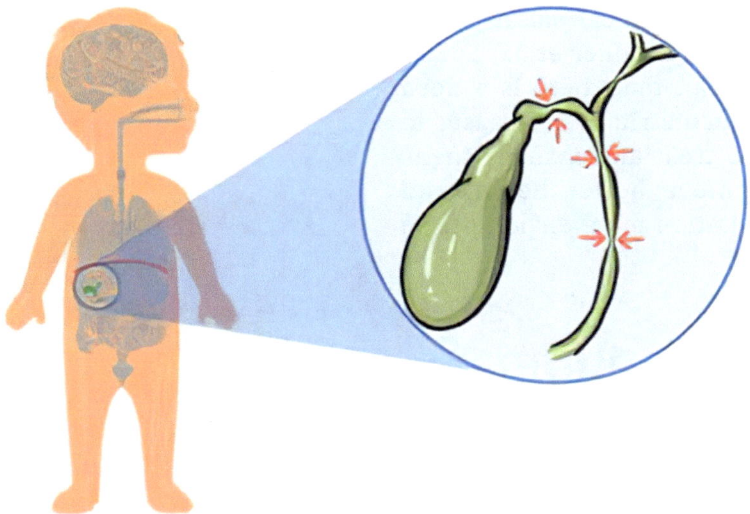

Figure 11.1. Biliary disorders in pediatrics

Source: https://santripty.com/wp-content/uploads/2024/10/biliary-atresia-1.jpg.

Importance of Studying Pediatric Liver Diseases

It is essential to study pediatric liver diseases, mainly biliary atresia, because the number of liver disorders in children is on the rise. Because of these diseases, patients can develop serious health problems such as liver failure, which often calls for liver transplantation. Biliary atresia, which stops the flow of bile in newborns, is one of the main reasons for liver disease that leads to transplantation in early childhood. It is very important to understand how these diseases develop and progress to create effective treatment plans that help children live longer and better. Finding and treating liver diseases in children as early as possible can greatly impact their health, so research on pediatric liver diseases is critical for pediatric healthcare. Also, studying pediatric liver diseases helps us understand the special immune responses seen in children. How children react to infections and treatments differs from how adults react, which greatly influences the management and outcomes of liver diseases in children. For instance, research indicates that post-operative infections, particularly those caused by cytomegalovirus (CMV), pose a substantial risk for pediatric liver transplant recipients. Knowing how inherited metabolic diseases and similar conditions make a person more prone to infections can improve clinical care. For instance, in pediatric liver transplantation, those with biliary atresia exhibit different infection rates compared to other metabolic disorders, underscoring the necessity for tailored treatment protocols and monitoring strategies in managing these patients (Ushijima *et al.*, 2025). Efforts in education and research about pediatric liver diseases may result in new technology and treatment methods. Because of continuous research, surgeons can now use minimally invasive procedures for biliary atresia, which helps patients recover faster and with better results. Also, looking into post-transplant issues, for example leukocytosis, helps us improve care for children. In one study, leukocytosis was prevalent post-transplantation, yet only extreme leukocytosis was associated with confirmed infections, highlighting the nuanced clinical picture faced by healthcare providers (Shanker *et al.*, 2025). Such research points out that there is a need to continue studying pediatric liver diseases to develop new ways to treat and manage them, helping children achieve better health and offering useful information for their long-term care.

11.1. Understanding Biliary Atresia

Biliary atresia is a major problem in children's liver diseases caused by the complete blockage of the bile ducts outside the liver, which leads to severe liver damage. If chronic inflammation is not treated promptly, it can cause cholestasis, cirrhosis, and liver failure. A good knowledge of biliary atresia's pathophysiology helps doctors identify and treat the condition quickly. Doctors do not know for sure what causes it, but different theories connect it to factors such as the environment, infections, and genes. Recent genetic studies have pointed out that certain genes may increase the risk of biliary atresia. Blocked bile flow causes toxic substances to build up, which makes liver damage worse and adds to the difficulty of treating the infants. People understand this condition more fully by also looking at the factors that make it more severe. Jaundice, pale stools, and dark urine are common signs of biliary atresia, and these usually appear in the first few months of a baby's life. Swift diagnosis is necessary because immediate surgery, most often the Kasai procedure, can lead to much better results. This method tries to get bile back to the small intestine by connecting the liver directly to the intestine, bypassing the blocked ducts. Still, the results are not always good, and many babies must have a liver transplant as the disease continues. When bile duct atresia is treated promptly, studies suggest that the patient has a better chance of long-term health, proving that quick recognition is very important. For this reason, knowing the clinical details of biliary atresia is very important for pediatric healthcare providers.

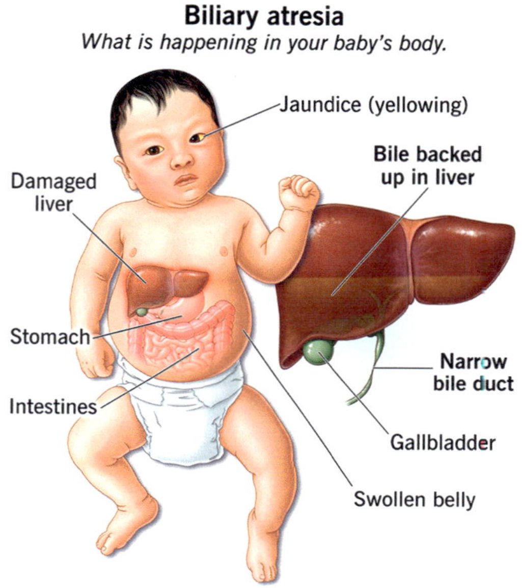

Figure 11.2. Biliary atresia.

Source: https://my.clevelandclinic.org/-/scassets/images/org/health/articles/21076-biliary-atresia.

New findings in genetics could provide more information on the causes and development of biliary atresia. A genome-wide association study identified significant single-nucleotide polymorphisms (SNPs) associated with the condition, particularly those linked to the EFEMP1 gene, which is implicated in extracellular matrix remodeling and cell proliferation (Bailey-Wilson *et al.*, 2018). It may suggest that the person is genetically more likely to develop this disease, so further study is needed, especially for personalized medicine. This knowledge can guide doctors to better treat and manage biliary atresia by using therapies that target the real causes instead of just the symptoms. At the same time, as biliary atresia is better understood, progress in liver transplantation continues, since this is the only cure for advanced liver disease from the condition. (Clemente *et al.*, 2016) (Figure 11.2).

11.1.1. Pathophysiology of Biliary Atresia

The pathophysiology of biliary atresia is a complex interaction between developmental defects and immune responses that ultimately lead to obstructive cholestasis. It typically occurs in infants with progressive inflammation and fibrosis of the extrahepatic bile ducts. Obstruction in biliary atresia prevents bile flow into the intestine, causing the accumulation of toxic substances within the liver, which exacerbates hepatocellular injury and cirrhosis.

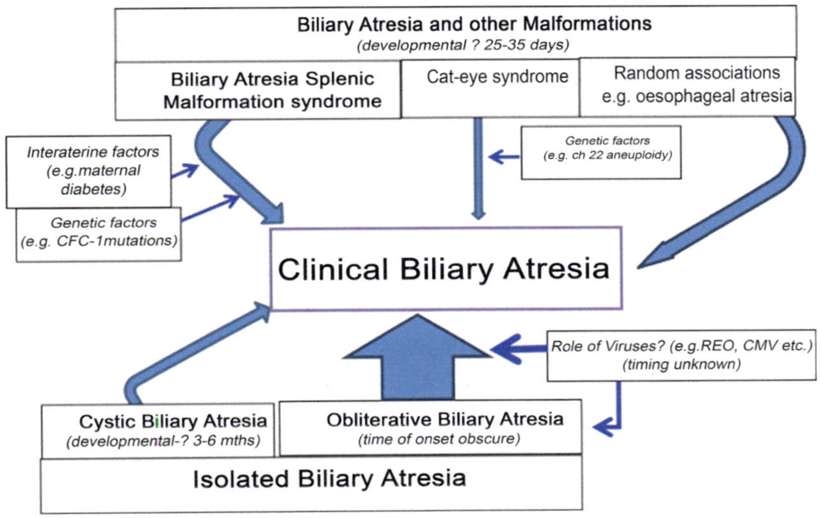

Figure 11.3. Patterns of clinical biliary atresia.

Source: https://www.researchgate.net/profile/Claus-Petersen-4/publication/256288529/figure/fig1/AS:202840329986051@1425372311518/Patterns-of-Clinical-Biliary-Atresia.png.

This process ultimately underlies the pathogenic cycle leading to cholestatic liver disease, significantly compromising hepatic function. Prompt recognition of biliary atresia is critical, as early surgical intervention can slow the progression of liver damage to such an extent that long-term prognosis is improved in children with this condition. Recent studies have analyzed many putative biomarkers that may provide insight into the pathophysiological processes underlying biliary atresia, paving the way to improved diagnosis and treatment. Of these biomarkers, the increase in growth differentiation factor 15 (GDF15) and fibroblast growth factor 21 (FGF21) is of particular interest. In pediatric patients, these biomarkers have shown elevated levels in conditions such as biliary atresia, which distinguishes this disease from other pediatric liver diseases. Identification of biliary atresia using non-invasive testing would provide a fundamental prognostic insight and enhance clinical management protocols. Moreover, research highlights the prognostic relevance, since their levels were determined to be increased in relation to disease severity and indication for liver transplantation, thereby paving the way for their potential application in personalizing best patient management (Hove *et al.*, 2024). Another paradigm of biliary atresia pathophysiology complexity is participation by microRNAs, primarily miR-122, in the pathogenesis of the disease. miR-122 is the most abundant microRNA in the liver and has also been reported to be linked with a number of hepatic pathologies. Elevated serum miR-122 levels have been demonstrated in studies of patients with biliary atresia, suggesting its value as a biomarker. While the expression level of miR-122 may be implicated in pathological processes, its sensitivity and specificity as a biomarker must be confirmed by large-scale studies. The study of miR-122 offers a possible avenue for the elucidation of molecular biliary atresia changes, highlighting the usefulness of subsequent investigation into diagnostic markers that can maximize early detection and improve patient prognosis (Motazedian *et al.*, 2024) (Figure 11.3).

11.1.2. Symptoms and Clinical Presentation

Presentation of biliary atresia most often happens in the first few weeks of life, and jaundice is the most important clinical presentation. Jaundice is generated by the accumulation of bilirubin due to bile flow obstruction, which impairs appropriate hepatic function. Aside from jaundice, the majority of infants with this condition usually experience pale or clay-colored stools with a lack of bile in the intestine, leading to fat malabsorption and fat-soluble vitamins. This presentation is followed by dark urine, pruritus, and abdominal distension as the liver begins to show signs of compromised function. Early diagnosis and treatment are important because delayed intervention can lead to permanent liver damage. Thus, being aware of these presenting signs is important in differentiating biliary atresia from other neonatal jaundice etiologies, which may not be surgical. Other important symptoms of biliary atresia apart from jaundice include ascites, weight loss, and hepatomegaly. Ascites is the unexplained accumulation of fluid in the abdominal cavity that usually indicates severe liver dysfunction and portal hypertension. Babies with biliary atresia also usually fail to thrive due to inadequate nutrition intake secondary to malabsorption caused by bile obstruction. Hepatomegaly, or liver enlargement, is frequently present and may be suggestive of inflammation and increased workload on the liver as it attempts to make up for the loss of biliary function. These clinical presentations are indicative of the insidious nature of the disease, with the focus being on early diagnosis and recognition. If not treated, infants develop complications such as cirrhosis and portal hypertension, making the clinical picture and management more complex. Clinical presentation of biliary atresia presents significant challenges not just to diagnosis but also to management of the disease. Delayed diagnosis can exacerbate the risk of complications like hepatic failure and the requirement for liver transplantation. The complexities that are involved in biliary tract complications in pediatric liver transplantation further add to these problems. Research states that biliary tract complications are a major cause of morbidity and mortality following liver transplantation, with obstructions and leaks from the biliary tree common occurrences (Gordon *et al.*, 1987). Collaborative studies by scientists and health care practitioners have facilitated advancements in the understanding of the natural history of the condition and treatment responsiveness (van Wessel *et al.*, 2020). Cross-disciplinary collaboration is necessary to advance outcomes in individuals affected, as it provides the basis for the development of individually tailored treatment plans addressing the variability of biliary atresia and its associated symptoms and thus improving prognosis in patients (Figure 11.4).

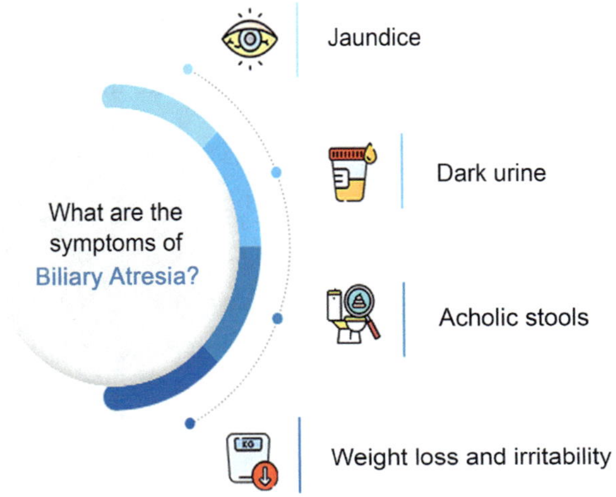

Figure 11.4. Symptoms of biliary atresia.

Source: https://www.ailbsindia.com/wp-content/uploads/2023/04/what-are-the-symptoms-of-biliary-atresia.jpg.

11.1.3. Diagnosis and Imaging Techniques

Early detection of biliary atresia and similar pediatric liver diseases is very important for the best treatment results and to avoid serious complications. The use of imaging has made it possible to see important details in the hepatobiliary system. US, CT, and MRI are the most important imaging tests, and US and MRI are preferred because they do not use ionizing radiation. The US allows the detection of gallbladder, biliary tree abnormalities, and liver shape, but MRI is better for seeing soft tissue, which is important for biliary structures. Both tests are important for telling apart biliary atresia from choledochal cysts, which can look the same. As imaging modalities continue to advance, their diagnostic utility in detecting anatomical variations and potential complications in pediatric liver diseases becomes increasingly valuable, enhancing the overall management approach (Nydegger *et al.*, 2010). In cases of choledochal cysts, a type of biliary malformation, MRI and magnetic resonance cholangiopancreatography (MRCP) are the gold standards for diagnosis. They allow doctors to clearly see the biliary tree, which helps them spot cystic dilations accurately. Asian populations are more likely to have choledochal cysts, which can cause jaundice in infants and abdominal pain in older children. Because the symptoms of these conditions are often vague, imaging tests are very important in the diagnosis. MRCP helps doctors see the entire biliary system clearly, which helps them decide on treatment and plan surgery quickly. Furthermore, understanding the implications of delayed diagnosis, such as increased morbidity from complications like cholangitis and pancreatitis, underscores the importance of precise imaging techniques in pediatric hepatobiliary conditions (Gezer *et al.*, 2019). Better imaging tools have helped doctors diagnose pediatric liver diseases, especially biliary atresia. New approaches, such as elastography and CEUS, have appeared to measure liver stiffness and blood flow in the liver. These approaches are very useful when evaluating liver fibrosis and managing chronic liver disease in children. The use of advanced imaging methods with traditional techniques improves the accuracy of finding liver diseases and helps create personalized treatment plans. In addition, new developments in imaging help with the initial diagnosis and are important for checking up and monitoring patients after surgery. Ultimately, the continuous advancements in imaging modalities reflect a commitment to improving patient outcomes in those afflicted by biliary atresia and other pediatric liver diseases, emphasizing the need for ongoing research and development in this domain (Figure 11.15).

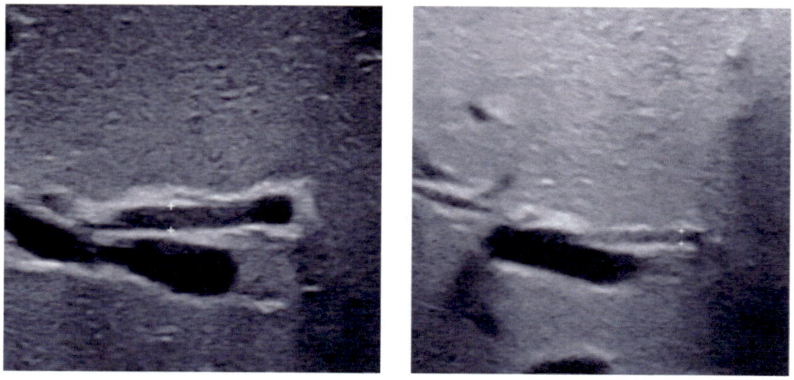

(a) (b)

Figure 11.5. Hepatic artery measurement images of infants with (a) and without biliary atresia (b).

Source: https://www.mdpi.com/diagnostics/diagnostics-12-00051/article_deploy/html/images/diagnostics-12-00051-g005.png.

11.2. Causes and Risk Factors

The etiology of biliary atresia (BA) remains largely enigmatic, complicating efforts to develop targeted preventive measures. Though the exact reasons are not completely known, most researchers believe that a combination of genetic, environmental, and infectious factors may be involved in its development. In particular, recent findings show that BA may be linked to certain genetic markers, which suggests it can be passed down in families. For instance, recent genome-wide association studies (GWAS) identified significant SNPs associated with BA, implicating the EFEMP1 gene, which plays a role in extracellular matrix remodeling and cholangiocyte function, as a potential susceptibility locus. Also, environmental factors during pregnancy might worsen these genetic issues, making BA more likely in infants who are genetically at risk. Apart from genetics, people have looked at different environmental and infectious factors as possible causes of biliary atresia. Pregnant women who have CMV or rubella infections have a higher risk of their child developing BA, which suggests that viruses may play a part in the disease. Investigations into what toxins or medications a pregnant woman takes play a role in this discussion. Studies suggest that exposure to certain chemicals or medications may disrupt fetal biliary tract development, thereby heightening the risk of BA (Borel *et al.*, 1985). Because of many factors being involved, it is difficult to fully understand this condition, which highlights the importance of research that explores all the ways these different but linked factors contribute to it. Also, the process from when biliary atresia is first identified to liver failure has major effects on the health of children. Symptoms usually appear within the first few months, and fast treatment is very important to control the condition. When the extrahepatic bile ducts are destroyed, cholestasis occurs, which may result in liver fibrosis and eventually cirrhosis if not managed quickly. If surgery such as the Kasai procedure is not done, the chance of CLD increases greatly. Subsequent liver transplantation has emerged as a critical treatment option for advanced cases; however, the survival rates post-transplantation demonstrate the complex challenge BA poses to health care systems (Borel *et al.*, 1985). Given that Biliary atresia is a leading indication for pediatric liver transplants, understanding its causes and risk factors remains imperative for developing enhanced therapeutic strategies (Figure 11.6).

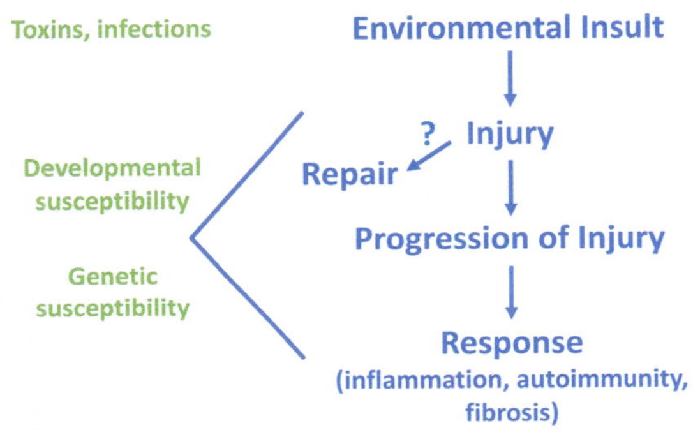

Figure 11.6. Schematic of hypothesis of biliary atresia etiology. Right side shows potential sequence of events, beginning with a prenatal bile duct injury, in biliary atresia. Left side highlights the potential contribution of developmental and genetic susceptibility to the injury and response.

Source: https://www.researchgate.net/publication/331329228/figure/fig1/AS:730245187514369@1551115428299/Schematic-of-hypothesis-of-biliary-atresia-etiology-Right-side-shows-potential-sequence.jpg.

11.2.1. Genetic Predispositions

In exploring the complexity of biliary atresia and pediatric liver disease, it is important to comprehend genetic predispositions in their etiology. Genetic predispositions can be a major contributing factor in biliary atresia, where bile ducts become obstructed, thereby resulting in the ultimate cause of severe liver injury. Research suggests that certain genetic mutations or syndromes may conceal the normal physiological pathways necessary for liver development and function. For instance, studies have hypothesized a correlation between genetic abnormalities and the clinical presentation of biliary atresia, and therefore, genetic screening in high-risk individuals is indicated. The awareness of these predispositions enables better detection of affected infants and enhances the critical early interventions required to effectively manage this disease. Besides, genetic predispositions to biliary atresia are not unique and encompass a broad spectrum of pediatric liver disorders. Disease severity and progression influence genetic mutations predisposing children to various liver disorders. Because CLD in children has been found to increase in prevalence, genetic factors need to be acknowledged in addition to environmental exposure. For example, genetic differences in the metabolic pathway may lead to conditions such as nonalcoholic fatty liver disease, which is increasingly diagnosed in children. Additionally, family predispositions of the occurrence of liver disease, coupled with emerging genetic discoveries, seem to advocate for the reality that pathologies of the liver in children serve as prognosticators for CLD in adults, and thus, full genetic analysis must be undertaken in a bid to offset future health outcomes (Alisi *et al.*, 2015). The interplay between genetic predispositions and liver disease also highlights the importance of targeted research and tailored therapeutic regimens. Information regarding the genetic basis of pediatric liver diseases can be a window through which custom-made treatments can be developed according to an individual's genetic makeup. As the medical community advances further in its attempts to identify specific genetic markers, targets for treatment have become more apparent, as have new modes of intervention precisely calibrated to address the individualized demands of each child. Remarkably, aggressive focal liver lesions that are found in children, though rare, also carry distinct genetic mutations in comparison to adult forms of the same diseases (Augustiniene *et al.*, 2023). Accordingly, management and treatment of genetic predisposition are part of the general management and treatment of biliary atresia and other childhood liver diseases, thus equipping practitioners to handle these complex conditions more efficaciously.

11.2.2. Environmental Influences

The etiology of biliary atresia (BA) in infants entails several environmental variables that extend beyond mere genetic predispositions. Even though the exact etiology of BA remains, to a large extent, unidentified, studies are leading toward an emerging role for environmental agents in initiating and causing disease. For instance, prenatal exposures to either maternal infection or toxins have been implicated as having the potential to trigger inflammatory pathways that disrupt cholangiocyte development in a normal fashion. This disturbance can trigger the fibrosclerotic obliteration of bile ducts and result in the cholestasis seen in BA. Additionally, maternal nutrition and the perinatal milieu have also been incriminated in other pediatric liver diseases and indicate that an approach involving multiple factors is needed to understand the pathogenesis of BA in its complete sense. Thus, environmental exposure surveillance is significant to identify vulnerable populations and set up preventative measures in the management of pediatric liver disease. Moreover, the impact of prenatal environmental exposure carries over into neurological sequelae, which may result from BA and its treatment. Children with BA often experience a cascade of health complications, from the physical effects of liver damage to neurodevelopmental ones, as highlighted by existing research. Research points out that vulnerability to inflammatory processes at times of brain development might reroute neurodevelopmental pathways, linking BA with results such as Autism Spectrum Disorder (ASD). These correlations need an even broader understanding of how the systemic impact of liver disease can interact with neurodevelopmental differences. Environmental determinants, thus, particularly those affecting cognitive and emotional development in children with BA, need to be considered with attention to detail in order to optimize clinical outcomes and improve long-term quality of life in such patients (Earl *et al.*, 2024). The environmental setting for children with biliary atresia is not only constrained to influences of the mother during pregnancy but also transcends to the socioeconomic factors influencing postnatal environments. Children with BA tend to experience enormous inequalities in access to health resources, which can impact their outcomes. For instance, children who have minimal access to specialized medical care or rehabilitative services may experience prolonged recovery and heightened risk for neurodevelopmental delay. Moreover, the emotional and psychological burden that comes with dealing with family dynamics around chronic disease may further exacerbate developmental disorders. Familiarity with the critical intersection of socioeconomic status, healthcare access, and the environment is essential to optimizing treatment strategies. By integrating these parameters into patient care, clinicians can better help children with BA achieve the optimal developmental milestones, leading to superior long-term health outcomes (Earl *et al.*, 2024).

11.2.3. Associated Congenital Anomalies

The occurrence of concomitant congenital malformations in children with biliary atresia (BA) is a major area of investigation in the context of pediatric liver disease. Biliary atresia is primarily defined as the obliteration of the extrahepatic bile ducts, and it has significant clinical connotations, such as liver failure. But there is a need to keep in mind that BA patients have a wide range of concomitant congenital malformations. These abnormalities can affect numerous systems and thus complicate the clinical course and the prognostic outcome. Structural cardiac defects, splenic pathology, and gastrointestinal pathology have been identified in patients with BA and indicate that the disease is not an isolated occurrence but part of a larger syndrome of developmental dysplasias. Understanding the incidence and pattern of associated congenital malformations is fundamental to tailoring surgical operations and other treatments to optimize survival rates and enhance quality of life in involved children. Research has provided evidence of an alarming correlation between biliary atresia and complex vascular malformations, which pose particular problems for management. Studies have demonstrated that a considerable proportion of infants undergoing liver transplantation for extrahepatic biliary atresia had noteworthy vascular anomalies, including absent inferior vena cava (IVC) and abnormal hepatic artery anatomy. Such complex vascular malformations may complicate transplants and contribute to heightened mortality when not appropriately identified prior to surgical operations. This finding further emphasizes the importance of preoperative diagnosis and early assessment of vascular anomalies in this specific patient population. Identification of such anomalies prior to transplantation may allow clinicians to determine candidacy and formulate appropriate surgical approaches, ultimately impacting the overall success rates of transplant operations in pediatric patients with biliary atresia and associated vascular anomalies (Lilly *et al.*, 1974). The genetic underpinnings of biliary atresia may also help us understand its associated congenital anomalies. Genome-wide association studies carried out in the recent past have brought evidence to light of significant loci that suggest the potential of an inherited component in this condition. Certain SNPs have been implicated with biliary atresia and its association with other anomalies. The EFEMP1 gene, associated with various cellular processes like extracellular matrix remodeling, has its expression altered in BA and other cholestatic disease patients. This correlation suggests the likelihood of genetic impact not just upon the underlying disorder but upon its associated anomalies as well, suggesting an interplay between heredity and environment. Further research into these genetic links may reveal further insight into the multifactorial conditions of biliary atresia and provide a pathway towards higher diagnostic and therapeutic interventions in treating similar cases in pediatrics (Bailey-Wilson *et al.*, 2018).

11.3. Treatment Options for Biliary Atresia

The management of biliary atresia is a multifaceted one with a focus on reversing bile flow and preventing further liver disease progression. The most prevalent type of management is the Kasai procedure, whereby the small bowel is surgically connected to the liver in a bid to create an alternative route for bile drainage. This procedure is typically performed within the first few months of life to maximize its effectiveness, as earlier intervention generally correlates with better outcomes. The success of the Kasai procedure, however, is variable; approximately 50% of patients will achieve sufficient bile flow to avoid liver transplantation at five years post-operation. Despite this surgery, many patients subsequently require hepatic transplantation due to ongoing cholestasis and liver damage, indicating the importance of total medical care throughout their illness. As research continues, other treatment options are being explored to better treat children with biliary atresia. Pharmacologic intervention advancements, such as the use of ursodeoxycholic acid, have been investigated to enhance bile flow and reduce liver inflammation after the Kasai procedure. Furthermore, the identification of genetic factors, as recent GWAS have underscored, may offer possibilities for therapy aimed at the pathophysiologic mechanisms of the disease. Information on the role of some genes, like EFEMP1, being implicated with the structural function of the biliary tree, can lead to the creation of new therapeutic approaches. Therefore, continuous investigation into the pathophysiology and evolution of biliary atresia is crucial in order to direct future therapy and improve patient outcomes, as part of the dynamic state of pediatric liver disease treatment. Along with drug and surgical therapy, supportive management is important for the total care of biliary atresia. Nutritional support is crucial for the involved children, who tend to be malnourished as a result of impaired bile secretion. Prevention of complications like growth retardation and vitamin deficiency is of prime importance to ensure the best possible state of these patients. Regular monitoring allows for early intervention when complication like liver failure or portal hypertension arises, again underscoring the necessity of multidisciplinary care by pediatric gastroenterologists, surgeons, and nutritionists. In addition, understanding the regenerative properties of the liver and the involvement of stem/progenitor cell niches, as proposed in recent literature, suggests potential avenues for future research in pursuing recovery and regeneration in pediatric liver disease, including biliary atresia (Alvaro *et al.*, 2018; Bailey-Wilson *et al.*, 2018).

11.3.1. Surgical Interventions (e.g., Kasai Procedure)

Among the list of surgical interventions used in the treatment of biliary atresia, the Kasai procedure has emerged as the main primary intervention. The operation seeks to restore bile flow by removing the atretic bile ducts and anastomosing the liver to a loop of intestine directly, creating an anastomosis for bile drainage purposes. Timing of the surgery is critical; it is generally performed before the infant reaches three months of age due to the fact that results have been proven to significantly deteriorate if delayed. A successful outcome from the Kasai procedure can lead to enhanced liver function as well as a late requirement for liver transplant. The surgery is not a promise of success for all patients, and the majority will continue to require a liver transplant as the disease progresses. Understanding the multifaceted role of the Kasai procedure in biliary atresia is essential to improving clinical outcomes for infants with the disease. Postoperative monitoring is an essential part of assessing the effectiveness of the Kasai procedure and informing subsequent treatment. Research shows that serum total bilirubin level during the initial three months following the procedure is an essential biomarker for assessing clinical improvement. Specifically, infants with bilirubin levels below 2 mg/dL are associated with significantly improved transplant-free survival at age two compared to their peers who cannot achieve this level. Conversely, elevated bilirubin levels are associated with a greater risk for developing complications in the form of increased rates of ascites, hypoalbuminemia, and coagulopathy. These complications need early management, possibly even liver transplant, and therefore highlight the importance of monitoring and prompt decision-making in the case of children afflicted with biliary atresia (Arnon *et al.*, 2016). While the Kasai procedure is a critical intervention, its shortcomings are such that it needs a prolonged surgical method of addressing biliary atresia. Liver transplant has become the treatment of choice in infants and children who progress to end-stage liver disease, particularly in the setting of failure of surgical operations like the Kasai procedure. Liver transplant in children is complicated due to children's delicate anatomy. Strategies for minimizing operative risks and managing complications are crucial to ensuring good results. Advances in operative technique and post-operative management have improved performance in this area. Moreover, understanding the overall prognosis of biliary atresia is also a global outlook covering not only surgical outcomes but even long-term management and planning in individuals who may possibly need a transplant in the future (Wiederkehr *et al.*, 2016) (Figure 11.7).

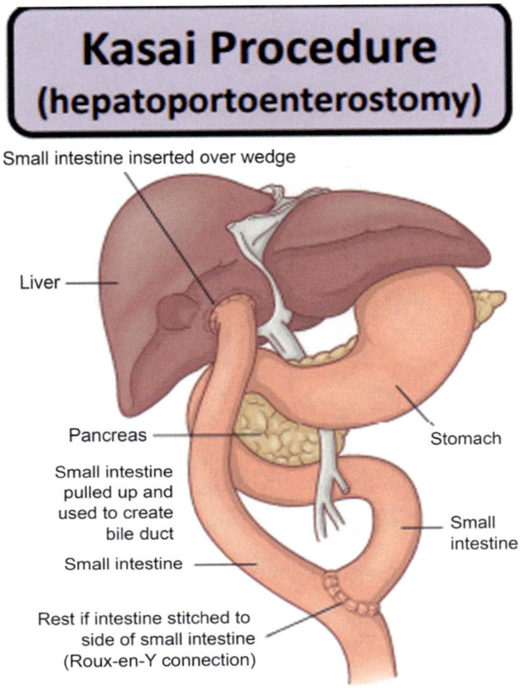

Figure 11.7. Kasai procedure.

Source: https://myanes.ca/wp-content/uploads/2021/12/image-2.png.

11.3.2. Liver Transplantation Considerations

The choice of liver transplantation for the child with biliary atresia and other disorders hinges heavily on the timing of treatment and the determinants. Biliary atresia is a syndrome of steadily progressing obstructed bile drainage that leads to liver damage and ultimately cirrhosis if left untreated. Traditionally, portoenterostomy has been a treatment option that, while beneficial for some newborns, is successful in only about 25% of patients. Thus, the majority of patients ultimately require liver transplantation as a last resort for end-stage liver disease. Candidate assessment for transplantation involves careful assessment processes to determine liver function, growth measurements, and psychosocial factors, to guarantee that the procedure offers the most available chance for improved quality of life and longevity. This comprehensive pre-transplant assessment is essential in addressing the unique challenges of the special needs of pediatric patients, most of whom have vastly different issues than adults. Logistical and technical issues of liver transplantation in infants and children are significantly affected by organ availability and graft size. Because of the stringent requirements for donor livers that can accommodate small patients, transplant units have increasingly modified their approach, wherein partial or smaller liver grafts are commonly used. This innovation encourages a more proactive response to address waiting lists while maximizing the utilization of available organs. Technological innovations are also complementarily enhancing the transplantation procedure, particularly with minimally invasive laparoscopic surgery that reduces recovery time and complications of traditional open surgery. The combination of such methods in children's liver transplantation is not just a significant advancement in surgical technique but also sensitive to the paramount goal of improving post-surgery results in high-risk populations of child patients (Berloco *et al.*, 2012). Post-transplant care remains a critical determinant of the success of liver transplantation in children with biliary atresia. Immunosuppression is vital in preventing organ rejection but has potential risks of severe side effects, such as nephrotoxicity and opportunistic infections, which need to be closely monitored. The use of cyclosporine, supplemented with low-dose prednisone, has been standard, though evolving treatment protocols are increasingly using triple or quadruple drug therapy to diminish these risks effectively. Additionally, the risk of graft reinfection reinforces the importance of individualized follow-up and includes the ongoing surveillance of immunosuppressive regimens. With ongoing research to develop new therapies like human monoclonal antibodies, the future for pediatric liver transplantation is bright to enhance patient prognosis and ensure long-term graft survival (Gordon *et al.*, 1988) (Figure 11.8).

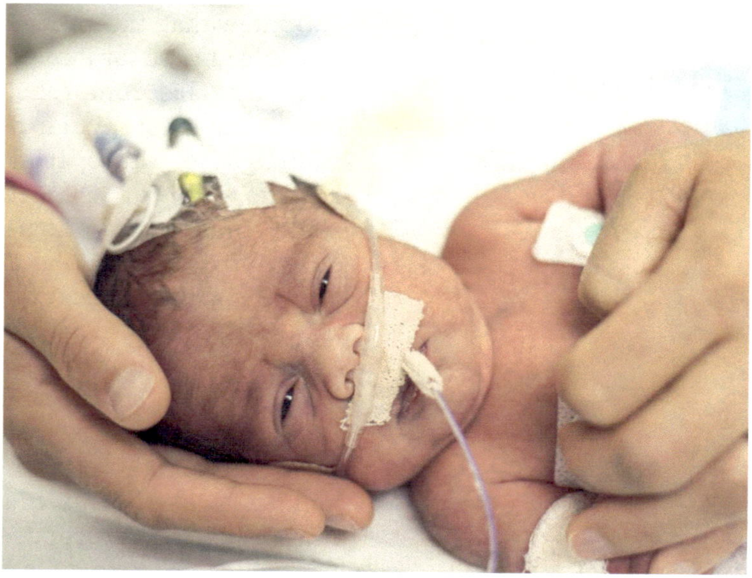

Figure 11.8. Four-month-old baby born with biliary atresia undergoes liver transplant.

Source: https://images.medindia.net/health-images/1200_1000/baby-ryan-mi.jpg.

11.3.3. Post-Operative Care and Management

Post-surgical care and management following liver surgery, particularly in children with biliary atresia, is necessary to ensure optimal recovery and avoid complications. After a procedure like a liver transplant, one has to be very careful about monitoring the vital signs and liver function. This includes close monitoring of bilirubin and coagulation profile because these are indicative of hepatic function and rejection or otherwise of the graft. As well, clinicians must carefully monitor for signs of infection because the surgical site can be a portal of entry for organisms, especially in immunocompromised children. Multidisciplinary teams made up of surgeons, nurses, and nutritionists have an important role in post-operative care on an individualized basis to make certain that each child's unique needs are addressed in recovery. In the case of biliary atresia, the fine points of recovery after surgery are complicated by the possibility of vascular malformations, which can exert a profound impact on results. Evidence shows that children with severe vascular anomalies, such as missing IVC or ectatic hepatic artery origin, have higher risks during and after transplantation. In these children, recognition of the same pre-operatively is relevant, allowing specific surgical techniques and better post-operative precautions. Consideration of these risks early in the evaluation is an indication of the importance of rigorous imaging and diligent pretransplant planning in order to ensure that the patient is adequately prepared for what they are going to endure following transplant. Management of these risks not only improves outcomes in the early recovery period but also increases long-term survival rates within this high-risk group (Lilly *et al.*, 1974). Furthermore, technological advancements in minimally invasive techniques, such as laparoscopic surgery, have revolutionized the post-operative care for liver procedures. Laparoscopy has proven to reduce pain, reduce hospital stays, and have lower infection rates around the wound than standard open surgery, which is a significant benefit for children. For children with liver transplantation, the use of laparoscopic techniques can help streamline their surgical procedure and enhance recovery outcomes. The transition to laparoscopic methods has further added to the increased outcomes in the aspect of exposure to heat and general surgery stress, making them an established practice in the treatment of liver pathologies. With developments further on, the addition of laparoscopic approaches to post-surgery care regimens is poised to remain in the limelight, highlighting increased demands for change and innovation in managing children's livers (Berloco *et al.*, 2012) (Figure 11.9).

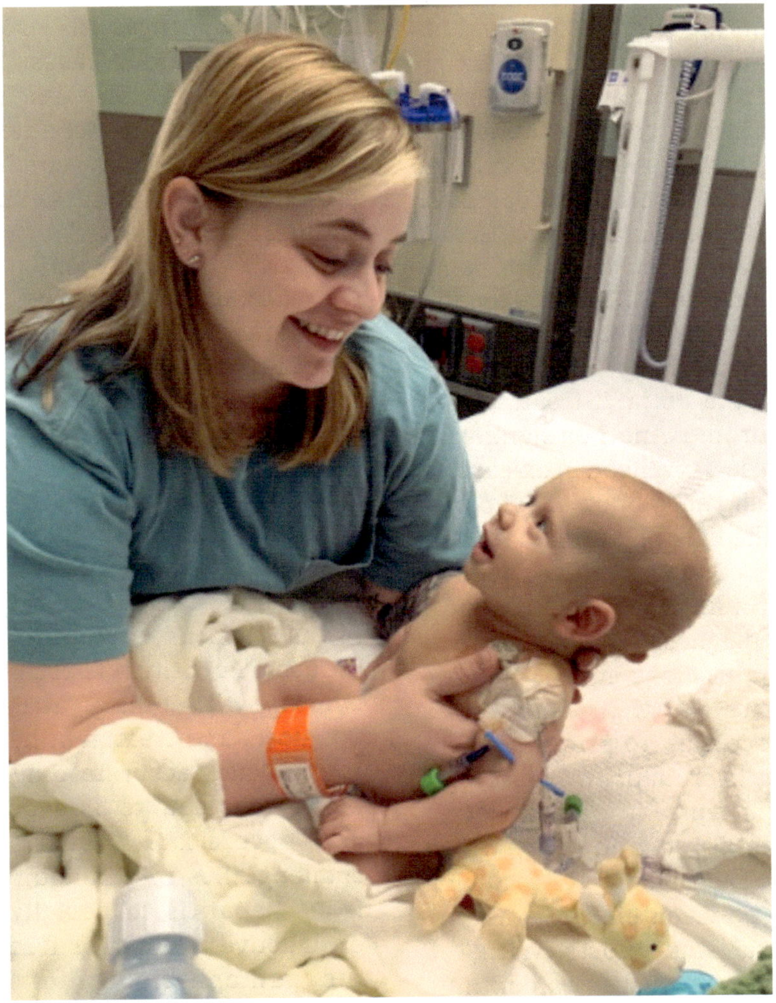

Figure 11.9. Post-operative care.

Source: https://www.reddit.com/media?url=https%3A%2F%2Fpreview.redd.it%2Fmy-tough-guy-and-his-mom-after-his-kasai-procedure-v0-0zmkkqv1oowa1.jpg%3Fwidth%3D1080%26crop%3Dsmart%26auto%3Dwebp%26s%3Daae2699bf68d504ef7f735a64416f7946bd13ad1&rdt=37562.

11.4. Other Pediatric Liver Diseases

The range of pediatric liver disorders goes much further than biliary atresia and includes a host of conditions that may greatly compromise liver function in infants and children. One such disease is hepatic encephalopathy (HE), a neuropsychiatric illness frequently encountered in CLD-affected children. It is caused by the buildup of toxins in the circulatory system due to the liver's inability to detoxify toxins effectively. This syndrome can also manifest as changes in conscious state, cognitive function, and behavior, highlighting the liver's critical role in maintaining metabolic homeostasis. Therapy for HE is based on numerous methods, with dietary manipulation and lactulose being effective in reducing ammonia. Early detection and treatment are crucial to prevent irreversible neurological injury, highlighting the importance of future research in the optimal treatment of this challenging syndrome. Another significant pediatric liver disease is Wilson's disease, a genetic disorder causing deposition of copper in tissues, particularly the liver and brain. Wilson's disease in children can present as hepatic failure, psychiatric findings, and neurological decline, which makes diagnosis and management difficult. The genetic etiology means genetic counseling of patients and their families, as early treatment is necessary to prevent severe consequences such as liver failure or neurologic damage. Treatment is typically with chelating drugs like penicillamine or zinc salts, which reduce copper levels. The challenge is achieving the delicate balance between effective therapy and limiting potential side effects. With the progress of research, new therapies continue to arise with the aim of enhancing patient outcomes and improving the quality of life for those suffering from this disorder. Cirrhosis, an outcome of many chronic liver diseases, is also a serious pediatric condition, perhaps secondary to the conditions of biliary atresia, metabolic disturbances, and viral hepatitis. This end-stage liver disease manifests as multifactorial liver dysfunction and portal hypertension with serious complications. Growth retardation, ascites, and the possibility of the development of hepatic encephalopathy (HE) are frequent abnormalities in the pediatric population with cirrhosis and require specialized care for nutritional adaptation and prevention of complications. Liver transplantation in children remains the last resort in end-stage liver disease, although challenges arise from the limited donor pool for pediatric cases. Moreover, children with congenital diseases like biliary atresia usually experience challenges to successful transplantation if concomitant vascular anomalies complicate surgical correction (Lilly *et al.*, 1974). The frequent occurrence of graft reinfection and post-transplantation complications also requires continuous follow-up and individually directed therapeutic measures in this high-risk group (Gordon *et al.*, 1988).

11.4.1. Hepatitis in Children

Hepatitis in children is a significant problem in the context of pediatric liver disease, and particularly that of biliary atresia. Hepatitis, an inflammation of the liver, presents in several forms, such as viral, autoimmune, and drug-induced hepatitis. These illnesses commonly overlap with biliary atresia, and therefore, diagnosis and treatment become cumbersome. Prompt and accurate diagnosis is crucial, as delay can lead to irrevocable liver damage and necessitate liver transplantation. The challenge lies in distinguishing biliary atresia from hepatitis, especially in infancy when obstructive jaundice is frequent. Furthermore, the pathophysiology of hepatitis has the tendency to exacerbate pre-existing diseases like biliary atresia by interfering with hepatic function and bile secretion, speeding up the disease process and its effects. The diagnostic approach to hepatitis in children is conservative assessment with the application of many imaging modalities and laboratory assessments. Even though ultrasound is commonly employed in primary assessments, more sophisticated patterns such as ultrasound elastography (USE) have also gained popularity, particularly in distinguishing between biliary atresia and hepatitis. USE sensitivity and specificity, indicated by a high area under the summary receiver operating characteristic curve, to validate it as a diagnostic tool for children that is non-invasive (Li *et al.*, 2022). The challenge continues to be in interpreting results because of overlapping clinical presentations of hepatitis and biliary atresia. It is hence necessary for pediatric clinicians to remain vigilant and aware of the latest diagnostic procedures and criteria in order to enable the optimal management of these liver diseases. Therapeutic strategies in the treatment of hepatitis in children, especially those with underlying biliary atresia, need to be balanced. Treatment may comprise antiviral treatment in the case of viral hepatitis or immunosuppressants for autoimmune types. Where liver function is largely affected by these conditions, patients are potential candidates for a liver transplant. Astoundingly, research has identified that growth hormone (GH) levels may be utilized as a prognostic factor during liver transplantation in children, indicating the interrelated dynamics between hepatitis, biliary atresia, and liver functionality (Kurabekova *et al.*, 2023). Therefore, an ongoing investigation exploring the interaction between such conditions is necessary because they can influence clinical practice and improve treatment outcome in affected children. On this basis, a proper comprehension of hepatitis and biliary atresia is critical for enabling personalized interventions and improving management of pediatric liver disease as a whole (Figure 11.10).

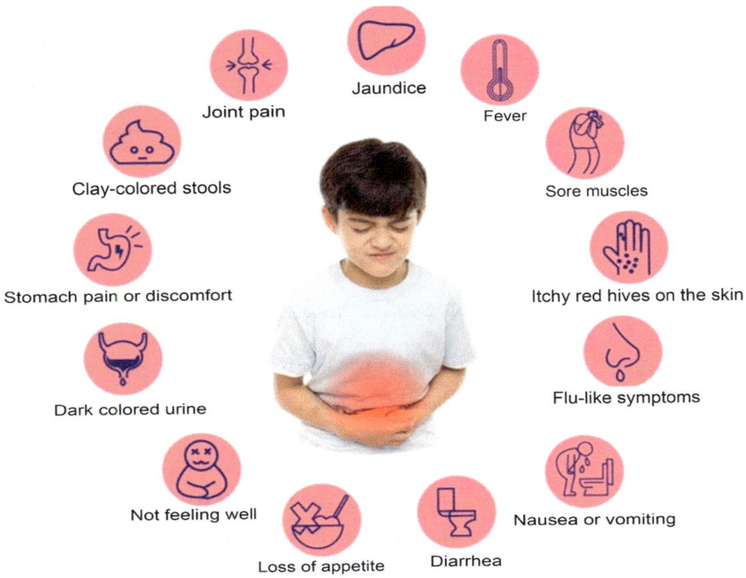

Figure 11.10. Hepatitis in children.

Source: https://scontent.fdel11-2.fna.fbcdn.net/v/t39.30808-6/274186056_4864850940271792_8893025994976886421_n.png?_nc_cat=107&ccb=1-7&_nc_sid=127cfc&_nc_ohc=ppljTbioPQQQ7kNvwEY1ybq&_nc_oc=AdkpTxKopzJpl8wx4ibX5-Yyom9e-aSdnFHAjepDnHx6oMZCQqSm6FCkW9jz0DVzy233RFPJgQFpwNYNQO3Ok08Q&_nc_zt=23&_nc_ht=scontent.fdel11-2.fna&_nc_gid=e4U90R1Lueu2Yt5A30mDcw&oh=00_AfKJWO6rW4TE74tmb1XBGM7j-x6ZV2PvPFLKjqAf2oSv7w&oe=6828AFD3.

11.4.2. Fatty Liver Disease in Pediatrics

The increasing prevalence of fatty liver disease in pediatric populations has significant public health and pediatric medical implications. The disease, which is characterized by the abnormal accumulation of lipids within hepatocytes, has emerged as a leading etiology of liver disease among children, which is most frequently linked to obesity, insulin resistance, and metabolic syndrome. While in the past it was thought to be a predominantly adult disease, studies indicate NAFLD is now impacting an enormous percentage of children.

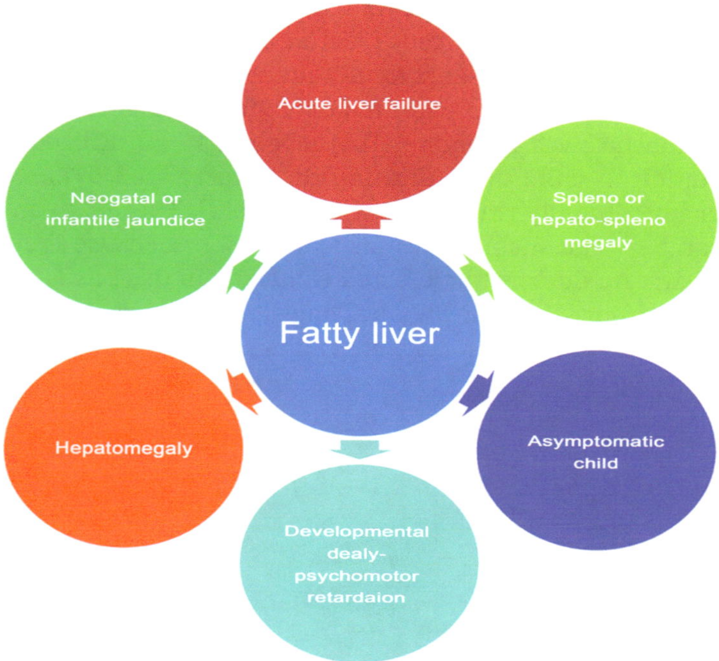

Figure 11.11. Clinical presentation of liver steatosis in children.

Source: https://www.researchgate.net/profile/Pietro-Vajro/publication/353952915/figure/fig1/AS:1057798678913024@1629210266248/Clinical-presentation-of-liver-steatosis-in-children-2.png.

The nonmetabolic presentation of infantile fatty liver disease is challenging for early diagnosis, typically resulting in late-stage presentations such as cirrhosis. Information about this illness is highly crucial because rising instances of obesity among children are directly contributing to the rising incidence of hepatic steatosis and related illnesses, making it mandatory to perform wide-ranging screening and preventive measures among children. Another important consideration for treating pediatric fatty liver illness is that one should be aware of its long-term consequences. CLD, of which types caused by conditions like fatty liver are some examples, are not merely temporary states; they may be precursors to more dire states like cirrhosis and HCC in later years. There is some emerging evidence that indicates children with fatty liver disease are at risk of later developing chronic liver disease, something that speaks to the need to act early and alter lifestyle. As discussed in the literature, children's liver diseases are often underdiagnosed since their presentation is insidious in the initial stages, and late intervention and diagnosis are the consequences (Alisi *et al.*, 2015). These problems need to be addressed since proper management can alter the natural history of liver diseases and produce more favorable outcomes for the diseased children (Alisi *et al.*, 2015). In the course of acquiring understanding and treating fatty liver disease, pediatricians, hepatologists, and pathologists must communicate. Proper diagnosis is highly reliant on clinical evaluation concordance, imaging studies, and histopathological findings, particularly where LBx needs to be used for determining hepatic steatosis severity and associated inflammation. Recent developments in liver pathology have yielded crucial insight into histopathologic features of fatty liver disease, enhancing diagnosis and guiding the appropriate therapeutic intervention. Pediatric liver transplantation, being a potential option in end-stage liver disease, is compounded by the complexity of the spectrum of conditions that need intervention; thus, identification of the histological features of fatty liver is crucial in optimizing the management of the patient (Alaggio *et al.*, 2022). This model of collaboration not only enables successful treatment modalities but also forms a greater understanding of evolving pediatric liver disease, strengthening the merit of early detection and intervention strategies (Figure 11.11).

11.4.3. Wilson's Disease and Its Implications

Wilson's disease is an autosomal recessive condition due to a mutation in the ATP7B gene that leads to copper deposition in the body. Wilson's disease is mainly hepatic and leads to hepatic failure, hepatocellular damage, and cirrhosis if left untreated. Wilson's disease in children may manifest as ALF or CLD, making differential diagnosis in pediatric practice challenging. Due to its genetic etiology, early diagnosis and treatment are very important, as ongoing accumulation may result in severe neuropsychiatric manifestations in addition to hepatic involvement. The interaction of hepatic health with neurological function makes it imperative that there should be wide-ranging management plans that address hepatic as well as extrahepatic symptoms, including appropriate emphasis on genetic counseling and family screening among involved groups. The implications of Wilson's disease extend past the immediate physical health of affected children; they also involve significant psychosocial elements affecting overall quality of life. Young patients often acquire a number of issues stemming from the chronic nature of the disease, including anxiety, depression, and social stigmatization of outwardly visible health challenges. Moreover, the regimen of treatment—increasingly extended to lifelong chelation therapy—may also be costly to both patients and their families. These regimens require strict adherence, regular monitoring by physicians, and robust support systems to offset the psychological costs. Notably, the emerging paradigm for Wilson's disease as one of the hereditary liver disease spectrum needs to have a greater focus on inclusive care models with the integration of mental health services and traditional medical management for optimal patient outcomes (Adams *et al.*, 2013). Liver transplant is an available curative option for advanced Wilson's disease, thereby revealing the intersection of surgical skill with gene disease therapy. By substituting the defective organ, OLT not only remedies the complications of copper deposition but also puts in a normal organ that will normalize copper metabolism. The intervention is a part of the broader context of organ transplantation in the treatment of genetic disease, particularly those diseases that have hepatic manifestations. One needs to remember, however, that although transplantation can remedy hepatic abnormalities, it will not remedy systemic manifestations related to the genetic defect. In accordance, further research is required in an attempt to further elucidate the complexities of Wilson's disease, our knowledge of its molecular pathogenesis, and its facilitation of improved therapeutic care for liver diseases in children that, as with biliary atresia, might also benefit from surgery (Hartley *et al.*, 1992) (Figure 11.12).

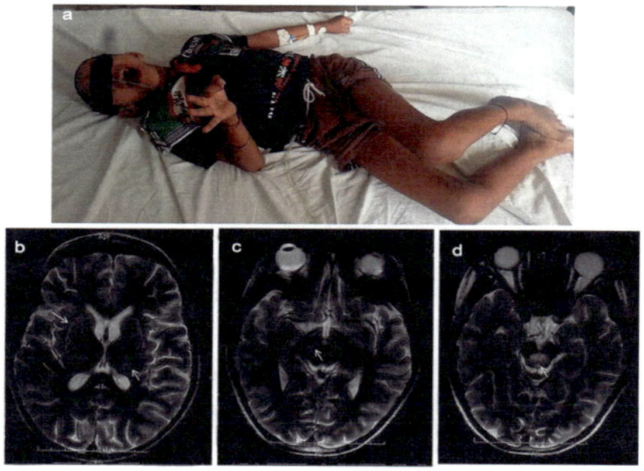

Figure 11.12. Clinical photograph and cranial MRI of a child with Wilson disease. (a) The clinical photograph shows severe generalized dystonia. There are mouth open, limb and truncal dystonia leading to bedridden state, nasogastric feeding, and anarthria. His MRI shows T2 hyperintense signal changes in (b) corpus striatum, thalamus, (c) substantia nigra, and (d) red nuclei bilaterally.

Source: https://www.researchgate.net/publication/342905395/figure/fig1/AS:962705838067712@1606538366682/Clinical-photograph-and-cranial-MRI-of-a-child-with-Wilson-disease-a-The-clinical.jpg.

11.5. Long-Term Outcomes and Prognosis

The prognosis for children diagnosed with biliary atresia (BA) can be significantly influenced by the degree of liver fibrosis evident at the time of follow-up LBx. Research indicates that patients presenting with mild fibrosis (F0-F2) tend to experience better long-term native-liver survival (NLS) compared to those with severe fibrosis (F3, F4). BA progress causes more problems and happens more quickly in children with advanced fibrosis, which is a worrying sign. Also, severe fibrosis brings more problems than just a low survival rate, as these children often have more complications that can reduce their well-being and physical health. This underscores the importance of regular monitoring and intervention strategies that can preemptively address and mitigate the complications associated with advanced liver disease in BA patients (Takase *et al.*, 2025). The role of liver transplantation (LT) emerges as a critical avenue for managing pediatric liver diseases, including BA. Liver transplantation is shown to be very helpful in the long run for patients whose liver function does not improve with Kasai portoenterostomy. Patients who receive LT tend to have good survival rates, which highlights LT as a good option when standard treatments do not work. Five years after LT, most pediatric patients with BA and similar liver diseases survive, which makes LT a good option for treating their end-stage liver disease. Continued research and data collection are essential to enhance understanding and improve protocols surrounding LT in this vulnerable demographic (Kar *et al.*, 2025). In addition, the long-term results for kids with biliary atresia and other liver diseases depend greatly on their ongoing medical care and monitoring. After the Kasai procedure and other initial surgeries, patients need ongoing care to monitor their liver health and manage any problems that come up. Using this complete approach is very important for improving how well these children live and for their survival. Various findings show that patients who get regular check-ups and early help for complications do better than those who do not. Because of this, it is important to focus on educating patients, including caregivers, and to bring together different specialists in pediatric care to manage biliary atresia better. By refining approaches to secondary diseases and complications, healthcare professionals can significantly affect the long-term prognosis of this patient population (Takase *et al.*, 2025).

11.5.1. Quality of Life Post-Treatment

Quality of life after biliary atresia treatment and other liver diseases in children mostly determines long-term outcomes for children affected. Following diagnosis and treatment that can involve surgery or liver transplant, most patients recover significantly in their health status. For instance, research indicates that a liver transplant can effectively cure end-stage liver disease, with significant relief from chronic liver disease signs and symptoms. Above all, in survivors of child liver transplantation, most of them have general health improvements, including normal development and enhanced liver function. Such changes tend to have a major impact on the daily life of the affected children, allowing them to engage in activities that are typical for their age and, therefore, bringing an element of normalcy to their childhood lives (Gartner *et al.*, 1984). But even though physical benefits after treatment are noteworthy, neither can the psychosocial quality of life after treatment be overlooked. Those patients who undergo exhaustive medical intervention are equally likely to suffer from emotional and psychological distress caused by the illness process, repeated hospitalization, and the altered pace of their daily routines. These factors can cause stress and anxiety, not only in the patients but also in their families. Support networks, including educational interventions, counseling, and peer support groups, can provide necessary coping mechanisms that enhance resilience and quality of life following treatment. Incorporating physical recuperation with emotional well-being is a holistic approach to taking care of biliary atresia patients, in that quality of life is more than just physical (Bailey-Wilson *et al.*, 2018). As a consequence of the above-stated multifaceted aspect of post-treatment quality of life, ongoing monitoring and follow-up are vital aspects of care for children with liver disease. Follow-up should not only analyze liver function and other physiological parameters, but also emotional and psychological health. Incorporating quality of life assessment into routine clinical practice allows physicians to detect areas where patients may need additional support, hence rectifying potential problems before they escalate. Besides, research on long-term conditions of children who have been treated for biliary atresia has provided insights into patterns of quality of life that inform future care management. As medical technology continues to improve, it is important to understand the long-term effect of treatment on quality of life among such patients in a bid to improve their overall health trajectories (Gartner *et al.*, 1984) (Figure 11.13).

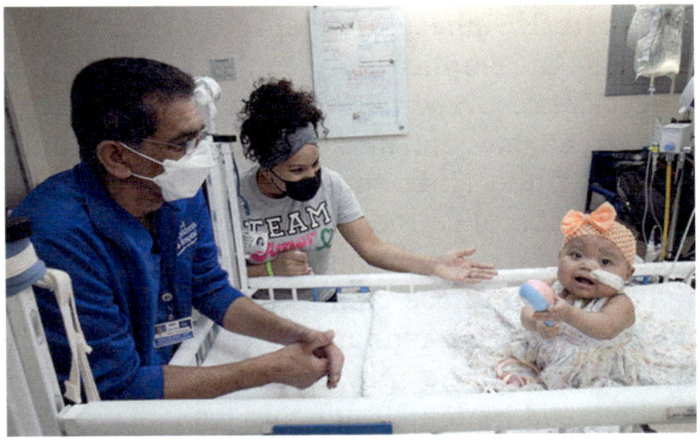

Figure 11.13. Quality of Life Post-Treatment

Source: https://storage.googleapis.com/jacksonh/1/Danilia_Liver-Disease-8.jpg.

11.5.2. Potential Complications and Follow-Up Care

Treatment of biliary atresia also requires a precise balancing of disease and treatment complications. Post-operative biliary obstruction is one of the complications, which is the biliary obstruction resulting from the narrowing of hepatic bile ducts. This complication carries a serious risk during the months following surgical interventions such as the Kasai operation, aimed at restoring bile flow. According to recent findings, postoperative problems in the early phase typically lead to increased morbidity and further surgery, which can result in patient interactions that long-term follow-up will have to handle (Putnam *et al.*, 1976). Therefore, follow-up imaging studies and evaluation, particularly within the first two years following surgery, are crucial in maintaining close monitoring of the liver's function and early identification of obstructions, thus allowing for timely interventions that could prevent serious outcomes for the pediatric patient. Transplantation, particularly if biliary atresia progresses to end-stage liver disease, is a significant part of follow-up management. After liver transplantation, complications may include rejection phases, biliary leaks, and vascular complications, which are usual in the postoperative phase after surgery (Gartner *et al.*, 1984). Complications can complicate the process of recovery, and thus, strict monitoring of liver enzymes and also bilirubin levels should be carried out since these levels may indicate possible complications of graft function. The success of transplantation in children can highly rely on these complications, and hence, close long-term management is necessary. Furthermore, the psychosocial impact on families and patients following transplantation must be taken into consideration, as dealing with the facts of chronic illness and the need for life-long immunosuppressive therapy can be challenging. Both medical and behavioral health support systems must be included in the follow-up care plan. Prognosis for long-term survival among children with biliary atresia can be significantly enhanced through proper follow-up management, meeting the physical as well as psychological needs of these patients. Survivorship in pediatric patients following liver transplantation, for instance, has been associated with a high survival rate of over 50% on the anniversary date in patients under optimal medical observation (Gartner *et al.*, 1984). Continuous follow-up care permits intervention to be tailored to repeated reevaluation of liver function and overall health status. Additionally, education of caregivers for signs of potential complications and compliance with follow-up appointments aids in the preservation of health impacts. With the increasing age of patients, transition planning is crucial to ensure the provision of age-appropriate care and support services for a healthy life span. Hence, a multimodal and holistic approach is required to minimize complications and maintain long-term health in children with biliary atresia.

11.5.3. Importance of Early Detection and Intervention

The significance of prompt detection and intervention of biliary atresia (BA) cannot be overstated, as it is central to improving patient outcomes. BA is the leading cause of liver transplantation in children and rapidly evolves to severe complications if not timely diagnosed and treated. Early detection allows for surgical interventions, like the Kasai portoenterostomy, to be implemented that are much more effective when done during the early months of life. Delayed detection can lead to permanent impairment of liver function and to the need for transplantation later on, when it is more risky and complex. Thus, raising the level of public awareness and educating medical practitioners about BA symptoms is important towards enhancing early detection rates and facilitating early medical intervention. Focus on early intervention also has backing from the extreme consequences of late treatment. Late diagnosis after the window period of optimal time for surgery drastically decreases the likelihood of restoring biliary flow successfully. Thus, untreated BA or delayed treatment results in progressive liver damage, cirrhosis, and eventually death in early life. It is reported that many cases of BA are diagnosed late, as parents and general practitioners are unaware of the signs and symptoms of the disease. By integrating education and support into community health programs, we can increase awareness and provide children with BA timely surgical care. Increasing the knowledge base of providers and families about BA is crucial to reducing the number of delayed diagnoses and enhancing the quality of care for affected infants. Education programs for healthcare providers and the public have been demonstrated to have a dramatic increase in knowledge and awareness about biliary atresia. Pre- and post-test evaluation in one study revealed that education caused dramatic knowledge increases in the audience, emphasizing the effect of targeted education. By empowering parents and healthcare professionals with knowledge about BA, we can introduce earlier diagnosis and, subsequently, earlier treatment. Because treatment regimens are crucial to avoiding the life-threatening consequences of biliary atresia, a culture that greatly values education and health-seeking behavior is also essential. Not only are such interventions worthwhile for survival, but also for enhancing the quality of life in children suffering from this volatile condition, highlighting the key role played by early detection and intervention in breaking pediatric liver disease (Aji *et al.*, 2020; Lachaux *et al.*, 2005).

SUMMARY

By and large, the complexity of biliary atresia and liver disease in children underscores the imperative need for early detection and intervention. The relationship between these ailments and the long-term health of the children highlights a developing issue of concern for pediatricians as well as parents. As suggested by the technology in surgical techniques, such as delayed primary closure and microsurgical anastomosis, there have in fact been revolutionary developments in optimizing post-operative conditions. Above all, the provision of new immunosuppressants and frequent anti-coagulation procedures has been positively contributing to the overall prognosis, emphasizing the importance of continuous innovation in surgical treatment and post-operative treatment as a contributor towards patient survival and quality of life improvement (Ziaziaris *et al.*, 2017). Furthermore, the psychosocial effects of diseases of children's livers, like biliary atresia, should never be underestimated. Studies indicate that such children are often characterized by educational difficulties, psychopathology, and interrupted neurodevelopmental trajectories. The findings that imply early intervention, particularly in the form of immediate surgical treatment, as a means to achieve better development outcomes further underscore the necessity of a multi-aspect intervention. Addressing both the physical and the neurodevelopmental aspects can radically change a child's development and adjustment in living with a chronic condition (Earl *et al.*, 2024). Therefore, the inclusion of neurodevelopmental assessments in the routine treatment of biliary atresia in children can provide crucial information regarding their developmental course and permit interventions in advance to avoid adverse outcomes. Therefore, the management of biliary atresia and other pediatric liver diseases in their entirety comprises a multidisciplinary approach encompassing surgery, monitoring, and preemptive neurodevelopmental treatment. The implications of such complex disorders extend beyond the immediate clinical needs; they include the general development and health of those involved. Continued research and clinical advancement are necessary to enhance treatment protocols and achieve better holistic outcomes. By fostering an interdependent system of collaboration between medical teams, families, and support systems, we are better suited to enhance the opportunities and general quality of life for children battling the challenges of biliary atresia and other liver diseases in children, ultimately enabling them to thrive early in life and beyond.

Biliary atresia (BA) is a serious liver disease of infancy characterized by increasingly severe inflammation and ultimate obliteration of the biliary tree. The disease leads to bile drainage obstruction, cholestasis, and ultimately liver failure without intervention. The urgency of surgical intervention, in the form of the Kasai procedure, is the most critical to avoid the severe effects of BA, as nonintervention of this leads to a very poor prognosis during the early years of life. The most common indication of liver transplantation in children throughout the globe, BA is particularly challenging and highlights the significance of early diagnosis and intervention as part of an attempt to improve long-term results. Recent research also indicates that the impact of BA does not just extend to hepatic failure but also encompasses significant neurodevelopmental complications arising in infancy, a time frame for brain growth, which is evidence of the multidimensional nature of the disease (Earl *et al.*, 2024). The interconnectedness of biliary atresia with other pediatric liver diseases is evidenced by the findings that show how initial interventions determine neurodevelopmental status. Research illustrates a startling prevalence of neurodevelopmental disorders and autism spectrum disorder (ASD) in children with BA, illustrating how CLD may undermine cognitive as well as social function. Kasai procedure timing and early surgical interventions appear to be decisive factors in developmental outcomes for children with BA. This suggests that not only does the disease itself pose a threat to physical health, but it also poses a high risk to cognitive and social development—key factors in a child's overall health and resultant quality of life (Earl *et al.*, 2024). Therefore, increasing surgical timing and monitoring of developmental outcomes would enhance the quality-of-care plans in this vulnerable population. Furthermore, the study of the genetic underpinnings of biliary atresia has been demonstrated to yield clues that may represent vital bridges to its pathogenesis. Investigations have revealed the presence of potential genetic susceptibilities, such as certain mutations in the PKHD1 gene, which have been implicated in both biliary atresia as well as overlapping conditions such as autosomal recessive polycystic kidney disease. Discovery of the molecular pathways that tie these disorders together could allow for targeted genetic therapy and early screening regimens. Evidence suggests that dysregulation of epithelial cell proliferation might be involved in the pathology of both BA and renal disease secondary to it, and thus, investigation into shared pathways that these diseases may utilize becomes even more critical. Lastly, the integration of current knowledge regarding genetic markers and liver function can contribute to improved diagnostic and treatment plans, validating the utility of an integrated care model in treating biliary atresia and child health.

CLOSER LOOK

CYTOMEGALOVIRUS (CMV)

CMV is a common herpesvirus that often causes no symptoms in healthy individuals, but can be serious in newborns and those with weakened immune systems. CMV is a ubiquitous infection, with most people acquiring it early in life, often without knowing it. While many remain asymptomatic, some may experience mild, flu-like symptoms, while individuals with weakened immune systems or pregnant women may face more serious complications (Figure 11.14).

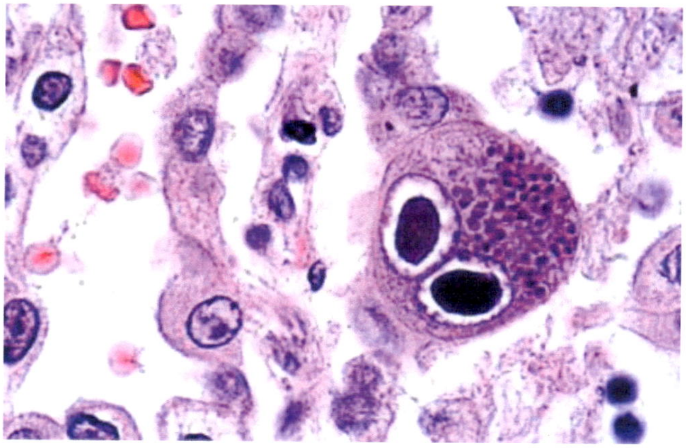

Figure 11.14. Cytomegalovirus (CMV)

Source: https://img.medscapestatic.com/pi/meds/ckb/33/37033tn.jpg.

- **Transmission:** CMV is spread through body fluids like saliva, urine, blood, and breast milk, as well as through sexual contact and during childbirth.
- **Latent Infection:** Once infected, CMV remains in the body for life, often dormant, and can reactivate under certain circumstances.
- **Symptoms:** Healthy individuals may be asymptomatic or experience mild symptoms like fever and fatigue. However, in those with weakened immune systems, CMV can cause serious complications like pneumonia, blindness, or encephalitis.
- **Pregnancy:** CMV infection during pregnancy can lead to serious health problems in the baby, including hearing loss and developmental delays.
- **Congenital CMV:** Newborns infected with CMV before or during birth can experience serious health problems, with hearing loss being the most common long-term issue.
- **Diagnosis** Diagnosis can be made by blood tests, tissue biopsy samples, or direct examination.
- **Treatment:** Treatment is generally not needed for healthy individuals with mild symptoms. However, antiviral medications may be used to treat severe cases in immunocompromised individuals or newborns.

References

1. Adams, A., Ajioka, Y., Alagille, D., Ambrosino, G., Araki, T., Arias, I. M., *et al.* (2013). *Monogenic Diseases That Can Be Cured by Liver Transplantation*. https://core.ac.uk/download/589954856.pdf.
2. Aji, A., Safira, A., Amaliah, R., Ismet, M., Febriadi, M., Kurnia, D., *et al.* (2020). *Analysis of Knowledge Regarding Biliary Atresia Among Healthcare Providers and Laypersons in East Jakarta After Educational Intervention*. https://core.ac.uk/download/639378387.pdf (accessed on 24 May 2025).
3. Alaggio, R., Caporalini, C., Ferro, J., Francalanci, P., *et al.* (2022). Not only a small liver – The pathologist's perspective in the pediatric liver transplant setting. https://core.ac.uk/download/512042380.pdf (accessed on 24 May 2025).
4. Alisi, A., Alterio, A., Della Corte, C., Mosca, A., *et al.* (2015). *Pediatric Liver Diseases: Current Challenges and Future Perspectives*. https://core.ac.uk/download/84688423.pdf (accessed on 24 May 2025).
5. Alvaro, D., Cardinale, V., Carpino, G., Franchitto, A., *et al.* (2018). Contribution of resident stem cells to liver and biliary tree regeneration in human diseases. https://core.ac.uk/download/188824417.pdf (accessed on 24 May 2025).
6. Arnon, R., Bass, L. M., Bezerra, J. A., Haber, B. A., *et al.* (2016). Total serum bilirubin within 3 months of hepatoportoenterostomy predicts short-term outcomes in biliary atresia. https://core.ac.uk/download/84831921.pdf (accessed on 24 May 2025).
7. Augustiniene, R., Cao, J. Y., Cekuolis, A., Chen, W., *et al.* (2023). Review on pediatric malignant focal liver lesions with imaging evaluation: Part I. https://core.ac.uk/download/596417762.pdf (accessed on 24 May 2025).
8. Bailey-Wilson, J. E., Chen, Y., Devoto, M., Gilbert, J. R., *et al.* (2018). A genome-wide association study identifies a susceptibility locus for biliary atresia on 2p16.1 within the gene EFEMP1. https://core.ac.uk/download/160649031.pdf (accessed on 24 May 2025).
9. Berloco, P. B., Di Laudo, M., Frattaroli, F. M., Guglielmo, N., *et al.* (2012). Laparoscopy in liver transplantation: The future has arrived. https://core.ac.uk/download/154948504.pdf (accessed on 24 May 2025).
10. Blair-Reid, S. A. (2010). *An Investigation of The Ciliary Protein PKHD1 in Cyst Development in Liver Disease: Clues to The Pathogenesis of Biliary Atresia*. Centre for Liver Research School of Immunity and Infection College of Medical and Dental Sciences University of Birmingham https://core.ac.uk/download/75865.pdf
11. Borel, P., Shaw, B. W., Calne, R. Y., Esquivel, C. O., Hanto, D. W., Hume, D. M., Iwatsuki, S., *et al.* (1985). *Indications for Liver Transplantation in The Cyclosporine Era*. https://core.ac.uk/download/12204044.pdf (accessed on 24 May 2025).
12. Clemente, M. G., & Dessanti, A. (2016). Emergencies in neonatal management: Jaundice and biliary atresia. https://core.ac.uk/download/33724315.pdf (accessed on 24 May 2025).
13. Earl, M. (2024). An investigation into the neurodevelopmental profile of infants and children with chronic liver disease. https://core.ac.uk/download/603255692.pdf (accessed on 24 May 2025).

14. Gartner, J. C., Iwatsuki, S., Malatack, J. J., Shaw, B. W., *et al.* (1984). *Orthotopic Liver Transplantation in Children: Two-Year Experience With 47 Patients*. https://core.ac.uk/download/12203968.pdf (accessed on 24 May 2025).
15. Gezer, H. Ö. (2019). *Pediatric Choledochal Cysts: Unknowns are Decreasing*. https://core.ac.uk/download/322443267.pdf (accessed on 24 May 2025).
16. Gordon, R. D., & Starzl, T. E. (1988). *Changing Perspectives on Liver Transplantation In 1988*. https://core.ac.uk/download/12204389.pdf (accessed on 24 May 2025).
17. Gordon, R. D., Iwatsuki, S., Lerut, J., Starzl, T. E., *et al.* (1987). Surgical complications in human orthotopic liver transplantation. https://core.ac.uk/download/12204197.pdf (accessed on 24 May 2025).
18. Hartley, J. L. (1992). *The Molecular Genetic Investigation of Pediatric Liver Disease* [Doctoral dissertation, University of Birmingham]. https://core.ac.uk/download/pdf/40029640.pdf (accessed on 24 May 2025).
19. Kar, H. D. D., Aydın, H. İ., Özçay, F., Sezer, O. B., Baskın, E., Şahin, F., Terzi, Y., *et al.* (2025). Short and long-term outcomes of liver transplantation in pediatric patients with inborn errors of metabolism: A single-center study. *Pediatric Transplantation, 29*(3), e70067. https://www.semanticscholar.org/paper/22cf52000b79ae812ea56b9bac8c2bd661aca93d (accessed on 24 May 2025).
20. Kerola, A. (2019). *Native Liver Fibrosis in Biliary Atresia: From Pathobiology to Clinical Outcomes* [Doctoral dissertation, University of Helsinki]. https://core.ac.uk/download/224641302.pdf (accessed on 24 May 2025).
21. Kurabekova, R., Silina, O., Tsirulnikova, O., Pashkova, I., Gichkun, O., Olefirenko, G., Oleshkevich, S. Y., *et al.* (2023). Prognostic significance of growth hormone in pediatric liver transplantation. *Russian Journal of Transplantology and Artificial Organs*. https://www.semanticscholar.org/paper/a907a8aca1b8e5b1398b4628abf18012a727feb2 (accessed on 24 May 2025).
22. Lachaux, A., Strickland, A. D., Abuhamad, A. Z., Bangaru, B., Fischler, B., Gridelli, B., *et al.* (2005). *Biliary Atresia*. https://core.ac.uk/download/pdf/4041581.pdf.
23. Li, Y. q., Jiang, J. q., & Wang, H. (2022). Ultrasound elastography in the diagnosis of biliary atresia in pediatric surgery: A systematic review and meta-analysis of diagnostic test. *Translational Pediatrics, 11*, 748–756. https://www.semanticscholar.org/paper/42c1927604bc4b619ddc215298f40bbe968517db (accessed on 24 May 2025).
24. Lilly, J. R., & Starzl, T. E. (1974). Live transplantation in children with biliary atresia and vascular anomalies. https://core.ac.uk/download/12203758.pdf (accessed on 24 May 2025).
25. Madadi-Sanjani, O., Uecker, M., Thomas, G., Fischer, L., Hegen, B., Herrmann, J., Reinshagen, K., & Tomuschat, C. (2024). Optimizing Post-Kasai Management in Biliary Atresia: Balancing Native Liver Survival and Transplant Timing. European Journal of Pediatric Surgery. https://www.semanticscholar.org/paper/Optimizing-Post-Kasai-Management-in-Biliary-Native-Madadi-Sanjani-Uecker/8a50b7646d11fd004bb69c316caeff2bfe356547
26. Motazedian, N., Azarpira, N., Falamarzi, K., Dehghani, S., Ataollahi, M., Esfandiari, E., Dara, M., *et al.* (2024). Comparison of Mir122 expression in children with biliary atresia and healthy group. *Molecular Biology Research Communications, 13*, 147–154. https://www.semanticscholar.org/paper/291d7db799f71a922517f22b1e7cc67998db8a0a (accessed on 24 May 2025).

27. Nydegger, A., Sevilla, A., Gillams, A. R., Gaines, B. A., Colombo, C., Metreweli, C., Sivit, C. J., *et al.* (2010). *Hepatobiliary and Pancreatic Imaging in Children—Techniques and An Overview of Non-Neoplastic Disease Entities*. https://core.ac.uk/download/pdf/8510110.pdf (accessed on 24 May 2025).

28. Parmar, A., Miethke, A., Feldman, A., Lowichik, A., Klipsch, A., Rutherford, A., Sherker, A., *et al.* (2022). *Serum Biomarkers Correlated with Liver Stiffness Assessed in A Multicenter Study of Pediatric Cholestatic Liver Disease*. https://core.ac.uk/download/643777678.pdf.

29. Putnam, C. W., DeShazo, R. D., Porter, K. A., Lilly, J. R., Weil, R., Starzl, T. E., *et al.* (1976). *Transplantation in Children*. https://core.ac.uk/download/12203776.pdf (accessed on 24 May 2025).

30. Shanker, A. I., Maloney, L. T., & Boster, J. M. (2025). Leukocytosis is common following pediatric liver transplant for biliary atresia but should be interpreted with caution. *OBM Transplantation*. https://www.semanticscholar.org/paper/cda2975e4e5101e0857d64af2cc7f5dc76e10689 (accessed on 24 May 2025).

31. Takase, K., Ueno, T., Matsumoto, S., Uga, N., Deguchi, K., Nomura, M., Watanabe, M., *et al.* (2025). Impact of follow-up liver biopsy on long-term outcomes post-Kasai procedure in patients with biliary atresia. *Pediatric Surgery International, 41*. https://www.semanticscholar.org/paper/a9d19faa7794d93ff53724ca1c54c9cce5cdd7d9 (accessed on 24 May 2025).

32. Ushijima, K., Sanada, Y., Otomo, S., Ogaki, K., Wakiya, T., Okada, N., Hirata, Y., *et al.* (2025). Inherited metabolic diseases are a potent risk factor for cytomegalovirus infection in pediatric living donor liver transplantation. *BMC Infectious Diseases, 25*. https://www.semanticscholar.org/paper/4ba7f2ec37408496f7695e866f2c42e5e4362d70 (accessed on 24 May 2025).

33. Hove Van , J. V., Friederich, M. W., Strode, D. K., Van Hove, R. A., Miller, K. R., Sharma, R., Shah, H., *et al.* (2024). Protein biomarkers GDF15 and FGF21 to differentiate mitochondrial hepatopathies from other pediatric liver diseases. *Hepatology Communications, 8*. https://www.semanticscholar.org/paper/08d74975d021e55f736c89c84c0aabe5c06ca873 (accessed on 24 May 2025).

34. van Wessel, D. (2020). *Rare Cholestatic Childhood Diseases: Advances in Clinical Care* [Doctoral dissertation, University Medical Center Utrecht]. https://core.ac.uk/download/519034534.pdf.

35. Wiederkehr, B. de A., Wiederkehr, H. de A., & Wiederkehr, J. C. (2016). *Pediatric Liver Transplantation*. https://core.ac.uk/download/322427360.pdf (accessed on 24 May 2025).

36. Ziaziaris, W. A. (2017). *Pediatric Liver Transplantation: Improvement in Outcomes* [Master's thesis, University of Sydney]. https://core.ac.uk/download/212688772.pdf (accessed on 24 May 2025).

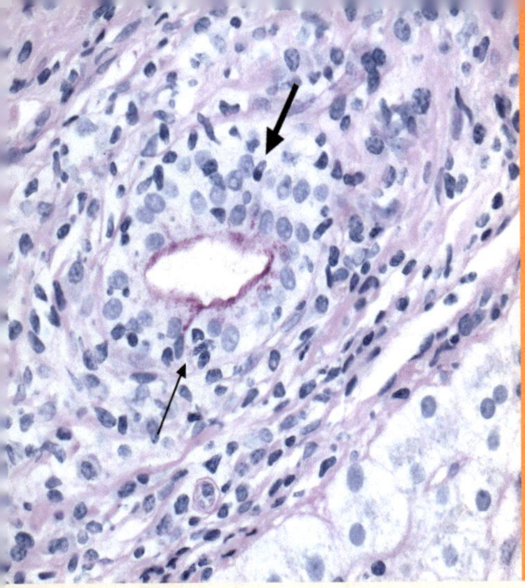

Chapter 12

PRIMARY BILIARY CHOLANGITIS (PBC) AND PRIMARY SCLEROSING CHOLANGITIS (PSC)

Contents

Introduction

The study of liver diseases has assumed more importance with their complex pathophysiology and the development of illnesses such as Primary Biliary Cholangitis (PBC) and Primary Sclerosing Cholangitis (PSC). Both conditions have cholestasis, a disruption of bile flow, as the shared characteristic, leading to liver damage and a set of disabling manifestations. PBC is most common in women and is believed to be of autoimmune origin, where the immune system of the body acts against the bile ducts. PSC, however, is associated strongly with IBD and occurs more frequently in men. Both of these conditions need to be recognized due to their role extending beyond the physical sphere to impact the patient's quality of life and necessitate multidisciplinary management plans addressing clinical as well as psychosocial factors. The intricate interaction between BAs and cholestatic liver conditions necessitates the identification of new treatment strategies. BAs are not just digestive enzymes but also signaling molecules that can regulate liver pathology and disease aetiology. Alterations in bile acid composition and flow in patients with PBC and PSC have been noted, influencing pathology and symptom expression, such as severe pruritus. Previous research has determined that pharmacological blockade of the apical sodium-dependent bile acid transporter (ASBT) could potentially have therapeutically valuable implications for these conditions. By altering the circulating bile acid pool, there is a potential for clinicians to improve symptom management and potentially avoid disease progression, providing an interesting area for further research (Hegade *et al.*, 2017). Treatment regimens for PBC and PSC have previously focused on immunosuppressive treatment aimed at slowing disease activity and symptom relief. With the exception of liver transplantation, definitive options are limited, making it critical to continue research into effective medical management. The intricacy involved in the treatment of autoimmune liver diseases like PBC and PSC underlines the necessity for individualized, patient-centered treatment regimens that account for variability in individual patient requirements and therapeutic response. Current literature provides a critical review of the merits and limitations of various immunosuppressive therapies, providing an impetus for an understanding of their role within the global management of autoimmune liver disease (Abhyankar *et al.*, 2013). This chapter will also provide an elaboration of the pathophysiology, diagnosis, and new therapeutic strategies of PBC and PSC to enhance understanding and effectiveness of treatment regimens.

Definition of Primary Biliary Cholangitis (PBC)

The term PBC designates a chronic autoimmune liver disease characterized by the progressive destruction of the small bile ducts within the liver. This condition predominantly affects middle-aged women, manifesting through bile accumulation that ultimately leads to cholestasis, fibrosis, and, in advanced cases, cirrhosis. While the precise etiology of PBC remains to a large extent unknown, it is considered to be a complex interplay of genetic predisposition and environmental exposures, in addition to dysregulated immune responses to the cholangiocytes—the epithelial cells of the bile duct. Symptoms are usually nonspecific in presentation and include fatigue, pruritus (pruritus sicca), and jaundice, which can significantly impair quality of life. Also, the disease may persist for years without symptoms, highlighting the importance of early diagnosis and follow-up for proper control. Research work has clarified some of the pathologic mechanisms present in the course of PBC, with a focus on the epigenetic alterations seen in PBC patients. Epigenome-wide association studies, such as those with the Illumina MethylationEPIC Bead Chip, have found notable variation between patients in methylation levels and suggested that there is an association between these alterations and disease expression. For instance, increased epigenetic age acceleration mirrors that PBC can lead to premature cellular aging. Besides, these studies have mentioned specific genes involved in immunity, such as the NOD-like receptor family and human leukocyte antigen, which play an essential role in understanding how the disease progresses and potential therapeutic measures. The studies have indicated that abnormal immune signaling may be responsible for the death of cholangiocytes, further attesting to the autoimmune basis of PBC and calling for more research into its mechanisms (Juran *et al.*, 2024). By way of comparison, it is important to distinguish PBC from Primary Sclerosing Cholangitis (PSC), a second autoimmune liver disease of distinctive characteristics. While PBC tends to target small bile ducts and is strongly female-dominated, PSC involves medium to large bile ducts and is strongly male-dominated. PSC patients have a much increased risk of cholangiocarcinoma (CCA), which is a carcinoma arising in bile duct cells. This inequality underscores the importance of understanding the unique immune surveillance mechanisms of each disease. For instance, it has been suggested that PBC autoimmune processes confer a certain protection against CCA, whereas chronic inflammation in PSC promotes cancer risk. This observation fosters the understanding of liver-related complications developed due to these diseases and emphasizes the necessity for personalized therapeutic treatments in affected individuals (Nanjundappa *et al.*, 2023) (Figure 12.1).

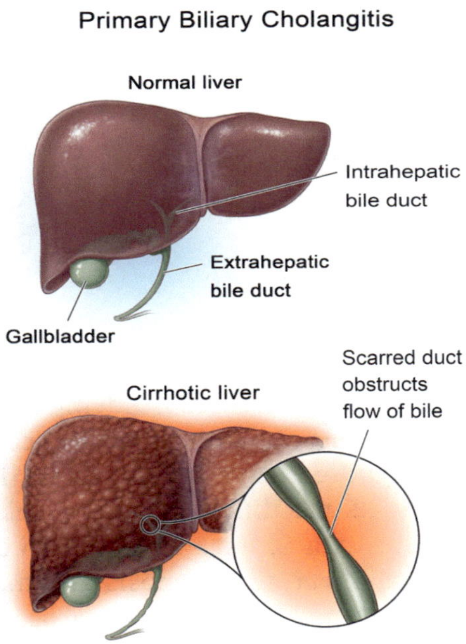

Figure 12.1. Primary biliary cholangitis (PBC).

Source: https://my.clevelandclinic.org/-/scassets/images/org/health/articles/17715-primary-biliary-cholangitis.

Definition of Primary Sclerosing Cholangitis (PSC)

The definition of PSC revolves around its characterization as a chronic liver disease (CLD) primarily affecting the bile ducts. In this disease, the cholangioles are damaged by progressive inflammation and scarring, which causes them to narrow and finally be destroyed. Because of this process, bile flow is blocked, causing cholestasis, and this leads to more BAs in the liver and blood. The cause of PSC is still not well understood, though it is often found together with IBDs, mainly ulcerative colitis. Since there is a link, PSC is generally thought of as an immune-mediated disease, which puts it in the same group as other autoimmune disorders. Such complexity in its definition highlights the multifactorial nature of the disease, further complicating the understanding of its clinical implications (Leuschner *et al.*, 2013). It is thought by researchers that both autoimmune responses and problems with bile acids may be important in PSCs, but there is no clear agreement among experts. It is thought that PSC can be caused by a variety of factors, especially in cases linked to IBD, which makes its clinical definition more complex. Because the disease can be unpredictable and may lead to LC or cholangiocarcinoma, it is important to keep studying its causes. Looking into these pathophysiological insights is necessary to improve the way patients are managed and treated. With no definitive therapy currently available to impact clinical endpoints, understanding the definition and implications of PSC becomes integral to informing future research directions and treatment strategies (Boberg *et al.*, 2015).

Also, diagnosing and monitoring PSC can be quite complex. Diagnosis often relies on a combination of imaging studies, liver function tests (LFTs), and the presence of characteristic bile duct irregularities. These criteria help doctors tell PSC apart from other liver diseases, for example, PBC. There are major difficulties in managing PSC because there are not many effective treatments, and the course of the disease is unpredictable. Because PSC raises the risk of hepatobiliary malignancies, regular monitoring for these diseases is very important for patients. As ongoing research efforts seek to demystify the pathophysiology of PSC and its relationship with other diseases, a clearer understanding of its definition will be pivotal in advancing treatment paradigms and improving patient outcomes (Boberg *et al.*, 2015; Leuschner *et al.*, 2013) (Figure 12.2).

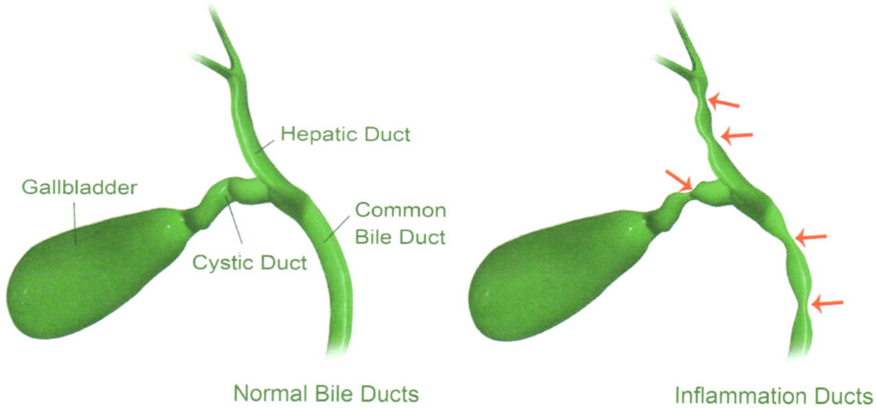

Figure 12.2. Primary sclerosing cholangitis (PSC).

Source: https://ai-care.id/photos/Folder%20Apri/Bilier/62ba5983666ab.jpg.

Importance of Studying PBC and PSC

Because it is difficult to diagnose and manage these autoimmune liver diseases, studying PBC and PSC is very important. Both PBC and PSC may result in serious health problems and death, as patients usually have complex symptoms that make it hard to diagnose them promptly. In particular, the OS, which features symptoms of both PBC and PSC, highlights the difficulties clinicians have in making a diagnosis. The case in the research tells of a patient with Crohn's disease who ended up with PBC-PSC OS, so doctors had to use thorough tests to confirm the diagnosis and manage the condition properly. Understanding the nuances and interrelations between these diseases can greatly enhance clinical decision-making, ultimately leading to better patient outcomes, as evidenced by the successful treatment response to ursodeoxycholic acid (UDCA) in the stated case (Souissi *et al.*, 2024). Also, looking into PBC and PSC can lead to finding new treatments that can greatly improve care for patients. Studies have recently focused on finding targets in these diseases that can be treated with drugs, which is necessary for treating the disease itself instead of only managing the symptoms. The study showed that LEFTY2 and HSPB1 for PBC and FCGR3B for PSC are good candidates for treatment. The results underline why it is important to join genetic research with medical knowledge to develop new treatments. By identifying specific genetic markers and their associations with disease progression, researchers can create targeted therapies, offering hope for improved clinical outcomes (Dai *et al.*, 2024). It is also very important to point out that studying PBC and PSC has major public health significance, given the rising number of autoimmune liver diseases worldwide. As more people become aware of these conditions, learning about their causes, how common they are, and how to manage them is very important. Looking at the comparison of PBC and PSC cases and their results helps healthcare systems decide how to use resources and create screening programs for people who may be affected. Also, because studies suggest genetics may play a role in both diseases, public health strategies can benefit from this knowledge and improve prevention. So, ongoing research on PBC and PSC helps develop a better understanding of autoimmune liver diseases and supports the creation of effective public health strategies for those affected.

12.1. Pathophysiology of PBC

The pathophysiology of Primary Biliary Cholangitis (PBC) is a complex interaction between immune dysregulation, genetic predisposition, and environmental factors that underlie the progressive injury of small bile ducts of the liver. PBC is largely defined as an autoimmune disorder, where the body's immune system inappropriately attacks its own biliary epithelial cells. These dysfunctions lead to chronic injury and inflammation of the cholangiocytes, resulting in cholestasis, interrupted bile flow, and hepatic tissue fibrosis that develops progressively. BA accumulation due to defective biliary secretion exacerbates hepatocellular injury, perpetuating a vicious cycle that ultimately leads to cirrhosis and complications in the form of liver failure (Leuschner *et al.*, 2013).

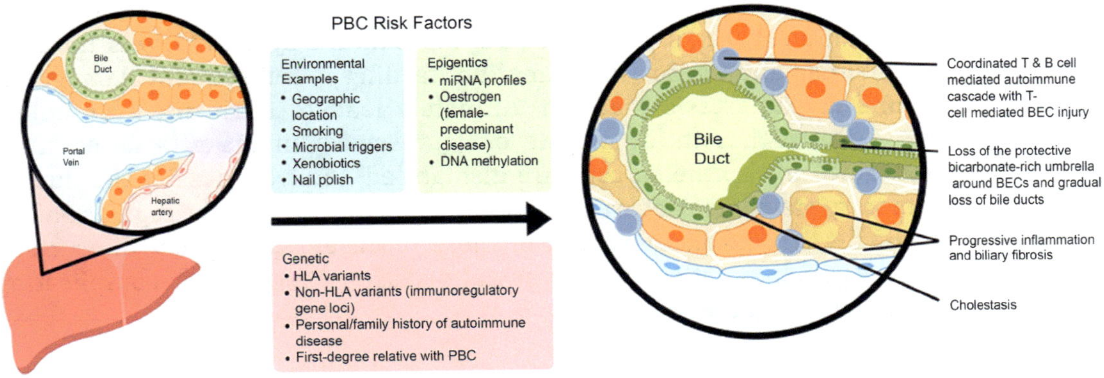

Figure 12.3. Pathophysiological processes involved in primary biliary cholangitis. HLA, human leukocyte antigen; miRNA, micro-ribonucleic acid molecules; PBC, primary biliary cholangitis.

Source: https://www.researchgate.net/publication/343815246/figure/fig2/AS:11431281173649867@1689006525917/Pathophysiological-processes-involved-in-primary-biliary-cholangitis-HLA-human.png.

Explanation of these pathological processes is significant as it allows the identification of potential therapeutic targets and management strategies for PBC. New research has revealed valuable information regarding mechanisms of inflammation in PBC. There is a notable presence of specific autoantibodies, such as antimitochondrial antibodies (AMA), which are a hallmark of the disease. These antibodies, along with other immune mediators, create an inflammatory environment that sustains cholangitis through the activation of immune cells and cytokines. Furthermore, the association of PBC with certain genetic factors identifies that patients with certain genetic backgrounds are more likely to present increased susceptibility to the disease (Alpini *et al.*, 2019). Such genetic susceptibility, combined with environmental precipitants like infection or exposure to certain chemicals, establishes the complex nature of PBC. As the science evolves, the interconnections can yield new therapies that act on both gene action and immune dysregulation. The resulting chronic cholestasis of PBC often leads to advanced liver fibrosis and, in turn, cirrhosis and constitutes a critical endpoint for disease evolution in these illnesses. Fibrotic tissue, the product of persistent inflammation, disrupts the normal structure and function of the liver. It is also crucial to comprehend the fibrogenic pathways, as well as the functions of hepatic stellate cells and the extracellular matrix, to devise potential interventions. Present treatments are primarily focused on minimizing the progression of liver damage by the administration of medications like UDCA, which promotes bile acid circulation and stability (Leuschner *et al.*, 2013). However, a compelling need persists for the creation of new treatments to abrogate the underlying pathophysiologic processes of PBC. Experimental innovative strategies, such as immunomodulation and stem cell therapy, present potential therapeutic avenues in the ongoing battle against this challenging liver disease (Alpini *et al.*, 2019) (Figure 12.3).

12.1.1. Immune-Mediated Destruction of Bile Ducts

Immune-mediated bile duct damage is the core pathology shared by PBC and PSC in the pathophysiology of autoimmune liver diseases. In PBC, the immune system targets the small bile ducts in an abnormal manner and causes inflammation, leading to subsequent damage. Chronic bile duct damage results in cholestasis that can ultimately lead to cirrhosis, liver failure, and related complications. PSC also has its own cycle of aggressive immune attacks on intra- and extrahepatic bile ducts. Since the epithelial cells are dismantled, the weakness of the ducts makes the developing inflammatory state one of scarring and fibrosis. This immune dysregulation is central to the understanding of the clinical presentation of these diseases, specifically their association with autoimmune diseases such as inflammatory bowel disease (IBD), further complicating their management and treatment (Grama *et al.*, 2023).

The immune-mediated injury underlying PBC and PSC is suggestive of a multifactorial aetiology involving genetic predisposition, environmental triggers, and immune regulatory disturbances. Studies have identified some human leukocyte antigen (HLA) haplotypes to confer risk, indicating the genetic component of susceptibility to such disorders. The environment, in the form of infections and toxins, may also augment immune stimulation, leading to increased inflammation and subsequent damage to the ducts. These interactions could also alter the intestinal microbiota, resulting in the emergence of cholangiopathies. These complex interactions demand an integrated appreciation of disease progression. Understanding these factors with new therapies might give new treatment paradigms, hopefully containing the immune-mediated mechanisms of both PBC and PSC (Alkhatib, 2023). Therapeutic strategies for modulating the immune-mediated bile duct damage in PBC and PSC are undergoing a shift, with an aim to prevent inflammation and preserve bile duct integrity. Immunosuppressive therapies like corticosteroids and biologics have emerged as first-line treatments aiming to inhibit the pathologic immune response. However, treatment efficacy is often unpredictable, necessitating individualized therapy in accordance with the individual disease presentation in each patient. Moreover, more recent studies have suggested the potential for liver transplant in advanced disease, based on the progressive nature of both diseases. Although not curative, transplantation is an option that is necessary in patients with extensive liver impairment, again reflecting the utility of multimodal management strategies. Advances in understanding of immunologic mechanisms governing biliary injury are promising for new treatment approaches that will enhance patient outcomes in the future (Grama *et al.*, 2023).

12.1.2. Role of Autoantibodies in PBC

Investigating autoantibodies in PBC has become very important, helping to explain how the disease develops. Autoantibodies are produced by the immune system and can attack self-antigens, which leads to swelling and harm to tissues. In PBC, a key sign of the disease is the presence of AMA, and this also points to the immune system attacking the bile duct cells. The ways these antibodies act, such as by triggering inflammation and supporting apoptosis, demonstrate the complexity of the immune system in PBC. More research is needed to understand how these autoantibodies are involved in the progression of cholestasis. Autoantibodies that have been identified are linked to the symptoms seen in PBC. Studies also suggest that AMA can cause mitochondrial pathways to malfunction, which harms cholangiocytes and worsens bile accumulation. Other immunological studies have found that certain autoantibodies can bind to parts of the biliary epithelium, which may add to the pathological picture of PBC. Learning more about how autoantibodies work with target antigens could lead researchers to find new therapeutic options to stop the immunological attack on cholangiocytes. This information may guide unique treatment plans for patients, which could improve their results and control the ongoing progression of PBC. Besides using autoantibodies to diagnose, they can also help predict how severe and how fast a disease will progress. New studies indicate that the type of autoantibodies present can be a sign of liver damage, which helps clinicians choose the right treatment for each patient. In PSC, the presence of autoantibodies against integrin $\alpha v\beta 6$ has been found, and this suggests that PBC and PSC have similar pathways leading to disease, even though the targets are not the same. Exploring how these mechanisms are alike and different could improve our general understanding of cholestatic diseases, leading to new ideas in research and treatment. Ultimately, the role of autoantibodies in PBC and PSC encapsulates a vital intersection of immunology, pathology, and clinical practice that continues to evolve as research advances (Figure 12.4).

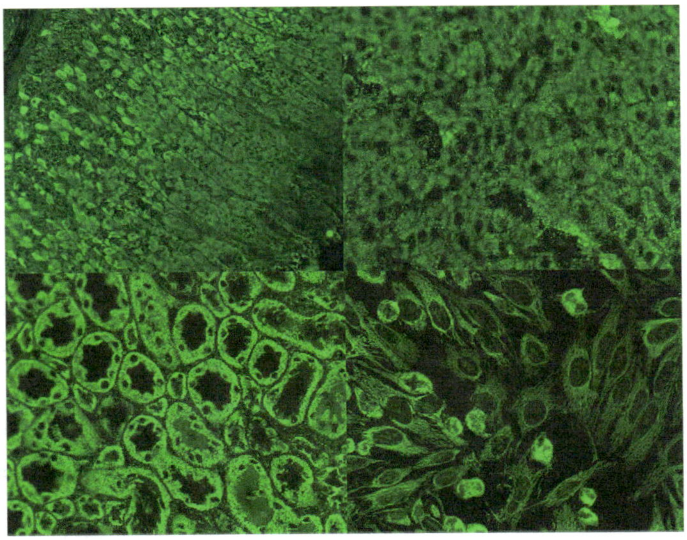

Figure 12.4. Immunofluorescence staining pattern of antimitochondrial antibodies (AMA) shown on stomach (top left), liver (top right), kidney (bottom left) and hep-20-10 cells (bottom right).

Source: https://upload.wikimedia.org/wikipedia/commons/thumb/a/af/AMA_ANTIBODIES.jpg/800px-AMA_ANTIBODIES.jpg.

12.1.3. Genetic Predisposition and Environmental Factors

The complex interplay between genetic predisposition and environmental factors is pivotal in understanding the onset and progression of chronic liver diseases (CLD) such as PBC and PSC. Some genetic studies have found that those with certain genetic markers, mainly those linked to autoimmune diseases, have a greater chance of getting PBC or PSC. For example, the presence of specific HLA (human leukocyte antigen) alleles has been correlated with increased risks of developing these conditions, indicating a strong hereditary component. Even so, genes alone do not fully explain why diseases are more common or severe in some populations, which shows that environmental factors can strongly influence both susceptibility and the immune system. A person's environment, which includes lifestyle and location, has a strong effect on developing autoimmune liver diseases. Evidence points out that PBC and PSC are more common among people exposed to smoking and socioeconomic deprivation. Higher chances of PBC are linked to being a woman, smoking, and having a lower socioeconomic status, which proves that these external factors can affect how diseases are passed down in families. Moreover, the epidemiological analysis indicates that geographical latitude has important implications, with variations in PBC and Autoimmune Hepatitis (AIH) incidence strongly correlating with being positioned farther from the equator. They reveal that environmental factors interacting with genetic vulnerability are important in causing these diseases.

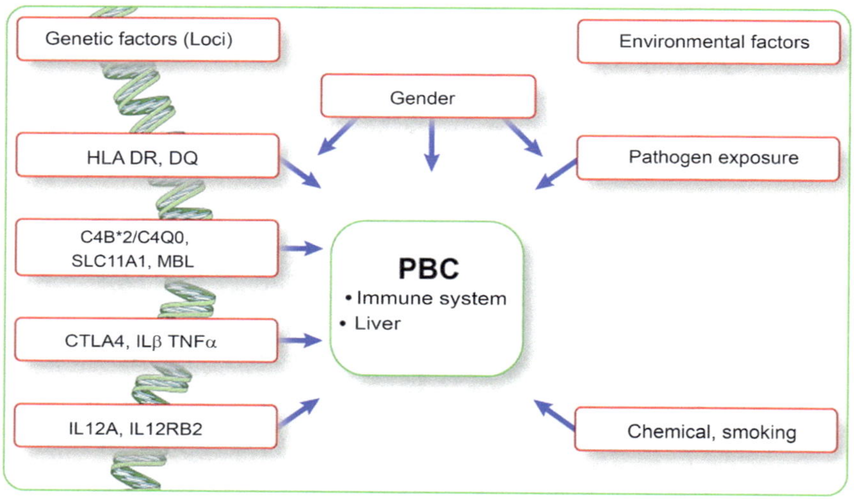

Figure 12.5. PBC results from a combination of multiple genetic and environmental factors that may affect the immune system and the liver.

Source: https://www.researchgate.net/publication/42609899/figure/fig4/AS:267751356891138@1440848306164/PBC-results-from-a-combination-of-multiple-genetic-and-environmental-factors-that-may.png.

PBC and PSC are complex, which raises the question of whether they should be seen as separate diseases or as a range influenced by both genes and environment. It is still controversial how PSC develops, as there is ongoing debate about whether immune problems or bile acid changes are more important. Recent studies try to explain these issues by connecting new findings about pathogenesis with the symptoms and treatment options seen in patients. The absence of effective medical therapies and the unpredictability of disease progression raise critical questions about patient monitoring and treatment approaches, bringing to light the challenges posed by the interplay of genetic predisposition and environmental factors in understanding the full scope of PBC and PSC as formidable clinical entities in hepatology, as emphasized in Boberg *et al.* (2015) (Figure 12.5).

12.2. Pathophysiology of PSC

The pathophysiology of PSC is complex and multifactorial, with a highly complex relationship between immune dysregulation and genetic susceptibility. In PSC, the inflammatory process initially affects intra- and extrahepatic bile ducts, later fibrosis ensues, and finally, obliteration of these structures. The pathological course of this process begins with cholestasis, which is bile obstruction, culminating eventually in biliary cirrhosis and profound impairment of liver function. The immune-mediated pathogenesis of PSC is accentuated by its tight association with IBD, suggesting parallel pathophysiologic processes that may drive the disease process. Such an association suggests potential dysfunctions in autoreactive immune mechanisms that underlie chronic inflammation and bile duct damage. This complexity demands that not only the immune components but also the genetic components behind PSC be well studied, by observation, such as the heterogeneity of clinical presentation. PSC has been explored to clarify significant pathophysiologic factors behind the course of PSC, like genetic predispositions and environmental stimuli that can possibly trigger disease progression. Genetic influences, including certain human leukocyte antigen (HLA) haplotypes, have been implicated in the modulation of immune responses resulting in inflammation of the bile ducts. Additionally, the contribution of intestinal dysbiosis to the stimulation of an immune reaction against bile duct cells has become a high-priority area of research. Hydrophobic BAs' cytotoxic effect also causes damage to cholangiocytes, which enhances inflammation and creates a cycle of bile duct injury (Pak *et al.*, 2024). The repetitive cycle is not only the cause of decreasing liver function but also increases the risk of developing complications in large folds, such as cholangiocarcinoma, thus creating serious challenges for long-term management in patients.

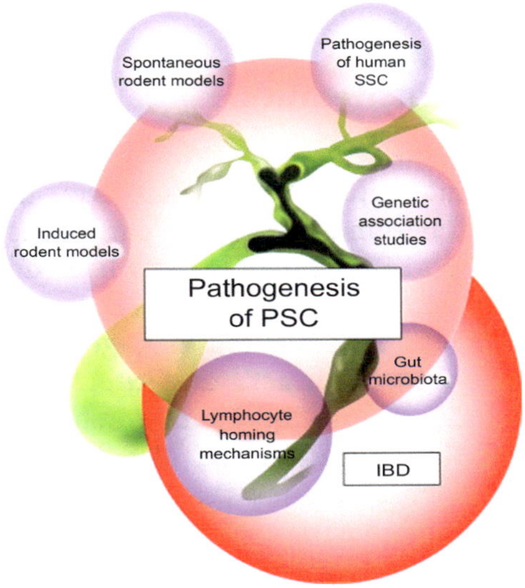

Figure 12.6. Pathogenesis of primary sclerosing cholangitis.

Source: https://www.researchgate.net/publication/278725191/figure/fig2/AS:267779278372905@1440854963785/Relationship-between-pathogenesis-of-primary-sclerosing-cholangitis-PSC-and-ongoing.png.

Lastly, the management of PSC is hindered by its mysterious pathophysiology and absence of curative long-term therapies. Current therapies, such as the administration of UDCA to monitor serum alkaline phosphatase (ALP) levels, allow for symptomatic improvement but do little to influence disease progression. Moreover, despite treating clinically significant bile duct strictures with interventional endoscopy, liver transplantation remains the sole potentially curative treatment. It is worth carrying out ongoing research trying to elucidate the various aspects of PSCs' pathophysiology, as elucidation of such mechanisms will be important for the design of targeted therapies. Tailored therapies addressing the specific immune-mediated processes involved in PSC can enhance patient results and likely reduce the likelihood of relapse after liver transplant, highlighting the need for further studies within this complex field (Grama *et al.*, 2023) (Figure 12.6).

12.2.1. Inflammation and Fibrosis of Bile Ducts

The intricate interaction of bile duct fibrosis and inflammation is key to the pathogenesis of both PBC and PSC. In cholestatic liver disease, inflammation of the bile ducts follows as a result of immune-mediated damage that leads to damage in the ducts and their eventual fibrosis. Dysregulation is characterized by lymphocytic infiltration and elevation of pro-inflammatory cytokines that are involved in injurious mechanisms affecting the bile duct epithelium. Along with disease progression, this inflammatory milieu promotes fibrogenesis, where there is a hyperplastic deposition of collagen, causing obliteration of the bile duct and impaired bile flow. This pathological transformation favors the necessity to regulate inflammation as a therapeutic option to avoid the complications of chronic cholestatic liver diseases. Moreover, recent findings on bile acid signaling pathways have also elucidated the role of BAs toward inflammation in the setting of liver injury in PBC and PSC. BAs have the potential to induce cytotoxicity in cholangiocytes, which promotes inflammation and fibrosis by a number of molecular mechanisms. In particular, dysregulation of bile acid levels catalyzes the chronic stimulation of inflammatory pathways, which augment liver injury.

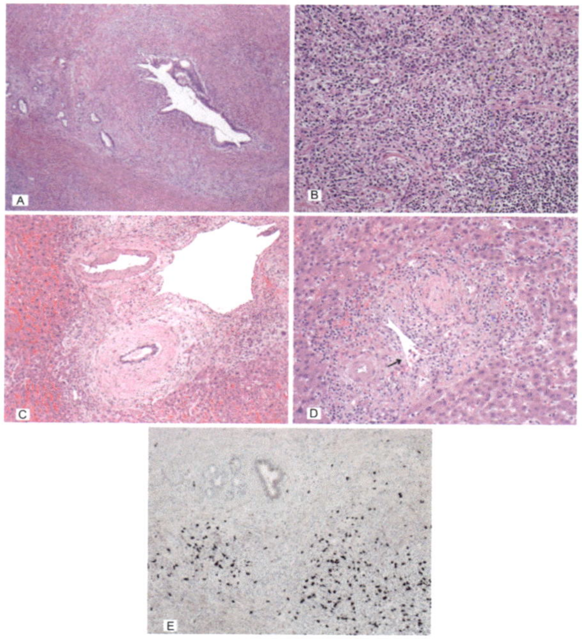

Figure 12.7. (A) Large bile duct with marked fibrotic thickening and inflammation of the wall. Storiform fibrosis extends beyond the bile duct wall. (B) The inflammatory infiltrates consist of abundant plasma cells, some lymphocytes and eosinophils. (C) Onion-skin periductal fibrosis and narrowing of the bile duct lumen are seen in this portal tract. (D) Portal tract with mild inflammation and obliterative phlebitis (arrow), and bile duct loss. (E) Abundant IgG4 plasma cells are present in the inflammatory infiltrate.

Source: https://www.researchgate.net/profile/Danya-Rosen-2/publication/271595979/figure/fig2/AS:601762562048008@1520482783331/A-Large-bile-duct-with-marked-fibrotic-thickening-and-inflammation-of-the-wall.png.

Notably, clinical trials that have investigated modulating bile acid receptors, such as the Farnesoid X receptor, have been promising in reducing bile acid synthesis and suppressing inflammation. A novel therapeutic approach to treatment of the inflammatory mechanisms that drive PBC and PSC is offered by modulating these bile acid pathways. Thus, understanding bile acid kinetics has the potential to unveil novel therapies for bile duct integrity and function.

The role of stem/progenitor cell populations in the course of the regenerating response of chronic injury cannot be overstressed in bile duct processes of inflammation and fibrosis. Biliary Tree Stem/Progenitor Cells (BTSCs) and Hepatic Stem/progenitor Cells (HpSCs) contribute to bile duct repair but are inherently linked with the degree of inflammation and fibrosis within the liver. Although adult hepatocytes and cholangiocytes generally dominate regenerative responses, marginal involvement of stem cell niches is clear in the case of chronic inflammation with extensive injury. Activation of stem cell niches may lead to the increased fibrogenesis that once again fuels injury-repair cycles. Thus, the elucidation of the mechanisms underlying stem cell activation and regulation serves not only to advance insight into disease progression in PSC and PBC but also highlights potential avenues for therapeutic intervention aimed at halting fibrosis and facilitating functional regeneration of the bile ducts (Figure 12.7).

12.2.2. Association with Inflammatory Bowel Disease

In recent times, there has been a lot of interest in the link between IBD and autoimmune liver diseases, mainly PBC and PSC. Studies show that patients with ulcerative colitis have a high risk of getting PSC which can make their health outcomes more complex. A big study found that 6.8% of children with IBD had autoimmune liver disease, and there was a strong link between severe ulcerative colitis and issues in the bile ducts. Because of this evidence, it is important to keep a close eye on these patients, as early treatment and management can make a big difference in their lives. The interplay between chronic inflammation in the gut and biliary tract pathology suggests a shared pathophysiological mechanism that warrants further exploration within both clinical and research settings (Alexopoulou *et al.*, 2016). People with IBD are more likely to develop liver diseases because of their genetic background. Changes in the IL2/IL21 gene area are thought to affect the risk of PSC in people with ulcerative colitis. A group of affected individuals and healthy controls were studied, and it was found that some SNPs in this region are linked to a major decrease in PSC risk. They show that both genetic and environmental factors play a role in causing autoimmune diseases. Furthermore, the presence of other autoimmune disorders within this population emphasizes the importance of understanding shared genetic markers, which may aid in predicting disease progression and tailoring therapeutic interventions for patients afflicted by such dual-pathology conditions (Albers *et al.*, 2011).

Healthcare providers need to be aware of liver complications in patients with IBD. Because autoimmune liver diseases, especially PSC, are more common in IBD patients, doctors should include regular liver function tests in their usual care. Problems such as cholestasis and damage to the liver can develop silently and become serious if they are not found early. Learning about these associations should be offered to patients so they can recognize new symptoms and encourage the right tests. While the coexistence of PBC, PSC, and IBD may not always present as a direct clinical correlation, the intertwined nature of these diseases beckons further research and clinical vigilance to optimize patient care and outcomes (Alexopoulou *et al.*, 2016) (Figure 12.8).

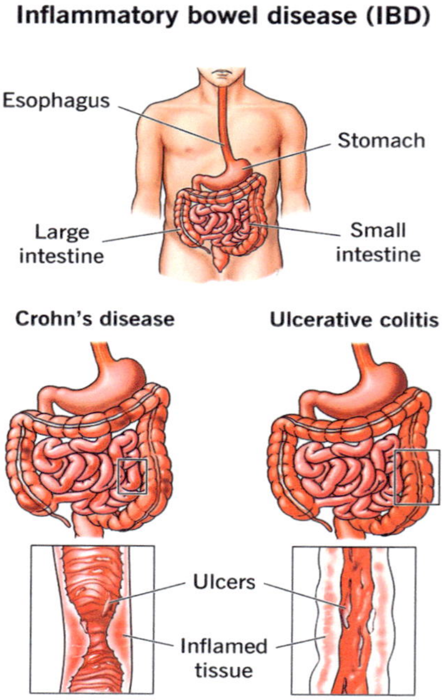

Figure 12.8. Inflammatory bowel disease (IBD).

Source: https://my.clevelandclinic.org/-/scassets/images/org/health/articles/15587-inflammatory-bowel-disease-ibd.jpg.

12.2.3. Genetic and Environmental Risk Factors

Both PBC and PSC develop because of the interaction between genetic and environmental risks. Certain alleles in the genes are linked to autoimmune reactions, which increase the risk of getting these forms of cholangitis. It has been shown that some genetic variants are linked to autoimmune diseases, for example, rheumatoid arthritis and IBD, which can also make PBC and PSC more likely. Studies indicate that genetically predicted rheumatoid arthritis is significantly linked to a heightened risk of PBC, suggesting common immunological pathways that may lead to liver damage and cholangitis development in predisposed individuals (Gao *et al.*, 2024). Because of this genetic background, we can better understand how family background can affect the risk of these liver diseases. Environmental causes also play a big role in increasing the risk of PBC and PSC, usually in combination with genetic factors. Taking up smoking increases the chances of getting these diseases. It is noted in research that people who start smoking are more likely to develop PBC, which suggests that certain environmental factors can trigger the disease in those who are genetically predisposed. Additionally, dietary factors, such as low coffee intake and vitamin D levels, reveal interesting protective correlations, further emphasizing how environmental contexts shape health outcomes (Gao *et al.*, 2024). Also, when there are changes in gut microbiota, known as dysbiosis, it is now recognized as a negative environmental factor that ties gut health to both liver problems and the immune system. Because there are many different risk factors, it is important to use a wide range of strategies to deal with cholangitis. Studying genetic and environmental causes continues to add new ideas to the way PBC and PSC are managed and prevented. Using sophisticated methods such as GWAS, scientists are now revealing the genetic reasons behind these diseases, pointing out new risk factors that were not known before. When knowledge increases, it becomes possible to use specific treatments, such as using probiotics to regulate the gut microbiota. Some of these new approaches are intended to fix dysbiosis and may help the liver while reducing inflammation. For this reason, using both genetic and environmental factors is essential for building models that can direct doctors in treating patients with PBC and PSC, which leads to better outcomes.

12.3. Clinical Presentation of PBC

The presenting features of PBC are a wide range of symptoms, usually evolving over time and thus often difficult to diagnose in the early stages. Fatigue and pruritus are common presenting complaints and have an important effect on the quality of life. Fatigue tends to be severe, sometimes unrelieved by rest, and may predate other clinical symptoms by many months or even years. Pruritus, or itching, can be intense and worsen at night, resulting in nocturnal disturbances. Soon, other signs may develop, including jaundice, abdominal pain, and xanthelasmata, yellowish fatty deposits about the eyelids. Such physical findings point to cholestasis, the pathophysiologic process of PBC in which bile flow is impeded, with resultant liver damage and progression to cirrhosis if not properly treated. With the progression of the disease, PBC patients can have serious complications due to its chronic nature. Destructive cholangitis is a characteristic of this illness that affects the small bile ducts and leads to fibrosis and inflammation. These changes can cause portal hypertension and liver failure. Biochemical and laboratory investigations typically reveal elevated levels of ALP, indicative of cholestasis, while AMA occurs in the majority of patients and constitutes a vital serological indicator of the disease. According to future epidemiological information, the prevalence of PBC has been found to be associated with several demographic parameters, including sex and geographic latitude. There have been recent studies that the prevalence of PBC increases with higher northerly latitude, and gender and smoking status have been found to be demographic variables in its incidence, pointing to the polyfactorial etiology of the disease (Hirschfield *et al.*, 2021). The clinical presentation of PBC has also been associated with extrahepatic disease expression, which contributes to the general picture of the disease. Patients may have a range of autoimmune disorders, so diagnosis and treatment become complex. Such comorbidities may be Sjögrens syndrome, autoimmune thyroid disorders, and rheumatoid arthritis and lead to more systemic disease requiring holistic management. Detection of such overlapping conditions is extremely critical to clinicians because they may decide whether multimodal therapeutic maneuvers are needed. Treatment is largely based on the use of UDCA, with the intent of restoring liver function and arresting the evolution of the disease. With early treatment, the prognosis has now become better, but constant surveillance and individualized therapy are still crucial because of the unpredictable clinical course followed by patients (Akbar *et al.*, 2011).

12.3.1. Common Symptoms and Signs

The clinical presentation of PBC and PSC involves overlapping but distinctive symptoms that can complicate diagnosis and treatment. PBC is generally accompanied by fatigue and pruritus that are often the first symptoms to be reported by patients. The fatigue is severe and affects quality of life by compromising activities of daily living. Pruritus or intense itching is due to the accumulation of BAs as a consequence of disrupted bile flow, and it can seriously disrupt sleep and daily activities. The patient can also get features of jaundice and other cutaneous signs such as xanthomas. These symptoms need to be recognized at an early stage to treat them, since if left untreated, these would lead to severe hepatic complications and are thus targeted towards therapeutic goals to preserve liver function and overall health. PSC, however, has a different set of symptoms with predominantly inflammatory and fibrotic bile duct alterations. The usual presenting symptoms of PSC include right upper quadrant pain, pruritus, and fatigue, but it can be asymptomatic on presentation. Jaundice occurs as the disease progresses, indicating severe impairment of bile drainage. PSC is frequently associated with other autoimmune diseases, such as IBD, thus complicating the clinical picture. Overlapping conditions require a comprehensive clinical assessment to differentiate PSC from other liver diseases. As PSC is also linked with a higher risk of colorectal cancer, recognition of its symptoms is important for early detection and intervention to prevent complications and improve patient outcomes in at-risk populations. Detection of the typical symptoms and signs of PBC and PSC not only aids in clinical diagnosis but also highlights the importance of patient education and follow-up. These signs and symptoms, like pruritus and fatigue, can be non-specific and should be managed cautiously to enhance the quality of life in the patient. As more is learned about these diseases, scientists are attempting to understand pathogenic mechanisms of these symptoms, like genetic backgrounds and gut microbiota imbalances, as recent research suggests. Knowledge of these mechanisms will inform crucial therapeutic development, highlighting symptomatology's role in steering research towards more effective therapies for PBC and PSC. As critical treatments enhance patient outcomes by alleviating common symptoms, they inform strategies for subsequent clinical research to better the lives of individuals affected by these chronic ailments (Bhushan *et al.*, 2024; Trivedi *et al.*, 2024) (Figure 12.9).

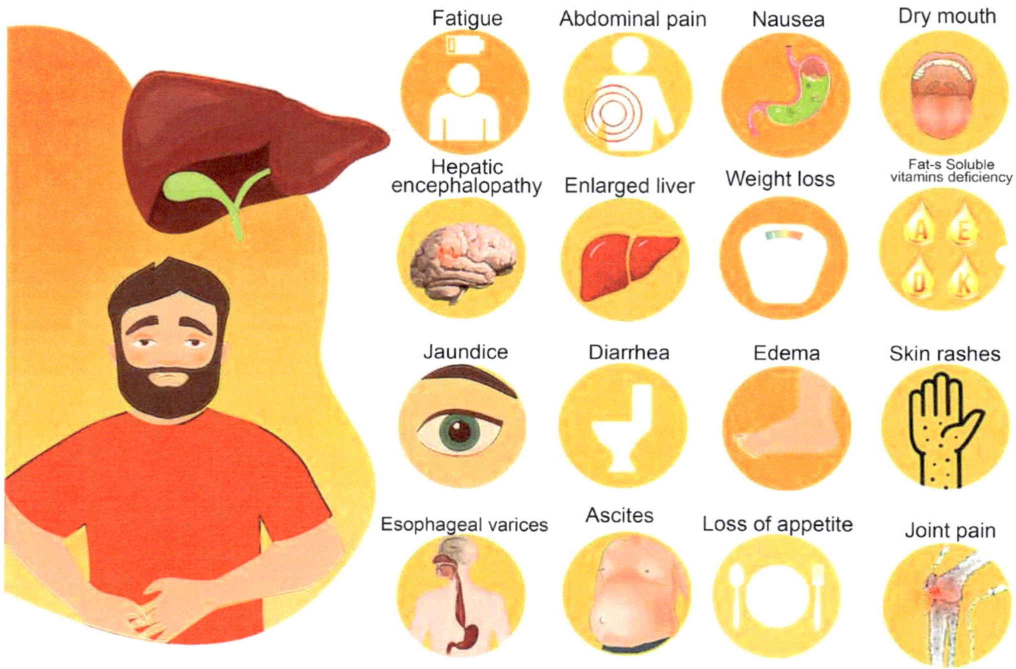

Figure 12.9. Primary biliary cholangitis (PBC) symptoms.

Source: https://a2zhealthy.com/primary-biliary-cholangitis/2/.

12.3.2. Diagnostic Criteria and Tests

Serological tests, mainly looking for AMA, are the main basis for diagnosing PBC. AMA is always seen in PBC, and more than 90% of patients with symptoms have a positive test. So, doctors check enzyme levels, including ALP, to detect cholestasis, and LBx is usually not needed for a definite diagnosis. Also, using clinical, biochemical, and histological characteristics in scoring helps determine how severe the disease is and what treatment plan to use. Laboratory findings about the liver allow doctors to identify issues early and begin the right treatments, which is important for a patient's overall recovery. Ultimately, the integration of clinical assessments with serological findings constitutes the cornerstone of PBC diagnosis as it helps distinguish PBC from other cholestatic liver diseases (Akbar *et al.*, 2011). Unlike other conditions, PSC is diagnosed in a more complicated way because it can affect many parts of the body, and there are no special blood tests to identify it.

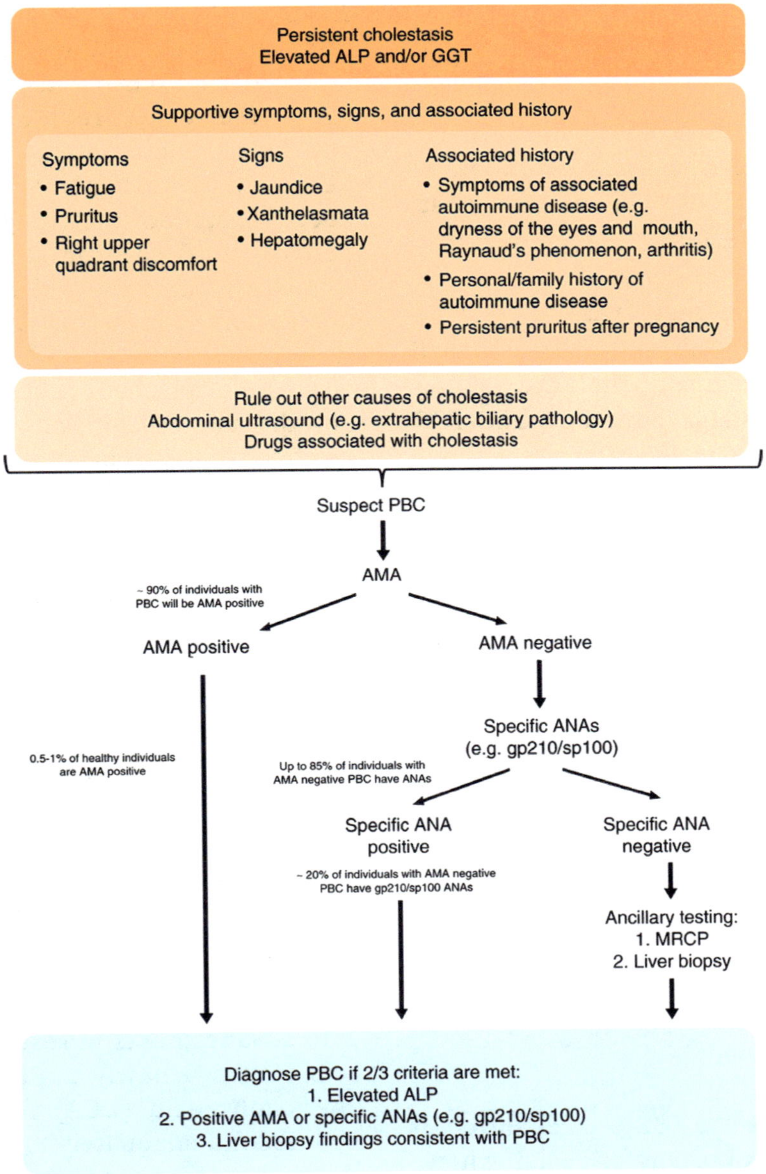

Figure 12.10. Proposed diagnostic algorithm for the assessment of a patient for suspected primary biliary cholangitis.

Source: https://www.researchgate.net/publication/343815246/figure/fig1/AS:11431281173666003@1689006524491/Proposed-diagnostic-algorithm-for-the-assessment-of-a-patient-for-suspected-primary.png.

The first step is often to do LFTs, and these often reveal that ALP is higher than normal, suggesting cholestasis. Magnetic resonance cholangiography (MRCP) is the most effective imaging modality employed to visualize the characteristic bile duct strictures and dilatations associated with PSC. Although PSC may sometimes be related to autoimmune diseases, as the literature states, it does not have AMA, which sets it apart from other cholestatic diseases. Biopsy may be performed in some cases to rule out other pathologies, providing valuable histological data that can aid in confirming the diagnosis, as well as assessing the extent of liver damage (Forenc *et al.*, 2024). Better diagnostic tools are helping doctors find and manage both PBC and PSC earlier. New ways to detect liver fibrosis without surgery, such as using elastography, are being investigated. Such new tools may change the way doctors diagnose, which can make it easier to treat patients promptly and effectively. In addition, understanding the impact of genetics on disease risk and progression is growing, which is broadening the usual ways diseases are diagnosed. Therefore, ongoing research aimed at refining these diagnostic criteria is necessary for optimizing individualized patient care, ensuring that therapeutic strategies are implemented effectively based on timely and accurate diagnoses of PBC and PSC (Akbar *et al.*, 2011) (Figure 12.10).

12.3.3. Staging and Progression of the Disease

The way liver diseases like PBC and PSC develop and progress is very important for deciding how the disease will be treated and for the patient's outlook. Chronic bile duct inflammation is the cause of both conditions, which results in biliary damage and cirrhosis. In the first stages, PBC may not cause any symptoms, but as time goes on, patients usually feel tired, itchy, and have liver problems. Staging systems, such as the Model for End-Stage Liver Disease (MELD), help quantify liver impairment, but they are not always fully predictive of the disease trajectory. Without staging systems, it is more difficult to assess and treat PSC, but age, liver function tests, and the presence of complications can show how serious the disease is and if it might get worse, which requires close monitoring and quick action, mainly for those who may need a liver transplant. Both PBC and PSC need a detailed knowledge of the processes that cause disease progression. The immune system attacking small bile ducts in PBC causes cholestasis, which may lead to fibrosis and cirrhosis. Detecting changes in DNA methylation, which is an epigenetic process, helps understand how diseases develop and which treatments may be effective. It has been found in recent studies that patients with PSC have different epigenetic changes than those with PBC. These results indicate that epigenetic changes could be very important in how diseases start and advance, as seen by their links to immune signaling and the activation of macrophages and T-cells. Such detailed investigations into the epigenome of affected patients elucidate significant variations in immune cell composition and suggest that tailored therapeutic approaches may enhance patient outcomes (Juran *et al.*, 2024). Treatment and management methods are being updated as doctors learn more about the stages and causes of PBC and PSC. UDCA is the primary first-line treatment for PBC, and it is given to prevent the disease from advancing. However, with advancements in research, physicians can now leverage newly approved therapies like obeticholic acid (OCA) for patients who do not respond adequately to standard treatment. Unlike the other conditions, PSC does not have approved medications, so transplantation is usually the only treatment for advanced cases. Experts should continue to look for new treatments for PSC and also keep studying the causes and mechanisms of both diseases. Improving our understanding of the staging and progression of PBC and PSC is paramount to enhancing therapeutic outcomes and ensuring personalized patient care (Bhushan *et al.*, 2024) (Figure 12.11).

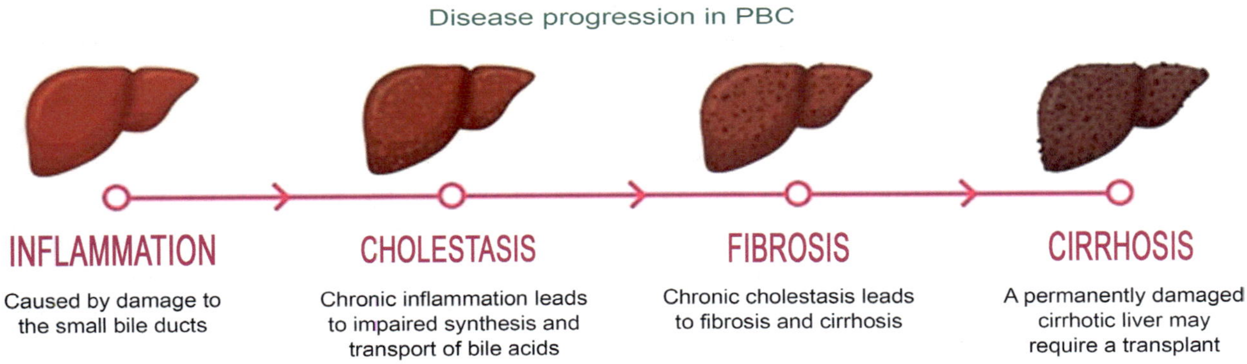

Figure 12.11. Disease progression in PBC.

Source: https://labmedicineblog.com/wp-content/uploads/2025/04/pbc1.jpg.

12.4. Clinical Presentation of PSC

The clinical presentation of PSC is often with a variety of diverse symptoms in severity and type, making early diagnosis challenging. Patients may present with nonspecific symptoms such as fatigue, pruritus, and jaundice initially, and the resulting diagnosis is delayed regarding the underlying condition. As the disease progresses, more sinister complications can happen, including biliary obstruction and cholangitis, which may present with fever, chills, and right upper quadrant pain. The association of PSC and IBD, particularly ulcerative colitis, is important and helps to further complicate the presentation because gastrointestinal symptoms can overwhelm the presentation. These varied presentations should alert clinicians to a high degree of suspicion during evaluation of patients with atypical hepatic complaints or accompanying gastrointestinal disease and therefore emphasize the benefit of early diagnosis and intervention to prevent long-term consequences (Semlali *et al.*, 2024). Diagnosis in PSC is also supported by imaging studies such as magnetic resonance cholangiopancreatography (MRCP), which can reveal characteristic features such as strictures and beading of bile ducts, and is useful in the diagnosis of extrahepatic complications. These imaging results are essential to the differential diagnosis of PSC from other cholestatic liver diseases, e.g., PBC. ERCP not only aids in diagnosis in the scenario of PSC but can also be used as a source of therapeutic interventions, particularly with biliary obstructions. Regular follow-up with scheduled use of ERCPs has been found to enhance transplant-free survival for patients, emphasizing the significance of continued monitoring and management strategies (Özdirik *et al.*, 2024). The interplay of endoscopic therapy and imaging in the management of PSC merely mirrors the clinical presentation's complexity, whereby prompt intervention may be pivotal to shaping patient outcomes. Furthermore, PSC may evolve insidiously, with patients remaining asymptomatic for decades, such that early diagnosis may prove elusive. Upon progression of the disease, conditions such as hepatic decompensation and hepatobiliary malignancy may emerge, with the incidence of cholangiocarcinoma of special concern. Chronic cholestasis can lead to systemic complications like fat-soluble vitamin deficiency and osteoporosis. This demands a multi-disciplinary approach that encompasses not just hepatological management but also advises lifestyle modification and nutritional supplementation. Appreciation of the complete spectrum of PSCs' clinical presentation and potential complications is necessary for healthcare providers. Such awareness can enable early diagnosis and intervention, ultimately enhancing quality of life and survival chances for individuals so affected (Özdirik *et al.*, 2024; Semlali *et al.*, 2024).

12.4.1. Symptoms and Complications

PBC and PSC symptoms can significantly impact the quality of life of the affected individuals. Most characteristically, patients with PBC have fatigue, pruritus, and jaundice, which can gradually increase as the disease process prolongs. Debilitating fatigue from PBC has been described to impair everyday function and overall feeling of well-being. In some cases, the patient may be completely asymptomatic until the latter part of the disease course.

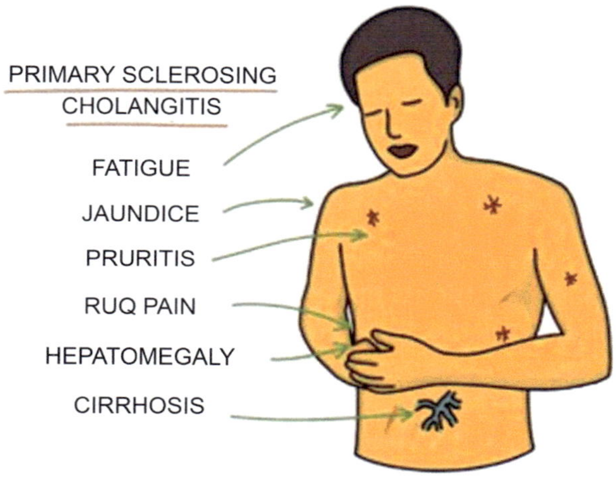

Figure 12.12. Primary sclerosing cholangitis (PSC) symptoms.

Source: https://zerotofinals.com/wp-content/uploads/PSC-Presetnation-300x236.jpg.

PSC, however, is usually linked to IBD, primarily ulcerative colitis, and further complicates symptomatology. PSC may present symptoms of abdominal pain, weight loss, and fever that reflect intrahepatic and extrahepatic complications and should therefore be approached cautiously in handling and follow-up. Complications of PBC and PSC are multifaceted and are prone to diverge due to the varying disease mechanisms. In PBC, cholestasis may lead to chronic liver fibrosis that goes on to cirrhosis with the resultant complications such as portal hypertension and HE. The high risk of developing HCC in patients with PBC also puts such patients in the spotlight for regular screening throughout the disease. In PSC, association with IBD further complicates the disorder; more than 30% of patients with IBD develop liver dysfunction, which can lead to chronic cholestatic liver disease and transmit liver-related symptoms. These complications underscore the interdependence of the hepatobiliary system and the GI tract in these conditions and highlight the importance of a multidisciplinary approach to management. Both PBC and PSC have systemic features that go beyond hepatobiliary manifestations, thus complicating the clinical presentation. For instance, osteoporosis, vitamin deficiency, and other autoimmune disorders are some of the extrahepatic manifestations, reflecting the autoimmune nature of PBC and the immunological associations of PSC. Furthermore, chronicity of these disorders contributes to psychological complications like depression and anxiety as a result of the psychosocial effects of chronic disease. For PSC, the overlap with ulcerative colitis will further exacerbate these complications to develop resistant forms, and young patients will become disabled in otherwise productive working ages. This hepatic and gastrointestinal overlap in complications mandates a holistic approach to address both the physical and mental health issues that are encountered by patients with PBC and PSC (Leuschner *et al.*, 2013; Nurmukhamedova *et al.*, 2023) (Figure 12.12).

12.4.2. Diagnostic Imaging Techniques

Diagnostic imaging is very important for assessing and managing liver diseases, mainly in patients with PBC and PSC. Imaging modalities such as ultrasound, CT, and magnetic resonance imaging (MRI) serve as non-invasive tools that allow for the assessment of liver morphology, bile duct integrity, and the presence of complications associated with these conditions. Because ultrasound is easy to use and can detect liver problems like cirrhosis and enlarged bile ducts, it is often the first test chosen. MRI and CT allow healthcare providers to study the liver's structure in detail, which helps them tell PBC and PSC apart by looking for bile duct problems and changes in liver texture that are typical of each disease.

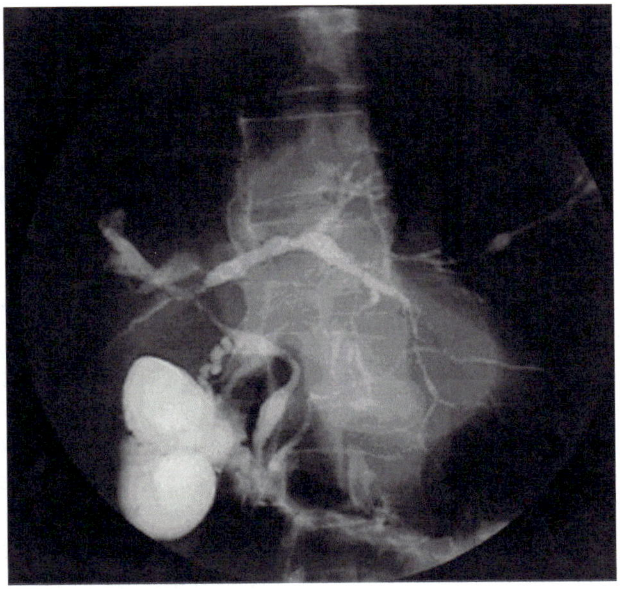

Figure 12.13. Cholangiogram of primary sclerosing cholangitis.

Source: https://upload.wikimedia.org/wikipedia/commons/3/37/Cholangiogram_of_primary_sclerosing_cholangitis.jpg.

Using transient elastography has become a useful method for checking liver stiffness, which is connected to the stage of fibrosis in liver diseases. In the case of autoimmune liver diseases, including PBC and PSC, it is highly accurate in making a diagnosis. A recent study highlighted that the area under the receiver operating characteristic curve (AUROC) values for transient elastography in PBC patients ranged from 0.91 for cirrhosis to 0.93 for advanced fibrosis. They prove that using new imaging techniques is very important for monitoring the course of a disease and its response to treatment. Furthermore, other noninvasive indices, such as the aspartate aminotransferase (AST) to platelet ratio index, have shown lower accuracy, emphasizing the necessity of integrating transient elastography as a standard tool in managing patients with PBC and PSC, especially in determining advanced fibrosis stages (Chen *et al.*, 2023). Using both diagnostic imaging and clinical evaluation for PBC and PSC helps with the correct diagnosis and also directs the treatment plan. Thanks to new imaging methods, it is now possible to find liver problems early, which is very important for these autoimmune liver diseases. For example, imaging studies often reveal concentric lamellar fibrosis and other abnormalities that can inform the clinical management of OS between PBC and PSC, as detailed in specific case studies (Souissi *et al.*, 2024). With such a clear diagnosis, clinicians are able to prescribe UDCA which studies have found can improve liver function in appropriate patients. Thus, the ongoing development and application of sophisticated imaging techniques significantly enhance the comprehensive care of individuals affected by PBC and PSC, ultimately leading to improved patient outcomes (Figure 12.13).

12.4.3. Differentiating PSC from Other Cholestatic Liver Diseases

To tell apart PSC from other cholestatic liver diseases, like PBC, one needs to be aware of their specific symptoms and how the diseases work. PSC is marked by changes in the biliary tree and inflammation, which result in cholestasis, but PBC mainly involves the immune system attacking the small bile ducts. A main difference is the demographic; most PSC cases happen in young men and are linked to IBD, whereas PBC is more common in older women. Furthermore, serological markers such as AMAs are specific to PBC, while PSC typically presents with perinuclear anti-neutrophil cytoplasmic antibodies (pANCA). This separation of clinical and laboratory findings is very important for making the right diagnosis and choosing the right treatment for patients with cholestatic liver diseases. Many cholestatic liver diseases have similar biochemical and histological features, which makes it necessary to use advanced tests to tell PSC apart from PBC and other conditions. Using serum metabolomics, recent research has found profiles that can help doctors accurately tell PSC apart from PBC. For instance*et al.*, Bell *et al.* (2014) demonstrated that a mass spectrometry-based profiling approach revealed 56 metabolites that significantly differed between PSC and PBC groups. It helps doctors make more accurate diagnoses and also teaches us more about the metabolic problems in these diseases. With this kind of metabolic analysis, clinicians can more easily tell apart cholestatic conditions, which is important for managing and treating patients properly. Because the course of PSC varies and its response to treatment is not always the same, it is important to clearly tell it apart from other cholestatic liver diseases. Due to the unpredictable course of PSC and the possible complications like fibrosis and cirrhosis, managing these patients can be difficult because of the variable symptoms. Because biomarkers for measuring disease activity are not well-established, it has been hard to assess risk and choose effective treatments. Research into prognostic biomarkers, such as the enhanced liver fibrosis test (ELF), has indicated potential improvements in risk stratification in PSC, as highlighted by *et al.*Fossdal *et al.* (2023). Using several biomarker panels together, doctors can improve their ability to predict outcomes in PSC patients, which allows for more individualized treatment than what is used for other cholestatic liver diseases. These advancements in biomarker identification are crucial in streamlining clinical decision-making and improving patient outcomes across the spectrum of cholestatic liver diseases (Figure 12.14).

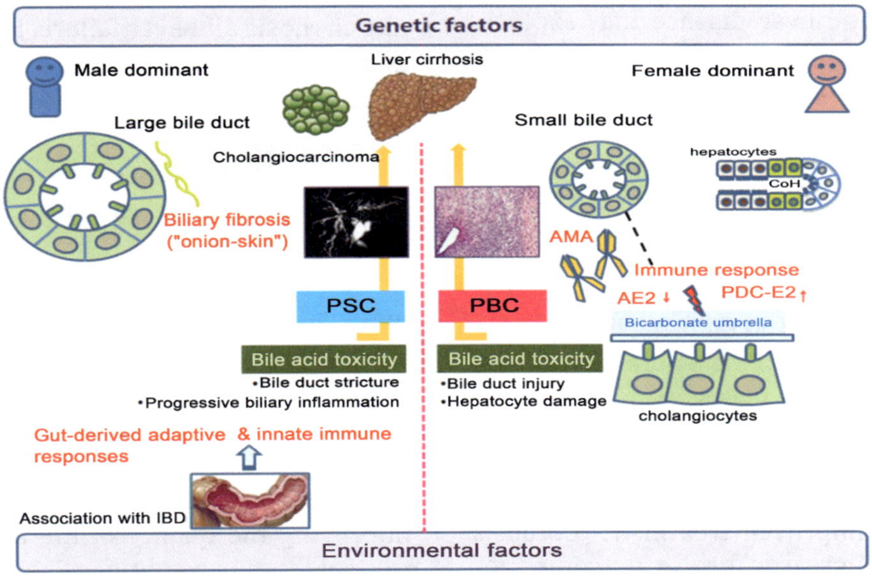

Figure 12.14. The comparison between PBC and PSC.

Source: https://www.researchgate.net/publication/360988410/figure/fig1/AS:11431281210341619@1702045344059/The-comparison-between-PBC-and-PSC-This-is-a-figure-highlighting-the-differences-between.tif.

12.5. Treatment Options for PBC

The management of PBC mainly relies on UDCA, which has also been established as the treatment milestone. Clinical trials have demonstrated that UDCA has a positive impact on biochemical tests and also retards disease evolution, and thus it is obligatory in PBC patients. Nonetheless, it is to be understood that close to 40% of the patients treated with UDCA can be classified as incomplete responders and hence need other or additional treatments. Against the backdrop of this clinical fact, new pharmacologic agents are the focus of ongoing research aimed at enhancing outcomes for such suboptimal responders. Research into novel therapy is a testament to an evolving paradigm in the management of PBC, testifying to the utility of personalized medicine in addressing the range of patient responses to therapies available (Mukewar, 2025). One of the emerging treatment options for PBC is the research on peroxisome proliferator-activated receptors (PPARs) since they play a vital role in regulating bile acid metabolism. Novel second-line therapies, particularly for non-respondee to UDCA alone, have recently been identified as PPAR agonists. Particular drugs such as elafibranor and seladelpar are in the spotlight, with the former recently acquiring accelerated approval from the United States Food and Drug Administration. These compounds have the potential to improve biliary function and decrease symptoms of cholestasis, including pruritus, which is a disabling and common feature in PBC. Progress in such new treatments serves to underscore the continuous evolution of therapeutic strategies for the improvement of patient quality of life and clinical outcomes in PBC (Hayes *et al.*, 2024). The therapeutic landscape for PBC is also complemented by research on chronic cholestatic liver disease that explores the implications of gut microbiome modulation as well as bile acid synthetic pathway effects. Current clinical research also continues to try to better understand how these biological systems interact and might potentially be targeted therapeutically. The use of non-invasive quantification of liver fibrosis, such as FIB-4 and transient elastography, also plays a key role in stratifying patient risk and tailoring intervention effectively. As researchers enter these new fields of research, the necessity for complete clinical trials to assess the safety and efficacy of emerging and existing therapies remains. This sustained investment in research verifies the commitment to improved treatment protocols and eventually increased health outcomes for PBC patients (Mukewar, 2025).

12.5.1. Pharmacological Therapies

Pharmacological therapies for PBC and PSC have evolved significantly, although challenges remain. In PBC, the primary treatment options include UDCA, which is effective in slowing disease progression in early-stage patients. However, approximately 40% of individuals exhibit an incomplete response to UDCA, necessitating alternative treatments such as obeticholic acid (OCA). While OCA represents an advancement in therapy for PBC, it is significant that its therapeutic efficacy in PSC remains modest, highlighting the importance of sustained research and development efforts in the area of pharmacological management of cholestasis-related liver disease.

As highlighted in current studies, various pharmacological mechanisms are being explored to enhance the current therapy available to such patients, particularly those that are poorly responsive to current treatments (Elzubeir *et al.*, 2025). The lack of a successful pharmacological treatment licensed for PSC constitutes a significant treatment problem, as the disease has a high tendency to lead to severe complications like cirrhosis and liver failure. Fresh evidence of immunologic mechanisms of pathogenesis of PSC has implicated a central role for T helper 17 cells (Th17) and their interleukin 17 (IL-17) signaling pathway. This fresh evidence has prompted studies of novel therapeutic agents targeting these pathways. For instance, brodalumab, an IL-17RA-targeted monoclonal antibody, is being tested in clinical trials to determine its safety and potential therapeutic efficacy in the treatment of PSC. These treatments are a departure from the paradigm of personalized medicine, not just extending the duration of the disease but also lessening symptoms and improving the quality of life for patients with this debilitating condition (Elzubeir *et al.*, 2025).

Research on peroxisome proliferator-activated receptors (PPARs) as therapeutic targets for the management of PBC and PSC is another promising avenue in drug therapy. PPARα, in particular, has been noted since it is involved in the detoxification and metabolism of bile acids. PPARα agonists such as fenofibrate have been reported to have potential in lowering cholestatic markers in patients who are resistant to UDCA and therefore serve as a useful adjunct treatment. In addition, newer PPAR agonists targeting more than one isoform (e.g., PPARβ/δ and PPARγ) are being developed that could provide additional therapeutic alternatives for promoting improved patient outcomes while treating the underlying biochemical dysregulation of cholestatic liver diseases. Continued investigation of such new pharmacologic agents is needed to progress therapy for PBC and PSC toward the goal of improving survival and quality of life in such patients (Gallucci *et al.*, 2024) (Figure 12.15).

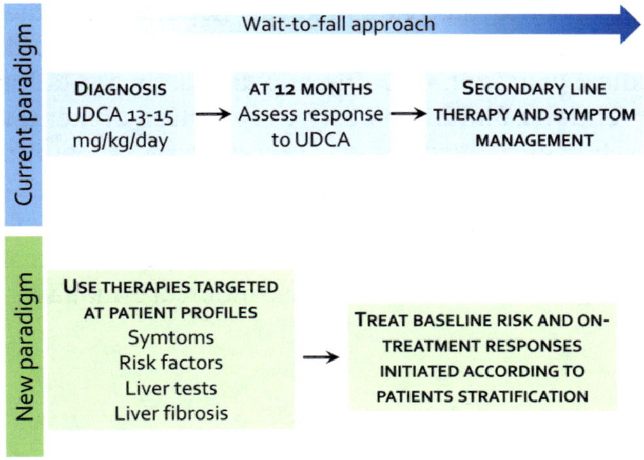

Figure 12.15. Comparison between current and new paradigms of PBC treatment. Current approaches include initiation of UDCA with assessment after 1 year of therapy and eventual shift to a second-line therapy in case of insufficient response to UDCA chosen on the basis of existing symptoms, comorbidities and drug availability. In contrast, the new paradigm is based on a more personalized approach that takes into account individual risk assessment since the beginning of the therapy.

Source: https://www.mdpi.com/cells/cells-13-01580/article_deploy/html/images/cells-13-01580-g003.png.

12.5.2. Lifestyle Modifications and Supportive Care

Lifestyle modification is also at the core of chronic liver disease (CLD) management, such as PBC and PSC. A well-balanced, high-nutrient diet is recommended, which plays a significant role in symptom relief and aiding in liver function. A diet low in saturated fats and high in omega-3 fatty acids can produce an anti-inflammatory effect, and the addition of fruits and vegetables ensures adequate vitamins and minerals. In addition, healthy weight through exercise can increase the metabolic capacity as well as reduce the progression of liver disease. Through lifestyle promotion on the basis of dietary health, patients can have an improved quality of life as well as possibly reduce the risk of complications related to their liver conditions, which therefore emphasizes the need for changing lifestyle in coping with PBC and PSC. Supportive therapy is a crucial component of symptom management in relation to PBC and PSC. Patients frequently complain of severe fatigue, potentially significantly influencing life quality. According to Kośnik and Wójcicki (2022), specific management aimed at reducing fatigue is essential in CLD patients. This can include the development of a structured daily routine that blends periods of rest with exercise intervals, as daily exercise is found to promote energy and mood. Moreover, psychological support, including counseling or support groups, can help deal with the emotional consequences of chronic illness. These supportive interventions should be given priority by clinicians together with medical intervention to ensure that the patient receives a total care approach to encompass that the patient not only deals with the disease but also with enhancing his/her life satisfaction and general well-being. Multidisciplinary interventions for patients with PBC and PSC are increasingly being identified as critical for these patients, especially since their conditions are likely to require complex management regimens. Integrated care involving hepatologists, dietitians, and mental health professionals can best utilize both lifestyle intervention and supportive therapy. Hepatologists, for instance, can treat the medical condition of CLD while dietitians can tailor nutrition programs that complement medical interventions. Simultaneously, the addition of mental health intervention is an acknowledgment of the psychological burden that CLD creates, with emotional well-being translated into better treatment compliance and outcomes. Besides, a well-coordinated optimal care plan can foster the patients' degree of understanding of their ailments and enable them to become active participants in their own health care, leading to better long-term outcomes as demonstrated by the necessity of holistic methods behind modern chronic care management (Aśnik *et al.*, 2022; Fuochi E *et al.*, 2023).

12.5.3. Liver Transplantation Considerations

The demand for liver transplantation is particularly high in patients with end-stage PBC and PSC, diseases that are marked by chronic inflammation and ultimate fibrosis of the liver. The conditions need to be diagnosed and treated early because they tend to progress to cirrhosis, which is marked by irreversible damage to the liver and faulty function. In PBC patients, standard treatment such as UDCA can slow down the progression of the disease, but if the liver fails to respond, only a transplant is a curative option.

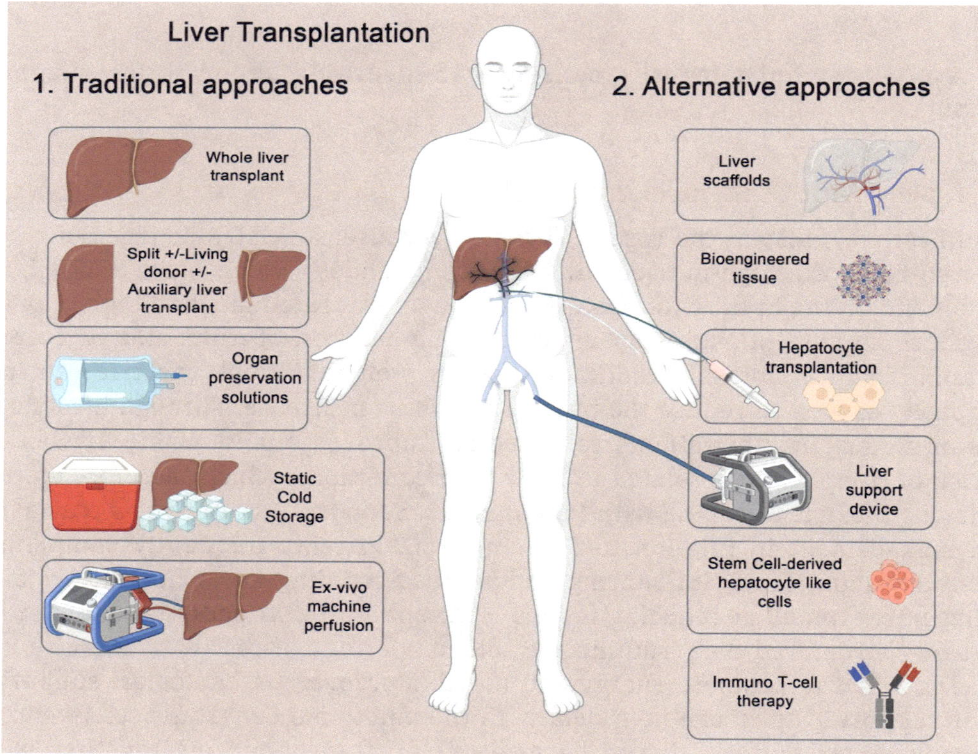

Figure 12.16. Liver transplantation.

Source: https://pub.mdpi-res.com/jcm/jcm-12-05586/article_deploy/html/images/jcm-12-05586-ag.png?1693204626.

In contrast, PSC also has increased complexity due to association with IBD and recurrent cholangitis, and thus management as well as timing of transplant is tricky. To manage the complex interplay of these conditions is key to the optimization of transplant candidacy and readiness for post-operative care in these patients (Trivedi *et al.*, 2024). Evaluation of a candidate's health status and response to treatment is also given careful consideration. In PBC, mortality without effective management strategies is high, and therefore careful monitoring of disease activity by repeating liver function tests, imaging, and symptom management is required. Although PSC lacks effective medical therapies apart from transplantation, new information suggests that newer agents may be possible that can modify disease progression. Ideal selection criteria for transplant must take into consideration such differences in disease processes. The special issue of PSC, too, with risks of post-transplant complications like re-recurrence of disease, demands multidisciplinary management, showing the necessity to monitor liver status as well as that of any concomitant disease (Bhushan *et al.*, 2024). Post-transplant results for the PBC and PSC patients are quite disparate, on the basis of pre-transplant disease severity and the presence of comorbid conditions. For PBC patients, transplant is worthwhile with excellent results, with most living with nearly normal liver function and improved quality of life post-surgery. PSC involves an increased risk of complications, including recurrence of disease in the grafted liver. Thus, long-term follow-up regimens are imperative for survivors, such as continued monitoring of liver function and management of complications. Researchers are studying ways to enhance post-transplant outcomes by employing new therapeutic approaches to mitigate disease recurrence and improve patients' overall survival. As the understanding of these autoimmune liver disorders advances, individualized therapy and postoperative care will remain integral components of follow-up care of patients who have received liver transplantation for PBC and PSC (Trivedi *et al.*, 2024) (Figure 12.16).

12.6. Treatment Options for PSC

Because PSC is a complex and progressive disease, the treatment choices have not been very broad in the past. Because it is an immune disorder that affects bile flow, PSC can seriously harm the liver and calls for a variety of treatments. The main focus now is on reducing symptoms and handling any complications. UDCA seems to help with liver biochemistry and may slow the progress of disease in a group of patients, but its effects on clinical outcomes are still being studied. Recent studies indicate that the utilization of new immunomodulatory therapies could represent a potential advancement in treatment strategies, particularly in light of the findings regarding the cellular environment in PSC-affected livers, where dysfunctional immune responses predominate (Andrews *et al.*, 2024). Developing and testing these new treatments depends on continuous clinical trials. Because PSC is commonly linked to problems like IBD, gastroenterologists and hepatologists need to work together for the best care of patients. Those with advanced liver disease to be closely watched for liver cancer and the related risk of cholangiocarcinoma. Regular surveillance through imaging and serum biomarkers, such as CA19-9, is recommended to detect malignancies at an early stage, particularly given the strong association of PSC with cholangiocarcinoma (L-Sánchez *et al.*, 2022). Liver transplantation is still considered the best treatment for people with severe liver disease, yet there are not enough donors, and patients must take immunosuppressants for life, which causes many difficulties. Therefore, understanding diseases better and finding better ways to treat them helps people affected by them live better and longer. Researchers are now discovering how cells are involved in PSC pathology, which can lead to new treatments. Recent findings, such as the hyper-activation and exhausted states of myeloid cells in PSC tissue, highlight how these immune profiles can inform targeted drug development aimed at restoring immune balance (Andrews *et al.*, 2024). Also, the presence of cholangiocyte-like hepatocytes in fibrotic areas suggests that there may be different ways the liver tries to repair itself in PSC. This new information might result in treatments that handle PSC symptoms and also change the way the disease progresses. When precision medicine is used with patient biomarkers, it may make treatments more effective, which underlines the need for a strong and flexible approach to PSC.

12.6.1. Current Medical Therapies and Their Efficacy

Because the causes of PBC and PSC are not fully known, managing these diseases is still difficult. At present, doctors mainly manage symptoms and try to slow the disease, rather than provide a cure. UDCA is now considered a main treatment for PBC, as it effectively improves liver function and delays the development of cirrhosis. According to recent studies, UDCA improves bile production and also guards against liver cell damage. Also, more agents are being studied to make UDCA therapy more effective, as knowledge about cholestatic liver diseases continues to advance. Still, for PSC, the absence of effective treatments highlights the importance of finding new approaches to deal with the special immune and fibrotic changes in this disease, as is being studied by researchers. Because of new treatments, BAs and the pathways they use have become attractive targets for treating cholestatic liver diseases such as PSC. Investigations have shown that problems with bile acid regulation result in cell damage, inflammation, and scarring, which has encouraged researchers to focus more on bile acid receptor mediators. Bile acid synthesis and circulation are mainly regulated by the Farnesoid X receptor and the apical sodium-dependent bile acid transporter. There are now new methods to manage these receptors, which help lessen liver injury and inflammation in PSC. Clinical studies are being done to test how these bile acid receptor modulators work, which may bring a new option for treating CLD that has been hard to manage effectively, highlighting the role of diet and the gut-liver connection.

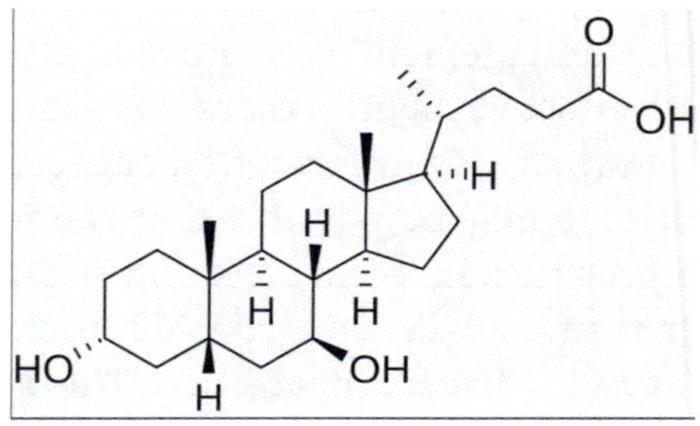

Figure 12.17. Chemical structure of ursodeoxycholic acid.

Source: https://upload.wikimedia.org/wikipedia/commons/thumb/6/6b/Ursodeoxycholic_acid_acsv.svg/1024px-Ursodeoxycholic_acid_acsv.svg.png.

Because reactions to therapies differ, a personalized method is still required for managing PBC and PSC. Monitoring a disease by doing LFTs, imaging, and endoscopic exams is considered important in current medical practice. This way of managing patients points out that these diseases are not the same for everyone, and their treatment outcomes may vary a lot. As a result, combining lifestyle changes such as eating healthy and exercising with medications may give the best results. As research on the underlying processes and new drugs goes on, there is a chance for creating better and more targeted treatments. Ultimately, the pursuit of individualized treatments for PBC and PSC is crucial for improving patient quality of life and long-term liver health, paving the way for future advancements in therapeutic efficacy (Figure 12.17).

12.6.2. Role of Endoscopic Interventions

Endoscopic therapy is the key to the treatment of PBC and PSC. Though these conditions inherently affect bile duct function and liver quality, endoscopic interventions such as Endoscopic Retrograde Cholangiopancreatography (ERCP) are necessary for the diagnosis and management of cholestasis-related complications. ERCP allows for bile duct imaging, and it becomes feasible to differentiate PSC from other biliary diseases, such as cholangiocarcinoma. With the procurement of tissue samples and the use of techniques to relieve bile duct obstructions, ERCP also enhances symptoms arising from stricture formations and enhances patient outcomes in the long term. The procedure is especially vital in patients who may not be candidates for liver transplantation because maintenance of bile flow will prolong survival and enhance the quality of care in this group of patients (Mizuno *et al.*, 2025). The value of planned follow-up interventions with ERCP has been highlighted by recent studies, emphasizing proactive PSC management. Retrospective analysis confirmed that patients who underwent planned ERCPs had higher transplant-free survival (TFS) rates than those who underwent ERCP on a purely clinical basis. Specifically, the analysis indicated that median TFS was notably longer in patients who were subjected to routine monitoring and intervention. Such ongoing monitoring allows for early identification and management of biliary obstruction-related exacerbations, as well as reducing the incidence of recurrent cholangitis and other undesirable complications. Thus, this proactive strategy not only enhances patient welfare but also highlights the imperative to integrate endoscopic interventions into routine care protocols for PSC patients (Özdirik *et al.*, 2024). Integration of endoscopic ultrasonography (EUS) into the care of PBC and PSC is a developing area with the potential for improved patient outcomes. Although its role in PSC has yet to be determined, it provides a minimally invasive imaging modality that can provide a worthwhile benefit in the diagnosis of pancreatic and biliary illness. EUS can potentially detect the very subtle changes in biliary architecture that will not be evident on conventional imaging modalities and thus provide additional diagnostic certainty. As the literature continues to establish the role of EUS and its potential benefits when applied in conjunction with ERCP, it is imperative to explore how these combined endoscopic methodologies can optimally maximize outcomes in the management of patients afflicted with these multifactorial cholestatic disorders. This new approach can shape the future of interventional gastroenterology, advocating personalized treatment based on the individual pathophysiology of PBC and PSC.

12.6.3. Liver Transplantation as a Treatment Option

Liver transplantation becomes a pressing intervention in situations involving patients with severe PBC and PSC, particularly when conventional treatments are not sufficient. Being cholestatic chronic illnesses, both PBC and PSC can lead to severe liver damage, progressing to cirrhosis and threatening liver failure. In these situations, transplantation is not just a therapeutic intervention but also, in most situations, a requirement to improve survival and reestablish the quality of life. With the limitations of present-day medical therapy, such as UDCA and more recently introduced agents like obeticholic acid (OCA) for PBC, liver transplantation is a more long-term outcome for patients who have progressed to end-stage liver disease. The problem lies in the consideration for liver transplantation, taking on significance in the management of the long-term outcomes in patients with these autoimmune liver diseases (Trivedi *et al.*, 2024). Furthermore, suitability for transplantation is a judicious assessment of numerous varied clinical parameters, including the severity of liver damage and the general health of the patient. Transplantation in patients with PBC and PSC is typically reserved for patients who develop decompensated cirrhosis, intractable pruritus, or other disabling manifestations that are not controlled by pharmacologic measures. The intricacies of autoimmune liver diseases, coupled with the heterogeneity in their presentations, require patient-specific deliberation to determine the timing and appropriateness of transplantation. Moreover, as these diseases also increase the risk for complications such as cholangiocarcinoma, monitoring over time and early intervention form an essential part of the care plan. Last but not least, the decision to even entertain transplant is a multidisciplinary one involving hepatologists, transplant surgeons, and even the patients themselves to provide the optimal outcome (Trivedi *et al.*, 2024). Despite advances in medical treatment of PBC and PSC, liver transplantation remains the only therapeutic option for end-stage liver disease caused by these conditions. Post-transplantation, the patients enjoy improvement in liver function and symptom relief for the disease, a welcome milestone in their medical trajectory. But transplantation success entails a lifetime of immunosuppressive therapy to prevent graft rejection, as well as ongoing monitoring for potential recurrence of autoimmune disease. Therapeutic avenues and advances in immunosuppression regimens will further optimize the post-transplant experience, highlighting justification for continued research along such lines. With evolutions in the terrain, understanding of the interface between novel treatments and liver transplantation will be important to further enhance survival and quality of life in patients with PBC and PSC (Bhushan *et al.*, 2024).

SUMMARY

The intricacies of PBC and PSC highlight the need for a multi-pronged approach towards understanding and managing these autoimmune liver conditions. The two diseases, though uncommon, are challenging to diagnose and treat because they are chronic in nature and also carry the potential to develop into liver failure. As can be seen from recent publications, although giving important insights into the etiological pathological processes, the dynamic interaction between genetic susceptibility, environmental factors, and homeostasis of gut microbiota remains pivotal to the identification of targeted treatment modalities. Studies must uncover these complexities further, thereby enabling the implementation of more potent treatment regimens capable of directly acting on the paradigm of the conditions and improving the outcomes in patients (Trivedi *et al.*, 2024). Furthermore, while treatment of PBC has become better with newer therapy agents being licensed, PSC remains with limited intensive therapy other than liver transplant. This stark difference highlights the necessity for more clinical research and creativity in treating PSC. Despite recent developments such as the inclusion of obeticholic acid and promising investigational treatments, neither disease group has a panacea for all. The worth of a therapeutic regimen tailored to the individual is its potential to halt disease progression and alleviate symptoms, thus enhancing the quality of life in patients with these conditions (Bhushan *et al.*, 2024). As research becomes ever more sophisticated, joint efforts by clinicians, researchers, and patients are becoming more critical. Stakeholders must advocate for more funding and support of research, which can usher new treatments to market sooner. Knowledge of PBC and PSC in depth not only assists those diagnosed but also lays the groundwork for prevention in at-risk populations. In the years to come, there is a need to foster awareness, early detection, and continuous education regarding these rare autoimmune diseases, while promoting an open environment for innovation in treatment modalities, and closely monitoring their clinical efficacy and safety. The commitment to learn more about our knowledge and treatment will ultimately have long-term impacts on improved patient management and outcomes in PBC and PSC patients.

The autoimmune pathogenesis of PBC and the immunological involvement in PSC highlight similarities and differences between these two cholestatic liver illnesses. PBC primarily involves small intrahepatic bile ducts and is characterized by lymphocytic damage, which is believed to be an autoimmune response leading to progressive cholestasis and ultimate hepatic failure. Evidence points toward diminished lymphokine production, namely tumor necrosis factor, as key to the pathogenesis of PBCs, with evidence pointing toward complex interaction between immune mechanisms and tissue damage (Eisenburg *et al.*, 1992). On the other hand, PSC is defined by intrahepatic and extrahepatic bile duct fibrosis, with significant prevalence among patients with IBD. While PSC describes a typical pathophysiological picture, the common immune dysregulation is the basis for the disorders. Although the pathologies are distinct, general similarities between PBC's clinical presentation and course and those of PSC are appreciated. Both illnesses typically manifest with cholestatic symptoms such as jaundice, fatigue, and pruritus secondary to bile flow disruption. Patients typically experience a gradual deterioration of liver function, eventually leading to cirrhosis, although the rate of progression may be extremely variable between patients and diseases. Both PBC and PSC also share connections to other autoimmune diseases, pointing to potential similarities in immune mechanisms. PBCs are female predominant compared with the male profile of PSC, establishing a significant demographic distinction; however, both conditions affect middle-aged adults. This symptom overlap and complication further contribute to the necessity of extensive diagnostic work-ups to better differentiate these diseases. Treatment management of PBC and PSC illustrates both convergence and divergence in clinical practice, particularly in therapeutic approaches. UDCA is currently considered the treatment of choice for PBC, improving liver function and hindering disease progression in the majority of patients. In contrast, no therapeutic regimens for PSC have been developed, a finding necessitating emphasis on the management of such complications as biliary strictures and cholangiocarcinoma risk (Bergquist *et al.*, 2009). Such therapeutic inadequacy suggests a necessity for immediate innovative research with the aim of finding effective PSC treatments. Both conditions can, further, necessitate liver transplantation as a last resort for end-stage liver disease. Lastly, recognition of the finer differences and similarities in pathophysiology, presentation, and management of PBC and PSC is necessary to optimize patient outcome and guide research in the future."

CLOSER LOOK

ANTIMITOCHONDRIAL ANTIBODIES (AMAS)

AMAs are autoantibodies that target mitochondria, the powerhouses of cells. They are particularly associated with PBC, a liver disease, and can also be found in other autoimmune conditions. AMAs are detected through blood tests, and elevated levels can indicate PBC or other autoimmune disorders (Figure 12.18).

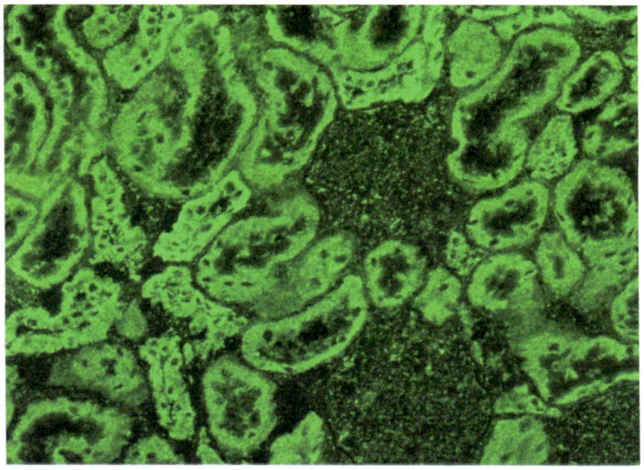

Figure 12.18. **Antimitochondrial Antibodies (AMAs)**

Source: https://www.launchdiagnostics.com/wp-content/uploads/2015/09/AMA.png.

- **Mitochondria and Autoantibodies:** Mitochondria are essential for cellular energy production. AMAs are autoantibodies that mistakenly attack these organelles.
- **Primary Biliary Cholangitis (PBC):** AMAs are a hallmark of PBC, a chronic autoimmune disease that damages the bile ducts in the liver. About 90-95% of individuals with PBC have detectable AMAs.
- **AMA Types:** Several AMA subtypes exist, with M2 and M9 being particularly associated with PBC.
- **Blood Test:** A blood test measures the amount of AMAs in the blood.
- **Clinical Significance:** High levels of AMAs, especially AMA-M2, strongly suggest PBC. Lower levels may be found in other autoimmune diseases or liver conditions.
- **Other Conditions:** AMAs can also be found in autoimmune diseases like Sjögren's syndrome, systemic sclerosis, and autoimmune thyroid disease, as well as in inflammatory myopathy and even heart disease.

Diagnosis and Monitoring: AMAs are a valuable tool for diagnosing PBC and monitoring its progression. Decreasing AMA titres over time may indicate successful treatment, according to a study published in the National Institutes of Health (NIH).

References

1. Abhyankar, A., Bonder, A., & Tapper, E. (2013). *Immunosuppressive Therapy in Immune-Mediated Liver Disease in the Non-Transplanted Patient.* https://core.ac.uk/download/28947826.pdf (accessed on 24 May 2025).
2. Akbar, H. O., & Fallatah, H. I. (2011). *Autoimmune Liver Disease–Are There Spectra that We do not Know?* https://core.ac.uk/download/pdf/8620050.pdf.
3. Albers, H. M., Barrett, J. C., Bergquist, A., Bo, X., Göke, B., *et al.* (2011). *Analysis of IL2/IL21 Gene Variants in Cholestatic Liver Diseases Reveals an Association with Primary Sclerosing Cholangitis.* https://core.ac.uk/download/16432732.pdf (accessed on 24 May 2025).
4. Alexopoulou, A., Alvarez, F., Block, J., Boonstra, K., Deneau, M., Dotson, J. L., Faubion, W. A., *et al.* (2016). *Clinical Features and Risk Factors of Autoimmune Liver Involvement in Pediatric Inflammatory Bowel Disease.* https://core.ac.uk/download/74318847.pdf (accessed on 24 May 2025).
5. Alkhatib, A. J. (2023). Autoimmunity and liver disease: Updates of the literature. *New Medical Innovations and Research.* https://www.semanticscholar.org/paper/ad15ec150520a9daf8604b01ff32a352f54cb137 (accessed on 24 May 2025).
6. Alpini, G., Francis, H., Glaser, S., Kennedy, L., *et al.* (2019). Preclinical insights into cholangiopathies: disease modeling and emerging therapeutic targets. https://core.ac.uk/download/344336420.pdf (accessed on 24 May 2025).
7. Alpini, G., Francis, H., Kennedy, L., Kundu, D., *et al.* (2020). Bile acid receptor therapeutics effects on chronic liver diseases. https://core.ac.uk/download/299809078.pdf (accessed on 24 May 2025).
8. Alvaro, D., Cardinale, V., Carpino, G., Franchitto, A., *et al.* (2018). Contribution of resident stem cells to liver and biliary tree regeneration in human diseases. https://core.ac.uk/download/188824417.pdf (accessed on 24 May 2025).
9. Andrews, T., Nakib, D., Perciani, C. T., Zhong, X., Liu, L., Winter, E., Camat, D., *et al.* (2024). Single-cell, single-nucleus, and spatial transcriptomics characterization of the immunological landscape in the healthy and PSC human liver. *Journal of Hepatology, 80*, 730–743. https://doi.org/10.1016/j.jhep.2023.12.023.
10. Bell, L. N., Chalasani, N., Comerford, M., Vuppalanchi, R., *et al.* (2014). Serum metabolic signatures of primary biliary cirrhosis and primary sclerosing cholangitis. https://core.ac.uk/download/46963417.pdf (accessed on 24 May 2025).
11. Bergquist, A., Escorsell, A., Karrar, A., Lopez-Vazquez, A., Shorbagi, A., Spurkland, A., Stiehl, A., *et al.* (2009). *The Immunobiology of Primary Sclerosing Cholangitis.* https://core.ac.uk/download/pdf/8336461.pdf.
12. Bhushan, S., Sohal, A., Kowdley, K. V., *et al.* (2024). Primary biliary cholangitis and primary sclerosing cholangitis therapy landscape. *The American Journal of Gastroenterology.* https://www.semanticscholar.org/paper/2033a0279d24ac75b5eb077d7e39896768d7db3e (accessed on 24 May 2025).
13. Boberg, K. M., & Karlsen, T. H. (2015). Update on Primary Sclerosing Cholangitis. https://core.ac.uk/download/479088936.pdf (accessed on 24 May 2025).

14. Chen, H., Shen, Y., Wu, S. D., Zhu, Q., Weng, C. Z., Zhang, J., Wang, M. X., *et al.* (2023). Diagnostic role of transient elastography in patients with autoimmune liver diseases: A systematic review and meta-analysis. *World Journal of Gastroenterology, 29*, 5503–5525. https://www.semanticscholar.org/paper/f8dca206b84652285c111d4d2da4fcafe07e6915 (accessed on 24 May 2025).

15. Yoshida, Hiroyuki ...[et al]. Anti-integrin αvβ6 autoantibodies in patients with primary sclerosing cholangitis. Journal of Gastroenterology 2023, 58(8): 778-789 https://core.ac.uk/download/587263704.pdf (accessed on 24 May 2025).

16. Dai, L., Ye, Y., Mugaany, J., Hu, Z., Huang, J., & Lu, C. (2024). Leveraging pQTL-based Mendelian randomization to identify new treatment prospects for primary biliary cholangitis and primary sclerosing cholangitis. *Aging (Albany NY), 16*, 9228–9250. https://www.semanticscholar.org/paper/349e4a929c59107881545a58bb4811156917c55a (accessed on 24 May 2025).

17. Eisenburg, J., Hoffmann, R. M., Jung, M. C., Messer, G., *et al.* (1992). T lymphocytes from patients with primary biliary cirrhosis produce reduced amounts of lymphotoxin, tumor necrosis factor and interferon-gamma upon mitogen stimulation. https://core.ac.uk/download/12163939.pdf (accessed on 24 May 2025).

18. Elzubeir, A., High, J., Hammond, M., Shepstone, L., Pond, M., Walmsley, M., Trivedi, P., *et al.* (2025). Assessing brodalumab in the treatment of primary sclerosing cholangitis (SABR-PSC pilot study): Protocol for a single-arm, multicentre, pilot study. *BMJ Open Gastroenterology, 12*. https://www.semanticscholar.org/paper/4315243fbaab975f4da2cfbdf5636cd81f6cc6be (accessed on 24 May 2025).

19. Forenc, T., Kaczorowska, A., Kaczorowski, R., Krupa, R., *et al.* (2024). Clinically oriented look into diagnostics and therapy of primary sclerosing cholangitis: Review of literature. https://core.ac.uk/download/620863367.pdf (accessed on 24 May 2025).

20. Fossdal, G. (2023). Primary sclerosing cholangitis: Surrogate markers of natural history, disease severity, and prognosis. https://core.ac.uk/download/596353721.pdf (accessed on 24 May 2025).

21. Fuochi, E., Anastasio, L., Lynch, E. N., Campani, C., Dragoni, G., Milani, S., Galli, A., *et al.* (2023). Main factors influencing long-term outcomes of liver transplantation in 2022. *World Journal of Hepatology, 15*(3), 321–352. https://doi.org/10.4254/wjh.v15.i3.321.

22. Gallucci, G., Hayes, C. M., Boyer, J. L., Barbier, O., Assis, D. N., & Ghonem, N. S. (2024). PPAR-mediated bile acid glucuronidation: Therapeutic targets for the treatment of cholestatic liver diseases. *Cells, 13*. https://www.semanticscholar.org/paper/d652c07f2363d107d3cc417da40ec6d89f1592d2 (accessed on 24 May 2025).

23. Gao, W., Peng, C., Wang, Z., Li, Y., & Liu, M. (2024). Genetic association and causal relationship between multiple modifiable risk factors and autoimmune liver disease: A two-sample Mendelian randomization study. *Journal of Translational Medicine, 22*. https://www.semanticscholar.org/paper/b0e9e05e60d7dc48c2d452125f506c5879f571b0 (accessed on 24 May 2025).

24. Grama, A., Mititelu, A., Sîrbe, C., Bența, G., & Pop, T. (2023). Immune-mediated cholangiopathies in children: The need to better understand the pathophysiology for finding the future possible treatment targets. *Frontiers in Immunology, 14*. https://www.semanticscholar.org/paper/a2fd220751683423824b786d7ceb05c3e006ec80 (accessed on 24 May 2025).

25. Hayes, C. M., Gallucci, G., Boyer, J. L., Assis, D. N., & Ghonem, N. S. (2024). PPAR agonists for the treatment of cholestatic liver diseases: Over a decade of clinical progress. *Hepatology Communications, 9*. https://www.semanticscholar.org/paper/b12d8a04ba4e85487b87b9c9cfbd3cdb792d135d (accessed on 24 May 2025).

26. Hegade, V. S., Hirschfield, G. M., & Jones, D. E. J. (2017). Apical sodium-dependent transporter inhibitors in primary biliary cholangitis and primary sclerosing cholangitis. https://core.ac.uk/download/pdf/267299827.pdf (accessed on 24 May 2025).

27. Hirschfield, G., Marshall, T., Ryan, R., Webb, G., *et al.* (2021). The epidemiology of UK autoimmune liver disease varies with geographic latitude. https://core.ac.uk/download/426751311.pdf (accessed on 24 May 2025).

28. Izquierdo-Sánchez, L., Lamarca, Á., La Casta, A., Buettner, S., Utpatel, K., Klümpen, H. J., Adeva, J., *et al.* (2022). Cholangiocarcinoma landscape in Europe: Diagnostic, prognostic and therapeutic insights from the ENSCCA Registry. *Journal of Hepatology, 76*, 1109–1121. https://doi.org/10.1016/j.jhep.2021.12.010.

29. Juran, B., McCauley, B. M., Atkinson, E. J., Schlicht, E., Bianchi, J. K., Vollenweider, J. M., Ye, H., *et al.* (2024). Epigenetic disease markers in primary sclerosing cholangitis and primary biliary cholangitis—Methylomics of cholestatic liver disease. *Hepatology Communications, 8*. https://www.semanticscholar.org/paper/992a77cea8d660f5d021bc87f11844797769a4a6 (accessed on 24 May 2025).

30. Kersten, R. H. J. (2024). Cholangiocellular defense mechanisms in IgG4-related cholangitis: Role of autoantigens and autoantibodies. https://core.ac.uk/download/604744591.pdf (accessed on 24 May 2025).

31. Kośnik, A., & Wójcicki, M. (2022). Fatigue in chronic liver disease patients: Prevalence, pathophysiology, and management. *Gastroenterology Review, 17*, 21–27. https://doi.org/10.5114/pg.2022.114594.

32. Leuschner, U., & Schlichting, J. (2013). Drug therapy of primary biliary diseases: Classical and modern strategies. https://core.ac.uk/download/14526202.pdf (accessed on 24 May 2025).

33. Miteva, D., Peshevska-Sekulovska, M., Snegarova, V., Peruhova, M., Vasilev, G., Sekulovski, M., *et al.* (2023). Microbiome and genetic factors in the pathogenesis of liver diseases. *Gastroenterology Insights*. https://www.semanticscholar.org/paper/6618d8840ec2b32c933655cc5a4a046a8314f204 (accessed on 24 May 2025).

34. Mizuno, S., Uchida, Y., Ando, S., Nakao, M., Sugawara, K., Nakayama, N., Imai, Y., *et al.* (2025). Endoscopic management of primary sclerosing cholangitis. *Digestive Endoscopy: Official Journal of the Japan Gastroenterological Endoscopy Society*. https://www.semanticscholar.org/paper/130c5667842341297827fabe441ac9e4be3a9d9f (accessed on 24 May 2025).

35. Mukewar, S. (2025). Recent advances in diagnosis and management of chronic cholestatic liver diseases: Expert consensus. *International Journal of Research in Medical Sciences*. https://www.semanticscholar.org/paper/eb16fa42970246141e2f934751ded5fd927951be (accessed on 24 May 2025).

36. Nanjundappa, R. H., Christen, U., & Umeshappa, C. S. (2023). Distinct immune surveillance in primary biliary cholangitis and primary sclerosing cholangitis is linked with discrete cholangiocarcinoma risk. *Hepatology Communications, 7*. https://www.semanticscholar.org/paper/526f789d52fcfa39cc3a359b240c17297edfccef (accessed on 24 May 2025).

37. Nurmukhamedova, N. S., Sharopov, Z. A., & Xudoynazarov, A. A. (2023). Review on hepatobiliary disorders and complications of ulcerative colitis. https://core.ac.uk/download/591387690.pdf (accessed on 24 May 2025).

38. Özdirik, B., Veltzke-Schlieker, W., Nicklaus, J., Berger, H., Schmidt, D., Leonhardt, S., Penndorf, V., *et al.* (2024). Long-term impact of scheduled regular endoscopic interventions for patients with primary sclerosing cholangitis. *Hepatology Communications, 8*. https://www.semanticscholar.org/paper/5fc4331be953658e6ab39ecf42b5b4c0b2db047f (accessed on 24 May 2025).

39. Pak, E., Petrova, T. M., Korobka, R. V., Ushakov, A. A., Kucherenko, O. B., Katsiyaev, V. Y., & Bukhtin, O. V. (2024). Recurrence of primary sclerosing cholangitis in the graft. *Medical Herald of the South of Russia*. https://www.semanticscholar.org/paper/fcf705c85a29ec7fcad1e3fbbd12eb64a73c882c (accessed on 24 May 2025).

40. Semlali, R., Handa, A., Chakor, F., Nacir, O., Lairani, F., Ait Errami, A., S., O., *et al.* (2024). Uncommon association of primary biliary cholangitis and ulcerative colitis in a male patient, cirrhosis as a presenting feature: A case report. *Scholars Journal of Medical Case Reports*. https://www.semanticscholar.org/paper/909818c928b989789fe1ee60e7972efbc2000d06 (accessed on 24 May 2025).

41. Souissi, S., Laabidi, S., Mustpha, N. B., Chelly, I., Serghini, M., Fékih, M., Laabidi, A., *et al.* (2024). Overlap syndrome of seronegative primary biliary cholangitis and small duct primary sclerosing cholangitis: A first case report and literature review. *Future Science OA, 10*. https://www.semanticscholar.org/paper/4ec2d0aaf30d4775236c85c891193c5f4f25bf53 (accessed on 24 May 2025).

42. Trivedi, P., Hirschfield, G. M., Adams, D. H., & Vierling, J. M. (2024). Immunopathogenesis of primary biliary cholangitis, primary sclerosing cholangitis and autoimmune hepatitis: Themes and concepts. *Gastroenterology*. https://www.semanticscholar.org/paper/a7321926f05831df9c52524849076678d9ae33c1 (accessed on 24 May 2025).

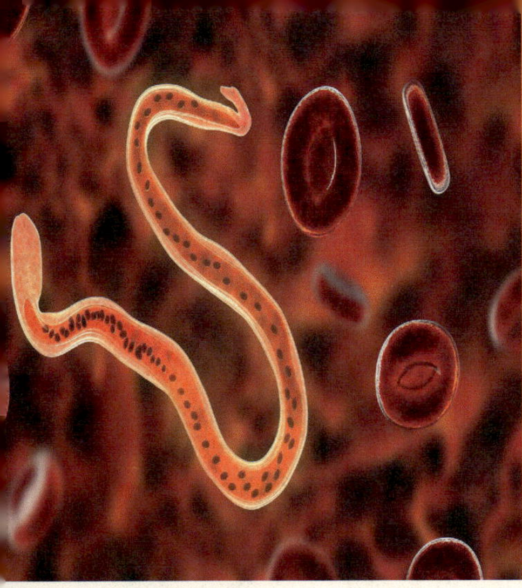

Chapter 13

PARASITIC AND INFECTIOUS DISEASES OF THE LIVER

Contents

Introduction

The liver plays a vital part in keeping the body's metabolism stable and also detoxifying other substances in the body. At the same time, the liver can be affected by many parasitic and infectious diseases that can cause serious problems for the organ. Examples are viral hepatitis, which may result in cirrhosis and liver cancer if not treated. Understanding these diseases, researchers have pointed out that the environment and, in particular, water quality, is a major cause of liver problems. For instance, more than 80% of human activity-generated sewage is discharged without treatment, contributing to excessive health risks resulting from water pollution, one being liver-altering diseases (Lin *et al.*, 2022). Thus, the reaction to infectious agents' influence on the liver is of utmost importance in matters of public health mitigation and prevention. Since liver diseases are increasing around the world, it is now important to study how these diseases are spread and what effects the parasites and pathogens have on the liver. Hepatitis viruses can multiply where clean water is not available, and a lot of research has found that poor sanitation is linked to these infections. Because of these findings, it is now clearer that environmental health is important for liver disease, so more extensive research is needed. In addition, there is interest in looking at how flavonoids in food interact with liver health. Flavonoids possess potential liver disease-protective effects due to their anti-inflammatory and antioxidant action (Ullah *et al.*, 2020). For this reason, both the environmental and nutritional factors that cause liver disease should be studied together. It is important to be aware of how to prevent and treat liver disease, mainly in places where it is common. Improving how people wash their hands can play a big role in stopping parasitic infections that lead to liver diseases. Besides prevention, more studies should focus on finding effective treatments, especially on how different drugs can affect the liver. Further studies should focus on how substances found in nature, such as flavonoids, can help prevent and treat liver disease. Having a clear idea of parasitic infections and the benefits of some food ingredients, medical professionals are able to manage liver diseases and introduce helpful public health policies.

Definition of Parasitic and Infectious Diseases

Both parasitic and infectious diseases are major threats to health worldwide, and they mainly impact the liver. Parasitic diseases happen when parasites need another organism to complete their life cycle. The liver's ability to support growth is used by parasites, which results in diseases such as schistosomiasis and echinococcosis. Trematode (blood fluke)-induced schistosomiasis can cause widespread liver fibrosis and portal hypertension, while echinococcosis caused by the Echinococcus species can cause cysts in the liver, followed by complications of bile duct obstruction. Some bacterial and viral infections may seriously affect the liver's function. Hepatitis viruses, like their affinity for liver cells, have the ability to bring about chronic infection, cirrhosis, and hepatocellular carcinoma (HCC) that reflect the importance of early diagnosis and effective treatment strategies towards limiting the adverse effects of these conditions on liver functions. Also, parasitic and infectious diseases develop through various factors and can cause many physical reactions in the body. An example is that a parasitic infection can cause inflammation, which leads to hepatocyte damage, and this can result in immune-related injury. Infections similar to leptospirosis, such as BI, can also lead to hepatic cholestasis and inflammation, which makes the disease more complicated. It is important to know these mechanisms to create interventions that protect the liver. Also, this complexity is shown in the way infections like hepatitis are influenced by other infections or diseases they share. Good health care strategies need to include both ways to prevent illness and ways to treat it.

To be specific, more attention should be given to preventive steps to fight the high rate of liver health problems in areas where infections are common. It is also important for management to understand how these liver diseases spread, what their symptoms are, and which social and economic factors contribute to their transmission. Endemic areas for schistosomiasis are often marked by poor hygiene and scarce clean water, which greatly affects the prevalence and severity of cases. Moreover, global health programs should focus on the dependency between infection and nutrition; anemia from various causes, including parasitic infection, is prevalent and a large public health risk, especially among vulnerable groups (Chaparro *et al.*, 2019). Also, community-based efforts can help control these diseases and show the benefits of using education, better sanitation and available healthcare services together. Thus, understanding the precise definitions and processes of infectious and parasitic diseases is essential to crafting effective control measures that target liver health at the population and individual levels (Figure 13.1) (Bowlus *et al.*, 2022).

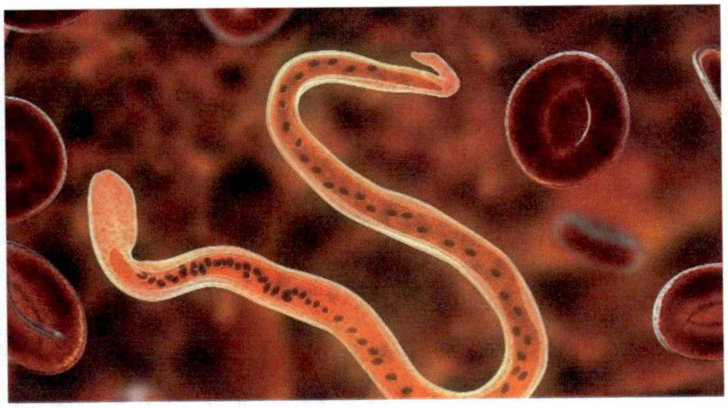

Figure 13.1. Parasitic and Infectious Diseases

Source: https://www.cdc.gov/yellow-book/media/images/2025/02/10.6-Post-Travel-Parasitic-Disease-Including-Evaluation-of-Eosinophilia.jpg.

Importance of the Liver in Human Health

The liver is necessary for maintaining good health in people. Among its key roles are processing nutrients, eliminating dangerous substances, and making important proteins such as albumin and clotting factors. The body's ability to handle nutrients, keep blood sugar under control, and remove waste is influenced by the health of the liver. Parasitic or infectious diseases can damage the liver, which may result in poor liver function. LC or hepatitis can interrupt normal liver activities, which leads to health issues that may harm the function of a single organ and have an adverse effect on the body as a whole. So, knowing what the liver does is important for understanding the broader effects of liver diseases on people. In addition to its role in metabolism, the liver is important for the immune system. It keeps infections away by filtering blood and taking out bacteria and viruses. Because of this, the immune response is very important when dealing with liver infections, for example, schistosomiasis or hepatitis. When the liver is chronically inflamed because of these infections, it can cause scarring and fibrosis, which makes the immune system react more strongly and increases the risk of cancer. Inflammation triggered by these infections may lead to more harm and make people more likely to get other diseases. Therefore, maintaining liver health is not only essential for metabolic harmony but also for safeguarding the body against infectious diseases that could arise from liver dysfunction (Zhao *et al.*, 2021). Moreover, the liver's role in detoxification cannot be understated. It handles toxins from the environment, from what we eat, and from our body's waste. The liver makes these substances less dangerous so they can be removed from the body. However, if the detoxification process is affected by infection or disease, more toxic substances can build up, which leads to oxidative stress and more liver damage. This situation creates a vicious cycle, where the liver's compromised state exacerbates its ability to detoxify, allowing for the progression of infectious diseases, such as those caused by poor drinking water quality and subsequent diarrhea, which can drastically impact public health (Lin *et al.*, 2022). So, the liver, being so important for the body's health, especially when it is attacked by parasites or infectious diseases, is demonstrated by its many functions.

13.1. Common Parasitic Diseases Affecting the Liver

Schistosomiasis is a major parasitic disease of the liver because it is found in many parts of the world and affects public health. In tropical and subtropical areas, this disease is common because it is caused by the Schistosoma fluke. Liver fibrosis and portal hypertension are possible complications if the parasites settle in the hepatic portal system. Because adult worms live in mesenteric veins, their eggs can trigger major inflammation and result in the growth of granulomas, which can damage the liver. A big worry is that this disease keeps going, which can cause cirrhosis or make someone more prone to liver cancer. Hence, proper diagnosis and treatment are necessary to manage schistosomiasis, especially in places where medical resources are limited, which makes it challenging to prevent and control the disease. Liver flukes *Fasciola hepatica* and *Fasciola gigantica* cause fascioliasis, which can also result in liver complications. Mostly, these parasites infect sheep and cattle, though people can also get them if they consume water or plants that are contaminated. When the liver is infected, the larvae move through the liver cells, causing cell damage, blockage of the bile ducts, and inflammation. Fever, abdominal pain, and jaundice can appear in severe cases, which greatly affect how the liver functions. If chronic fascioliasis is not treated, it can bring about bile duct fibrosis and cholangitis, which can result in biliary obstruction. It is clear that we need to pay more attention, screen people, and support public health, mainly where livestock farming is common and can lead to zoonotic infections. Also, Clonorchis sinensis and *Opisthorchis viverrini* are parasites that can damage the liver and should not be ignored. In Southeast Asia, these liver flukes are common because many people eat raw or undercooked freshwater fish. Infections with clonorchiasis and opisthorchiasis can block the bile ducts and harm the liver, which often leads to cholangiocarcinoma. Long-term infection with these parasites causes the bile ducts to be inflamed, which raises the chance of cancer. Due to the serious health issues and the chance of zoonotic infection, informing the public about safe food handling and the need for early diagnosis is crucial for preventing these infections. Ensuring proper monitoring and control measures could significantly reduce the incidence of these diseases and their associated liver complications (Bowlus *et al.*, 2022; Sonne *et al.*, 2020).

13.1.1. Schistosomiasis

Schistosomiasis is very important to public health because millions of people globally are affected by it, mainly in Africa, the Middle East, Asia, and South America. Schistosomiasis is mostly acquired when people are exposed to water containing larvae of Schistosoma trematodes that come from snails. The transmission emphasizes the fundamental connection between disease prevalence and the quality of water because more than 80% of human-made sewage is discharged into aquatic ecosystems untreated, and this results in widespread environmental pollution that favors the development of conditions for schistosomiasis and other diseases (Lin *et al.*, 2022). It is very important to use programmatic approaches to ensure safe water and sanitation, as this helps stop the spread of schistosomiasis and also addresses the health risks of using contaminated water. Pathologically, Schistosomiasis is very detrimental to the liver. If Schistosoma eggs are not controlled, they can cause continuous inflammation and fibrosis in the liver, which might result in cirrhosis. This is made possible through a complex interaction between parasite life cycle and host immunity such that portal tract egg deposition initiates an immune reaction to heighten hepatic fibrosis and inflammation (Liu *et al.*, 2022). The inflammatory process is important in causing liver-related complications and this is typical in most parasitic and infectious diseases. It is important to deal with schistosomiasis by using effective treatments and also by preventing liver damage from persistent infections. Schistosomiasis is best controlled using medical care and public health steps that lower the chance of infection. Praziquantel is the main medicine used to treat schistosomiasis, and it is highly effective in killing adult worms. Still, because the disease is present in endemic areas, it is important to use preventive methods such as health education, cleaner water, and controlling snails. It is also helpful to know the details of liver fibrosis caused by schistosomiasis when designing new treatments and strategies. The long-term consequences of schistosomiasis on liver function are a paradigm of the relationship between parasitic infection and the entire spectrum of liver disease, necessitating continued investigation of potential treatments and prevention strategies against the health burden of liver disease due to this so-called neglected tropical disease (Liu *et al.*, 2022) (Figure 13.2).

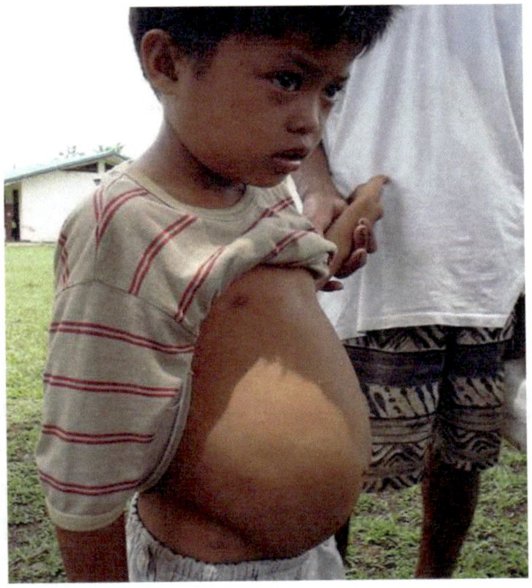

Figure 13.2. 11-year-old boy with ascites and portal hypertension due to schistosomiasis.

Source: https://upload.wikimedia.org/wikipedia/commons/4/43/Schistosomiasis_in_a_child_2.jpg.

13.1.2. Liver Flukes (Fascioliasis)

Liver flukes from the genus Fasciola are a major cause of parasitic infections in both humans and animals, and this condition is known as fascioliasis. Larvae usually grow in freshwater snails, and after that, they infect cattle and sheep, usually through water or plants that have been contaminated. The disease spreads mainly due to environmental factors, so poor hygiene and wrong livestock management can make areas more susceptible to outbreaks, which may result in more sickness and financial problems for farmers. The World Health Organization has categorized liver flukes as foodborne trematodes of public health importance, hence the importance of public awareness and preventive measures (Chai *et al.*, 2022). The symptoms of fascioliasis can be very different, from no symptoms at all to serious problems in the liver or bile ducts. The main symptoms are abdominal pain, fever, and jaundice because the flukes in the bile ducts cause inflammation, which may bring on cholangitis or block the bile ducts. Chronic fascioliasis also makes the disease more complicated by causing the liver to swell or raising the risk of bile duct cancer, which means early detection and care are more important. Most of the diagnostic methods are serology tests and ultrasonography, which can find the eggs in bile or the flukes in the biliary tract. The diagnosticity is crucial for effective treatment, which continues to be the center of research in parasitic diseases (Chai *et al.*, 2022). Over the years, fascioliasis has been treated with praziquantel and triclabendazole, becoming the main anthelmintics used in hospitals. Because triclabendazole can treat both the young and adult forms of Fasciola hepatica, it is now an important option for treating the infection. Therapeutic regimens should consider possible side effects, as while most cases are well managed, some unusual cases of liver toxicity have been seen, and extra care is needed when giving these drugs. Other drugs, such as albendazole, have been examined, but their effects on liver flukes are not as strong as those of triclabendazole. This underscores the necessity for ongoing research into drug resistance and novel therapeutic agent design, especially now that new findings point to broader uses of such agents than initially envisioned (Figure 13.3).

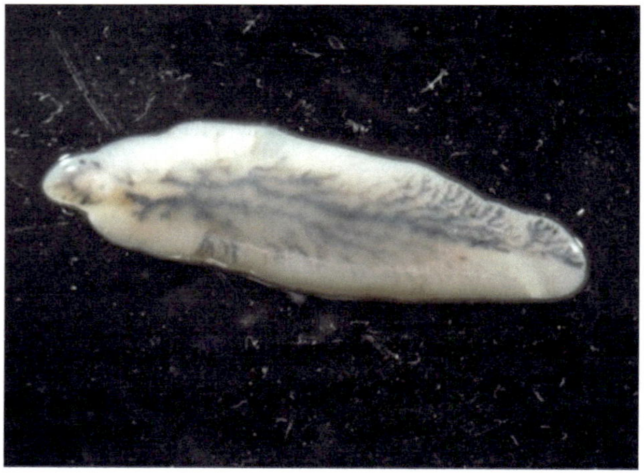

Figure 13.3. Fasciola hepatica.

Source: https://upload.wikimedia.org/wikipedia/commons/3/30/Fasciola_hepatica.JPG.

13.1.3. Echinococcosis

In many parts of the world, especially where there is a lot of livestock, echinococcosis, which is caused by Echinococcus tapeworms, is a major public health problem. Usually, dogs are the definitive hosts for these parasites, and sheep and other ungulates can have larval cysts in their livers. The disease manifests primarily as cystic echinococcosis (CE) or alveolar echinococcosis (AE), with the liver being the most commonly affected organ. If eggs from contaminated food or water are eaten, the larvae move and form cysts, which can cause many problems as they gradually harm the liver. A cystic structure can expand a lot, which may result in abdominal pain, nausea, and jaundice, showing how veterinary medicine and human health are related. Because the symptoms of echinococcosis are often similar to those of other liver diseases, it is often hard to diagnose. Using ultrasound, MRI, and CT scans is important for finding cysts and determining their size and any possible problems. These tests can support the diagnosis, but sometimes they can give a false-negative result. The choice of treatment depends on how severe the disease is, and surgery is usually recommended for large or bothersome cysts. Albendazole or mebendazole are examples of anti-parasitic drugs that are used, but with different results. Because there is no effective vaccine, it is still important to keep educating people and using preventive actions to control this zoonotic disease, combining veterinary and public health approaches. Echinococcosis has effects that go beyond personal health, since it also points to problems in the environment and society. How people manage livestock and develop cities is very important for the spread of the Echinococcus species. For this reason, using the One Health approach, which looks at human, animal, and environmental health together, is necessary for managing and preventing diseases. Improved sanitation, proper care of pets, and public education about infection should be included in preventive measures. Dealing with the factors that lead to echinococcosis is also very important. Such multifaceted interventions are echoed in other public health strategies, underlining the importance of proactive measures to curb infectious diseases, particularly as highlighted in contemporary discussions surrounding global health challenges (Brindha *et al.*, 2021; Ellwanger *et al.*, 2021) (Figure 13.4).

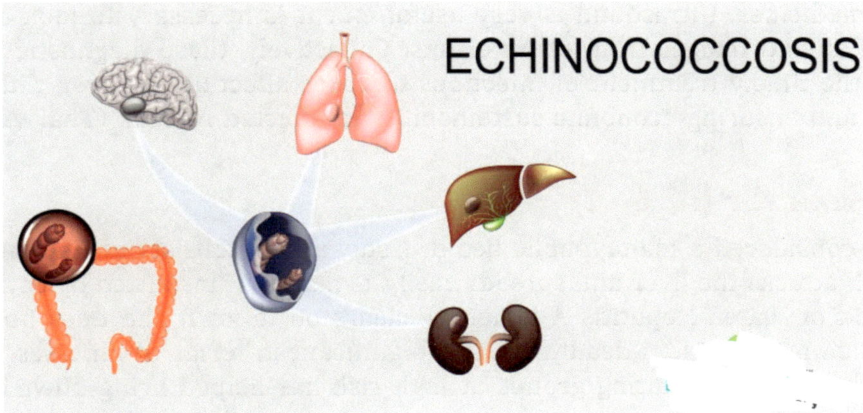

Figure 13.4. Echinococcosis.

Source: https://www.netmeds.com/images/cms/wysiwyg/blog/2021/02/1612249362_Echinococcosis_big_450.jpg.

13.2. Common Infectious Diseases Affecting the Liver

Many infectious diseases can harm the liver, which is in charge of many metabolic activities. Viral hepatitides are among the most important, and these include hepatitis A, B, and C. Such viral infections may result in acute inflammation, CLD, cirrhosis, and finally liver failure. Hepatitis B and C are major concerns because they are linked to serious health problems and HCC. Besides viruses, bacteria and parasites are also a major cause of concern. For example, BI can cause liver abscesses and echinococci, and different kinds of protozoa each have their own set of problems. It is very important to be aware of and diagnose these infections early, because the liver plays a key role in keeping the body healthy and in balance. Hepatobiliary diseases are often severe, for example, fascioliasis and hepatic coccidiosis, which are both parasitic infections of the liver. The liver fluke Fasciola hepatica in fascioliasis can cause major liver damage by moving through the liver, which results in inflammation and fibrosis. Hydraulic pressure and tissue death can also happen, which adds to the difficulties in diagnosis. In addition, infections with *Eimeria stiedae* in rabbits, which is the main cause of hepatic coccidiosis, can harm the liver. Studies have found that *Eimeria stiedae* may cause changes in liver biomarkers, showing that liver enzymes are increased, which suggests that hepatocytes are being damaged. These findings underscore the importance of veterinary and medical interventions to address both prevention and treatment of parasitic liver infections, which can otherwise result in considerable economic losses in agriculture, particularly in livestock farming and wild animal populations (Athanasiou *et al.*, 2023). Ultrasonography is an important test for finding liver infections, since it is non-invasive and can show any structural changes. It makes it possible to see if the echogenicity or echotexture of the liver has changed, which is important for telling different hepatic conditions apart. Mass lesions, effusions, and other signs of infection can be seen on ultrasound examinations. Images from these tests are used to distinguish between bacterial abscesses and hydatid cysts that need surgery from those that can be treated with medicines. Ultrasound is very useful, but it is necessary to look at the patient's history, test results, and images from other exams. Collectively, these diagnostic strategies play a crucial role in the timely treatment of infectious diseases affecting the liver, thus safeguarding health outcomes and ensuring economic sustainability in affected regions (Tharwat *et al.*, 2024).

13.2.1. Viral Hepatitis (A, B, C)

Viral hepatitis is considered a major public health issue, and it consists of Hepatitis A, B, and C. Hepatitis A, which attacks the liver and spreads easily, is mainly transmitted by eating or drinking contaminated food or water. Hepatitis A generally clears on its own and does not lead to long-term disease, which makes it less deadly but still significant in terms of illnesses, particularly in areas with poor hygiene. Vaccinating groups at high risk has helped bring down the number of infections. Thus, sanitatory and campaign-based vaccination public health interventions continue to be crucial in preventing Hepatitis A epidemics as well as containing the transmission of the infection among susceptible groups, thus commanding focus within broader infectious liver disease dynamics (Converse *et al.*, 2018).

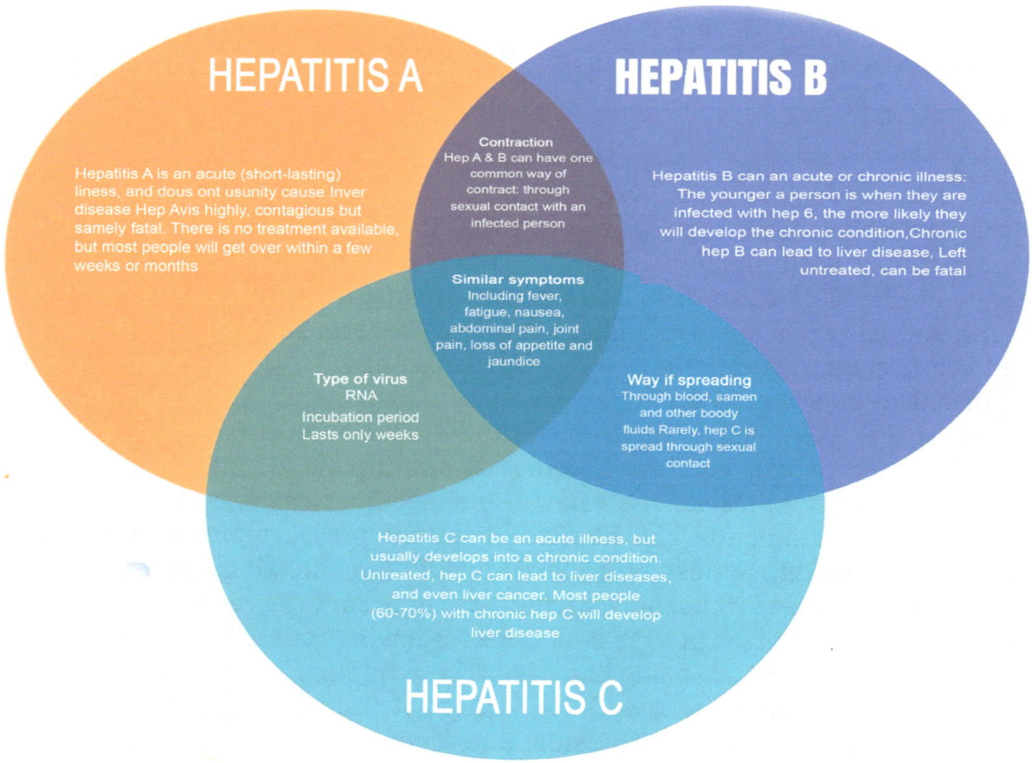

Figure 13.5. Hepatitis diagram.

Source: https://phadkelabs.com/blog/wp-content/uploads/2020/03/5611896-scaled.jpg.

Hepatitis B and C are more difficult because they can cause chronic infection and lead to serious problems. Hepatitis B, which you can get from contaminated body fluids, can result in

CLD, cirrhosis, and later HCC. Where vaccination against Hepatitis B is not given to all, the disease is still a major problem. Strong immunization programs have caused incidence rates to go down, proving that vaccination is a useful way to prevent disease. Most cases of hepatitis C, which are caused by blood-to-blood transmission, turn into a long-term infection in millions of people worldwide. DAA therapies have made a big difference, offering high chances of cure and improving Hepatitis C treatment. However, continued efforts toward making these treatments available to more people, especially in low-resource settings, are critical to battling this powerful infectious disease (Dhanya *et al.*, 2024). Because viral hepatitis is linked to other health factors, it is not always easy to fight these infections. How many people get viral hepatitis, and their outcomes are affected by social and economic conditions, access to health care, and the health system. Disease incidence is higher than normal in resource-limited low- and middle-income nations. Being infected with HIV at the same time can make liver disease from hepatitis worse and more severe. Using education, vaccination, and ensuring fair access to healthcare is still the main way to reduce the impact of viral hepatitis. By realizing the social and environmental determinants that have served as the cause of transmission as well as the outcomes of the infections, there is a possibility of creating more targeted interventions that can enhance liver health among various communities (Converse *et al.*, 2018) (Figure 13.5).

13.2.2. Bacterial Infections (e.g., Leptospirosis)

Many zoonotic diseases have their underlying interplay with the nature of BI and liver health. Among the diseases, leptospirosis is particularly significant. Leptospirosis is caused by the bacterium Leptospira, which primarily proliferates in water contaminated with the urine of infected animals. This infection usually occurs in several stages, beginning with a flu-like illness and potentially developing into more significant complications such as liver dysfunction. The liver is a location of essential metabolic activities, and interference by BI can result in serious health outcomes. The role of the liver highlights the necessity for epidemiological research to evaluate the effect of leptospirosis on hepatic health, especially among individuals at high risk due to environmental factors, e.g., inadequate sanitation and proximity to animal feces (Rahman *et al.*, 2020).

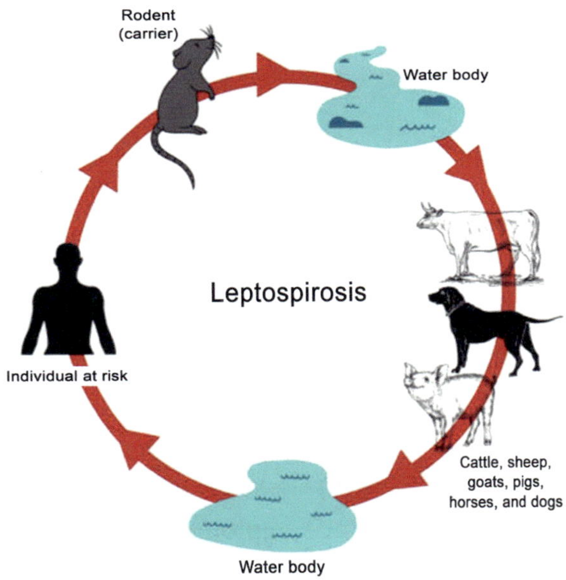

Figure 13.6. Leptospirosis.

Source: https://microbiologyjournal.org/wp-content/uploads/2022/05/fg01-1-399x420.jpg.

Other than leptospirosis, bacterial pathogens cause infectious diseases that disrupt liver function. On some occasions, infections are known to cause acute pancreatitis, which is due to microbial reasons, among them some bacterial pathogens. Such mechanisms indicate a significant but often overlooked correlation between infections such as *Mycoplasma pneumoniae* and leptospirosis and acute pancreatitis, both of which may be related to involvement of the liver (Rawla *et al.*, 2017). The processes by which such infections impact liver health tend to include an inflammatory process, which may also result in hepatic damage. When these bacteria infect, they can also trigger a series of immune reactions that may further worsen liver conditions and complicate existing liver diseases. It is thus important to comprehend such linkages in order to devise entire treatment regimens for such affected patients (Figure 13.6).

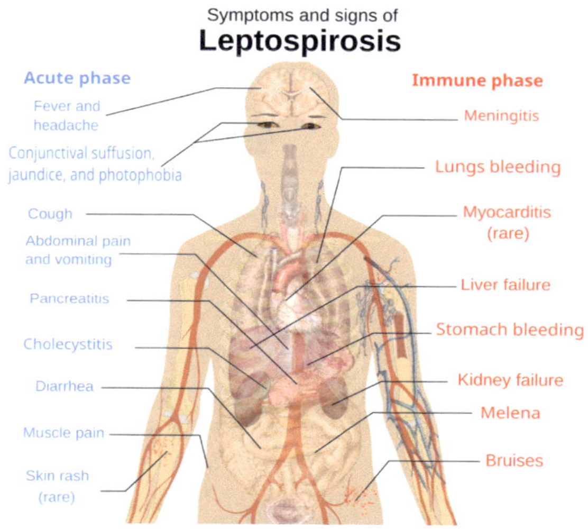

Figure 13.7. Signs and symptoms of leptospirosis.

Source: https://upload.wikimedia.org/wikipedia/commons/4/43/Signs_and_symptoms_of_leptospirosis.svg.

In addition to individual health effects, BI imposes a burden on public health systems with its zoonotic nature. Zoonoses refer to diseases that transfer from animals to humans, which constitute a large percentage of emerging infectious diseases; such diseases account for more than 60% of human pathogens (Rahman *et al.*, 2020). Factors driving these infections are climate change, urbanization, and increased human-animal interactions, which elevate the risk of transmission. It underscores the need for an integrated One Health approach that combines strategies of human, animal, and environmental health in combating the emergence of infections such as leptospirosis. Improvement of surveillance and preventive measures promoted against these infections will be essential in containing their adverse effects on the liver, achieving integrated public health results. A comprehensive strategy has to be employed in controlling the spread of the infections that remain a challenge in health care among most nations in the world (Figure 13.7).

13.2.3. Fungal Infections (e.g., Aspergillosis)

Fungal diseases, especially Aspergillus infections, have significant implications in the context of parasitic and infectious illnesses involving other organs, such as the liver. Aspergillus, which is a ubiquitous mold in the environment, has the potential to cause serious health issues, most importantly in immunocompromised patients. The liver can be involved indirectly through dissemination of such fungal pathogens via systemic circulation after pulmonary infection or due to contaminated foodstuffs. After the liver is damaged, it can serve as a favorable substrate for the implantation and growth of fungi, worsening the general clinical profile and making treatment plans more difficult. Understanding the interactions between fungal infections and liver health is essential for formulating effective management plans, as the liver plays a crucial role in immune response and filtering pathogens from the bloodstream, which can affect the severity and progression of fungal diseases, including those linked to zoonotic transmission (Rahman *et al.*, 2020). The clinical presentations of Aspergillus infection vary, usually presenting as allergic reactions, localized pulmonary infections, or invasive aspergillosis. In cases of patients presenting with hepatic involvement, the presentation of such an infection would be a combination of respiratory and hepatic failure. The diagnostic work for such infections must be carried out very carefully since presentation may often mimic other infectious or inflammatory processes involving the liver. The increasing prevalence of these infections, particularly among those with pre-existing liver conditions or compromised immunity, highlights the importance of recognizing and diagnosing Aspergillus infections promptly. Innovative diagnostic approaches, including the use of serological tests and imaging techniques, have enhanced our ability to detect aspergillosis, allowing for timely therapeutic interventions. However, failure to accurately diagnose can result in poor outcomes, emphasizing the need for heightened awareness in clinical settings (Góralska *et al.*, 2018). Treatment for fungal infections, including those caused by Aspergillus, poses challenges, particularly given the intricacies of liver function in drug metabolism and clearance. Therapeutic regimens commonly involve antifungal agents, with a focus on those that can penetrate well into the central nervous system and other critical areas. Effective management of concomitant liver disease necessitates careful selection of antifungal treatments that consider potential hepatotoxicity and drug interactions. For instance, amphotericin B and voriconazole are frequently employed, but their dosing may need adjustment based on liver function parameters. In addition, public health measures can better manage risk factors emerging with zoonotic fungal pathogens, responsible for a large fraction of new infections. This is critical in understanding better with One Health approaches these interactions in the complexities between environmental, animal, and human health that lead to healthier results for individuals who face simultaneous challenges of both fungal and parasitic etiologies of liver disease (Rahman *et al.*, 2020) (Figure 13.8).

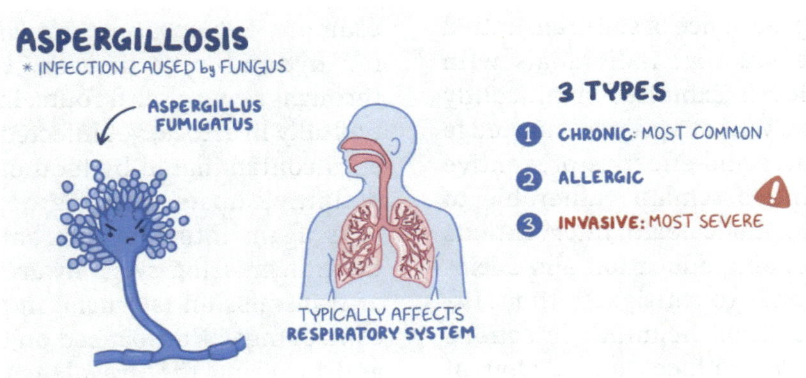

Figure 13.8. Aspergillosis.

Source: https://d16qt3wv6xm098.cloudfront.net/WVt_KTlwSvKZp1H5B7EbYiGEQL_IvZ_W/_.jpg.

13.3. Transmission and Risk Factors

Knowledge of the parasitic and infectious disease transmission mechanisms involving the liver is crucial in developing effective control measures. Most of these diseases exhibit intricate life cycles involving two or more hosts, and the importance of environmental and socio-economic determinants in the spread of disease. For example, where there is poor sanitation, direct contact with the polluted water sources can be used as a mechanism of parasite transmission, for example, schistosomiasis. The incidence of schistosomiasis in endemic communities, such as those examined in the Philippines, illustrates an association between environmental factors and health issues. People tend to indulge in dangerous habits, like bathing or wading in rivers, which considerably raises their infection risk. Addressing these behaviors requires an integrated approach that encompasses health education and improvement of local sanitation infrastructure, thereby targeting one of the key drivers of disease transmission and enhancing public health outcomes (Paller *et al.*, 2024). Risk factors associated with intestinal helminth infections further compound the complexities surrounding liver diseases caused by parasitic infestations. Various studies have shown that socio-economic conditions greatly influence the prevalence of these infections. Particularly in low-income communities, factors such as limited access to clean water, inadequate sewage systems, and a lack of health education exacerbate the risk of infection. The investigation concerning the association between educational attainment and the prevalence of soil-transmitted helminthiases revealed that individuals with lower educational levels exhibited significantly higher infection rates. Without proper knowledge of transmission routes and effective preventive measures, communities remain vulnerable to these diseases. Thus, public health interventions must focus on improving education and socio-economic conditions to mitigate the risk associated with intestinal helminth infections and, by extension, to reduce the burden of liver diseases stemming from these parasites (Paller *et al.*, 2024). The implications of these transmission dynamics extend beyond individual health, significantly impacting agricultural and economic productivity. As emphasized in veterinary medicine, cattle liver diseases can significantly impair agricultural yields. Cattle infectious diseases and parasitic infestations pose not only risks to animal health but also more general implications for food safety and economic stability in farming communities. Understanding the pathways and risk factors of these liver diseases is critical for the formulation of strategic prevention and control measures. Factors such as environmental contaminants, dietary issues, and veterinary care accessibility need to be examined thoroughly to formulate holistic strategies. By focusing on improving knowledge and awareness around these diseases, as well as addressing underlying socio-economic challenges, stakeholders can work toward safeguarding both animal and human health, ultimately leading to the enhancement of public and agricultural health systems.

13.3.1. Modes of Transmission for Parasitic Diseases

The transmission modes of parasitic diseases significantly influence the prevalence and management of these infections, particularly concerning the liver. Many common liver-affecting parasites, such as those belonging to the genus *Echinococcus* and *Fasciola*, utilize complex life cycles that often involve multiple hosts. For example, *Echinococcus granulosus*, responsible for hydatid cyst disease, typically spreads through the fecal-oral route. Intermediate hosts, typically livestock, get infected when they ingest eggs contaminated by food or water, while the definitive hosts, such as dogs, release these eggs again into the environment, completing the transmission cycle. Awareness of this mode of transmission is crucial in planning effective control measures focused on breaking the cycle and lowering the prevalence of liver diseases resulting from parasitic infection. In addition to the fecal-oral route of transmission, other means by which liver-affecting parasites disseminate include direct contact with the infected vectors. Schistosomiasis, caused by Schistosoma species, is a typical example of this. It spreads to humans through contact with freshwater sources contaminated with cercariae, the larval stage of the parasite. Upon skin penetration, the parasites migrate to the liver, where they mature and reproduce, significantly impacting hepatic function and leading to serious complications such as portal hypertension and liver fibrosis.

This direct mode of transmission highlights the importance of water safety and public health interventions in endemic regions. Effective educational campaigns about avoiding contact with contaminated water sources are essential for preventing schistosomiasis and protecting susceptible populations.

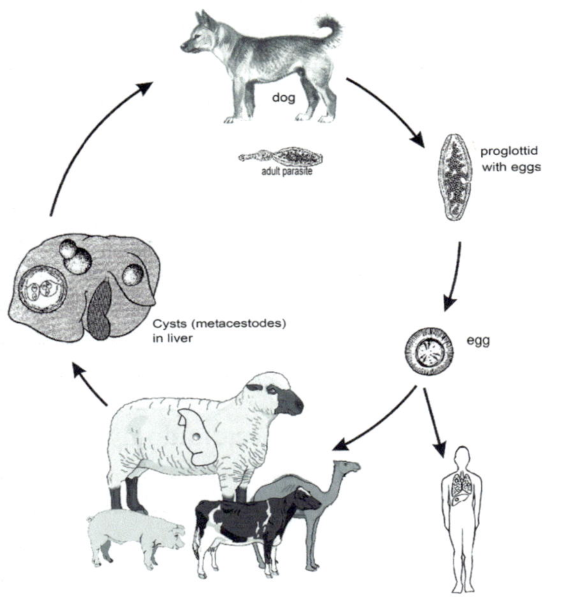

Figure 13.9. Life cycle of *Echinococcus granulosus* complex of genotypes frequently encountered in man.

Source: https://www.researchgate.net/profile/Paul-Torgerson/publication/280706498/figure/fig2/AS:667786896494603@1536224211435/Life-cycle-of-Echinococcus-granulosus-complex-of-genotypes-frequently-encountered-in-man.png.

Furthermore, globalization and environmental changes are reshaping the landscape of parasitic disease transmission. Increased human migration, tourism, and trade have amplified the risk of introducing parasites, which can lead to outbreaks in previously unaffected regions. For instance, the resurgence of parasitic infections in countries like Korea can be attributed in part to the re-entering of parasites through international travel and trade, despite improvements in sanitation and healthcare. As stated, the introduction of individuals from regions with a high prevalence of parasitic diseases raises awareness of potential threats to public health infrastructure. Consequently, it is imperative that surveillance systems adapt to monitor not only established but also emerging parasitic threats in the context of global movement patterns, thus ensuring that measures are in place to combat the transmission of these diseases effectively (Kim, 2024) (Figure 13.9).

13.3.2. Risk Factors for Infectious Liver Diseases

The emergence of infectious liver diseases is intricately linked to various risk factors that are largely socio-economic, environmental, and health-related. One significant risk factor is the prevalence of viral hepatitis, particularly types B and C, which are major contributors to liver disease globally. They are primarily transmitted through contaminated blood and bodily fluids, affecting populations in regions with inadequate healthcare systems. Studies suggest that hepatitis-related liver diseases are very concentrated in low-socioeconomic regions where access to health care is confined, which would further exacerbate the prevalence of these infections and contribute to the rising rates of liver cancer particularly within the Middle East and North Africa, where hepatitis C has historically burdened the countries, such as Egypt (Zhu *et al.*, 2024). This underscores the importance of access to comprehensive healthcare and targeted public health interventions to mitigate transmission risks. Environmental factors also play a critical role in the development of infectious liver diseases. Exposure to certain toxins, such as aflatoxins found in contaminated food and environments, can significantly increase the risk of liver disease, particularly HCC. Aflatoxins are produced by molds that thrive in warm, humid climates and often affect crops in low-income nations, adding another layer of vulnerability for populations already at risk due to health and socioeconomic factors. Moreover, vector-borne parasitic infections such as schistosomiasis, which can cause liver fibrosis and hepatic complications, are common in areas with poor sanitation and water management systems. One report mentioned that up to 400 million individuals are infected by schistosomiasis globally, mostly in areas with low socio-demographic indices, and this shows a direct relationship between environmental factors and the prevalence of infectious liver disease (Zhu *et al.*, 2024). Finally, lifestyle factors, especially dietary patterns and physical activity levels, play an important role in exposing individuals to the risk of contracting liver diseases. The increasing global epidemic of obesity, with its attendant metabolic disorders such as fatty liver disease, has emerged as an important risk factor for liver pathology. This is especially relevant in the developed world and some rapidly urbanizing regions where sedentary lifestyles and high-calorie intake are the norm. In addition, these lifestyle factors can synergize with viral hepatitis infections to increase the rate of liver damage. The MENA region, for instance, is facing a two-pronged threat of burgeoning rates of obesity coupled with a viral hepatitis burden contributing to escalating liver cancer incidence (Hosseini *et al.*, 2024). Intervention of such risk factors by public health programs based on the thrust of education, dietary modification, and the promotion of active lifestyles is a must to try and counteract the increase in infectious and parasitic liver diseases.

13.3.3. Geographic Distribution of Liver Diseases

The geographic distribution of liver diseases is significantly influenced by a variety of environmental, cultural, and socio-economic factors that vary across regions. In many developing countries, infections such as hepatitis B and C are rampant due to insufficient healthcare resources, inadequate vaccination programs, and widespread unsafe injecting practices. Zoonotic diseases, which are prevalent in rural settings, also contribute to the burden of liver diseases. For example, factors such as urbanization, climate change, and global travel enhance the spread of these infections, underlining human activity in relation to disease emergence. According to Rahman *et al.* (2020), these dynamics highlight the importance of handling environmental factors, mitigating impacts on human health from zoonotic diseases, such as those affecting the liver. Therefore, understanding the geographic distribution of liver diseases necessitates a comprehensive analysis that includes both infectious and parasitic dimensions. In Latin America, the landscape of liver diseases is notably shaped by endemic infections such as paracoccidioidomycosis. This systemic fungal disease, primarily associated with rural environments, drastically affects liver health through its various clinical manifestations. As reported in different regions of Brazil, notably Rondônia, the incidence of paracoccidioidomycosis has reached alarming levels, highlighting the need for increased awareness and investigation into its geographic patterns. Limited awareness and underreporting contribute to an underestimation of its prevalence, complicating efforts toward diagnosis and treatment. The geographic variability of this disease emphasizes the need for tailored public health initiatives. The development of evidence-based recommendations for managing paracoccidioidomycosis, as suggested by findings by Shikanai-Yasuda *et al.* (2017), is crucial for controlling its spread and mitigating its effects on liver health in endemic areas. Furthermore, the geographic distribution of liver diseases is influenced by healthcare infrastructure, education, and public health policies, which vary greatly between nations. In regions with limited healthcare access, such as parts of Sub-Saharan Africa and Southeast Asia, high infection rates of hepatitis and schistosomiasis contribute to liver disease burden, adversely affecting economic and social well-being. The complexities of diagnosing and managing these diseases are exacerbated in resource-limited settings, calling for a concerted emphasis on preventive measures and healthcare system improvements. Interventions such as immunization, blood transfusions from safe sources, and better hygienic conditions can prevent many cases of infectious liver diseases. According to Rahman *et al.* (2020), the distribution of liver diseases could be controlled geographically by being able to address sociological impacts with a One Health approach that integrates human, veterinary, and environmental health. This is one of the necessary interventions for effective prevention and management in cross-cutting geographic diversity.

13.4. Symptoms and Clinical Manifestations

The symptoms and clinical manifestations associated with parasitic and infectious diseases of the liver are diverse and can significantly vary depending on the causative agent. Initial symptoms often include fatigue, malaise, and loss of appetite, which are nonspecific but indicative of an underlying infection. As the disease progresses, patients may experience jaundice, characterized by yellowing of the skin and eyes, due to hepatic dysfunction and the consequent accumulation of bilirubin in the bloodstream. Additionally, abdominal pain and swelling may arise as the liver becomes inflamed or enlarged, reflecting the severity of the parasitic load or the acute nature of the infectious process. Recognizing these early signs is crucial, as delayed diagnosis and treatment can lead to more severe complications, including liver failure or cirrhosis, ultimately necessitating transplantation or leading to a critical health crisis (Crouser *et al.*, 2020). In cases of specific parasitic infections, more distinct clinical features emerge. For instance, schistosomiasis can cause portal hypertension, leading to esophageal varices and hematemesis, resulting in significant morbidity. Furthermore, infections like fascioliasis typically present with right upper quadrant pain and biliary obstruction due to the migration of parasites, which may also induce acute cholangitis. The clinical manifestations associated with leptospirosis may be similar, but they often come with a broader systemic involvement, including renal and pulmonary complications. All these cases require meticulous clinical evaluation and imaging diagnostics involving ultrasounds or CT scans to help diagnose, guide treatment, and prevent further complications (Butt *et al.*, 2017). Eosinophilia is also another notable feature of several parasitic infections, acting as a marker of an ongoing response. Elevated eosinophilic levels could be reflective of tissue inflammation, particularly where parasites invade or injure liver tissue. Eosinophilic response can lead to presenting complaints such as itching, rashes, or respiratory compromise, depending on the affected organ systems. Importantly, identification of the true parasitic illness requires correlation of eosinophilic levels with clinical presentation and relevant travel histories, underscoring the multi-faceted diagnostic process in parasitic liver disease. When untreated, such infections not only affect the function of the organ but also lead to systemic sequelae, thus requiring a comprehensive and prompt therapeutic approach (Crouser *et al.*, 2020).

13.4.1. General Symptoms of Liver Disease

The symptoms associated with liver disease can manifest in various forms, significantly depending on the underlying cause, such as parasitic or infectious infections. Among the most prevalent general symptoms are fatigue, jaundice, abdominal discomfort, and anorexia. Fatigue often arises due to diminished liver function, impacting the organ's ability to metabolize nutrients and store energy over time. Jaundice, a yellowing of the eyes and skin, results from an accumulation of bilirubin in the blood, which can signal dysfunctional liver metabolism. Pain in the upper right quadrant of the abdomen can be a sign of inflammation or swelling within the liver. It must be respected as an indicator of possible disease development. Such symptoms are early signs that must be recognized because they create a chance to approach the patient with medical services to help in diagnosing and addressing the causing factors, especially in cases of parasitic diseases that are likely to make the condition worse for the liver's functionality (Bowlus *et al.*, 2022). Besides the manifestation of these symptoms, emotional and psychological issues are increasingly receiving recognition among patients suffering from liver disease. Anxiety and depression may surface as a response to the chronic nature of the disease, often exacerbated by uncertainty around management and prognosis. The interplay between physical symptoms and psychological distress can create a cycle that hinders effective disease management. For instance, the experience of severe pruritus, often associated with cholestasis in liver disorders, can lead to significant lifestyle impairment, impacting sleep and daily activities. This emotional burden should not be underemphasized because it can ultimately add to the cumulative effect that liver disease will have on a patient's quality of life. A holistic approach, therefore, which will bring into focus psychological dimensions too, in addition to physical aspects, will be essential while treating liver diseases, especially those caused by parasitic infections (Butt *et al.*, 2017). Moreover, the evolving landscape of diagnostic criteria necessitates a heightened awareness of the diverse manifestations of liver disease symptoms among healthcare providers. Relying solely on classical symptomatology may lead to missed or delayed diagnoses, particularly in cases related to parasitic infestations like schistosomiasis or liver flukes. These infections can lead to liver damage and, over time, result in chronic conditions such as fibrosis or cirrhosis. Symptoms would be mild, warranting confusion with other benign diseases, but may indicate serious hepatic disease. A comprehensive medical history supported by specific serological and imaging studies can significantly help in the early detection of these infections and improve their therapeutic results. Thus, recognizing the nuanced symptoms of liver disease is vital for enabling timely and appropriate clinical responses, especially given the increasing prevalence of liver-affecting parasitic diseases globally (Bowlus *et al.*, 2022) (Figure 13.10).

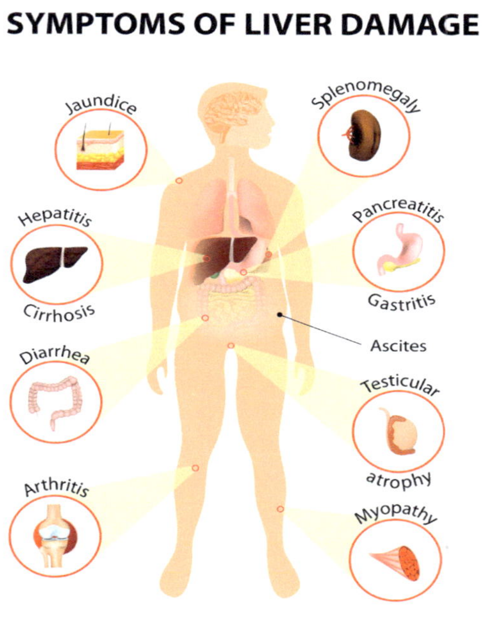

Figure 13.10. Symptoms of liver disease.

Source: https://cdn.apollohospitals.com/health-library-prod/2021/01/Factors-May-Damage-the-Liver-scaled.jpg.

13.4.2. Specific Symptoms of Parasitic Infections

Parasitic infections commonly show a variety of symptoms, mainly by disturbing the liver's normal role in the body. Jaundice, which is a yellowing of the skin and eyes, is one of the most common signs, caused by the liver being affected by parasites. An increase in parasites like protozoa and helminths may cause blockages in the bile ducts, resulting in more bilirubin in the blood. The liver can grow in response to parasites, which can cause the abdomen to swell and cause more pain. All of these symptoms together indicate major liver problems, which lead to further testing for parasitic infections as a possible cause of liver trouble. Many parasitic infections cause people to feel very tired, which can seriously weaken them. The tiredness is caused by the parasites and the immune system's reaction, which takes away important nutrients and causes inflammation. When these infections are severe, it is possible for more than one infection to happen, which can make the disease even more serious. Interestingly, research indicates that bacterial and viral co-infections can interact with parasitic infections, negatively impacting both the host's immune response and overall clinical outcomes (Okon *et al.*, 2023). This points out that noticing these symptoms along with the usual bacterial and viral infections in liver diseases can help develop better ways to diagnose and treat patients. Gastrointestinal problems are often seen in people with parasitic infections, and these may include diarrhea, nausea, and vomiting. The symptoms occur because the parasites take over the gastrointestinal tract and disrupt the usual digestive process. Parasites can cause inflammation, which results in increased permeability in the intestines and changes in the gut flora. These changes may also worsen malabsorption issues, which could lead to more infections or problems because the immune system is weakened. Water quality plays a crucial role in these scenarios, with poor sanitation contributing to the proliferation of enteric pathogens; it is reported that a majority of diseases linked to contaminated water are gastrointestinal in nature, which emphasizes the need for effective health interventions (Lin *et al.*, 2022). It is important to understand these symptoms to respond properly to liver-related parasitic and infectious diseases.

13.4.3. Specific Symptoms of Infectious Diseases

A variety of specific symptoms from infectious diseases can give important clues about their underlying causes, especially in conditions affecting the liver. Many people who have liver infections describe abdominal pain, which is usually caused by the liver becoming inflamed or swollen. Patients may say this pain comes and goes or is always there, and it may get worse after doing certain activities or eating certain foods. In addition, a person may have a fever and feel tired with abdominal discomfort, which adds to the difficulty of diagnosis. These systemic indicators not only suggest the presence of an infectious agent but also indicate the need for advanced diagnostic imaging techniques to assess the extent of liver involvement and the possibility of secondary infections or complications associated with liver disease, as emphasized in current guidelines for managing hepatobiliary disorders (Bowlus *et al.*, 2022). PSC and other infectious diseases of the liver can cause pruritus, which means an intense itchiness affecting many patients. The buildup of BAs in the blood is what causes this symptom, and this is usually caused by cholestasis or reduced bile flow. When patients have PSC, pruritus may become worse due to stress or changes in liver function, which suggests a connection between the liver and the nervous system. Chronic itching can also lead to anxiety and depression, which add more health problems for the patient. Recognition of this symptom is vital, as it not only affects quality of life but also serves as a clinical marker for monitoring disease progression and treatment efficacy, underscoring the multidimensional challenges posed by liver diseases (Bowlus *et al.*, 2022). Infections caused by parasites such as schistosomiasis show a distinct set of symptoms and may result in serious complications such as liver fibrosis. If Schistosoma eggs get lodged in the liver, people may have an enlarged liver, experience abdominal swelling, and feel tired and unwell for a long time. It means the immune system is responding very strongly to the presence of the parasites. If chronic inflammation persists, it can slowly harm the liver, which can result in cirrhosis and make a person more likely to get HCC. Both liver enlargement and abdominal pain are symptoms, and their presence together points to the complex nature of the disease and the importance of early detection and proper treatment. Failure to address these symptoms effectively can lead to life-threatening outcomes, reinforcing the imperative for targeted therapeutic interventions in addressing parasitic and infectious liver diseases (Figure 13.11).

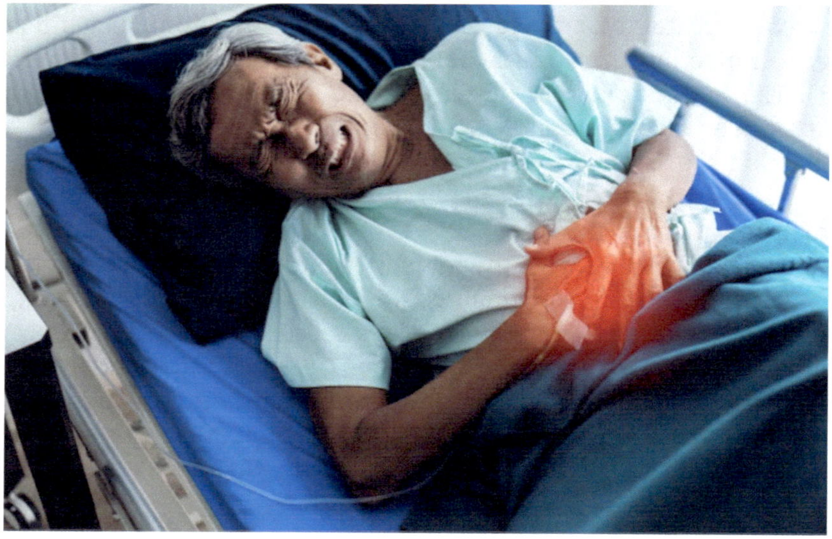

Figure 13.11. Symptoms of Infectious Diseases

Source: https://img.freepik.com/free-photo/pain-stomache-old-senior-asian-grandfather-patient-uniform-suffer-from-body-problem-health-ideas-concept_609648-2289.jpg?semt=ais_hybrid&w=740.

13.5. Diagnostic Methods

Lab diagnostic tests for infectious and parasitic liver ailments play a pivotal role in the proper identification and timely treatment of such conditions. An entire process generally begins with meticulous patient history and physical examination, which may manifest signs like jaundice, abdominal pain, or color change of stool. The laboratory tests then take over, following this initial evaluation. These are able to recognize indicators of liver inflammation or derangement, and some serological investigations identify antigens or antibodies to specific pathogens, i.e., hepatitis viruses. Imaging techniques like ultrasound, CT, and magnetic resonance imaging (MRI) aid in the detection of liver lesions, which could point towards infection or parasitic infestation. With these methods, physicians can limit the differential diagnosis to include only the most probable conditions that affect the liver, simplifying appropriate clinical care. Endoscopy is equally essential in the diagnostic protocol for liver disease. Upper GI endoscopy, for example, may be employed in assessing the esophagus and stomach for infection or bleeding, which indirectly affects the function of the liver. Where there is parasitic suspicion, endoscopic retrograde cholangiopancreatography (ERCP) will visualize the biliary tree directly and will be able to recover samples for pathological diagnosis. Biopsy procedures, drawn during endoscopy, will allow histological study, which will establish the true infectious agent or elf-pathological alteration in the liver. Discrimination between parasitic and non-parasitic liver diseases requires careful consideration of these findings, once more stressing the value of a multidisciplinary approach to diagnosis. Not only do these interventions contribute to the precision of the diagnosis, but they also direct the follow-up therapeutic action towards better management of these diseases. To augment imaging and laboratory diagnoses, the use of advanced molecular techniques has become a useful diagnostic tool in liver infections. Polymerase chain reaction (PCR) is particularly remarkable for its ability to amplify DNA or RNA of causative agents in order to effectively enable the detection of specific viral or parasitic organisms in the liver. This method greatly improves the speed and sensitivity of diagnosis compared to traditional culture methods, which may be slower to carry out and provide less definitive results. Furthermore, serological tests can provide more information regarding the immune response to infection and allow discrimination between active and resolved infection. Collectively, these advanced diagnostic methods play a critical role in managing parasitic and infectious liver diseases through the possibility of early diagnosis and tailored treatment, thereby improving patient care. As diagnostic technology continues to evolve, future research and coordination between health practitioners will be crucial in optimizing the diagnosis process (Adler *et al.*, 2015; Bernstein *et al.*, 2016).

13.5.1. Laboratory Tests for Liver Function

Liver function testing is critical in the diagnosis and management of parasitic and infectious illnesses that affect hepatic health. Laboratory liver function testing typically includes a series of biomarkers, including serum aminotransferases (AST and ALT), ALP, bilirubin, and albumin level. Elevated AST and ALT levels indicate hepatocyte injury, whereas ALP elevation can represent cholestasis or obstruction of the bile ducts that can be observed in parasitic infestations of the liver, like schistosomiasis or malaria. Also, bilirubin values indicate the efficiency with which the liver is eliminating waste products, and an increase in its value can represent acute hepatic dysfunction or hemolysis that is stressing the liver in infectious conditions. From these tests, clinicians can ascertain the degree of liver damage and steer treatment in order to facilitate infection control in cases that compromise liver function. In liver disease, particularly infection-related liver disease, the interpretation of liver function tests (LFTs) is more complex. For instance, candidates who need liver transplantation due to infectious complications should be thoroughly evaluated for liver function and infection susceptibility that can affect graft viability. As indicated in recent research, timely and precise microbiological diagnostics become critical in therapeutic planning, especially in immunocompromised patients such as transplant recipients. Lab testing dependence exceeds mere assessments of function because they guide therapeutic interventions that diminish drug toxicity and improve outcomes. In their treatment, the complexity of the liver's role in metabolizing and synthesizing drugs underscores the importance of routine liver function testing against the backdrop of rising challenges from emergent infections and resistant pathogens in transplant medicine (Fishman, 2017). Furthermore, the function of the liver in metabolism emphasizes the significance of exhaustive laboratory evaluation of patients suffering from parasitic disorders. Glycans, key molecules that are secreted by the liver, have multifarious biological roles ranging from cell signaling to detection of pathogens, demonstrating the complexity of organ interaction with the microbial and immune worlds. Elevated liver enzymes may not only signal liver injury but also represent a disruption in these metabolic processes, and it is enhanced by parasitic infections as the liver struggles to cope with inflammation and infection.

Analysis of LFTs reveals a broader impact on systemic health and implies the need for an inter-disciplinary approach to establish the extent to which parasitic diseases interfere with hepatic integrity and function within the host (Varki, 2016). Such efforts, therefore, call for continued research and innovation in laboratory procedures to facilitate the maximization of patient treatment and responding to the intricate interaction between parasitic pathogens and liver function (Figure 13.12).

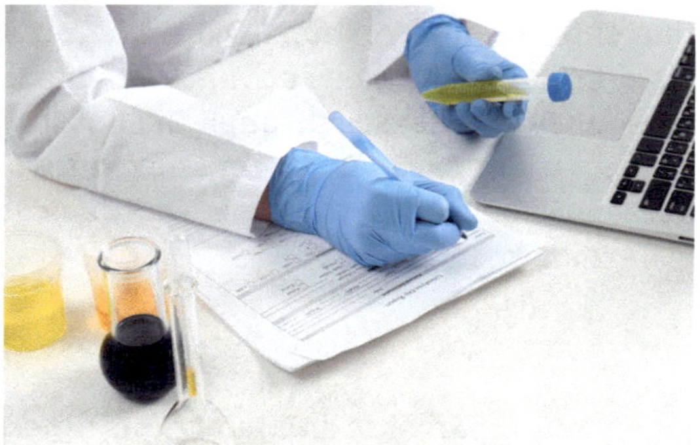

Figure 13.12. Testing for liver function.

Source: https://www.jariwalalab.com/wp-content/uploads/2023/09/lab-test.jpg.

13.5.2. Imaging Techniques (Ultrasound, CT, MRI)

Using advanced imaging methods has greatly improved how these diseases of the liver are diagnosed. Of these methods, US, CT, and MRI help to understand liver problems. Ultrasound stands out because it is non-invasive and can check liver conditions as they happen. It is usually the first method used to assess liver diseases because it is both easy to use and good at spotting cysts and abscesses, which are common in parasitic infections. The portability of ultrasound also facilitates its use in diverse clinical settings, including remote areas, where access to advanced imaging facilities may be limited (Crouser *et al.*, 2020). Because ultrasound is accessible, it is very useful for handling parasitic liver diseases such as CE. CT imaging, together with ultrasound, gives clear cross-sectional images of the liver and nearby organs, which helps make the diagnosis more accurate. Especially, CT is useful for spotting more complicated liver problems and assessing the severity of the disease. Because CT images are so detailed, doctors can more easily tell apart the various liver problems, including those caused by parasites.

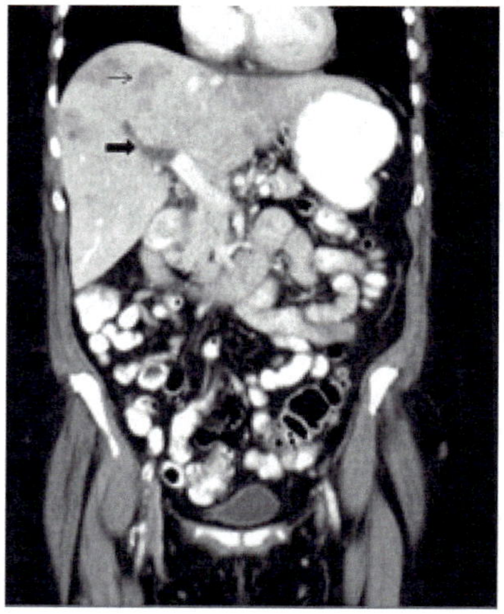

Figure 13.13. Computed tomography (CT) scan scout view showing right portal vein thrombus and liver abscess.

Source: https://www.researchgate.net/profile/Mahesh-Gajendran/publication/51707786/figure/fig2/AS:302076128186386@1449031969842/Computed-tomography-CT-scan-scout-view-showing-right-portal-vein-thrombus-and-liver.png.

Also, CT angiography helps to show if the blood vessels in the liver are affected by infection, which is important for planning and performing treatments. While CT provides superior anatomical detail compared to ultrasound, its use is associated with ionizing radiation, raising concerns about cumulative exposure, especially in populations requiring repeated assessments, such as those suffering chronic infectious conditions (Crouser *et al.*, 2020). Magnetic resonance imaging (MRI) represents another significant advancement in imaging techniques, particularly in the evaluation of liver diseases caused by parasites. MRI is especially good at showing soft tissue, which helps identify liver problems related to hydatid disease and amebic liver abscesses. MRI does not use ionizing radiation, which means it is safer for patients who might need to be scanned several times. MRI can be further improved with diffusion-weighted imaging to study changes in tissue that happen during infection. While the cost and availability of MRI can be limiting factors, its detailed imaging capabilities are unmatched for certain complex cases, facilitating more precise diagnosis and management of hepatic parasitic infections (Brunetti *et al.*, 2018) (Figure 13.13).

13.5.3. Serological Tests for Infectious Agents

Serological tests are very important for diagnosing liver infections and parasites because they can show if certain pathogens are present. Serological assays look for antibodies or antigens from infectious agents, which help identify hepatitis, schistosomiasis, and leptospirosis. For example, with HBV infection, clinicians use surface antigens and antibodies to determine the stage of the infection and choose the best treatment.

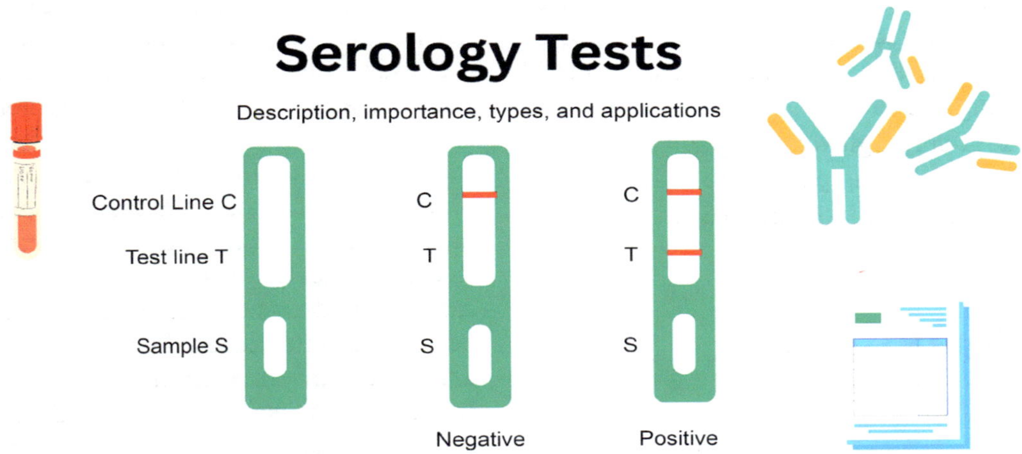

Figure 13.14. Serological tests.

Source: https://i0.wp.com/laboratoryintern.com/wp-content/uploads/2023/06/Serology-Tests.png.

This is very important for infections that can cause severe problems like cirrhosis or HCC in the liver. Beyond individual pathogens, these tests can also reflect immune responses influenced by co-infections, which are common in endemic regions, thereby highlighting the interconnected nature of these diseases (Bowlus *et al.*, 2022). Serological tests for liver-related infections are not always very sensitive or specific. For instance, while enzyme-linked immunosorbent assays (ELISA) are widely used for antibody detection, false negatives can occur, especially in immunocompromised individuals or in the early stages of infection when antibodies have yet to reach detectable levels. Also, understanding serological results requires doctors to look at the patient's symptoms and use imaging techniques such as ultrasound or MRI to understand the illness better. This multidimensional approach ensures that patients receive an accurate diagnosis, which is essential for effective management and treatment plans, particularly given the potentially severe outcomes associated with untreated liver diseases (Wilson *et al.*, 2019). Also, new ways of carrying out serological tests are helping to improve the diagnosis of liver infections. Today, rapid diagnostic tests and serological panels help detect several infectious diseases at once, which makes the process more efficient. Now, multiplex PCR along with serological tests allows scientists to detect co-infections, which are most common in places where infections from parasites and viruses are common. The combination improves our knowledge of what causes diseases, facilitates the detection of disease outbreaks, and supports public health plans. As new pathogens emerge and as existing ones evolve, maintaining a robust framework for serological testing will be crucial in effectively combating parasitic and infectious diseases affecting liver health (Bowlus *et al.*, 2022) (Figure 13.14).

13.6. Treatment Options

Treatment for parasitic and liver infectious diseases has improved a lot, just as dealing with many different pathogens is complex. There are three main forms of *leishmaniasis*: cutaneous, mucosal, and visceral, and every form needs different treatment approaches. Conventional first-line medications, like antimonials, have been the cornerstone but are linked with high side effects involving the heart, liver, and pancreas, making management challenging (eBioMedicine, 2023). As an alternative, liposomal amphotericin B and miltefosine are newer approaches, and miltefosine, which can be taken by mouth, shows differing results depending on the area where *Leishmania* species are found. Because people respond differently to treatments, it is important to have regional protocols and to look for new options that reduce dangers and tackle the disease. Treatment for malaria, especially cerebral malaria caused by Plasmodium falciparum, is also quite complex. This condition is particularly difficult because it has a high mortality rate and the rising challenge of developing resistance to drugs (Wei *et al.*, 2021). New methods for delivering dihydroartemisinin involve targeted nanoparticles, and these are showing good results. The new formulations help target the parasites found in red blood cells, making them more effective, and they also lower the risk of harming nearby organs such as the brain and liver. It helps treat both the parasite infection and the side effects of the disease, which could become a new standard method in the field. So, exploring advanced drug delivery methods could help find better treatments for malaria. Also, the range of treatment options should address the urgent need for therapies that are both affordable and sustainable in places where these parasitic infections are most common. International efforts are made to create effective plans for ensuring all people can get the drugs they need, as new treatments keep being introduced. For instance, initiatives driven by organizations like the Drugs for Neglected Diseases Initiative (DNDi) focus on the development of novel oral therapies for diseases such as *leishmaniasis* and malaria, which are particularly challenging due to their prevalence in impoverished regions (eBioMedicine, 2023). Since drug resistance is a major issue, scientists should focus on both creating new drugs and understanding the reasons for resistance. Taking a full approach to these issues is important for maintaining control and getting rid of hepatic parasitic diseases.

13.6.1. Antiparasitic Medications

Proper management of infectious and parasitic liver diseases depends on knowing about antiparasitic drugs. Treating diseases caused by parasites like amoebas, flukes, and protozoa, which damage the liver, relies on antiparasitic drugs. Their effectiveness is influenced by their ability to attack certain parasites as well as by their absorption, distribution, metabolism, and effects on the body. For example, metronidazole and albendazole have been found to be very effective in treating and managing hepatic complications caused by parasites. Moreover, the global rise in antimicrobial resistance brings forth the necessity of developing novel antiparasitic agents and expanding the scope of available treatment options among those affected by liver diseases, reinforcing the ongoing need for research in this field (Manganyi *et al.*, 2020). Natural products have become a promising area for finding new treatments for parasitic infections in the last few years. Endophytic fungi are famous for making chemicals that have strong antiparasitic effects. They live together with host plants without damaging them, which makes them valuable for finding new drugs. Studies have shown that metabolites from endophytic fungi are effective against bacteria, viruses, and parasites, and so they are promising candidates for discovering drugs to treat liver-related parasitic infections. The method is not only notable for its emphasis on biodiversity in drug discovery but also for the applicability of sustainable methods in the sourcing of therapeutic substances, especially with the increasing necessity of good antiparasitic drugs (Manganyi *et al.*, 2020). Also, progress in nanomedicine is leading to new developments in antiparasitic treatments. With nanotechnology, medicine can use new methods to help drugs reach parasites, which leads to better results from current antiparasitic treatments. Silver nanoparticles and other types of nanoparticles have been found to have special properties, like killing microbes and carrying drugs. Since liver diseases caused by parasites are a problem, this technology could help by increasing the absorption of antiparasitic drugs and reducing their side effects. As research continues to uncover the mechanisms underlying these nanoparticles, their integration into the therapeutic landscape for parasitic infections could provide new avenues for enabling timely and precise treatments, ultimately improving patient outcomes in the realm of parasitic and infectious diseases of the liver (Figure 13.15).

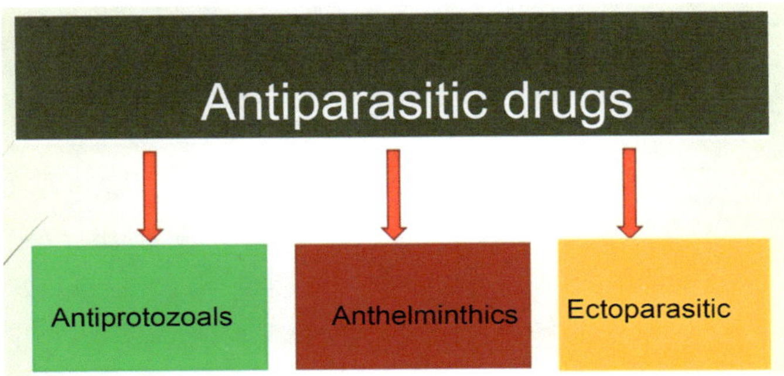

Figure 13.15. Antiparasitic drug.

Source: https://5.imimg.com/data5/SELLER/Default/2024/2/393950115/SW/II/UB/33400885/antiparasitic-drug.jpg.

13.6.2. Antiviral Therapies

The advent of antiviral therapies has transformed the landscape of treatment for CLD, particularly those caused by viral infections such as Hepatitis C. Direct-acting antivirals (DAAs) represent a significant breakthrough, offering patients a high chance of achieving a sustained virologic response

(SVR), which is critical in mitigating long-term liver damage and associated complications. A number of studies have found that patients who take DAA therapy not only get rid of the virus but also improve their liver health and overall metabolism. For instance, a recent investigation highlighted the role of DAAs in reversing insulin resistance among Hepatitis C genotype three patients, suggesting that effective antiviral treatment can lead to improved glucose metabolism and reduced risk of developing type 2 diabetes (Zubair *et al.*, 2025). It points out that antiviral therapies are helpful for liver diseases in several ways, not only by destroying the virus. In addition to their direct effects on viral clearance, antiviral therapies have been shown to enhance metabolic parameters in individuals with chronic Hepatitis C, particularly those with comorbid conditions such as type 2 diabetes mellitus (T2DM). Studies have found that using DAAs in patients with hepatitis C greatly reduces inflammation in the brain and scarring of the liver, which highlights the need for quick treatment. Improvements were noted not only in liver health markers but also in the BMI of treated patients, suggesting that SVR can play a crucial role in managing broader metabolic syndromes (Duport-Dodot *et al.*, 2024). Also, as hepatic inflammation and fibrosis decrease, the chance of getting severe problems like LC and HCC also decreases. Because of this evidence, it is important to use standard antiviral therapies as the initial treatment for chronic liver infections. It is very important to detect and treat viral hepatitis early, since early treatment with antiviral drugs can change the course of the disease. It has been proven that DAA treatment for SVR helps clear the virus in the short term and also improves a patient's long-term results, especially by decreasing the chance of death from liver disease. Because antiviral success is linked to better liver health and metabolism, it is important to keep researching and promoting efforts to make antiviral treatments more available to different groups. Ultimately, the integration of such therapies into standard care protocols for patients with CLD could foster significant advancements in managing parasitic and infectious diseases of the liver, heralding a new era of treatment possibilities (Figure 13.16).

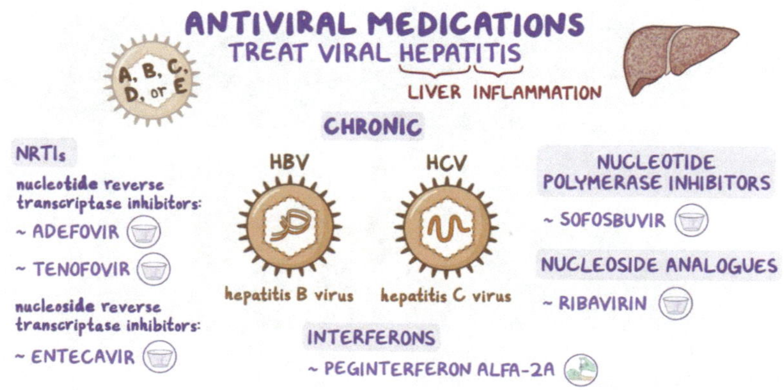

Figure 13.16. Antiviral medications.

Source: https://osmose-it.s3.amazonaws.com/PBP6NdsxRDWNSNt5XbXUyM33Tn6lOZr5/_.jpg.

13.6.3. Supportive Care and Management

Managing and supporting patients is very important for liver parasitic and infectious diseases since these conditions are not simple. Many patients have several symptoms that need to be managed well, such as pain, proper diet, and treatment of other infections. Supportive care can help reduce pain and improve daily life, which is necessary since many liver diseases may get worse if they are not treated. Working together, healthcare providers, dietitians, and mental health professionals can help create a complete treatment plan. Regularly checking liver function and assessing patients helps doctors adjust treatments according to each patient's needs, which improves outcomes when dealing with parasitic and infectious hepatitis. Supporting the immune system is very important in managing liver diseases because the liver is key to the body's immune response. Many studies demonstrate that sleep, which is often ignored, plays a major role in how well the immune system works. Sleeping enough helps the immune system, which makes the body better able to fight infections, including those in the liver. It shows that including good lifestyle habits in supportive care is important, and this should include enough rest. Also, sleep problems can have major effects, as chronic sleep deprivation can cause low-grade inflammation, which may worsen liver disease. So, a plan that includes good sleep habits could greatly help patients with liver infections improve their immune system and general health. Certain treatments are considered very important for the supportive care of liver diseases caused by parasites and infections. If antiviral therapies are suitable, they can reduce the number of viruses and support recovery, and antiparasitic drugs are designed to fight the underlying parasites. Complementing these treatments, supportive measures including hydration, optimal nutrition, and management of any complications, such as ascites or hepatic encephalopathy (HE), are crucial. Improving nutrition can support the immune system and help the liver recover, which makes the patient stronger. Even so, because infectious diseases are always changing, ongoing research is important to update these approaches and find new ways to manage them. As the field progresses, incorporating findings related to immune mechanism interactions, such as the role of sleep on immune support, can further enhance care strategies and patient outcomes (Besedovsky *et al.*, 2019; Crouser *et al.*, 2020).

13.7. Prevention and Control Measures

Effective prevention and control are key in the battle against parasitic and infectious liver diseases. One of the core methods entails having rigorous food safety protocols, which are critical given that most infections of the liver are initiated by foodborne pathogens. The WHO has highlighted the enormous global disease burden from foodborne diseases, particularly those resulting from contamination with viruses and bacteria such as hepatitis A and non-typhoidal Salmonella enterica. Through better food handling, public health campaigns, and proper sanitation habits, not only can the spread of such infections be prevented, but public education on the importance of eating safe food products can also take place. Therefore, measures to deal with food safety comprehensively at all levels from production right up to the plate could reduce the occurrence of liver diseases and safeguard public health in general (Havelaar *et al.*, 2015). Apart from food safety, immunization remains another central preventive mechanism for some infectious liver conditions such as hepatitis A and hepatitis B. The use of vaccination programs within public health has shown incredible outcomes, particularly in high-risk populations. By immunization against these conditions, the prevalence and incidence of viral pathogen-associated liver disease can be significantly reduced. In addition, these immunization programs must be complemented by education campaigns that inform communities about the benefits of vaccines and how they function to increase immune resistance against liver infection. Interagency efforts among healthcare providers, public health managers, and community organizations in this regard can maximize vaccine coverage and ultimately lead to lower rates of infection and improved liver health outcomes (Havelaar *et al.*, 2015). Aside from immunizations, healthcare systems must emphasize correct diagnosis, access to treatment, and disease control for those who are already infected with liver diseases. This can involve frequent screenings among those at risk, incorporating advanced diagnostic technology into medical practice, and providing timely and effective treatment for those who need it. In addition, the immunocompromised state that often results as a side effect of treatment regimens—e.g., those involving immunomodulatory therapies—must be monitored closely in patients in order to prevent opportunistic infections. In addition, education about the potential risks of immunosuppression will increasingly allow patients and doctors to proceed cautiously with measures of minimizing the risk of progressing liver disease and facilitating better health outcomes. Overall, a multifaceted preventive, educational, and low-cost health services-based approach can keep the burden of parasitic and infectious liver diseases under control.

13.7.1. Vaccination Strategies for Hepatitis

Vaccination for the prevention of hepatitis remains a key factor in the control of liver illness across the globe. Hepatitis viruses, particularly hepatitis A and B, are critical public health problems as they have the capacity to induce acute liver disease and chronic infection with profound implications for health. Vaccination plays a critical role in the control of these viruses. For instance, the hepatitis A vaccine has a high efficacy rate with rapid development of immunity and a highly widespread reduction in disease incidence among those populations in which it is administered. Similarly, the hepatitis B vaccine has dramatically decreased the prevalence of the viral infection. Vaccination protects not just the individuals but is also a component of herd immunity within populations, reducing overall virus transmission and epidemic control, which is of particular urgency in areas of high endemicity. The role of vaccination in the prevention of hepatitis is also accelerated through the successful incorporation of immunization interventions into overall public health strategies. Education efforts that generate an awareness about the spread of hepatitis, as well as the role of vaccination, are essential to ensure increased uptake levels. These interventions typically entail a focus on high-risk groups such as healthcare workers, individuals engaging in high-risk behavior, and those in poor sanitation zones. In these interventions, the medical community emphasizes a complete course of the vaccine schedule and booster shots where necessary, particularly in the case of the hepatitis B vaccine. Furthermore, the interface between sleep and immune response means that ensuring maximal health behavior also enhances vaccine efficacy, and hence the argument for integrated public health policy incorporating not only vaccination but also lifestyle intervention (Besedovsky *et al.*, 2019). New advances and ongoing research on vaccination techniques also provide optimism in fighting emerging strains of hepatitis C, a virus notoriously hard to fight with vaccination. There is no hepatitis C vaccine widely used at present, but ongoing research is focusing on understanding the virus's immune evasion mechanisms and the role of molecular mimicry in virus-specific immunity generation. Implications from the understanding of autoimmunity with hepatitis C can inform the design of vaccines that not only generate an optimal immune response but also suppress the risk of undesirable autoimmune manifestations with infection (Rojas *et al.*, 2018). As researchers continue to explore new vaccine prospects and delivery methods, the promise of successful vaccination against hepatitis is gradually increasing, holding prospects of broader disease control measures against liver disease due to hepatitis (Figure 13.17).

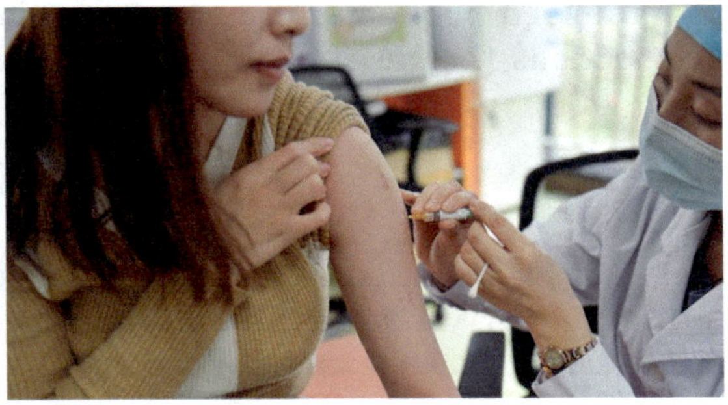

Figure 13.17. Hepatitis vaccination.

https://static01.nyt.com/images/2019/06/27/science/27HPV/27HPV-videoSixteenByNine3000.jpg?year=2019&h=1687&w=3000&sig=0x893145a4dc150768c6af62d9d17989fc&tw=1.

13.7.2. Public Health Initiatives for Parasitic Diseases

Public health efforts aimed at parasitic diseases are very important for reducing the health problems caused by these infections, especially in the liver, where Schistosoma and Echinococcus can bring about serious illness. A good intervention often includes teaching programs in the community about the ways to prevent and stop the spread of the disease. Many endemic areas have communities that lack proper hygiene, which makes them more likely to get infections. Workshops and information sharing with local people allow public health organizations to encourage better sanitation and hygiene, which leads to a decrease in infections. Educational efforts can also help people notice early signs of liver damage and get medical care, which is important for avoiding the serious problems that can result. Another cornerstone of public health initiatives for parasitic diseases is the implementation of mass drug administration (MDA) programs. Such programs, usually used together with local health departments, try to prevent diseases in groups of people, regardless of whether they are infected or not. Many parasitic infections have been shown to be significantly reduced by this approach. In places where many people have schistosomiasis, regular praziquantel treatment for at-risk groups can reduce the number of infections, which helps lessen the risk of liver complications over the years. Partnering with global health organizations to provide drugs and help improve local health systems is very important for these efforts. Bringing MDA into current healthcare systems fits with public health efforts, underlining the value of teamwork against infectious diseases. In addition, having surveillance and research programs is important for effective strategies to fight parasitic diseases. It is important to keep monitoring infections and the effectiveness of responses to make changes as situations change.

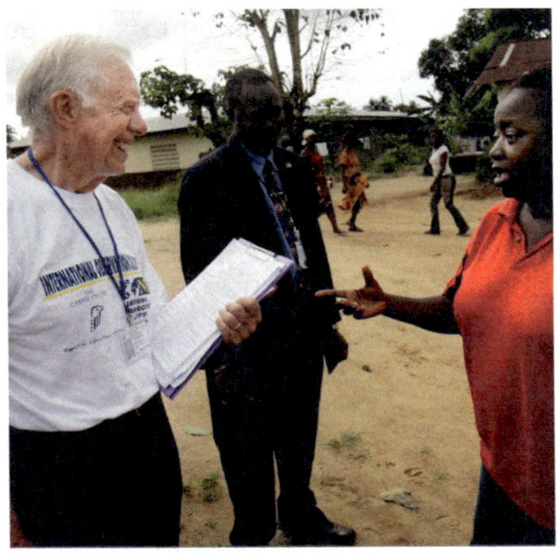

Figure 13.18. Public Health Iniciatives

Source: https://platform.vox.com/wp-content/uploads/sites/2/chorus/uploads/chorus_asset/file/15648311/GettyImages-55895815.0.1513808024.jpg?quality=90&strip=all&crop=16.666666666667,0,66.666666666667,100.

Stronger surveillance allows health officials to handle outbreaks fast, which helps keep parasitic infections from harming the liver. Also, finding new ways to diagnose, treat, and prevent diseases is very important for improving prevention efforts. When researchers, public health bodies, and communities join forces, these initiatives can help more effectively control parasitic diseases. Encouraging and coordinating interdisciplinary collaborations can not only enrich the scientific understanding of disease dynamics but also lead to well-rounded public health approaches that address the multifaceted challenges posed by parasitic infections (Ačiūtė *et al.*, 2020; Landrigan *et al.*, 2020) (Figure 13.18).

13.7.3. Personal Preventive Measures

To prevent liver problems caused by parasites and germs, it is mainly important to take personal preventive steps. Hygiene, mainly in what we eat and drink, is very important. Both hepatitis A and E are often spread through food and water that is not safe to consume and can cause serious problems if not treated. People should make sure their food is cooked properly and their water is safe, especially when visiting areas with a lot of these infections. When people follow these habits, they look after their own liver health and at the same time help reduce the spread of infectious agents, which helps to prevent outbreaks in vulnerable groups. In addition, vaccination is a key part of protecting yourself from liver infections. Many people can get vaccinated against hepatitis A and B, which greatly reduces the number of cases. Immunization plays a major role in lowering deaths and helps avoid the formation of serious liver diseases linked to hepatitis B, mainly in those who are highly at risk. Taking vaccinations regularly helps the immune system defend against certain viral infections. This active strategy matches public health efforts to stop infectious diseases, showing the role each person plays in keeping themselves and the community healthy. Knowing when vaccines are needed and being able to get them is very important for this preventive measure. Being aware of the risk factors is necessary to take personal steps to prevent liver diseases. People should know that some risky actions, such as having sex without protection and sharing needles, can make it easier for hepatitis B and C to spread. Teaching people about safe habits can greatly lower the number of liver infections. Regular check-ups help find viral infections early, which is important for quick treatment and control. By fostering a culture of health literacy and encouraging regular medical check-ups, communities can empower individuals to adopt preventive measures effectively, thus contributing to the decline of parasitic and infectious diseases affecting the liver (Chaparro *et al.*, 2019; Pallavi *et al.*, 2018).

SUMMARY

The importance of knowing about parasitic and infectious diseases of the liver is very high, especially because they cause so much harm to people around the world. The liver helps with many metabolic functions, detoxifies the body, and produces important proteins. If the liver is infected by hepatitis or parasites, the results can be very serious, sometimes resulting in liver failure or death. Furthermore, recent studies have pointed out that the patterns of these infections can change a lot because of external reasons such as lockdowns that were used during the COVID-19 pandemic. So, constant research and monitoring are needed to develop public health strategies that can help people at risk of liver diseases, given the variety of pathogens involved, such as viruses and parasites. The prevalence and outcomes of liver-related diseases depend greatly on the interaction of environmental, biological, and socio-economic factors. The study of infectious and parasitic diseases, which shows how rates can change during social upheaval, calls for a wide range of strategies to tackle these problems. Various studies on maternal health have shown that deaths from HIV/AIDS and malaria have decreased, which proves the success of targeted interventions. A major drop in pregnancy-related deaths has been noticed, thanks to better healthcare efforts that focus on mothers and controlling infectious diseases. Such evidence helps design treatments that are suited to liver diseases, showing the importance of healthcare policies that cover prevention as well as treatment. Handling parasitic and infectious diseases of the liver calls for worldwide efforts that involve helping communities and educating the public as well as treating individuals. As demonstrated by biliary atresia, it is important to learn about the reasons for infections, such as possible viruses and environmental factors, to develop good ways to prevent and treat them. Therefore, public health policy needs to use epidemiological data and note the social and economic factors that play a role in how these diseases affect people. Also, providing ongoing research money and ensuring proper healthcare facilities are necessary to battle liver diseases. Only through a unified and informed approach can healthcare systems effectively combat the persistent challenges posed by parasitic and infectious diseases, ensuring improved health outcomes for all populations at risk, as reflected in contemporary health studies and their implications for future interventions (Musarandega *et al.*, 2022; Nomden *et al.*, 2023).

It is important to mention that the immune system and sleep patterns have many interactions when it comes to parasitic and infectious diseases of the liver. It has been found that sleep and immunity influence each other, so infections can interfere with sleep, and better sleep quality helps the immune system. Not getting enough sleep can trigger low-grade inflammation, which increases the chance of diseases that harm the liver such as hepatitis and cirrhosis. Since the liver is important for immunity, knowing this relationship can help choose the best treatments for liver diseases. Thus, the intersection of sleep, immune response, and liver health emerges as a crucial factor that warrants further investigation as a potential area of therapeutic intervention (Besedovsky *et al.*, 2019). In addition, detecting liver diseases usually involves cooperation between healthcare providers and microbiology laboratories. The liver is affected by many different infections, so a system-based method for diagnosis is required because several pathogens can lead to liver complications. For example, viral hepatitis, leishmaniasis, and schistosomiasis are caused by unique agents, so patients need specific tests. When clinicians and microbiologists collaborate well, it becomes easier to find the cause of infections and pick the best treatment. Comprehensive guidelines, such as those outlined in expert documents, support physicians in choosing tests that improve diagnostic accuracy and patient outcomes (Miller *et al.*, 2018). So, having an integrated healthcare system is key to better handling liver infections. Managing diseases of the liver caused by parasites and infections mainly relies on learning about how hosts and pathogens interact and making use of new diagnostic tools. Current studies point out that it is important to continue research on how infections cause liver diseases to develop. They can explain how to stop or handle these diseases properly. Also, spotting key biomarkers in liver infections helps healthcare professionals choose the right treatments. Since infectious diseases are always evolving, new methods for diagnosis and treatment are still very necessary. By synthesizing current knowledge on infections affecting the liver, clinicians can be better equipped to both prevent and manage these conditions effectively and optimize patient care strategies (Besedovsky *et al.*, 2019; Miller *et al.*, 2018).

CLOSER LOOK

LIVER DYSFUNCTION

Liver dysfunction, also known as hepatic dysfunction, refers to any impairment of the liver's ability to perform its normal functions. These functions include filtering blood, metabolizing nutrients, producing proteins, and synthesizing bile. Liver dysfunction can be caused by various factors, including infections, alcohol consumption, certain medications, and underlying medical conditions. Symptoms of liver dysfunction can vary depending on the severity and underlying cause, and may include fatigue, jaundice, abdominal pain, and fluid retention (Figure 13.19).

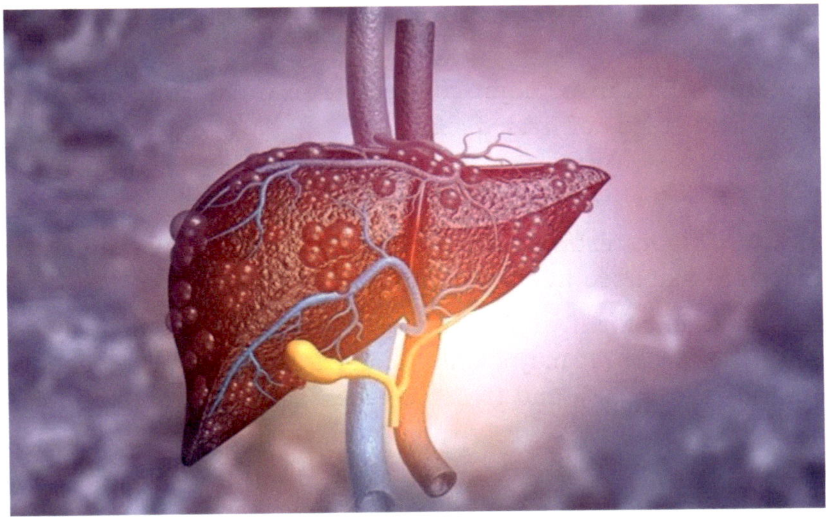

Figure 13.19. Liver Dysfunction

Source: https://d2jx2rerrg6sh3.cloudfront.net/image-handler/picture/2021/3/shutterstock_1118711141_(1).jpg.

Causes of Liver Dysfunction

- **Infections:** Viral hepatitis (A, B, C, D, E), parasitic infections, and BI can damage the liver and impair its function.
- **Alcohol Abuse:** Excessive alcohol consumption can lead to fatty liver disease, alcoholic hepatitis, and cirrhosis, all of which affect liver function.
- **Medications:** Some medications, such as certain antibiotics, statins, and pain relievers, can cause liver damage and dysfunction.
- **Underlying Medical Conditions:** Conditions like nonalcoholic fatty liver disease (NAFLD), diabetes, and autoimmune diseases can lead to liver dysfunction.
- **Other Factors:** Exposure to toxins, certain chemicals, and other environmental factors can also damage the liver.

Symptoms of Liver Dysfunction

- **Fatigue:** Persistent tiredness and lack of energy can be a sign of liver dysfunction.
- **Jaundice:** Yellowing of the skin and eyes due to the buildup of bilirubin in the blood.
- **Abdominal Pain and Swelling:** Pain and swelling in the upper right abdomen can indicate liver problems.
- **Fluid Retention:** Edema (swelling in the legs and ankles) and ascites (fluid buildup in the abdomen) can occur.
- **Easy Bruising and Bleeding:** Liver dysfunction can affect blood clotting factors, leading to increased bruising and bleeding.
- **Nausea and Loss of Appetite:** Digestive issues and a decrease in appetite can also be symptoms.
- **Other Symptoms:** Dark urine, light-colored stools, itchy skin, and brain fog (HE) can also occur in later stages of liver disease.

Diagnosis and Treatment

- **Diagnosis:** LFTs (blood tests), imaging tests (ultrasound, CT scan, MRI), and liver biopsies can help diagnose liver dysfunction.
- **Treatment:** Treatment for liver dysfunction depends on the underlying cause and severity of the condition. It may include medications to treat infections, lifestyle changes (diet and exercise), and in some cases, liver transplantation.

References

1. Adler, Y., Charron, P., Imazio, M., Badano, L. P., Barón-Esquivias, G., Bogaert, J., Brucato, A., *et al.* (2015). 2015 ESC guidelines for the diagnosis and management of pericardial diseases. *European Heart Journal, 36*, 2921–2964. https://doi.org/10.1093/eurheartj/ehv318.
2. Almatroudi A. Silver nanoparticles: synthesis, characterisation and biomedical applications. Open Life Sci. 2020 Nov 19;15(1):819-839. doi: 10.1515/biol-2020-0094. PMID: 33817269; PMCID: PMC7747521. https://pmc.ncbi.nlm.nih.gov/articles/PMC7747521/
3. Athanasiou, L., Tsokana, C., Doukas, D., Kantere, M., Katsoulos, P., Papakonstantinou, G., Katsogiannou, E., *et al.* (2023). Hepatic coccidiosis in wild rabbits in Greece: Parasite detection on liver imprints and the associated biochemical profile. *Veterinary Sciences, 10*. https://www.semanticscholar.org/paper/9de51f2b7f01ea420a5e4c09fe35e2d3b3be445b (accessed on 24 May 2025).
4. Bernstein, Ç. N., Eliakim, A. R., Fedail, S. S., Fried, M., Gearry, R. B., Goh, K. L., Hamid, S., *et al.* (2016). World Gastroenterology Organisation global guidelines inflammatory bowel disease. *Journal of Clinical Gastroenterology, 50*, 803–818. https://doi.org/10.1097/mcg.0000000000000660.
5. Besedovsky, L., Lange, T., & Haack, M. (2019). The sleep-immune crosstalk in health and disease. *Physiological Reviews, 99*(3), 1325–1380. https://doi.org/10.1152/physrev.00010.2018.
6. Bowlus, C. L., Arrivé, L., Bergquist, A., Deneau, M., Forman, L., Ilyas, S. I., Lunsford, K. E., *et al.* (2022). AASLD practice guidance on primary sclerosing cholangitis and cholangiocarcinoma. *Hepatology, 77*, 659–702. https://doi.org/10.1002/hep.32771.
7. Brindha, J., Balamurali, M. M., & Chanda, K. (2021). An overview on the therapeutics of neglected infectious diseases—Leishmaniasis and Chagas diseases. *Frontiers in Chemistry, 9*. https://doi.org/10.3389/fchem.2021.622286.
8. Brunetti, E., Tamarozzi, F., Macpherson, C. N. L., Fìlice, C., Piontek, M. S., Kabaalioğlu, A., Dong, Y., *et al.* (2018). Ultrasound and cystic echinococcosis. *Ultrasound International Open, 4*, E70–E78. https://doi.org/10.1055/a-0650-3807.
9. Budreviciute A, Damiati S, Sabir DK, Onder K, Schuller-Goetzburg P, Plakys G, Katileviciute A, Khoja S, Kodzius R. Management and Prevention Strategies for Non-communicable Diseases (NCDs) and Their Risk Factors. Front Public Health. 2020 Nov 26;8:574111. doi: 10.3389/fpubh.2020.574111. PMID: 33324597; PMCID: PMC7726193.
10. Butt, N. M., Lambert, J., Ali, S., Beer, P., Cross, N. C. P., Duncombe, A., Ewing, J., *et al.* (2017). Guideline for the investigation and management of eosinophilia. *British Journal of Hematology, 176*(4), 553–572. https://doi.org/10.1111/bjh.14488.
11. Chai, J. Y., & Jung, B. K. (2022). General overview of the current status of human foodborne trematodiasis. *Parasitology, 149*, 1262–1285. https://doi.org/10.1017/s0031182022000725.
12. Chai JY, Jung BK, Hong SJ. Albendazole and Mebendazole as Anti-Parasitic and Anti-Cancer Agents: an Update. Korean J Parasitol. 2021 Jun;59(3):189-225. doi: 10.3347/kjp.2021.59.3.189. Epub 2021 Jun 21. PMID: 34218593; PMCID: PMC8255490. https://pubmed.ncbi.nlm.nih.gov/34218593/
13. Chaparro, C. M., & Suchdev, P. S. (2019). Anemia epidemiology, pathophysiology, and etiology

in low- and middle-income countries. *Annals of the New York Academy of Sciences, 1450*, 15–31. https://doi.org/10.1111/nyas.14092.

14. Converse, P. J., Kaba, M., Kloos, H., *et al.* (2018). *Bibliography on HIV/AIDS in Ethiopia and Ethiopians in the Diaspora: The 2016 Update.* https://core.ac.uk/download/478298491.pdf (accessed on 24 May 2025).
15. Crouser, E. D., Maier, L. A., Wilson, K. C., Bonham, C. A., Morgenthau, A. S., Patterson, K., Abston, E., *et al.* (2020). Diagnosis and detection of sarcoidosis: An official American Thoracic Society clinical practice guideline. *American Journal of Respiratory and Critical Care Medicine, 201*, e26–e51. https://doi.org/10.1164/rccm.202002-0251st.
16. Dhanya, M. S., Anandhi, D., Roy, D. D., Alex, R. B., Karthick, S., Joseph, B., Renjith, K. R., *et al.* (2024). *The Influence of Maternal Infections on Congenital Heart Defect.* https://core.ac.uk/download/603897437.pdf.
17. Duport-Dodot, I., Olariu, C., Saran, A., Tilișcan, C., Stratan, L., Dodot, D. M., Aramă, V., *et al.* (2024). Evaluation of direct-acting antiviral agents' impact on liver biomarkers in patients with type-2 diabetes and hepatitis C virus infection. *Romanian Journal of Infectious Diseases.* https://www.semanticscholar.org/paper/1509b619da55b8d9ecffab0fd8a25ff2d2278b4d (accessed on 24 May 2025).
18. eBioMedicine. (2023). Leishmania: An urgent need for new treatments. *EBioMedicine, 87*, 104440. https://doi.org/10.1016/j.ebiom.2023.104440.
19. Ellwanger, J. H., da Veiga, A. B. G., Kaminski, V. de L., Valverde-Villegas, J. M., de Freitas, A. W. Q., & Chies, J. A. B. (2021). Control and prevention of infectious diseases from a One Health perspective. *Genetics and Molecular Biology, 44.* https://doi.org/10.1590/1678-4685-gmb-2020-0256.
20. Fishman, J. A. (2017). Infection in organ transplantation. *American Journal of Transplantation, 17*, 856–879. https://doi.org/10.1111/ajt.14208.
21. Góralska, K., Błaszkowska, J., & Dzikowiec, M. (2018). Neuroinfectious caused by fungi. *Infection, 46*, 443–459. https://doi.org/10.1007/s15010-018-1152-2.
22. Havelaar, A. H., Kirk, M., Torgerson, P. R., Gibb, H. J., Hald, T., Lake, R., Praet, N., *et al.* (2015). World Health Organization global estimates and regional comparisons of the burden of foodborne disease in 2010. *PLoS Medicine, 12*, e1001923. https://doi.org/10.1371/journal.pmed.1001923.
23. Hosseini, M. S., Khoshbaten, M., Kolahi, A. A., & Safiri, S. (2024). Liver cancer in the Middle East and North Africa: Epidemiology, trends, and risk factors. *International Journal of Aging.* https://www.semanticscholar.org/paper/dd60de7e29b9c9ff72c0b15baa6abcb02d5108d1 (accessed on 24 May 2025).
24. Kadesch, P., Quack, T., Gerbig, S., Grevelding, C. G., & Spengler, B. (2019). Lipid topography in *Schistosoma mansoni* cryosections, revealed by micro embedding and high-resolution atmospheric-pressure matrix-assisted laser desorption/ionization (MALDI) mass spectrometry imaging. *Analytical Chemistry, 91*(7), 4520–4528. https://doi.org/10.1021/acs.analchem.8b05440.
25. Kim, H. U. (2024). Parasitic diseases of upper gastrointestinal tract. *The Korean Journal of Helicobacter and Upper Gastrointestinal Research.* https://www.semanticscholar.org/paper/

dc98e3e19e1321aa76bb466d14f3491c0b49c3ba (accessed on 24 May 2025).

26. Landrigan, P. J., Stegeman, J. J., Fleming, L. E., Allemand, D., Anderson, D. M., Backer, L. C., Brücker-Davis, F., *et al.* (2020). Human health and ocean pollution. *Annals of Global Health, 86*, 151. https://doi.org/10.5334/aogh.2831.

27. Lin, L., Yang, H., & Xu, X. (2022). Effects of water pollution on human health and disease heterogeneity: A review. *Frontiers in Environmental Science, 10*. https://doi.org/10.3389/fenvs.2022.880246.

28. Liu, X., Wang, L., Tan, S., Chen, Z., Wu, B., & Wu, X. (2022). Therapeutic effects of berberine on liver fibrosis are associated with lipid metabolism and intestinal flora. *Frontiers in Pharmacology, 13*. https://doi.org/10.3389/fphar.2022.814871.

29. Manganyi, M. C., & Ateba, C. N. (2020). Untapped potentials of endophytic fungi: A review of novel bioactive compounds with biological applications. *Microorganisms, 8*(12), 1934. https://doi.org/10.3390/microorganisms8121934.

30. Miller, J. M., Binnicker, M. J., Campbell, S., Carroll, K. C., Chapin, K. C., Gilligan, P. H., Gonzalez, M. D., *et al.* (2018). A guide to utilization of the microbiology laboratory for diagnosis of infectious diseases: 2018 update by the Infectious Diseases Society of America and the American Society for Microbiology. *Clinical Infectious Diseases, 67*(6), e1–e94. https://doi.org/10.1093/cid/ciy381.

31. Musarandega, R., Ngwenya, S., Murewanhema, G., Machekano, R., Magwali, T., Nystrom, L., Pattinson, R., *et al.* (2022). Changes in causes of pregnancy-related and maternal mortality in Zimbabwe 2007–08 to 2018–19: Findings from two reproductive age mortality surveys. *BMC Public Health, 22*. https://www.semanticscholar.org/paper/ab0cee9fb0a557e4919001218200dbc154295f53 (accessed on 24 May 2025).

32. Nomden, M., Alizai, N., Betalli, P., Bruggink, J., Cananzi, M., Christensen, V., D'Antiga, L., *et al.* (2023). Incidence of isolated biliary atresia during the COVID lockdown in Europe: Results from a collaborative project by RARE-Liver. *Journal of Clinical Medicine, 12*. https://www.semanticscholar.org/paper/5b0bdc32ac581102d5702ea410ab027ac1a11d4e (accessed on 24 May 2025).

33. Okon, E. M., Okocha, R. C., Taiwo, A. B., Michael, F. B., & Bolanle, A. M. (2023). Dynamics of co-infection in fish: A review of pathogen-host interaction and clinical outcome. *Fish and Shellfish Immunology Reports, 4*, 100096. https://doi.org/10.1016/j.fsirep.2023.100096.

34. Pallavi, K., Sravani, D., Durga, S., *et al.* (2018). Hepatitis-A: Review on current and future scenario. *Journal of In Silico & In Vitro Pharmacology, 3*. https://doi.org/10.21767/2469-6692.100015.

35. Paller, V., Belizario, V., Ancog, R. C., Alonte, A. J., Jimenez, J. R. D., Corales, C. G., Divina, B. P., *et al.* (2024). Socio-economic risk factors for intestinal helminthiases in selected endemic communities in Mindanao, the Philippines: A cross-sectional study. *BMC Infectious Diseases, 24*. https://www.semanticscholar.org/paper/f0bb4f308f15fb4d3480a0e2855072b8b1cc2d02 (accessed on 24 May 2025).

36. Ponamarev, V., Popova, O., Kostrova, A., & Agafonova, L. (2024). Etiology and pathogenesis of non-infectious hepatopathy in cattle under industrial production conditions. E3S Web of Conferences. https://www.semanticscholar.org/paper/Etiology-and-pathogenesis-of-non-infectious-in-Ponamarev-Popova/87e3ea6e89589d87e254b16b580ec16faa7d0df5

37. Rahier JF, Magro F, Abreu C, Armuzzi A, Ben-Horin S, Chowers Y, Cottone M, de Ridder L, Doherty G, Ehehalt R, Esteve M, Katsanos K, Lees CW, Macmahon E, Moreels T, Reinisch W, Tilg H, Tremblay L, Veereman-Wauters G, Viget N, Yazdanpanah Y, Eliakim R, Colombel JF; European Crohn's and Colitis Organisation (ECCO). Second European evidence-based consensus on the prevention, diagnosis and management of opportunistic infections in inflammatory bowel disease. J Crohns Colitis. 2014 Jun;8(6):443-68. doi: 10.1016/j.crohns.2013.12.013. Epub 2014 Mar 6. PMID: 24613021. https://pubmed.ncbi.nlm.nih.gov/24613021/

38. Rahman, M. T., Sobur, M. A., Islam, M. S., Ievy, S., Hossain, M. J., El Zowalaty, M. E., Rahman, A. T., *et al.* (2020). Zoonotic diseases: Etiology, impact, and control. *Microorganisms, 8*(9), 1405. https://doi.org/10.3390/microorganisms8091405.

39. Rawla, P., Bandaru, S. S., & Vellipuram, A. (2017). Review of infectious etiology of acute pancreatitis. *Gastroenterology Research, 10*, 153–158. https://doi.org/10.14740/gr858w.

40. Rojas, M., Restrepo-Jiménez, P., Monsalve, D. M., Pachéco, Y., Acosta-Ampudia, Y., Ramírez-Santana, C., Leung, P. S. C., *et al.* (2018). Molecular mimicry and autoimmunity. *Journal of Autoimmunity, 95*, 100–123. https://doi.org/10.1016/j.jaut.2018.10.012

41. Shikanai-Yasuda, M. A., Mendes, R. P., Colombo, A. L., Queiroz-Telles, F., Kono, A., Paniago, A. M. M., Nathan, A., *et al.* (2017). Brazilian guidelines for the clinical management of paracoccidioidomycosis. *Revita da Sociedad Brasileira de Medicina Tropical, 50*, 715–740. https://doi.org/10.1590/0037-8682-0230-2017.

42. Sonne, C., Lakemeyer, J., Desforges, J. P., Eulaers, I., Persson, S., Stokholm, I., Galatius, A., *et al.* (2020). A review of pathogens in selected Baltic Sea indicator species. *Environment International, 137*, 105565. https://doi.org/10.1016/j.envint.2020.105565.

43. Tharwat, M., & Tsuka, T. (2024). Diagnostic utility of ultrasonography for thoracic and abdominal bacterial and parasitic diseases in ruminants: A comprehensive overview. *Frontiers in Veterinary Science, 11*. https://www.semanticscholar.org/paper/7bb93d5b0611db73b609 9fc53811b784180bd6d6 (accessed on 24 May 2025).

44. Ullah, A., Munir, S., Badshah, S. L., Khan, N., Ghani, L., Poulson, B. G., Emwas, A. H., *et al.* (2020). Important flavonoids and their role as a therapeutic agent. *Molecules, 25*, 5243. https://doi.org/10.3390/molecules25225243.

45. Varki, A. (2016). Biological roles of glycans. *Glycobiology, 27*, 3–49. https://doi.org/10.1093/glycob/cww086.

46. Wei, W., Cheng, W., Dai, W., Lu, F., Cheng, Y., Jiang, T., Ren, Z., *et al.* (2021). A nanodrug coated with membrane from brain microvascular endothelial cells protects against experimental cerebral malaria. *Nano Letters, 22*, 211–219. https://doi.org/10.1021/acs.nanolett.1c03514.

47. Wilson, M. R., Sample, H. A., Zorn, K. C., Arevalo, S., Yu, G., Neuhaus, J., Federman, S., *et al.* (2019). Clinical metagenomic sequencing for diagnosis of meningitis and encephalitis. *New England Journal of Medicine, 380*(24), 2327–2340. https://doi.org/10.1056/nejmoa1803396.

48. Zhao, H., Wu, L., Yan, G., Chen, Y., Zhou, M., Wu, Y., & Li, Y. (2021). Inflammation and tumor progression: Signaling pathways and targeted intervention. *Signal Transduction and Targeted Therapy, 6*. https://doi.org/10.1038/s41392-021-00658-5.

49. Zhu, Y. S., Sun, Z., Zheng, J. X., Zhang, S. X., Yin, J. X., Zhao, H., Shen, H. M., *et al.* (2024). Prevalence and attributable health burdens of vector-borne parasitic infectious diseases

of poverty, 1990–2021: Findings from the Global Burden of Disease Study 2021. *Infectious Diseases of Poverty, 13*. https://www.semanticscholar.org/paper/71d7bb10dbfd12e030ce0c0caa109954563d7bfd (accessed on 24 May 2025).

50. Zubair, M., Pasha, N. A., Khan, H., Rafique, K., Rao, M. A., & Sadiq, Z. (2025). Impact of direct-acting antiviral treatments on insulin resistance reversal in chronic hepatitis C patients. *Biological and Clinical Sciences Research Journal*. https://www.semanticscholar.org/paper/538fc60cfb12950226346a7278c107b3d551f16b (accessed on 24 May 2025).

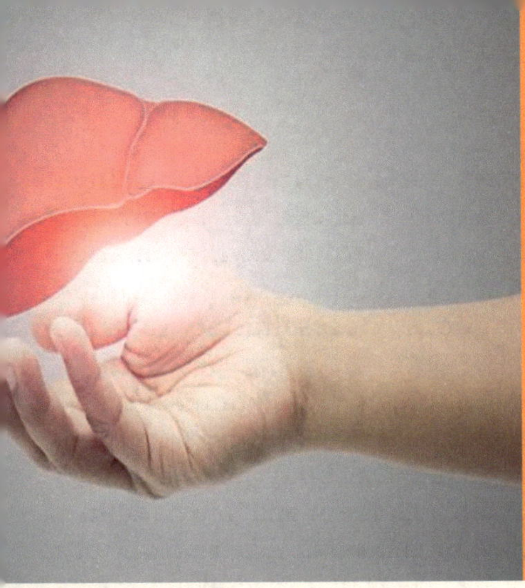

Chapter 14

DRUG-INDUCED LIVER INJURY (DILI)

Contents

Introduction

Liver, one of the organs responsible for several metabolic processes, is susceptible to injury by exogenous substances, primarily drugs. Drug-induced liver injury (DILI) has garnered tremendous interest owing to the pleiotropic mechanisms and multiform clinical manifestations. These range from bland, transitory elevations of liver enzymes to fulminant hepatic failure, defining the gravity of DILI as a public health problem. The multifactorial etiology makes it challenging to diagnose and treat, necessitating additional research to elucidate its mechanisms. As stressed in recent publications, a deepened understanding of DILI can optimistically lead to improved drug safety and public health outcomes, given its potential as a leading cause of drug withdrawal following approval and as a significant cause of adverse drug reactions (Guo *et al.*, 2024). Research into DILI has revealed its mechanisms to be classically classified as enzyme-mediated reactions that produce highly reactive metabolites. Highly reactive metabolites have the capability to cause cell damage and activation of key inflammatory pathways, which are normally mediated by enzymes belonging to the cytochrome P450 family. The intricacies associated with metabolism-dependent DILI have a tendency to render it unpredictable as to which drugs will cause hepatotoxicity, thus necessitating advanced methodology in preclinical screening. Thus, there is a pressing necessity for *in vitro* models that can effectively replicate the biochemical and structural features of human liver tissue. Existing literature emphasizes the inadequacies of traditional liver models towards testing the effect of chronic drug exposure and metabolism-dependent DILI, which do not maintain the crucial features of adult hepatocytes (Cox *et al.*, 2020). New technology is making it possible to develop more sophisticated *in vitro* models of the liver, such as three-dimensional (3D) culture systems. These novel approaches are intended to offer a more physiological environment, more appropriate to drug safety and hepatotoxicity testing. Through techniques like spheroids and organoids, researchers can support a mature hepatocyte phenotype and enhance cell lifespan, which allows for the performance of longer-term studies of drug action. These modeling progressions are critical in the preclinical identification of possible DILI before clinical trial. Lastly, the synergy between omics technologies and higher potency cellular systems will enable us to understand deeply molecular processes in DILI, thereby guiding safer drug creation and subsequent therapeutic intervention (Cox *et al.*, 2020; Guo *et al.*, 2024).

Definition of Drug-Induced Liver Injury (DILI)

Being aware of what DILI means is necessary to see how complex and important it is for health. DILI is when the liver is damaged by drugs or herbal supplements, which may cause inflammation and, in the most serious cases, lead to liver failure. This injury can present as an increase in liver enzymes, such as alanine aminotransferase (ALT) and aspartate aminotransferase (AST), often signifying hepatocellular injury. The clinical spectrum of DILI varies widely, from asymptomatic elevations in liver function tests (LFTs) to severe manifestations, necessitating careful monitoring of patients receiving potentially hepatotoxic medications. The risk and severity of DILI can be affected by genetics, how the drug is processed by the body, and patient characteristics, which makes managing patients with DILI complex for clinicians. After looking at how DILI occurs, it is clear that several different factors can make someone more susceptible. Certain genetic changes in drug-metabolizing enzymes can make it harder for patients to process some drugs, which can cause more liver damage. For example, some studies suggest that people with certain NAT2 gene variants are more likely to experience liver problems from isoniazid when treating tuberculosis, where 89 cases of anti-TB DILI were found. Specifically, the NAT2*5 genotype was associated with an increased likelihood of liver injury, highlighting the importance of understanding genetic factors in DILI scenarios. Therefore, recognizing these genetic variations not only aims at improving therapeutic outcomes but also offers strategies for personalized medicine approaches in treatment plans tailored to minimize the risks of liver injury (Tostmann *et al.*, 2014). Also, environmental risks and the use of several drugs can make DILI more likely and make it harder for healthcare providers to manage the case. Polypharmacy is more common in older adults and those with chronic diseases, which can lead to liver injury. Taking several medications at once can result in extra toxicity, which can increase the risk of liver damage. Also, diseases such as liver disease, which are present before treatment, can greatly affect how the liver responds and breaks down drugs. Because DILI is both complex and can vary, having clear rules helps doctors detect and treat it earlier, mainly in groups that are more likely to be affected. Continuing research into the genetic and environmental underpinnings of DILI is vital to developing effective prevention and management strategies, as evidenced by ongoing studies examining the broader implications of drug safety (Cunha *et al.*, 2010) (Figure 14.1).

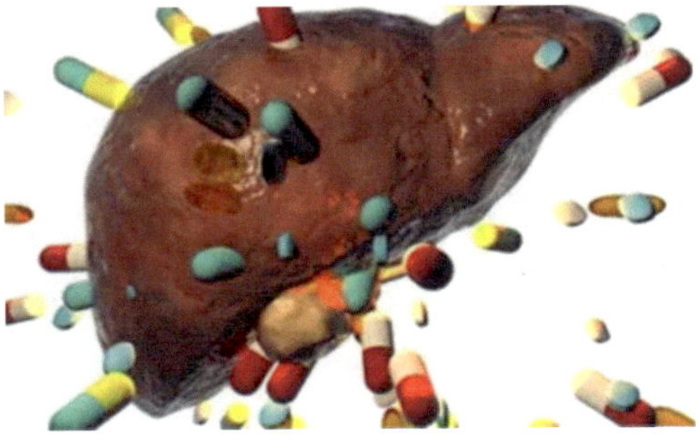

Figure 14.1. Liver Injury

Source: https://www.medtalks.in/faqhomebig/faqSquare-FAQ-_Drug_Induced_Li.jpg.

Importance of Studying DILI

It is significant to learn about DILI since it plays a vital role in public health and drug safety. DILI is held accountable for an appreciable percentage of market withdrawal of drugs and liver failure, which emphasizes the significance of a comprehensive study of this aspect. While formulating drugs, it is essential to take into consideration the risk of liver toxicity in order to limit adverse effects as early as the therapeutics are exposed to the patients. Understanding the mechanisms of DILI not only assures patient safety but also optimizes the overall success rate of drug development. Systematic investigations on structural determinants of DILI risk can provide important insights into how drugs interact at the molecular level and thus facilitate taking appropriately informed decisions while designing drugs. This proactive strategy is essential to the establishment of a culture of safety for healthcare. Furthermore, investigation of DILI has a broad impact on personalized medicine, for which the heterogeneity of drug reaction by individual patients is of utmost importance. Genetic, environmental, and lifestyle factors can exert remarkable influences on the incidence of DILI, and this requires more personalized prescribing regimens. By identifying specific biomarkers or susceptibility markers for liver injury, doctors can provide targeted therapies, thus reducing the possibility of side effects among susceptible populations. The development of machine learning (ML) techniques, as pointed out in recent literature, facilitates the prediction of the risk of DILI from chemical structure, thus enabling the identification of possible liver toxicity early in the process of drug discovery (Amin *et al.*, 2025). Inclusion of these strategies enhances the understanding of patient-related risks, further supporting the idea of personalized therapy in modern medicine. Apart from its use in personalized therapy, the study of DILI is very important for forming regulatory policy towards safeguarding public health. The regulatory agencies require clear evidence of the safety profiles of new drug candidates, as well as their ability to cause liver damage. In the past, the lack of predictive models for DILI has placed significant burdens on regulators and drug developers. Research in the current era targeting DILI not only helps in developing safer drugs but also enhances the regulatory criteria utilized for drug approval. Pre-therapy assessment and the identification of high-risk patients, as suggested in certain research (Maina *et al.*, 2024), emphasize the need to widen our understanding in this area. Improving our understanding of DILI will aid in formulating more efficient guidelines and policies such that new therapies are safe and work effectively for public use (Figure 14.2).

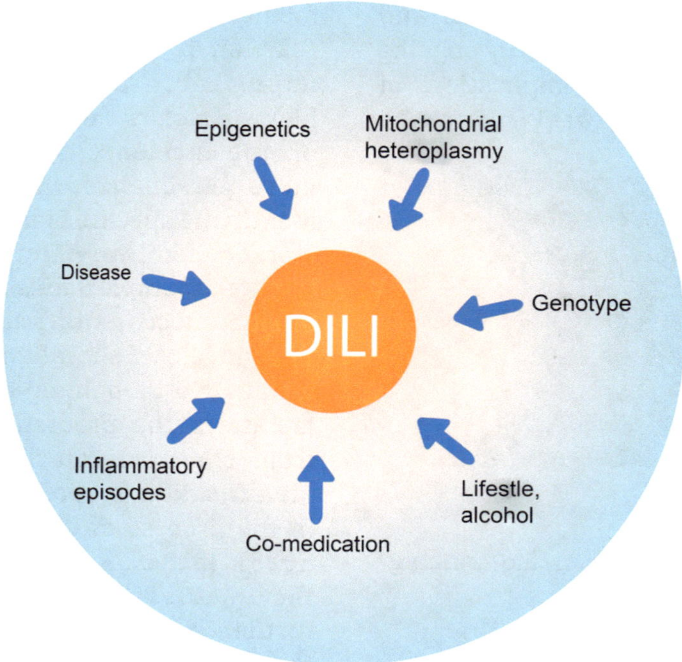

Figure 14.2. Determinants of susceptibility to drug-induced liver injury (DILI) A number of patient-specific (idiosyncratic) factors greatly modulate the sensitivity to the potential hepatotoxic effects of certain drugs.

Source: https://www.researchgate.net/publication/281682691/figure/fig2/AS:11431281276361881@1725629097784/Determinants-of-susceptibility-to-drug-induced-liver-injury-DILI-A-number-of.tif.

14.1. Mechanisms of drug-induced liver injury (DILI)

It is important to understand how DILI happens to spot those who may develop it and create ways to prevent it. DILI can happen via direct liver damage, allergic reactions, or unusual metabolic effects. When hepatocytes are damaged by an agent, it is called direct hepatotoxicity, and these changes are usually caused by the formation of reactive metabolites that cause stress and harm to the cells. For instance, certain herbal and dietary supplements (HDS) have been implicated in DILI, yet they remain largely unregulated, allowing for a greater potential for liver damage due to undetermined hepatotoxic mechanisms. The complexities of DILI mechanisms highlight the need for rigorous research into the safety profiles of HDS usage, as their clinical significance in liver injury increases alongside their popularity in the United States (Chauhan *et al.*, 2022). Certain drugs of abuse, especially when abused, often cause DILI by causing oxidative stress. The pathophysiological role of oxidative stress (OS) illustrates how drugs can lead to hepatocellular damage through the production of reactive oxygen species, which cause lipid peroxidation, protein oxidation, and DNA damage. This pathway has been investigated in relation to cocaine, and it has been demonstrated to cause both heart and liver problems. Research indicates that the modulation of oxidative stress pathways may provide therapeutic avenues for mitigating DILI; however, existing OS inhibitors have yet to demonstrate substantial clinical efficacy (Antonilli *et al.*, 2015). Because OS and drug metabolism are linked, it is difficult to fully understand DILI, which means more research is needed to explore its treatment and how it works. Because both genetic and environmental factors play a role, DILI becomes more complicated since people's differences in metabolism can be significant. Some genetic changes in the genes for drug-metabolizing enzymes can make a person more likely to experience hepatotoxicity from pharmaceuticals. Having alcohol with the medication or having a liver condition can further increase the chance of DILI by reducing blood flow and metabolism in the liver. Besides, some groups might be more sensitive to certain types of drugs because of these interactions. By knowing these mechanisms, clinicians can predict adverse drug reactions and also see why personalized medicine is important. Continued exploration of the multifactorial nature of DILI will enhance our capacity to implement effective preventive measures and therapeutic interventions (Figure 14.3).

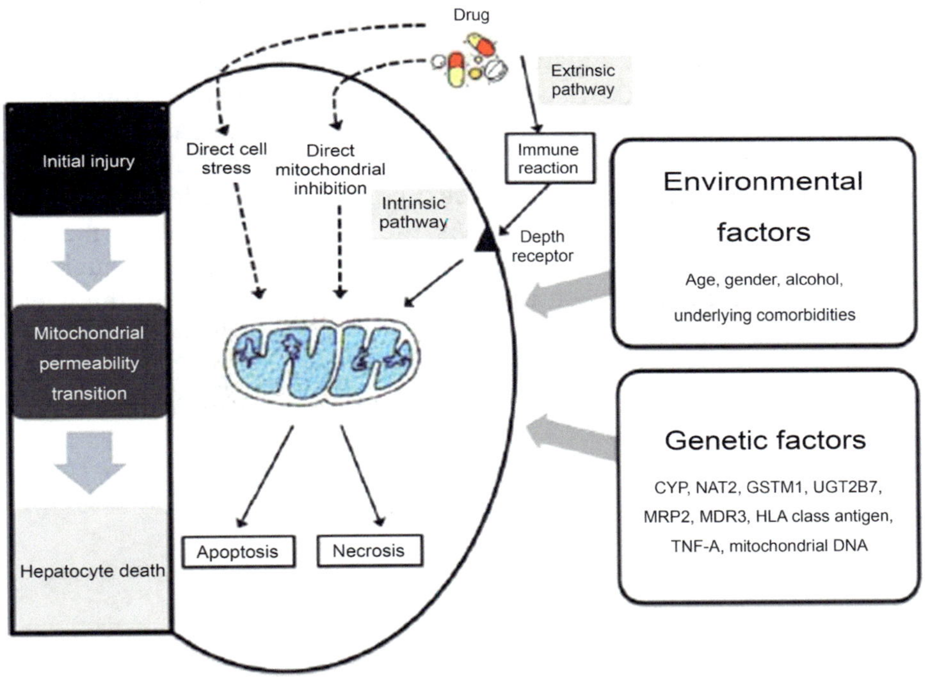

Figure 14.3. Three-step mechanism of drug-induced liver injury.

Source: https://www.researchgate.net/profile/Ki-Tae-Suk-2/publication/262041429/figure/fig2/AS:296917964738565@1447802167773/Three-step-mechanism-of-drug-induced-liver-injury.png.

14.1.1. Metabolic Activation of Drugs

Metabolic activation of the drugs is of utmost significance in the setting of DILI. The liver is responsible for the metabolism of a wide range of xenobiotics, including drugs, through enzymatic pathways involving mainly cytochrome P450 enzymes. While this process of metabolism is crucial for detoxification of the drugs and their excretion, it can also be responsible for the formation of reactive metabolites. These drug metabolites are usually more toxic than the parent drugs, inducing oxidative stress and cell damage that may result in liver injury. The unwanted effects induced by such reactive species vary widely with the chemical structure of the drug, the presence of cofactors, and the susceptibility of the individual based on genetic factors, thus rendering DILI a complex process requiring further exploration. Also, the possibility of such metabolites being hepatotoxic is proof of how it is important to understand the mechanisms of drug metabolism. For example, certain drugs will form metabolites that are covalently bound to cellular macromolecules, and this will disrupt normal cell function and start inflammatory processes. Activation of signaling pathways, such as the nuclear factor erythroid 2-like 2 (NRF2) pathway, may be able to protect against oxidative stress initiated by such reactive metabolites. Activation of NRF2 is the one that causes the cytoprotective gene expression to rise, leading to a decrease in cellular damage evoked by oxidative stress. Indeed, therapeutic impacts of natural agents, such as Sesamol, have been studied regarding their ability to influence these metabolic activities and give hepatoprotection (Mili *et al.*, 2023). The study of pharmacologic interventions with the potential to enhance liver protective mechanisms against DILI is suggested. Research into polyphenols, particularly in green tea, illustrates the possible bimodal activity of these compounds on drug metabolism and liver function. Epigallocatechin gallate (EGCG), a documented polyphenolic compound, has antioxidant and anti-inflammatory properties that enhance the body's resistance to hepatotoxic insult. Studies have indicated that EGCG can influence gut microbiota, with the result that it has broader implications for liver function and overall well-being, and hence a possible avenue for therapeutic intervention against DILI (Winiarska-Mieczan *et al.*, 2024). As the knowledge of drug metabolic activation increases, there is a greater need to consider both the pathologic consequences and also the protective measures that can be implemented in order to avert damage to the liver (Figure 14.4).

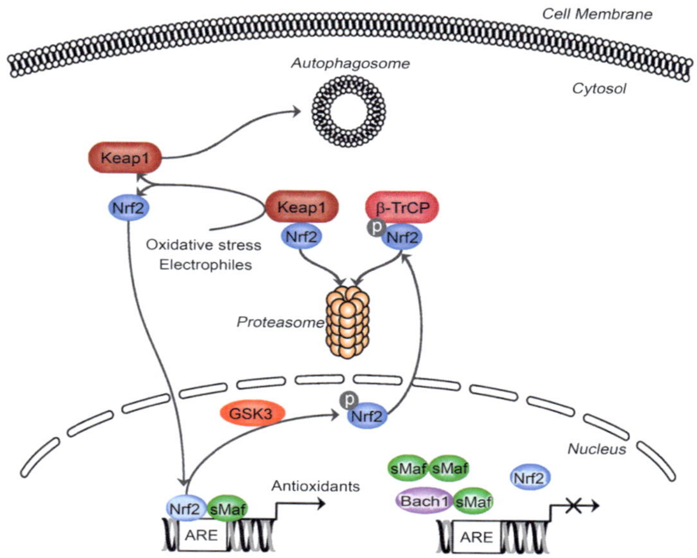

Figure 14.4. Mechanisms of nuclear factor erythroid 2-related factor 2 (Nrf2) regulation.

Source: https://www.researchgate.net/publication/319180604/figure/fig1/AS:114312813331733 98@1743276116148/Mechanisms-of-nuclear-factor-erythroid-2-related-factor-2-Nrf2-regulation-Under-normal.tif.

14.1.2. Immune-Mediated Liver Injury

Among the many causes of DILI, immune-mediated liver damage needs special attention. Such injuries occur when the immune system responds to some medicines, which causes inflammation and may harm liver cells. Immune-mediated reactions can appear without warning and may cause symptoms from slight liver problems to ALF. Usually, the reason for this reaction is that immune cells, mainly T-cells, see the drug-modified liver proteins as foreign and start attacking them. Because of this autoimmune response, liver cells are damaged, and the liver's important functions are changed, which results in complications throughout the body. Appreciating the part played by immune pathways in DILI is vital for learning about how liver damage occurs and for finding better treatments. Oxidative stress and immune system involvement in liver injury add to the difficulties of DILI. Inflammation causes ROS to increase, which can stress cells and result in hepatocellular apoptosis or necrosis. In light of this, controlling antioxidant enzymes is necessary, because they can help prevent harm to liver cells and sometimes even make inflammation worse. The level of oxidative stress in the body seems to affect how much and how fast immune-mediated liver damage develops. Seeing how antioxidants can be both helpful and harmful may lead to better ways to treat liver injury. As a result, we must study the interactions in redox biology that happen in the setting of immune-related liver damage to find new treatments for DILI. Moreover, the progression of immune-mediated liver injury can have dire implications for the development of conditions such as hepatocellular carcinoma (HCC). A long-lasting immune response can lead to chronic inflammation, which supports changes in cells and the formation of tumors. Having cirrhosis or fibrosis, which often develops from long-term liver damage, greatly raises the chance of HCC. Seeing how immune injury and cancer-causing factors affect DILI makes it clear that acting early is important in these cases. Applying therapies that address immune problems and the tumor environment may help patients and lower the number of HCC cases in those with drug-induced liver damage. Addressing these interrelated pathways not only enhances our understanding of DILI but also informs clinical practices and potential treatment paradigms (Figure 14.5).

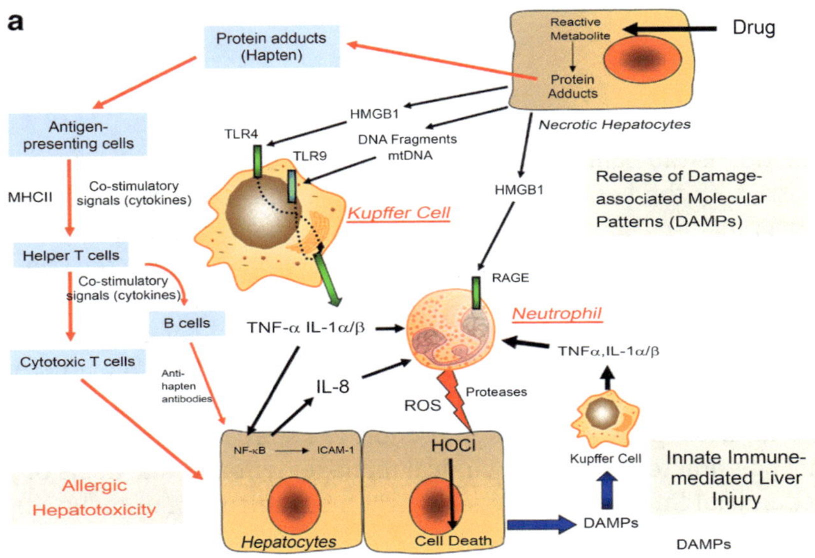

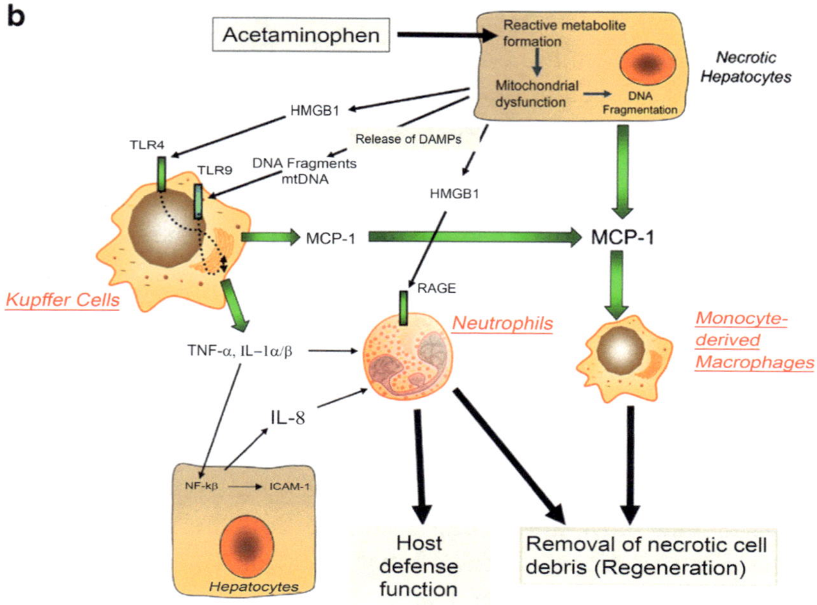

Figure 14.5. Mechanisms of drug-induced liver injury through innate or adaptive immune mechanisms. (a) General scheme of the drug-induced formation of reactive metabolites and protein adducts, which trigger necrosis and initiate a sterile inflammatory response by release of damage-associated molecular patterns (DAMPs), the promotion of cytokine and chemokine formation by activating pattern-recognition receptors, such as toll-like receptors (TLRs), and the consequent activation and recruitment of inflammatory cells, which can aggravate the initial injury (see text for details). (b) Sterile inflammatory response after acetaminophen-induced liver injury.

Source: https://www.researchgate.net/publication/326088179/figure/fig2/AS:963441032454197@1606713650785/Mechanisms-of-drug-induced-liver-injury-through-innate-or-adaptive-immune-mechanisms-a.png.

14.1.3. Mitochondrial Dysfunction

Mitochondrial dysfunction is the hallmark of DILI, as it can lead to energy production impairment and enhanced oxidative stress in the hepatocytes. Mitochondria play a crucial role in the process of ATP synthesis, and their dysfunction can lead to failure of cellular metabolic pathways, resulting in damage to the liver cells. Dysfunction in mitochondria is particularly observed when the liver is challenged with some drugs, which can interfere with mitochondrial function. For instance, it has been observed that exposure to linezolid may result in severe hepatotoxicity, as in a case of a patient who developed liver failure and lactic acidosis following long-term treatment. The establishment of microvesicular steatosis in this case gives weight to the observation that mitochondrial dysfunction is a central characteristic of drug-induced liver injuries' pathophysiology (Benoit *et al.*, 2010). Establishing this link is crucial because it will be in a position to direct both clinical management and diagnosis of patients with DILI. Beyond direct mitochondrial injury, pathophysiological mechanisms of mitochondrial damage have a tendency to conflate with other forms of cellular stress responses, exacerbating the pathophysiological burden of DILI. Oxidative stress is a significant contributor to this because drug perpetrators like cocaine have been directly linked to hepatic toxicity via mechanisms involving augmented oxidative damage. This oxidative stress results from an imbalance between ROS production and the antioxidant defense system at a crucial moment, leading to mitochondrial dysfunction and subsequent hepatocyte apoptosis (Antonilli *et al.*, 2015). When drugs induce oxidative stress, they possess the ability to overwhelm the liver's natural defenses and lead to widespread cellular damage. Understanding of the relationship between oxidative stress and mitochondrial dysfunction is key to deciphering the confusing etiology of DILI, highlighting the need for pharmacologic interventions that minimize oxidative injury to further improve patient outcomes.

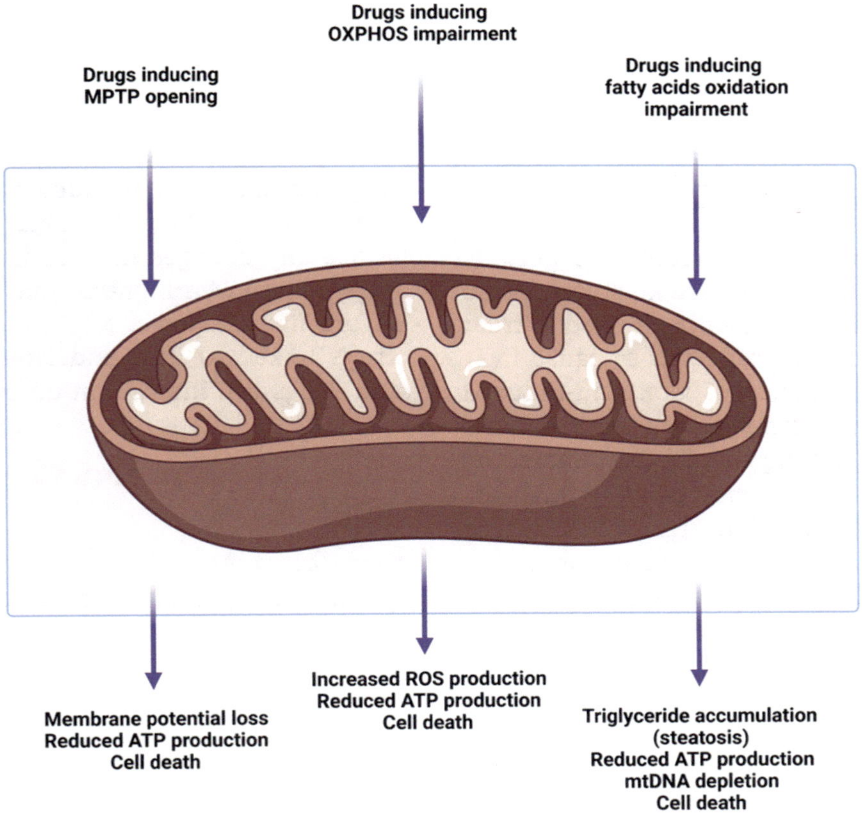

Figure 14.6. Schematic representation of the main mechanisms and consequences of drug-induced mitochondrial dysfunction.

Source: https://www.mdpi.com/ijms/ijms-23-03315/article_deploy/html/images/ijms-23-03315-g003.png.

Furthermore, understanding mitochondrial dysfunction in DILI presents opportunities for the use of new therapeutic strategies aimed at the restoration of mitochondrial function. Strategies to enhance the resilience of mitochondria may be through the use of mitochondrial-targeted antioxidants and oxidative stress modulators. These chemicals under investigation have the potential to prevent mitochondrial dysfunction and, by proxy, reduce liver injury resulting from drug toxicity. For example, agents like N-acetylcysteine (NAC) have been proposed to reverse oxidative stress and protect liver cells from DILI, showing an increasing recognition of the potential to modulate metabolic pathways affected by toxic insult (Antonilli *et al.*, 2015). With continued studies further clarifying the mechanisms of mitochondrial injury in drug exposure, hopefully one will eventually find a more effective and less cumbersome prevention regimen for DILI, ultimately providing greater therapeutic gains in vulnerable patients (Figure 14.6).

14.2. Common Drugs Associated with DILI

DILI is a major problem in medicine, especially because many medications are known to cause liver problems. Isoniazid, which is used to treat tuberculosis, has been reported to cause liver damage. The prevalence of isoniazid-induced liver injury (IILI) stems partly from genetic factors that affect drug metabolism, including polymorphisms in drug-metabolizing enzymes such as NAT2, CYP2E1, and GSTM1. Research has shown that patients with certain genotypes, specifically NAT2*5, exhibit a higher incidence of IILI, underscoring the importance of genetic investigation in predicting susceptibility to DILI (Tostmann *et al.*, 2014). The connection between pharmacogenomics and drug safety points out why personalized medicine methods are important for dealing with the risks of high-alert drugs such as isoniazid. Another class of commonly implicated drugs includes various nonsteroidal anti-inflammatory drugs (NSAIDs), which can also lead to liver injury. Although the use of drugs such as diclofenac and celecoxib has been linked to acute liver dysfunction, the chance of this happening can vary greatly among people. Some of these drugs may cause hypersensitivity or directly harm the liver, and the risk of liver damage usually goes up with higher doses and longer use. Even though the risk of DILI from NSAIDs is usually not high, it can have a major effect on people who already have liver disease. For example, in some groups, taking NSAIDs has been linked to more problems with the liver, which has led to advice to carefully monitor and assess the risks before prescribing these medications. Also, amoxicillin-clavulanate is commonly reported to be involved in DILI cases. Although this combination works against many infections, it has been related to liver harm, mainly in the first two months after starting therapy. The damage to the liver may occur from direct toxicity and also from hypersensitivity reactions, which highlights a bigger issue in the use of medicines. Liver response can also vary because of genetic factors, as is seen with isoniazid. It is very important to check and notice any changes in liver function regularly in patients given high-risk antibiotics to avoid severe liver damage. All in all, the variety of drugs linked to DILI underlines how patients and drugs can interact in different ways.

14.2.1. Over-the-Counter Medications

Over-the-counter (OTC) medicines are common and can be of great relief for a host of conditions, but they typically contain risks that will not be immediately visible to patients. Most individuals lose sight of the risk of adverse effects occurring due to their incorrect use, among which is the risk of DILI. Acetaminophen is a widespread over-the-counter medication that is usually safe if taken as directed. However, overuse or non-perceived interaction with other drugs or supplements can lead to significant hepatotoxicity. The increasing popularity of dietary supplements also raises other issues; a case in point is Garcinia cambogia, an appetite suppressant supplement, which has been associated with fulminant hepatic failure by hydroxycitric acid, pointing towards greater awareness of risks from apparently innocuous over-the-counter medicines (Bodzin *et al.*, 2016). Other than acetaminophen and weight-loss supplements, the OTC marketplace consists of a broad range of nonsteroidal anti-inflammatory drugs (NSAIDs). While useful for their pain-relieving and anti-inflammatory properties, excessive or chronic consumption may result in liver injury. Consumers must know about hepatotoxic potential with such ubiquitous drugs; case series involving DILI often highlight the importance of correct labeling and patient education. Furthermore, the interaction between OTC and prescription medications or other supplements increases these risks. For example, concomitant use of NSAIDs and alcohol will increase the risk of liver damage, illustrating the elaborate interaction between drug-induced causes of liver damage and the requirement for cautious management of medication in the case of DILI. Real-life observations illuminate the consequences of the misuse of OTC drugs when not monitored. For example, treatment with pexidartinib, an FDA-designated breakthrough therapy for some cancers, has been associated with severe DILI necessitating transplantation secondary to vanishing bile duct syndrome (Chien *et al.*, 2019). Such experience serves as a reminder to consumers that even drugs considered less active, such as OTC medications, have inherent dangers—particularly when used with other drugs. The rapidly evolving drug industry poses the necessity of ongoing education about the likely hazards of OTC medications, particularly in the context of their toxicities to the liver. As more consumers use these readily available aids for relief, sensitivity and understanding of the dangers of DILI must be accorded the highest attention so as not to precipitate harmful health outcomes (Figure 14.7).

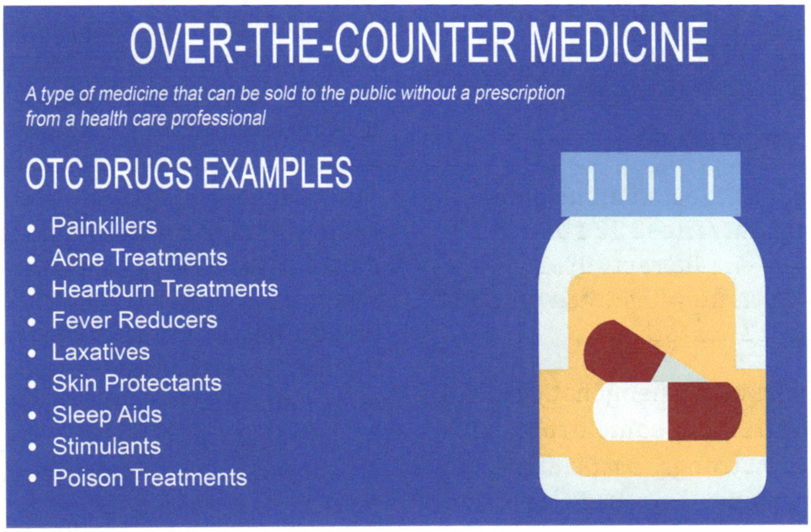

Figure 14.7. Over the counter medicine.

Source: https://www.retaildogma.com/wp-content/uploads/2023/11/over-the-counter-medicine.png.

14.2.2. Prescription Drugs

Prescription drugs are a main part of today's medical care, helping to treat many health problems. Even so, the possibility of causing DILI can be very risky and makes using these drugs more complicated. Some drugs, such as isoniazid, which is commonly used to treat tuberculosis, can harm the liver. Side effects can cause patients to stop taking important medications, which can result in the treatment not working or new strains of pathogens developing. For this reason, healthcare providers need to know how DILI happens so they can consider the risks and benefits of using medications. Studies keep finding new details about how certain genes and the risk of DILI interact for people taking specific drugs. Even though uncommon, some people react differently to drugs, which can lead to serious health problems, proving that personalized medicine is needed.

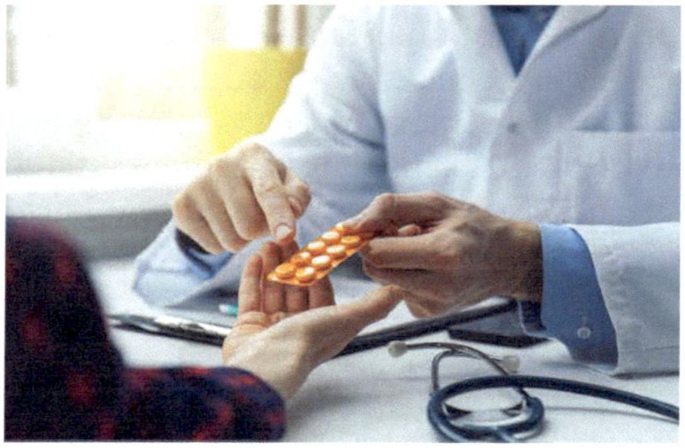

Figure 14.8. Prescription Drugs

Source: https://images.theconversation.com/files/424091/original/file-20210930-20-1owddsq.jpg?ixlib=rb-4.1.0&rect=0%2C0%2C2121%2C1412&q=20&auto=format&w=320&fit=clip&dpr=2&usm=12&cs=strip.

Specific HLA alleles and other genetic factors have been linked to DILI, but some drugs, such as isoniazid, are more strongly associated with genes that affect drug metabolism. Because of this, doctors may be able to use genetic information to guide prescribing, which could help avoid liver damage in at-risk patients and improve the effectiveness of the drugs. In trying to find protectants for DILI, scientists have studied the impact of plant-based therapies. One example is Livogrit Vital, which seems to be a promising option for addressing IILI. Investigations have found that this herbal mixture can boost the protection of liver cells, lower oxidative stress, and control apoptosis. Livogrit Vital works by modulating important molecules in the liver, which decreases the harmful effects of isoniazid and its toxic metabolites. This suggests that combining conventional prescription drugs with complementary herbal treatments could provide a dual benefit, enhancing drug efficacy while simultaneously preserving liver health, thus offering a holistic approach to managing conditions requiring long-term pharmacotherapy (Balkrishna *et al.*, 2024; Daly, 2022) (Figure 14.8).

14.2.3. Herbal Supplements

Widespread use of herbal supplements has created a huge interest in their potential to cause DILI. Many individuals are interested in these plant products in the hope that they are safer than conventional drugs. Data from an ever-growing literature, however, indicate that certain herbal supplements can result in severe hepatic injury. For example, green tea's EGCG, a well-documented dietary supplement, has been shown to have paradoxical effects on liver function. While there are studies demonstrating their protective action against liver damage in states of exposure to toxins, they create DILI when used under states of excessive dosing or co-administration with other hepatotoxins. This dualism underscores the necessity for increased comprehension of herbal supplement-related hepatotoxicity, especially as their safety and efficacy are often inadequately regulated about prescription drugs. Despite the popularity of herbal supplements, identification of their role in DILI is rendered challenging by a lack of uniform regulatory monitoring. Currently, an estimated over 100,000 HDS are available on store shelves and the internet, but their safety is not always adequately established. Consequently, diagnosis of DILI due to such products can be extremely challenging, as signs and symptoms are usually indistinguishable from other hepatobiliary diseases. The large number of herbal supplements makes it hard to isolate clear-cut clinical patterns, and common mechanisms of injury are therefore difficult to determine. Furthermore, studies have shown that despite the fact that most cases of DILI are due to pharmaceutical drugs, herbal supplements are becoming a significant percentage of cases, especially in some parts of the world where traditional medicine is the order of the day. This calls for increased scrutiny of the hepatotoxicity of such products.

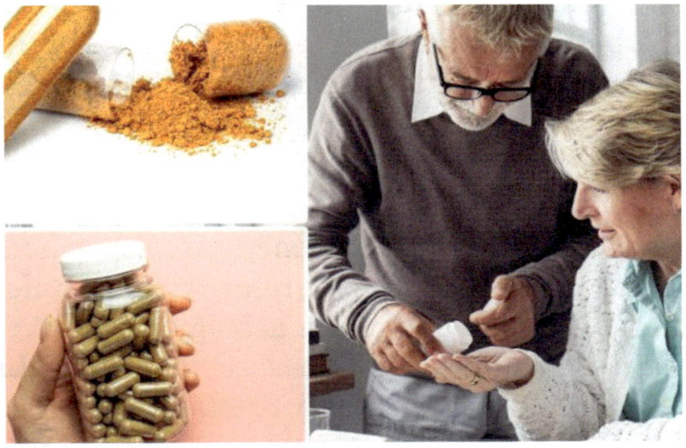

Figure 14.9. Herbal Supplements

Source: https://nypost.com/wp-content/uploads/sites/2/2024/08/senior-adult-taking-pills-medicine-87435332.jpg?quality=75&strip=all&w=1024.

It is critical to elucidate the mechanisms of herbal supplement-induced DILI to guide patient management and regulatory decision-making. It is proven that the liver's metabolic activity is central to this function, as many herbal compounds are intensely metabolized by enzymes present in the liver that possess the capability of generating toxic metabolites. For instance, idiosyncratic herbal responses can occur in a way with no apparent dose-response relationship, adding to the risk assessment complexity. Concurrently, genetic susceptibility of individuals can also affect the incidence and severity of DILI, suggesting heterogeneity of human response to herbal constituents. This information reaffirms the importance of personalized medicine that considers genetic, environmental, and lifestyle determinants in establishing risk. Since health practitioners are presently presented with the dilemma of herbal supplements, the integration of knowledge evolved from continuous research into clinical settings will be paramount to enhancing patient safety in light of DILI (A-Mieczan *et al.*, 2024; Fontana *et al.*, 2022) (Figure 14.9).

14.3. Risk Factors for DILI

It is very important to identify the causes of DILI to develop good prevention strategies and improve how patients are treated. A number of recent studies point out that traditional Chinese medicine is a major factor in DILI. One study showed that 62.5% of DILI cases involved drugs in this category. In addition, three-quarters (84.3%) of patients treated with herbal supplements experienced liver problems, which underlines the importance of being more aware of these treatments. It was found that DILI is more likely to be severe and long-lasting when it involves cholestatic liver injury, which suggests certain drugs can be more dangerous. Additionally, patients' preexisting conditions, such as gallbladder disease, have emerged as independent risk factors, indicating a need for thorough medical histories before initiating treatment with potentially hepatotoxic medications (Wei *et al.*, 2024). DILI is also notable because certain demographic and laboratory factors can influence how severe it is, mainly when related to anti-tuberculosis drugs. In a recent prospective study, various clinical and laboratory factors were examined to determine correlations with moderate to severe anti-tuberculosis drug-induced liver injury (ATB-DILI). Among the identified predictors, malnutrition (HR = 4.564) and low hemoglobin levels (HR = 2.825) significantly increased the risk of developing severe liver injury in the treated population. It shows that providing nutritional support and good care is important for tuberculosis patients on anti-tuberculosis drugs, since health problems may increase their risk of DILI. Multivariate analysis demonstrated that preemptive interventions targeting these factors may reduce the incidence of ATB-DILI, implying that comprehensive patient evaluations are essential (Liu *et al.*, 2024). Laboratory tests can help predict DILI, which is important for risk assessment. Baseline LFTs, especially the first total bilirubin, prothrombin time, and antinuclear antibody titers, can give important clues about the risk of chronic DILI. In clinical assessments, prolonged intervals in the normalization of indicators such as ALP and alanine aminotransferase (ALT) levels serve as valuable prognostic markers for chronic liver injury. They were linked to a higher risk of chronic DILI, and the cutoff points showed when care should be given. Understanding these relationships enables healthcare professionals to implement monitoring protocols that can promote early detection and prevent the progression of liver injury in susceptible populations (Wei *et al.*, 2024) (Figure 14.10).

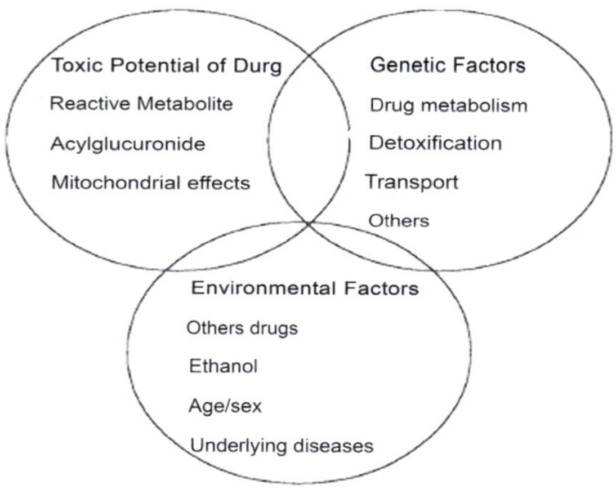

Figure 14.10. Risk factors for susceptibility to DILI.

Source: https://www.researchgate.net/publication/341933323/figure/fig1/AS:899050811449345@1591361825198/Risk-factors-for-susceptibility-to-DILI-16.ppm.

14.3.1. Genetic Predisposition

The genetic predisposition theory is crucial in the development of DILI, in which specific genetic characteristics may alter the reaction to pharmacological agents considerably. Genomic variations, particularly in genes responsible for drug metabolism, may result in susceptibility to drug-induced adverse effects, including hepatotoxicity. Polymorphism of cytochrome P450 enzymes, for instance, impacts the metabolic pathways of various drugs, both efficacy and toxicity. These genetic differences can lead to variations in drug bioactivation or detoxification and thus affect the likelihood of DILI occurrence among vulnerable individuals. Therefore, understanding genetic predispositions is important in demystifying the complex connection between pharmacology and patient profiles. Furthermore, the association of HLA alleles with hypersensitivity reactions is another area of genetic predisposition underlying DILI occurrences. Studies have identified that certain HLA haplotypes, such as HLA-B*1502, have a significant correlation with elevated risks of hypersensitivity syndromes, often manifesting as major cutaneous adverse reactions and also involving DILI features (Cohen *et al.*, 2011). The correlation emphasizes the importance of genetic screening, particularly among ethnically diverse populations in which some alleles occur more frequently. By genetic screening of susceptible patients, doctors can potentially respond by making prescribing changes ahead of time to prevent DILI and other life-threatening adverse effects. The idea of genetic susceptibility can also be extended to immune response interactions with drug-induced hepatotoxicity. Drug reactions by the immune system involve both genetic and environmental influences, such that the causation pathways of DILI are more complex (Andrade-Bellido *et al.*, 2007). For example, genetic determinants may influence the immune response to be one of tolerance or hypersensitivity towards drugs. Such calls for personalized medicine approaches considering individual genetics and also clinical history in the treatment of DILI. Detailed investigations of genetic markers of hepatotoxicity will enhance our capability to predict and prevent DILI and be the basis of optimal therapeutic strategies and patient safety during treatment with drugs.

14.3.2. Pre-Existing Liver Conditions

Having a pre-existing liver problem greatly increases the chances and seriousness of DILI. Patients with conditions such as alcoholic liver disease (ALD), non-alcoholic fatty liver disease (NAFLD), and chronic hepatitis pose unique challenges during pharmacological treatment. Many studies show that people with liver problems are more likely to experience liver damage from certain medicines, which might result in ALF or worsen their chronic liver condition. It is very important to know how these conditions affect the liver, since this knowledge guides the choice of treatment. For this reason, healthcare providers should check liver function before starting treatment to avoid using drugs that might harm the liver and to reduce the risk of adverse effects, mainly for people with existing liver problems. Studies have found that DILI is much more common in patients who already have liver problems. It was found in a study that patients who had liver disease before ICI treatment had a much higher chance of developing DILI. Among patients, those with a history of liver conditions had a higher rate of DILI (30.8%) than those who did not (17.8%). These data points out the need for careful monitoring and proactive actions designed for this group of people. When not observed, DILI can add to the liver's existing problems and make it harder to treat both the original illness and the complications caused by liver damage. Enhanced screening measures and tailored therapeutic interventions are, therefore, essential to address these increased risks related to pre-existing liver conditions (Elsaid *et al.*, 2024). DILI is especially significant in people whose liver is already impaired, such as patients dealing with SARS-CoV-2. There is now evidence that COVID-19 can cause transaminase levels to rise in people with pre-existing liver problems, which can increase the risk of severe outcomes. Because of this connection, healthcare workers are advised to watch for both pre-existing liver problems and liver injury from drugs, especially during the pandemic. Also, the drugs used to treat COVID-19 could cause side effects that are of special concern to people with a history of liver disease. The interaction of these factors necessitates a comprehensive approach focused on exploring safer therapeutic alternatives, such as phytochemicals known for their hepatoprotective properties (Balaji *et al.*, 2024). It points out that we must use combined approaches to keep patients safe and improve the effectiveness of drugs for those at high risk of DILI.

14.3.3. Age and Gender Differences

The interaction of gender and age variation in the presentation and outcome of DILI is a significant issue in clinical practice. It has been observed that certain age groups, particularly the elderly, exhibit enhanced susceptibility to DILI because of age-related biological changes. Liver function diminishes and drug metabolism is impaired with aging, thereby rendering the organ vulnerable to hepatotoxicity. Moreover, comorbidities associated with increasing age tend to necessitate polypharmacy, thereby again further propelling the risk of drug interaction capable of inducing liver injury. Representation of DILI in geriatric patients has been emphasized in studies, which report that the occurrences are not only more frequent but potentially more severe, thus making them even harder to treat and manage. Hence, the nuances of age-related susceptibility are paramount in outlining preventive strategies against DILI. Gender differences also find their way into the focus of the DILI spectrum, consistent with biological and hormonal variations in drug metabolism and toxicity. Epidemiologic evidence suggests that, on average, women are at greater risk for certain types of hepatic injury induced by specific drugs than men. A possible explanation for this gender difference is the action of estrogen, which has been shown to influence drug metabolism. In addition, social and clinical trends such as variations in drug prescription and adherence explain divergent outcomes associated with DILI. Women are also more likely to receive medications that are well-documented to cause liver damage, particularly for interventions in the area of reproductive health care, contributing to their risk exposure (Fu *et al.*, 2020). Hence, gender-drug exposure interaction brings to light the imperative for gender-sensitive interventions for DILI prevention and management. Age and gender variation influence extends beyond susceptibility to liver damage alone and is implicated in clinical outcomes and management. Detection of these variations is important for health professionals who are tasked with preventing the dangers of DILI. Individualized pharmacotherapy approaches considering a patient's gender, age, and overall health profile are essential to effectively tailor pharmacotherapy. Comprehensive assessments and monitoring are particularly significant for female patients and the elderly as they may exhibit different drug reactions and side effects. Additional investigations into biomarkers of age and gender-sensitive DILI reactions also hold promise for earlier recognition and better management approaches (Fu *et al.*, 2020). Through the integration of these factors into clinical practice, patient outcome and safety in the case of DILI can be maximized (Figure 14.11).

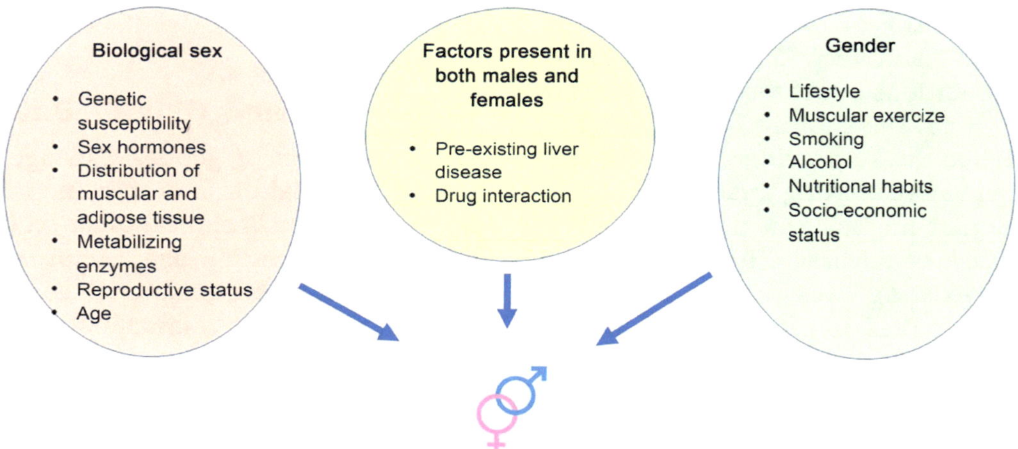

Figure 14.11. Gender and drug-induced liver injury (DILI).

Source: https://www.dldjournalonline.com/cms/10.1016/j.dld.2022.06.025/asset/96ee3523-8d41-4ccd-bc6c-1bdc24d232ad/main.assets/gr1_lrg.jpg.

14.4. Clinical Presentation of Drug-Induced Liver Injury (DILI)

The clinical presentation of Drug-Induced Liver Injury (DILI) is often multifaceted and can vary significantly among individuals. How much the liver is damaged can cause symptoms that vary from being mild to very severe. Some of the usual symptoms are jaundice, feeling tired, nausea and discomfort in the abdomen and these can be confused with other common illnesses. Since

DILI can show many different signs, doctors may not suspect it right away which causes delays in diagnosis. Sometimes, patients show unusual symptoms like fever and back pain which requires doctors to be especially attentive to prevent missing serious illnesses that can occur together with liver injury, for example iliopsoas abscess. Elevated liver enzymes are typically pivotal in diagnosing DILI, revealing hepatic injury through abnormal levels of ALT and aspartate aminotransferase (AST). Along with jaundice which results from elevated bilirubin, these biomarkers help tell DILI apart from other hepatobiliary disorders.

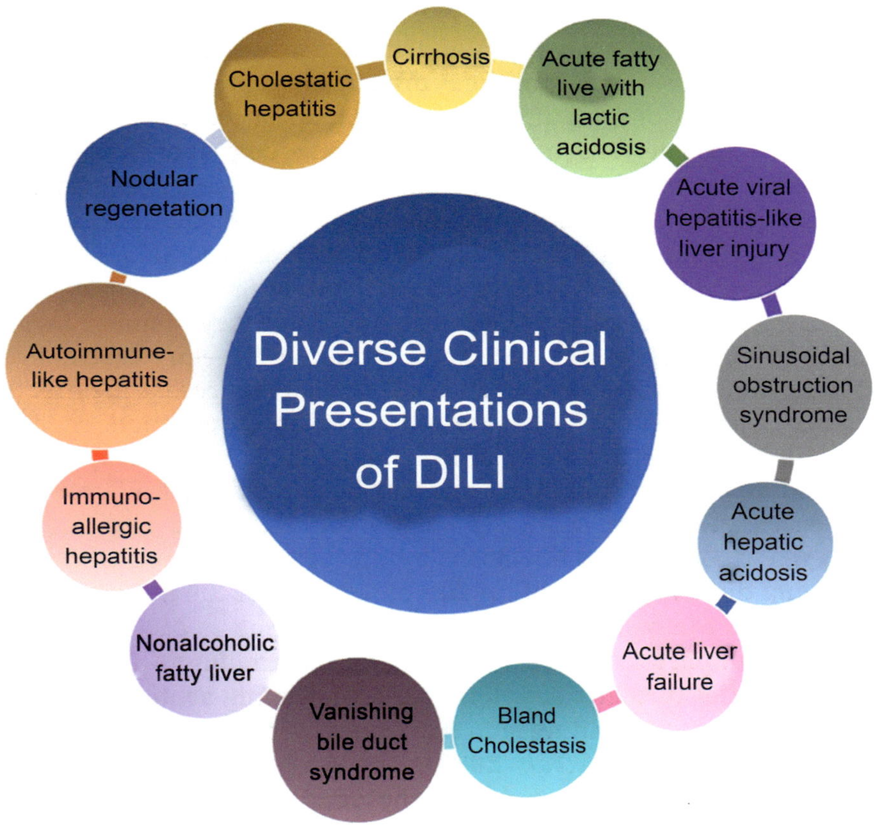
Diverse Clinical Presentations of DILI
Cirrhosis
Acute fatty live with lactic acidosis
Acute viral hepatitis-like liver injury
Sinusoidal obstruction syndrome
Acute hepatic acidosis
Acute liver failure
Bland Cholestasis
Vanishing bile duct syndrome
Nonalcoholic fatty liver
Immuno-allergic hepatitis
Autoimmune-like hepatitis
Nodular regenetation
Cholestatic hepatitis

Figure 14.12. Diverse clinical presentations of DILI.

Source: https://media.springernature.com/lw685/springer-static/image/art%3A10.1186%2Fs43094-025-00788-5/MediaObjects/43094_2025_788_Fig3_HTML.png.

This diagnosis is not simple since symptoms are present in different populations and because it is difficult to determine the causes. The revised Roussel Uclaf Causality Assessment Method (RUCAM) offers a structured approach to quantifying the likelihood of DILI, facilitating more accurate diagnoses. Changes to the system, for example, the RECAM-J 2023 made for Japanese patients, represent efforts to improve how DILI is detected in various medical situations. It is also important for clinicians to understand that some people may have unusual reactions to medications and these reactions might not appear for a long time after the drug is given. Healthcare professionals should check patients' medication histories carefully and carefully watch those at greater risk for DILI.

Those with liver problems, older people and those using several drugs may be more at risk. Since some drugs are more often related to DILI, finding out which ones can help doctors spot and treat the symptoms better. As case reports reveal atypical presentations, such as those highlighting the intricate connection between iliopsoas abscess and DILI, the importance of comprehensive clinical assessments becomes increasingly evident (Figure 14.12).

14.4.1. Symptoms and Signs

Knowledge of the signs and symptoms of DILI is important for early diagnosis and management. Clinically, patients can present with a variety of symptoms, such as fatigue, jaundice, abdominal pain, and unintended weight loss. Such symptoms are usually representative of the liver's impaired ability to carry out basic functions, resulting in the buildup of toxic compounds in the blood. In the majority of cases, the severity of symptoms parallels the degree of liver damage and is highly variable for a given drug. Certain drugs, for instance, will produce acute liver injury that causes symptom development quickly, while others will be the cause of insidious chronic liver dysfunction and therefore milder symptoms until a great deal of damage has accumulated. Therefore, clinicians should be vigilant in observing these symptoms, particularly in those patients receiving known hepatotoxic drugs. Laboratory aberrancies' detection is also a key element involved in the DILI evaluation. Classic LFTs—i.e., serum ALT, AST, and bilirubin levels—are crucial liver inflammation and injury parameters. Elevated levels of ALT and AST typically represent the first laboratory result that appears in cases of DILI, reflecting hepatocellular injury. In addition, changes in ALP levels can also indicate cholestatic injury, a form of DILI that can be induced by several medications. A nuanced understanding of such laboratory markers helps clinicians differentiate between DILI and other liver diseases and hence facilitates early intervention. As also observed with recent studies, some drugs like ribociclib and abemaciclib have been associated with unusual laboratory abnormalities, justifying the importance of regular monitoring of the liver of patients who receive these drugs, as justified in the research conclusions of *et al.*She *et al.* (2024). Patient reports of their symptoms are also important to the successful understanding of DILI. For example, recent literature refers to reports of turmeric supplements precipitating acute liver injury, as evidenced by presentations such as nausea, vomiting, and pain in the abdomen, leading to an acute hepatitis diagnosis in some instances (Smith *et al.*, 2023). The drug heterogeneity contributing to DILI substantiates the multidimensional character of the condition, requiring healthcare providers to conduct detailed evaluation when patients present with hepatic complaints. Along with that, detection of less common symptoms such as ascites or skin rashes will also identify drug-induced liver injury. Thus, recognition of common and uncommon presentations of DILI is essential for clinicians so that proper and timely treatment can be given to patients, resulting in improved outcomes.

14.4.2. Laboratory Findings

Laboratory tests are very important in helping to diagnose and manage DILI. ALT and AST are often used as indicators to show that the liver has been damaged. Although these enzymes may be raised for several reasons, major elevations, as seen in DILI, usually mean there is damage to the liver cells. An increase in alkaline phosphatase may suggest cholestasis, which helps in better diagnosing the patient. The meaning of these enzyme levels should be understood along with the patient's past health, when the drug was taken and any symptoms to tell DILI apart from other liver diseases. So, examining laboratory results carefully helps to confirm the cause and allows for prompt action to stop permanent liver damage. Additional lab tests are used along with transaminase levels to fully assess DILI. The level of total bilirubin can show how much liver function is impaired, since high levels, especially of conjugated bilirubin, may point to cholestatic damage. Furthermore, the presence of an elevated international normalized ratio (INR) signifies hepatic synthetic dysfunction, which can be critical in evaluating the extent of the injury. Spotting these laboratory abnormalities can back up the idea of DILI, but they should be considered carefully, as other conditions might have similar symptoms. Other tests, such as looking for autoantibodies or viral serologies, are important tools that help exclude other possible causes of liver injury. Using all the results from different laboratory tests, clinicians can make a better diagnosis of DILI and choose the best treatment. The complexities of diagnosing DILI are further compounded by the necessity for clear causality assessment, as outlined in established frameworks like the RUCAM (Maev *et al.*, 2023). This method points out that laboratory tests are important for seeing how certain drugs can cause liver damage. DILI is mainly diagnosed by excluding other causes, so laboratory tests are used to confirm liver damage as well as to exclude other causes. Recent advances in biomarker research are promising, aiming to refine diagnostic accuracy and facilitate a personalized medicine approach (García-Cortés *et al.*, 2024). Working together in international research helps to confirm and qualify the effectiveness of new biomarkers, which could lead to better ways to diagnose DILI. Strengthening our understanding of laboratory findings will ultimately lead to improved patient outcomes in those affected by this potentially fatal condition (Figure 14.13).

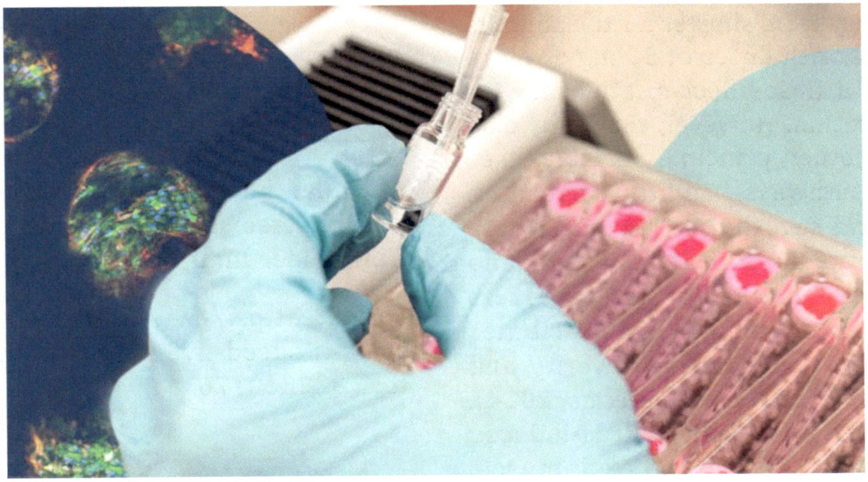

Figure 14.13. Analysis

Source: https://www.genengnews.com/wp-content/uploads/2024/04/CNBioInnovations_1089_gen_dili-featured-image_v1-768x432.jpg.

14.4.3. Severity Classification

Severity classification is relevant in the assessment of DILI since it gives information on clinical outcomes and shapes the course of treatment. All severity classification systems evaluate liver injury in terms of biochemical abnormalities, clinical presentation, and requirement for intervention. Proper classification of severity not only assists clinicians in managing patients but also gives valuable information about prognosis. The heterogeneity of DILI supports the urgency for a systematic approach; demarcating mild, moderate, and severe cases can affect the therapeutic approach taken. For instance, patients with severe DILI can require the offending agent to be immediately discontinued and closer clinical observation than in mild cases. The use of a consistent severity grading system is thus imperative for the improvement of patient outcomes and the harmonization of treatment regimens. Investigations have also highlighted important correlations between certain properties of drugs and the extent of DILI, further underscoring the need for personalized therapy strategies. In a comparison study involving 383 cases of DILI, clinical outcomes were investigated with respect to variables such as daily dose, hepatic metabolism, and the Biopharmaceutics Drug Disposition Classification System (BDDCS). Interestingly, the latency periods before the onset of liver injury were shorter for the patients exposed to drugs with doses of 50 mg or more daily, indicating a dose-effect relationship for severity classification. However, the study also discovered that other principal variables, i.e., the metabolism pathways, had little correlation with recovery and severity of outcome. These results demonstrate the complexity of DILI and highlight the need for healthcare providers to take a variety of medication attributes into account when categorizing severity and choosing interventions (Chalasani *et al.*, 2014). In addition, the idea of severity in drug-induced adverse effects, like statin-induced muscle toxicity, further demonstrates the difficulty inherent in classification systems. Current work in statin-induced myotoxicity has identified the need for making multifaceted phenotypic differentiation to explain the spectrum of toxicity from mild myalgia to rhabdomyolysis. A standardized nomenclature is essential in order to facilitate communication and clinical response for both DILI and other drug-induced damage. Utilizing systematic algorithms to define various phenotypes, healthcare providers can take an informed approach to treating patients with drug-induced side effects. This pharmacological property-patient response interaction is a reminder of the complexity of DILI and the requirement for top-level severity classification systems to enhance patient management (Alfirevic *et al.*, 2014) (Table 14.1).

Table 14.1. Drug-Induced Liver Injury Severity Index

Category	Severity	Descriptions
1	Mild	Elevated ALT/ALP concentration reaching criteria for DILI, but bilirubin concentration < 2× ULN
2	Moderate	Elevated ALT/ALP concentration reaching criteria for DILI and bilirubin concentration ≥ 2× ULN, or symptomatic hepatitis
3	Severe	Elevated ALT/ALP concentration reaching criteria for DILI, bilirubin concentration ≥ 2× ULN and one of the following: International normalised ratio (INR) ≥1.5, ascites and or encephalopathy, disease duration <26 weeks and absence of underlying cirrhosis/other organ failure considered to be due to DILI
4	Fatal/ transplant	Death or liver transplantation due to DILI

ALT, alanine aminotransferase; ALP, alkaline phosphatase; DILI, druginduced liver injury; ULN, upper limit of normal.

Source: https://www.researchgate.net/figure/Drug-induced-liver-injury-severity-index-14_tbl1_322360776.

14.5. Diagnosis of DILI

It is very hard to diagnose DILI in clinical practice, mainly because there are no specific signs or tests that can confirm it. DILI is hard to understand because its symptoms can be similar to those of other liver diseases, which means doctors must use a detailed approach, including the patient's medical records, drugs taken, and tests that rule out other conditions. Health professionals should look at both a patient's medication history and laboratory results to identify if DILI is the cause of liver problems. The RUCAM and similar approaches help doctors assess the chance that a drug has damaged the liver. Recent advancements, including the revised RUCAM and the Electronic Causality Assessment Method (RECAM), further enhance diagnostic precision but still necessitate validation through ongoing research (García-Cortés *et al.*, 2024). The main way to diagnose DILI now is by checking standard blood markers, which usually only appear when liver damage is advanced. Because of this, researchers and doctors are looking for new ways to find liver damage early and with more accuracy. New technologies, for example, persistent luminescent nanoprobes, are suggesting that they could greatly transform how diseases are detected. With these nanoprobes, which are attached to single-stranded DNA and used to find raised hydrogen peroxide levels in the body, it is possible to see liver damage as it happens. Preclinical findings suggest that this approach can yield results significantly faster than conventional serum-based methods, demonstrating a signal-to-noise ratio of 20.9 and highlighting the promise of this high-sensitivity technique for early diagnosis (Zhang *et al.*, 2024). Such technologies might help detect DILI earlier, before major symptoms are seen. It is very important to understand the ways in which DILI is diagnosed to prevent problems with drug therapy. Using both clinical assessment and advanced diagnostic methods helps doctors handle DILI in patients more effectively. Also, such networks between countries help in understanding DILIs and advance the development of personalized medicine. Since healthcare is now focused on personalized treatments, finding reliable ways to diagnose is very important. Regular research helps create better methods for diagnosing DILI, which in turn can lead to better patient outcomes. By bridging existing gaps in current medical practice, the evolution of DILI diagnosis holds the potential to significantly influence clinical pathways and therapeutic strategies in the management of drug-related liver injury (García-Cortés *et al.*, 2024).

14.5.1. Clinical Assessment

Clinical assessment of DILI is a critical process involving thorough assessment of patient history, clinical presentation, and biochemical indicators of liver function. Clinical assessment is particularly challenging in patients with underlying liver disorders such as nonalcoholic fatty liver disease (NAFLD) or nonalcoholic steatohepatitis (NASH). Patients with these conditions can have elevated liver enzymes, so altered thresholds for the diagnosis of DILI would be required. Recent evidence indicates that the practice of assessing DILI in NASH patients needs to involve best practice for detection and management and the use of monitoring liver tests, along with the application of standardized hepatic inclusion and exclusion criteria in clinical trials (Adams *et al.*, 2019). Through the application of patient-specific clinical evaluation, medical practitioners will be able to diagnose and treat better cases of DILI and ultimately offer improved outcomes to the patient while contributing to safer drug development processes. The essential component of the clinical assessment is the application of causality evaluation methods to determine the relationship between newly prescribed drugs and hepatotoxicity. This involves careful analysis of temporal associations, patient history, and current medication, and consideration of potential confounding factors of age, sex, and baseline disease. Individual drugs, like atorvastatin and simvastatin, have shown differential hepatotoxicity profiles that need careful comparative scrutiny (Clarke *et al.*, 2016). Elucidation of the differences in terms of liver enzyme monitoring and biochemical markers can guide clinicians in making rational choices in relation to the continuation or adjustment of treatment. Successful clinical assessment thus relies on the integration of various data sources and clinical signals, which aids in the differentiation of drug-induced liver injury from other liver ailments. Moreover, the implementation of systematic criteria for monitoring LFTs is part of clinical assessment in the case of DILI. Regular monitoring of biochemical markers like ALT, AST, and ALP helps identify early alterations that may indicate looming liver damage. Active monitoring in patients undergoing therapy using drugs known to be hepatotoxic lowers the risk of serious events. In addition, clinical assessment also has to consider the impact of dosage and treatment duration on liver function, as some drugs can be more hepatotoxic under some conditions. Being well-established with monitoring protocols, particularly in risk categories like those with pre-existing liver disease, can form part of drug intervention safety during clinical assessment of DILI (Adams *et al.*, 2019).

14.5.2. Liver Function Tests (LFTs)

Assessing DILI relies on LFTs, which give important information about the condition and function of the liver. Most of these tests check enzymes, proteins, and substances made or handled by the liver, for example, ALT, AST, ALP, and bilirubin. If these markers are higher than normal, it could show that the liver is being harmed by some medications. LFT results help find liver injury and also reveal whether it is hepatocellular, cholestatic, or a combination of both. Because hepatotoxic drugs can cause different liver problems, linking the test results to the patient's history and symptoms is necessary for proper treatment, which shows why LFTs are important in managing DILI. In clinical trials, especially those involving patients with pre-existing conditions such as nonalcoholic fatty liver disease (NAFLD) and nonalcoholic steatohepatitis (NASH), the assessment of LFTs becomes even more complex. Even without taking any drugs, patients with NASH may experience changes in liver enzymes, so their tests must be monitored and reviewed specially. There are not enough specific rules for understanding LFTs in this patient group, which means it is important to standardize practices to improve patient safety and the effectiveness of drugs. Recent publications have attempted to establish best practices for the detection and management of suspected DILI in patients with NASH, further emphasizing the need for clinicians to be familiar with the nuances of interpreting LFTs within this context (Adams *et al.*, 2019). Using new assessment tools for liver injury, such as eDISH, is a major step forward in understanding DILI. This program helps to see the changes in serum ALT and total bilirubin over time, which reflects how the liver is working. It enables doctors to spot significant liver lesions, and if these are ignored, they can have serious outcomes. Notably, the FDA has reported that, since the adoption of these comprehensive assessment strategies, there have been no drug withdrawals due to post-marketing hepatotoxicity, indicating a potential improvement in drug safety profiles (Senior, 2014). Thus, as DILI continues to be a prominent concern in pharmacotherapy, the critical interpretation of LFTs and the integration of advanced monitoring methods will remain essential in clinical practice, guiding clinicians in managing and mitigating risks related to liver injury (Figure 14.14).

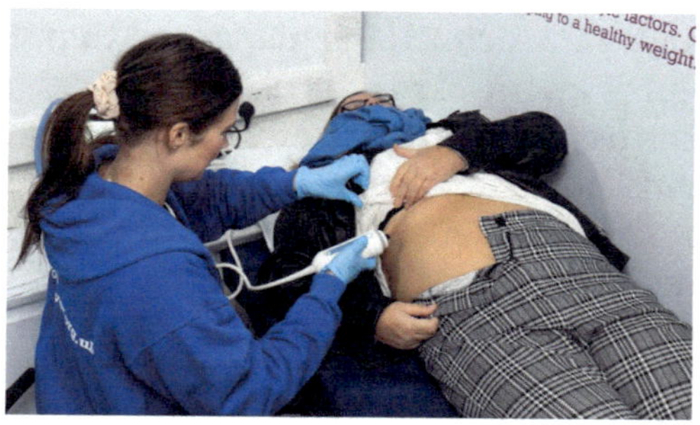

Figure 14.14. Liver Function Tests

Source: https://17xpvwx1p0y4h.cdn.shift8web.com/wp-content/uploads/LYL-corporate-Fibroscan.jpg.

14.5.3. Histological Evaluation

Histological analysis is significant in the diagnosis of DILI because it tells us about the cellular pathophysiology and patterns of injury involved in the condition. With LBx, tissue architecture can be assessed, and particular histopathological features that are associated with the clinician's presentation can be identified. These consist of such alterations as hepatocyte necrosis, portal inflammation, and cholestasis, each of which might be linked with a variant cause of liver damage. For instance, studies have shown that hepatocellular-injury-type DILI is typical for spotty or focal histological features of necrosis, while cholestatic type is marked by ductular reactions (Kawano *et al.*, 2024). The ability to classify these histopathological patterns allows clinicians to distinguish DILI from other liver disorders, thus influencing management and therapeutic interventions. Histological pattern assessment in DILI is paramount given the lack of definitive diagnostic markers. In suspected DILI, LBx is a valuable diagnostic tool that provides essential information with the potential to guide treatment (Venkataswamy *et al.*, 2024). Cholestatic hepatitis was found to be the most common histopathologic feature in patients with DILI by retrospective analysis and emphasized presentation variability and the commonality of herbal and traditional drugs as the cause. Furthermore, such features as eosinophilic infiltration and inflammatory portal tracts were found in a large proportion of cases and may offer clues to DILI diagnosis. By comparing these histological findings with clinical histories and biochemical tests, pathologists can significantly assist in the attainment of accurate diagnoses and best patient outcomes. Finally, a histological study aids in clarifying the prognosis of various types of DILI. For example, Kaplan–Meier analysis demonstrated that patients with hepatocellular-injury-type DILI are likely to demonstrate better overall survival compared to cholestatic injury types (Kawano *et al.*, 2024). This not only reinforces the necessity of histological findings in diagnosis but also in patient management. In addition, histological findings can also determine present risk factors such as lymphocyte count and ALP levels associated with a specific form of liver damage. It is along this line that an adequate conceptualization of histopathological patterns helps clinicians in formulating their treatment approach and improving prognosis in DILI patients.

14.6. Management and Treatment of DILI

Due to the complexity and variety of DILI, its management and treatment can be complicated. As soon as the condition is diagnosed, stopping the offending agent is very important, since continued exposure can worsen liver damage. In the clinic, doctors review a patient's medical history to find out if any drugs they are taking might be harmful to the liver. LFTs are needed to check levels of AST and ALT, which reflect damage to the liver. Sometimes, severe cases require hospitalization, since being closely watched and supported in a hospital can help reduce risks. Depending on the degree and reason for DILI, the therapy may change a lot, so doctors use personalized methods to help patients recover and avoid lasting liver issues. In some cases of DILI, medicines can be used to help lessen liver damage after the offending drug is stopped. As an illustration, using NAC has become important in treating liver damage caused by acetaminophen by increasing glutathione and helping the body get rid of toxins. Furthermore, studies indicate that alternative herbal treatments, like the ethanolic extract of *Amaranthus spinosus*, can exhibit hepatoprotective properties through antioxidant and anti-inflammatory effects, as demonstrated in various model systems, including rodent studies where significant biochemical improvements were noted after treatment with the extract (Yusuff *et al.*, 2025). Even so, these alternative strategies point to the possible use of additional therapies in DILI, but proper research is still needed to verify their safety and effectiveness in people. In chronic DILI cases, especially in areas of India where multiple health problems are common, the way treatment is handled needs more attention. Chronic cholestatic liver diseases (CCLD) frequently intersect with DILI, as seen in patients affected by cholestasis from hepatitis or other infectious agents. Establishing a comprehensive management framework is crucial, emphasizing regular non-invasive assessments of liver fibrosis alongside pharmacotherapy, such as UDCA for conditions like primary biliary cholangitis (Mukewar, 2025). Even though there are not many treatments for cholestatic liver diseases, new approaches that target gut microbes and bile acid production suggest new ways to control both cholestatic and DILI conditions. Thus, ongoing research and a multidisciplinary approach are vital for developing targeted interventions to enhance patient outcomes in DILI management (Figure 14.15).

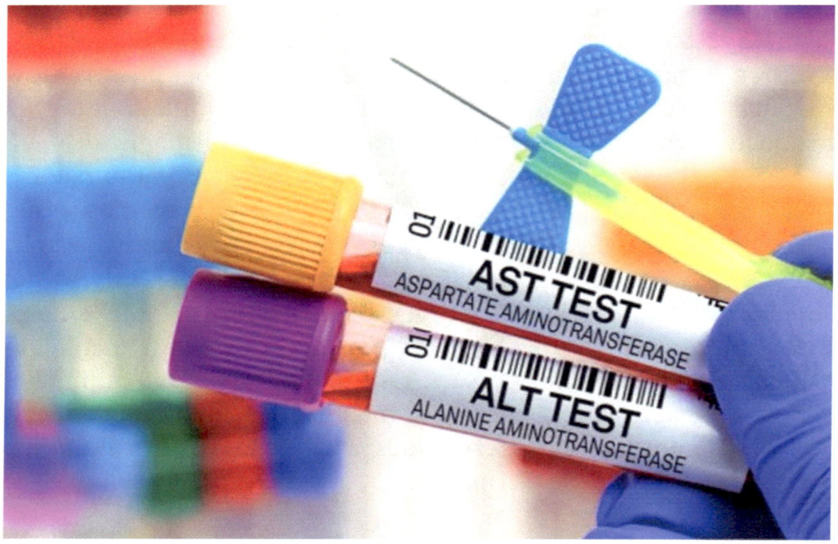

Figure 14.15. Aspartate aminotransferase (AST) test.

Source: https://facty.mblycdn.com/fh/resized/2022/05/730x487/GettyImages-1382922268.jpg.

14.6.1. Discontinuation of the Offending Drug

Discontinuation of the causative drug is a crucial intervention in DILI treatment. Because of the heterogeneity of DILI manifestations, ranging from asymptomatic elevations in transaminases to cases causing ALF, identification of the offending drug and its discontinuation becomes absolutely essential at the earliest. Clinicians are known to classify DILI based on the nature of injury—hepatocellular, cholestatic, or mixed—using the ratio of serum ALT and ALP as investigative markers. The spectrum of liver injury requires an individualized management plan, where the first step is the immediate discontinuation of the drug to avert further hepatotoxicity (Kozielewicz *et al.*, 2025). This action is essential because long-term exposure to the offending drug can exacerbate liver injury, making the patient's clinical picture more complicated and potentially causing irreversible damage. The effectiveness of the discontinuation strategy in DILI heavily rests upon the accurate determination of the offending drug. While most cases reveal recovery upon withdrawal, clinical outcomes also rely on certain factors such as the patient's health status, pharmacokinetics of the drug, and genetic factors of susceptibility to the liver (Roy *et al.*, 2024). Furthermore, certain classes of drugs, including antibiotics, have also been shown to be involved more frequently, highlighting a need for precaution from health practitioners when prescribing these drugs. Early recognition of evidence of systemic hypersensitivity may also direct the withdrawal procedure, as such presentations may complicate the clinical presentation and simulate other liver conditions. Withdrawal, thus, not only averts additional damage but also allows for a more accurate assessment of the condition and the potential path to recovery of the patients. Withdrawal of the offending drug is imperative in the course of DILI treatment, but supportive therapy also plays a vital role in facilitating recovery. Although final antidotes for DILI are scarce, symptomatic treatment may include therapeutic measures in the form of glucocorticosteroids and UDCA in severe conditions where inflammation and biliary dysmorphism are present (Kozielewicz *et al.*, 2025). Liver transplantation may ultimately be considered in ALF resulting from DILI. Follow-up regarding liver function post-withdrawal is essential in measuring the efficacy of the intervention and guiding follow-up treatment. Moreover, education about potential hepatotoxic agents must be emphasized in a manner that highlights the significance of informed choice in prescribing patterns, along with patient education to prevent recurrence of DILI. Therefore, de-escalation of the offending drug is a crucial initial step towards multi-pronged management of DILI.

14.6.2. Supportive Care and Monitoring

To deal with DILI, supportive care and monitoring are very important, mainly to prevent the harmful effects of hepatotoxic drugs. Upon suspicion of DILI, it is imperative to promptly discontinue the offending medication, which is supported by evidence showing that early intervention significantly improves patient outcomes (Pradhan *et al.*, 2025). After the drug is stopped, it is necessary to keep monitoring LFTs to see if the liver injury is getting better or worse. This approach not only allows healthcare providers to assess the effectiveness of supportive care interventions but also helps in determining the appropriate timeline for potential reintroduction of the antitubercular therapy, especially in cases of anti-TB DILI, as indicated in studies involving tuberculosis patients (Ozturk *et al.*, 2024). Supporting the patient with hydration, nutrition, and managing their symptoms speeds up recovery and lowers the chance of more problems. In the context of anti-TB treatment, the implementation of supportive care becomes even more significant as patients present with various symptoms such as nausea, vomiting, and anorexia, which can exacerbate liver injury (Pradhan *et al.*, 2025). Using diet to support nutrition can strengthen patients and help them recover. Therefore, because DILI patients have special symptoms, careful monitoring plans are needed to detect any worsening of liver function quickly. It includes both medical and psychosocial care, so that all the needs of the patients are met. A multidisciplinary approach improves the success of treatment because it enables healthcare professionals to work together and provide patients with the best possible care. In addition, teaching patients about their condition is very important during the monitoring stage of DILI. Telling patients about the symptoms of liver dysfunction allows them to get medical help when needed. Encouraging vigilance in observing symptoms such as jaundice or increasing abdominal discomfort can lead to early detection of recurrence or worsening of liver injury (Ozturk *et al.*, 2024). Also, explaining ways to modify lifestyle and why keeping follow-up appointments is important helps people take charge of their liver health. When people have to take many medications at once, these initiatives become very important, since knowing about drug interactions can help prevent DILI. Collectively, effective supportive care and monitoring not only prioritize patient safety but also enhance the overall efficacy of therapeutic interventions (Figure 14.16).

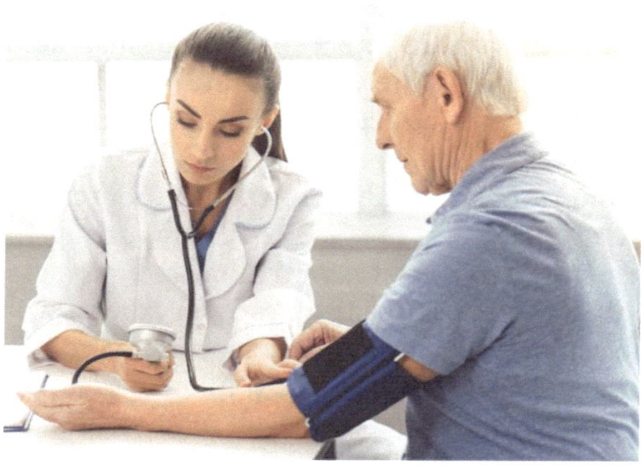

Figure 14.16. Discontinuation of the Offending Drug

Source: https://clincasequest.hospital/wp-content/uploads/sites/7/2023/12/doctor-medical-coat-is-testing-patient-blood-pressure-768x567.jpg.

14.6.3. Potential Use of Corticosteroids

The potential use of corticosteroids in the treatment of DILI has gained interest as clinicians seek promising therapeutic interventions. Corticosteroids have anti-inflammatory and immunosuppressive actions, which prove beneficial in cases of drug reaction-induced liver injury. The pathogenesis of DILI is usually linked with immune-mediated liver cell damage, and corticosteroids may arrest this inflammatory process. While empirical evidence supporting their utility in DILI keeps unfolding, some studies indicate favorable outcomes in patients with autoimmune-like symptoms or severe liver injury. This warrants further study on the timing, dosing, and formulation of the best corticosteroids to enhance therapeutic benefits and prevent potential side effects of steroid therapy. Recent research has suggested that the combination of corticosteroids with other protective substances may enhance their therapeutic effectiveness for treating DILI. For instance, polyphenolic substances such as EGCG have shown potential in promoting liver health through their antioxidant properties, potentially complementing corticosteroid treatment. Studies have established that modulation of gut microbiota by EGCGs may also help preserve liver function and suppress inflammation. Aside from corticosteroids, these drugs can also be included in a multidimensional treatment plan in order to reverse the effect of drug-induced liver injury. Scopoletin and other agents have also shown hepatoprotective activities in preclinical models, highlighting the importance of considering various pharmacological options. With ongoing research developments, the combination of corticosteroids with other drugs with hepatoprotective properties may reveal even more effective treatment of DILI. Despite the seeming advantages of corticosteroids for the treatment of DILI, judicious weighing of their risk is imperative. Corticosteroids are likely to introduce considerable side effects, particularly in those with pre-existing liver conditions or receiving hepatotoxic medications. Furthermore, induction of immunosuppression is a cause for concern regarding heightened infection and complication susceptibility. The emerging evidence addresses the need to stratify patients by their risk profiles before starting corticosteroid treatment. Regular measurement of LFTs is also important during treatment to assess therapeutic efficacy and prevent exacerbation of liver injury. Overall, while corticosteroids may be a valuable option to combat DILI, the development of effective guidelines with robust clinical evidence will play a vital role in standardizing their use in practice as well as ensuring patient safety (Sharma *et al.*, 2023; Winiarska-Mieczan *et al.*, 2024) (Figure 14.17).

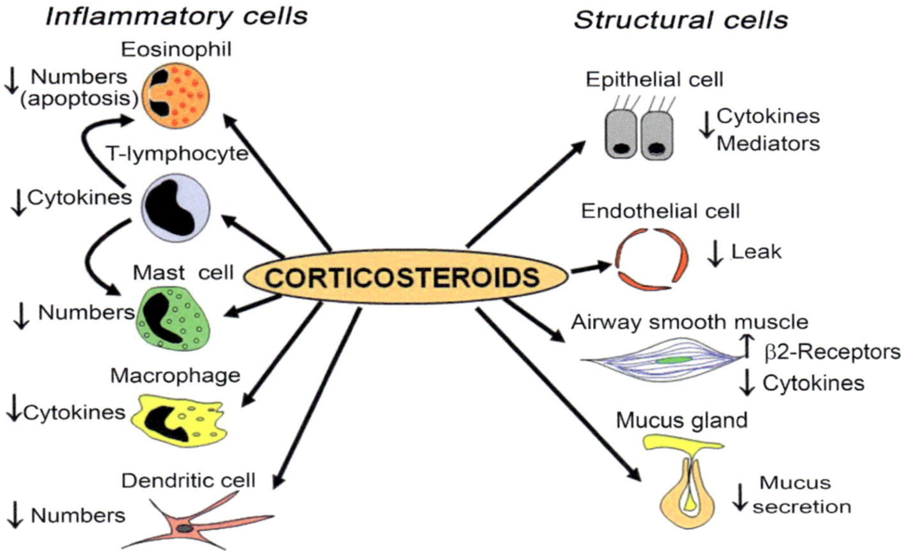

Figure 14.17. Corticosteroids.

Source: https://www.mdpi.com/pharmaceuticals/pharmaceuticals-03-00514/article_deploy/html/images/pharmaceuticals-03-00514-g001.png.

SUMMARY

DILI is a serious issue in the pharmaceutical sector that compromises the safety of patients and complicates the process of developing drugs. Because it is a multifaceted condition with various clinical manifestations, establishing the mechanisms responsible for DILI is essential in the development of effective preventive and curative interventions. Current advances in machine learning (ML) techniques, as witnessed with Amin *et al.* (2025), underscore the potential of computational models to identify structural determinants accountable for hepatotoxicity. These models assist in identifying DILI risk at the early stage, which is indispensable in making sound decisions during drug discovery. Emerging strategies must address coordination between researchers, clinicians, and regulatory bodies for enhancing DILI prediction potential and nurturing a culture conducive to DILI-safe drug development. The second distinguishing characteristic of DILI is the heterogeneity of factors that lead to its formation in different populations. Observations in distinct patient populations, such as children receiving chemotherapy for acute lymphoblastic leukemia, yield unique DILI predictors like BMI and vitamin D levels, as evidenced by Bai *et al.* (2024). Awareness of these independent predictors may not only enable risk stratification but also underscore the importance of individualized monitoring protocols. By clarifying the parameters of DILI, clinicians can apply proactive interventions that reduce risk, ultimately enhancing patient outcomes. Thorough education and training for healthcare providers on DILI is similarly important in facilitating timely recognition and management of this multifaceted condition. The implications of DILI are not limited to individual patient outcomes; they include public health concerns and pharmaceutical development as well. Addressing this phenomenon requires a multi-disciplinary answer that balances technological innovation, clinical expertise, and regulatory frameworks. The ongoing exploration of the chemical space to DILI, as mentioned in Amin *et al.* (2025), is a shining example of an informed effort toward achieving a diminution of the economic burden and health consequences of hepatotoxic medicines. Through encouraging collaborative research that enables the sharing of results and strategies between varied stakeholders, the scientific and medical communities will contribute to the creation of safer therapeutic drugs. Ultimately, a strategic plan for DILI research and management will not only protect patients but also create innovation for the pharmaceutical sector.

The multifactorial etiology of DILI continues to pose significant challenges in the fields of clinical medicine and pharmacology. Lack of predictability of DILI, as well as its capacity to manifest differently in different individuals, are some of the core issues of contention. Such unpredictability has complicated the diagnosis and management of patients. Recent research, however, showed that advancements in ML models are capable of simplifying this challenge. As an example, the development of pDILI_v1, which is a web application developed using an open-source, Python-based code, demonstrates how computational technologies can be employed to predict DILI risks systematically from chemical structures. This work not only enhances the number of DILI risk assessments available to researchers and practitioners but also emphasizes the importance of integrating computational methods into drug safety evaluations, ultimately aiming to develop safer drug compounds that lower hepatotoxic risks (Amin *et al.*, 2025). Apart from applying sophisticated computational models, the separation between idiosyncratic DILI and autoimmune hepatitis (AIH) is still a real concern among health professionals. A recent multicenter cohort study used a ML-based model called BJ-AID, which was capable of separating these two diseases based on the most crucial laboratory parameters. Having a high area under the receiver operating characteristic curve (AUROC), the BJ-AID model displays not only outstanding performance in typical cases but also in atypical ones, thereby facilitating better clinical decision-making. These innovations underscore the necessity for advanced diagnostic equipment, which enables hepatologists to provide more discerning treatment schemes to patients with ambiguous hepatic injury profiles (Wang *et al.*, 2025). Moreover, the introduction of predictive models grounded on ML into clinical practice brings an aspect of intelligence into DILI risk evaluation. Traditional methods are likely to make conclusions dependent on retrospective information and personal considerations, and in so doing, they are likely to omit critical information hidden within patients' profiles. However, with the creation of models like pDILI_v1 and BJ-AID, the field advances in leveraging big data and sophisticated algorithms to inform decision-making. This advancement not only has the promise to reduce incidences of DILI rates throughout drug development but also aims to optimize patient safety via early intervention and detection. Hence, investing in such advanced technologies is essential as they help medical professionals effectively cope with the complexities of DILI and improve overall liver health outcomes (Amin *et al.*, 2025; Wang *et al.*, 2025).

CLOSER LOOK

ASPARTATE AMINOTRANSFERASE

AST also known as SGOT, is an enzyme primarily found in the liver, but also present in heart, muscle, and kidney tissues. A blood test measuring AST levels is often used to assess liver health and can indicate liver damage or disease. High AST levels in the blood may suggest liver problems, though they can also be elevated due to other conditions or factors (Figure 14.18).

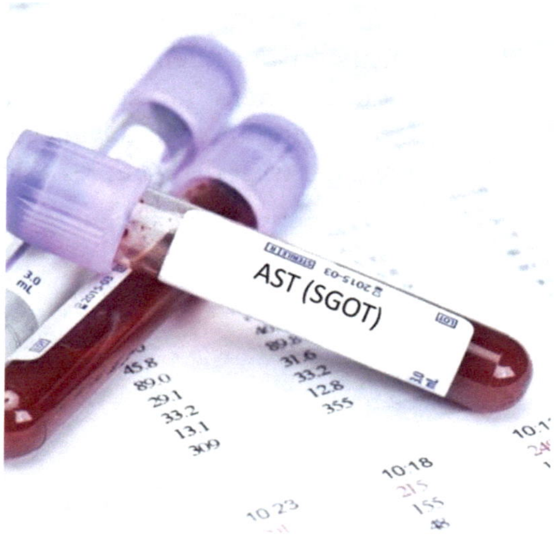

Figure 14.18. AST

Source: https://medical.thearcgroup.co.uk/wp-content/uploads/2024/12/AST-test.jpg.

Function:

- AST is an enzyme that plays a role in the metabolism of amino acids.
- It catalyzes the transfer of an amino group from aspartate to another molecule.

Role in Liver Function:

- AST is primarily found in the liver, but it can also be found in the heart, skeletal muscle, and kidneys.
- When liver cells are damaged, AST can leak into the bloodstream, leading to elevated levels.
- Elevated AST levels are often a sign of liver disease or damage.

AST Blood Test:

- An AST blood test measures the level of AST enzyme in the blood.

- It is commonly used to help diagnose and monitor liver conditions.
- The test is often included in a liver function panel or a comprehensive metabolic panel.

Normal Range:

- The normal range for AST levels can vary slightly between laboratories, but it's generally around 8 to 33 U/L.

Factors Affecting AST Levels:

- **Liver Disease:** Hepatitis, cirrhosis, and other liver conditions can cause elevated AST levels.
- **Muscle Damage**: Severe muscle injuries can also increase AST levels.
- **Heart Problems:** Heart attacks or HF can lead to elevated AST.
- **Medications:** Certain medications, including statins and some antibiotics, can affect AST levels.
- **Other Conditions:** Kidney or lung damage, mononucleosis, and some cancers can also cause increased AST.

Interpretation of Results:

While elevated AST levels may suggest liver problems, they don't always indicate serious issues.

A healthcare provider will consider other factors and test results to determine the cause of increased AST levels. It is important to discuss test results with a healthcare provider to understand their meaning and next steps.

References

1. Adams, L. A., Aithal, G. P., Andrade, R. J., Angulo, P., Armstrong, M. J., Arroyo, V., Athyros, V. G., *et al.* (2019). Consensus guidelines: Best practices for detection, assessment and management of suspected acute drug-induced liver injury during clinical trials in patients with nonalcoholic steatohepatitis. https://core.ac.uk/download/228066244.pdf (accessed on 24 May 2025).
2. Alfirevic, A., Armitage, J., Bloch, K. M., Carr, D. F., *et al.* (2014). Phenotype standardization for statin-induced myotoxicity. https://core.ac.uk/download/30662970.pdf (accessed on 24 May 2025).
3. Amicone L, Marchetti A. Microenvironment and tumor cells: two targets for new molecular therapies of hepatocellular carcinoma. Transl Gastroenterol Hepatol. 2018 May 2;3:24. doi: 10.21037/tgh.2018.04.05. PMID: 29971255; PMCID: PMC6002256.
4. Amin, S., Kar, S., & Piotto, S. (2025). pDILI_v1: A web-based machine learning tool for predicting drug-induced liver injury (DILI) integrating chemical space analysis and molecular fingerprints. *ACS Omega, 10*, 13502–13514. https://www.semanticscholar.org/paper/61e9cbbd310071cfea23fb3f6af59f9be98803d1 (accessed on 24 May 2025).
5. Andrade-Bellido, R. J., Carvajal, A., Cueto-Galán, R., & Lucena-González, *et al.* (2007). Genetic and molecular factors in drug-induced liver injury: A review. https://core.ac.uk/download/621566037.pdf (accessed on 24 May 2025).
6. Antonilli, L., Badiani, A., Grassi, M. C., & Graziani, *et al.* (2015). Cardiovascular and hepatic toxicity of cocaine: Potential beneficial effects of modulators of oxidative stress. https://core.ac.uk/download/30614196.pdf.
7. Bai, T., Hong, L., Na, L., Niu, Q., & Jiao, F. (2024). A single-center clinical analysis of drug-induced liver injury in children with acute leukemia. *Asian Journal of Pediatric Research*. https://www.semanticscholar.org/paper/14a8f7a2d03a670cee7d8f5db747fab1b276ba0c (accessed on 24 May 2025).
8. Balaji, D., Balakrishnan, R., Srinivasan, D., Subbarayan, R., Shrestha, R., Srivastava, N., & Chauhan, A. (2024). The impact of SARS-CoV-2 on liver diseases and potential phytochemical treatments. *Infectious Microbes and Diseases*. https://www.semanticscholar.org/paper/a78c63718ce90cda6b3132d01f737f4cd2ea3f3d (accessed on 24 May 2025).
9. Balkrishna, A., Gohel, V., Tomer, M., Dev, R., & Varshney, A. (2024). Herbo-vitamin medicine Livogrit Vital ameliorates isoniazid induced liver injury (IILI) in human liver (HepG2) cells by decreasing isoniazid accumulation and oxidative stress driven hepatotoxicity. *BMC Complementary Medicine and Therapies, 24*. https://www.semanticscholar.org/paper/48eef2b2b9f9c688de1b56d4405857ba519e4fd2 (accessed on 24 May 2025).
10. Benoit, D., De Bus, L., Depuydt, P., *et al.* (2010). Severe drug-induced liver injury associated with prolonged use of linezolid. https://core.ac.uk/download/55761329.pdf (accessed on 24 May 2025).
11. Bodzin, A. S., Busuttil, R. W., Lunsford, K. E., Reino, *et al.* (2016). Dangerous dietary supplements: Garcinia cambogia-associated hepatic failure requiring transplantation. https://core.ac.uk/download/323078129.pdf.

12. Chalasani, N., Fontana, R. J., Ghabril, M., *et al.* (2014). Relationship between characteristics of medications and drug-induced liver disease phenotype and outcome. https://core.ac.uk/download/46962330.pdf (accessed on 24 May 2025).

13. Chauhan, K., Erwin, R., Halegoua-De Marzio, D., *et al.* (2022). A comprehensive review on the use of herbal dietary supplements in the USA, reasons for their use, and review of potential hepatotoxicity. https://core.ac.uk/download/540858882.pdf (accessed on 24 May 2025).

14. Chien, A. J., Esserman, L. J., Hyland, C., *et al.* (2019). A case report of vanishing bile duct syndrome after exposure to pexidartinib (PLX3397) and paclitaxel. https://core.ac.uk/download/323072463.pdf.

15. Clarke, A. T., Ford, I., Hall, G. C., *et al.* (2016). High dose atorvastatin associated with increased risk of significant hepatotoxicity in comparison to simvastatin in UK GPRD cohort. https://core.ac.uk/download/42370116.pdf (accessed on 24 May 2025).

16. Cohen, L., Neuman, M. G., Hwang, P. A., & Nanau, R. M. (2011). Genetic and immune predictors for hypersensitivity syndrome to antiepileptic drugs. https://core.ac.uk/download/pdf/290366.pdf (accessed on 24 May 2025).

17. Cox, C. R., Lynch, S., Goldring, C., & Sharma, P. (2020). Current perspective: 3D spheroid models utilizing human-based cells for investigating metabolism-dependent drug-induced liver injury. *Frontiers in Medical Technology, 2*. https://www.semanticscholar.org/paper/1defab0f2a222e6ac9709a5ec5821e5ae83d1c68 (accessed on 24 May 2025).

18. Cunha, S. S., Merle, C. S. C., & Rodrigues, L. C. (2010). BCG vaccination and leprosy protection: Review of current evidence and status of BCG in leprosy control.

19. Daly, A. (2022). Genetics of drug-induced liver injury: Current knowledge and future prospects. *Clinical and Translational Science, 16*, 37–42. https://www.semanticscholar.org/paper/5930d15c5b4134c06d28665fce87f780a531d3e0 (accessed on 24 May 2025).

20. Elsaid, M. I., Meara, A. S., Owen, D. H., Manne, A., Tounkara, F., Mumtaz, K., Paskett, E., *et al.* (2024). Risk and impacts of drug-induced liver injury (DILI) due to immune-checkpoint inhibitors (ICI) on overall survival in patients with newly diagnosed cancer: A retrospective cohort study. *Journal of Clinical Oncology*. https://www.semanticscholar.org/paper/1618fcb83183a4d367abd4ace173596b10a6457a (accessed on 24 May 2025).

21. Fontana, R. J., Liou, I., Reuben, A., Suzuki, A., Fiel, M. I., Lee, W. M., & Navarro, V. J. (2022). AASLD practice guidance on drug, herbal, and dietary supplement–induced liver injury. *Hepatology, 77*, 1036–1065. https://doi.org/10.1002/hep.32689.

22. Fu, S., Wu, D., Jiang, W., Li, J., Jiang, L., Jia, C., & Zhou, T. (2020). Molecular biomarkers in drug-induced liver injury: Challenges and future perspectives. *Frontiers in Pharmacology, 10*. https://doi.org/10.3389/fphar.2019.01667.

23. García-Cortés, M., Matilla-Cabello, G., & Lucena, M. I. (2024). Methods for causality assessment of idiosyncratic drug-induced liver injury. *Liver International, 45*. https://www.semanticscholar.org/paper/2fd782c7e8501e2488d41ffa3109224a729ec87d (accessed on 24 May 2025).

24. Guo, K., & van den Beucken, T. (2024). Advances in drug-induced liver injury research: *In vitro* models, mechanisms, omics and gene modulation techniques. *Cell & Bioscience, 14*. https://www.semanticscholar.org/paper/b8f69d0259991e7a0f3274043387a377f5517900 (accessed on 24 May 2025).

25. Kawano, M., Yano, Y., Yamamoto, A., Yasutomi, E., Inoue, Y., Kitadai, J., Yoshida, R., *et al.* (2024). Risk factors for immune checkpoint inhibitor-induced liver injury and the significance of liver biopsy. *Diagnostics, 14*. https://www.semanticscholar.org/paper/eb03365a0b34bfec3cecbd851a7dcea7b9880ce4 (accessed on 24 May 2025).

26. Kozielewicz, D. M., Stalke, P., & Skrzypek, J. (2025). Drug-induced liver injury. Part I: Classification, diagnosis and treatment. *Clinical and Experimental Hepatology, 11*, 25–33. https://www.semanticscholar.org/paper/d51eb9c361495ac38d76f7a499579a79f8122e24 (accessed on 24 May 2025).

27. Lei XG, Zhu JH, Cheng WH, Bao Y, Ho YS, Reddi AR, Holmgren A, Arnér ES. Paradoxical Roles of Antioxidant Enzymes: Basic Mechanisms and Health Implications. Physiol Rev. 2016 Jan;96(1):307-64. doi: 10.1152/physrev.00010.2014. PMID: 26681794; PMCID: PMC4839492.

28. Liu, Q., Huang, L., Yan, H., Zong, Z., Chen, Z., Wu, X., Chen, L., *et al.* (2024). Clinical risk factors for moderate and severe antituberculosis drug-induced liver injury. *Frontiers in Pharmacology, 15*. https://www.semanticscholar.org/paper/7a80023a6bb7af917c597b3d598a6e43414d422c (accessed on 24 May 2025).

29. Maev, I., & Polunina, T. E. (2023). [Drug-induced liver injury: Diagnosis of exclusion]. *Terapevticheskii arkhiv, 95*(8), 611–620. https://www.semanticscholar.org/paper/153db2af4bdb05f8014eb0c9ebff26b62fa04e60 (accessed on 24 May 2025).

30. Maina, A., & Foster, G. R. (2024). Hepatitis after gene therapy, what are the possible causes? *Journal of Viral Hepatitis, 31*, 14–20. https://www.semanticscholar.org/paper/a9ca29889475ed0da9e043ef892607f98a318ef5 (accessed on 24 May 2025).

31. Mederle, O.A., Sima, L.V., Popa, D.I., Williams, C.G., Mîțu, D., Șutoi, D., Trebuian, C.I., Șelaru, M., Loloș, D., Pah, A.M., & Buleu, F.N. (2024). Primary Iliopsoas Abscess and Drug-Induced Liver Injury in the Emergency Department: A Case Report. Diseases, 12.

32. Mili, A., Birangal, S., Nandakumar, K., & Lobo, R. (2023). A computational study to identify Sesamol derivatives as NRF2 activator for protection against drug-induced liver injury (DILI). *Molecular Diversity, 28*, 1709–1731. https://www.semanticscholar.org/paper/253103f26d3b6919f6ac4e2d31373ae2552e42f1 (accessed on 24 May 2025).

33. Mukewar, S. (2025). Recent advances in diagnosis and management of chronic cholestatic liver diseases: Expert consensus. *International Journal of Research in Medical Sciences*. https://www.semanticscholar.org/paper/eb16fa42970246141e2f934751ded5fd927951be (accessed on 24 May 2025).

34. Ozturk, N. B., Uskudar, E., Toruner, M. D., Simsek, C., & Gurakar, A. (2024). Drug-induced liver injury: Diagnosis, management and the role of liver transplantation. *Hepatology Forum, 6*, 72–76. https://www.semanticscholar.org/paper/136527b93c98b7212868d600a1c045dc96e2fcda (accessed on 24 May 2025).

35. Pradhan, R. R., & Yadav, A. K. (2025). Incidence, clinical features, associated factors and outcomes of intensive phase antituberculosis drug induced liver injury among patients with tuberculosis at a tertiary care hospital in Nepal: A descriptive cross-sectional study. *Health Science Reports, 8*. https://www.semanticscholar.org/paper/7348fa17daffcb811cf8eba28954d4f43292dbcc (accessed on 24 May 2025).

36. Roy, S., Shah, Z., & Chakraborthy, G. S. (2024). A brief overview of drug-induced liver damage. *The Egyptian Journal of Internal Medicine*. https://www.semanticscholar.org/paper/71519e4ec922a4de01dbd3ff774769e3f5455d2c (accessed on 24 May 2025).

37. Senior, J. R. (2014). Evolution of the Food and Drug Administration approach to liver safety assessment for new drugs: Current status and challenges. https://core.ac.uk/download/189251303.pdf (accessed on 24 May 2025).

38. Sharma, S., Sharma, V., Taneja, S., Bhatia, A., Anand, A., Patil, A. N., & Banerjee, D. (2023). Scopoletin: A potential phytochemical therapy for antitubercular treatment drug-induced liver injury (ATT-DILI) model in Wistar rats. *Journal of Complementary and Integrative Medicine, 20*, 797–803. https://www.semanticscholar.org/paper/9a1bc13ea9d24132189bdcd8bc20472791999396 (accessed on 24 May 2025).

39. She, Y., Guo, Z., Zhai, Q., Liu, J., Du, Q., & Zhang, Z. (2024). CDK4/6 inhibitors in drug-induced liver injury: A pharmacovigilance study of the FAERS database and analysis of the drug–gene interaction network. *Frontiers in Pharmacology, 15*. https://www.semanticscholar.org/paper/db9d8962cd5e91dc89a42ce1e4d6117faab08503 (accessed on 24 May 2025).

40. Shen, T., Liu, Y., Shang, J., Xie, Q., Li, J., Yan, M., Xu, J., *et al.* (2019). Incidence and etiology of drug-induced liver injury in mainland China. *Gastroenterology, 156*, 2230–2241.e11. https://doi.org/10.1053/j.gastro.2019.02.002.

41. Smith, D. N., Pungwe, P., Comer, L. L., Ajayi, T. A., & Suarez, M. G. (2023). Turmeric-associated liver injury: A rare case of drug-induced liver injury. *Cureus, 15*. https://www.semanticscholar.org/paper/29d61444f6a811f62b61da2d4f6028cbc83c4dec (accessed on 24 May 2025).

42. Tanaka, A., Tsuji, K., Komiyama, Y., Tsuruya, K., Kakisaka, K., Tsutsui, A., Ichimoto, K., *et al.* (2024). RECAM-J 2023—Validation and development of the Japanese version of RECAM for the diagnosis of drug-induced liver injury. *Hepatology Research, 54*, 12–503. https://www.semanticscholar.org/paper/d36fca6c9ab240302a23a7e5a86e447254bbcb52 (accessed on 24 May 2025).

43. Tostmann, A., Wubuli, A., Roy, B., Roy, B., Benichou, C., Merle, C., Yee, D., *et al.* (2014). The incidence of liver injury in Uyghur patients treated for TB in Xinjiang Uyghur autonomous region, China, and its association with hepatic enzyme polymorphisms NAT2, CYP2E1, GSTM1 and GSTT1. https://core.ac.uk/download/19746989.pdf (accessed on 24 May 2025).

44. Venkataswamy, C., Thomas, E., & Kartikayan, R. (2024). Drug induced liver injury: A descriptive analysis of histopathological patterns and clinical outcomes. *International Journal of Advanced Medical and Health Research*. https://www.semanticscholar.org/paper/18c5b3a495e6e7d8fbeed0031e5504dea07878ef (accessed on 24 May 2025).

45. Wang, Y., Lin, X., Sun, Y., Liu, J., Li, J., Tian, Q., Guo, F., *et al.* (2025). Development and validation of a novel model to discriminate idiosyncratic drug-induced liver injury and autoimmune hepatitis. *Liver International, 45*(2), e16239. https://www.semanticscholar.org/paper/18ee7ecbeb2a4c1d98e5b34d3f313915341d980e (accessed on 24 May 2025).

46. Wei, Q., Li, L., Zeng, X. Q., Abidan, B., Yin, J., Gao, H., & Guo, J. S. (2024). An analysis on clinical characteristics and prognosis-related risk factors in patients with drug-induced liver injury. *Zhonghua Gan Zang Bing Za Zhi = Chinese Journal of Hepatology, 32*(3), 214–221. https://www.semanticscholar.org/paper/36311313bdec47506c7e037b1ff0ca78e6022208 (accessed on 24 May 2025).

47. Winiarska-Mieczan, A., Jachimowicz-Rogowska, K., Kwiecień, M., Borsuk-Stanulewicz, M., Tomczyk-Warunek, A., Stamirowska-Krzaczek, E., Purwin, C., *et al.* (2024). Regular consumption of green tea as an element of diet therapy in drug-induced liver injury (DILI). *Nutrients, 16*, 2837. https://doi.org/10.3390/nu16172837.

48. Yusuff, A. A., Ogunmoyole, T., & Johnson, O. D. (2025). Protective effects of Amaranthus spinosus leaf extract against CCl4-induced hepatorenal injury in rats: Insights from GC-MS analysis. *The Journal of Phytopharmacology*. https://www.semanticscholar.org/paper/728e574d0c47d5c3679eb212eba03f525b0a38c3 (accessed on 24 May 2025).

49. Zhang, F., Song, L., Lin, Y., Yang, Z. Z., Shi, J., Yuan, Q., & Zhang, Y. (2024). Smart persistent luminescence imaging for early diagnosis of drug-induced liver injury. *Chemical & Biomedical Imaging, 3*, 77–84. https://www.semanticscholar.org/paper/de76ab1b3c1588cb893cb44cada7df97fab9b483 (accessed on 24 May 2025).

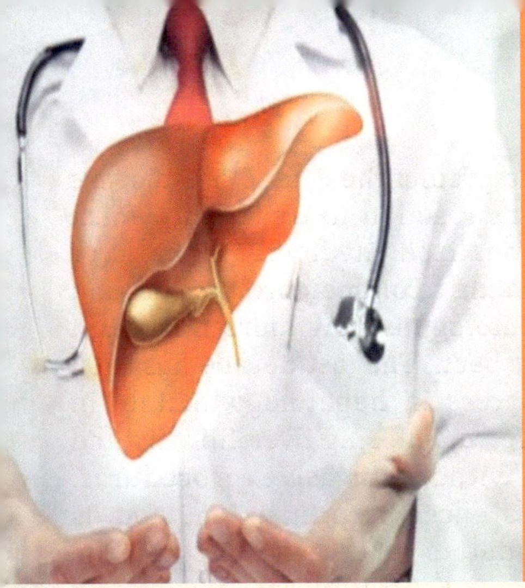

Chapter 15

ADVANCES IN HEPATOLOGY AND FUTURE PERSPECTIVES

Contents

Introduction

Hepatology has grown a lot because there is a need to manage serious liver problems that continue to affect many people. Close familiarity with liver pathologies like chronic hepatitis B (CHB) and hepatitis C virus (HCV) infection is required to develop sound therapeutic strategies. The pursuit of a functional cure of CHB is currently centered on the loss of hepatitis B surface antigen (HBsAg) as the primary priority, where the need for both viral suppression and immune modulation in treatment regimens is highlighted. Recent studies point to ways that current immunotherapies may be able to address the problem of immune deficiencies. Above all, understanding the intricacies of viral replication mechanisms holds the promise for indicating directions in future vaccine design and antiviral drug treatments that will result in new treatment protocols integrating various therapeutic modalities to enhance patient outcomes (Baumert *et al.*, 2023). Liver transplantation, especially concerning HCV recurrence, is a continuous cause for concern. After a liver transplant, the chance of HCV coming back is almost universal, so it is hard to predict how the disease will progress, and in some cases, the disease moves faster. Several factors have been found to influence post-transplant outcomes, and peak viral RNA early after surgery may be an important sign for both prognosis and choosing treatment. As has now been established by recent studies, identification of personalized immunological profiles prior to transplant can also inform personalized treatment regimens, indicating that personalized treatment modes according to each patient's underlying liver disease are needed (Rahman *et al.*, 2013). The main focus on personalized medicine shows that using biomarkers with treatment plans can greatly improve both a patient's survival and ongoing health. Technologies in development are helping to change hepatology by making it possible to monitor liver fibrosis and function without invasive methods. Biomarker exploration and other advanced methods have made it possible to assess the disease's severity without doing invasive liver biopsies. When knowledge about liver fibrosis improves, these non-invasive technologies can be used more often in regular clinical settings. Other new liver support methods, such as artificial liver systems and gene therapy, may greatly help people with advanced liver disease. Using these advanced strategies wisely, hepatology is on the brink of a major change to improve patient care worldwide and defeat liver diseases.

Overview of Hepatology

Because liver diseases are being seen more often around the world, hepatology has become more significant. Among these are viral hepatitis, LC, and HCC, which are hard to detect and manage. Hepatologists must be aware of the main changes in the body that lead to liver diseases to give the best care and treatment to patients. Earlier diagnosis of liver problems is now possible because of new diagnostic tools that aid in early treatment. In addition, scientists are finding new biomarkers that allow doctors to predict the course of a disease and the patient's reaction to treatment, which supports personalized medicine. Since liver disease is becoming a common problem around the world, hepatology is now more important than it has ever been. The last decade has seen important progress in hepatology, mainly in new methods for diagnosing liver fibrosis and inflammation without invasive procedures. LBx, which was once the primary method, is now less used due to its invasiveness and the problems it creates. For this reason, doctors rely on ultrasound elastography and serum markers, which are considered safer ways to examine the liver. They allow doctors to assess the extent of fibrosis and hepatic steatosis, without requiring invasive procedures. Because of these improvements, patients feel more comfortable and are more likely to stick to regular check-ups, which helps manage liver diseases better. As hepatology continues to evolve, these non-invasive assessments are likely to play an integral role in routine clinical practice, guiding therapeutic decision-making and monitoring disease progression over time (Press, 2019). Many studies have been done on antiviral and immunotherapy approaches, which have helped a lot in treating viral hepatitis, mostly hepatitis B and C. Due to direct-acting antiviral agents, hepatitis C can now be treated more effectively and with treatments that last less time and cause fewer side effects. In addition, scientists are working on new approaches like changing the immune response and making vaccines for hepatitis B, which may help control the disease. Studies on the immune system in the liver have inspired scientists to look into immunotherapy, which may use the immune system to treat liver cancers. Because of advances in hepatology, using these antiviral and immunotherapeutic approaches is crucial for handling liver disease problems worldwide and shaping future guidelines. The integration of these therapies represents a significant leap forward in treating liver diseases, with the potential to change the landscape of hepatology as we know it (Press, 2019) (Figure 15.1).

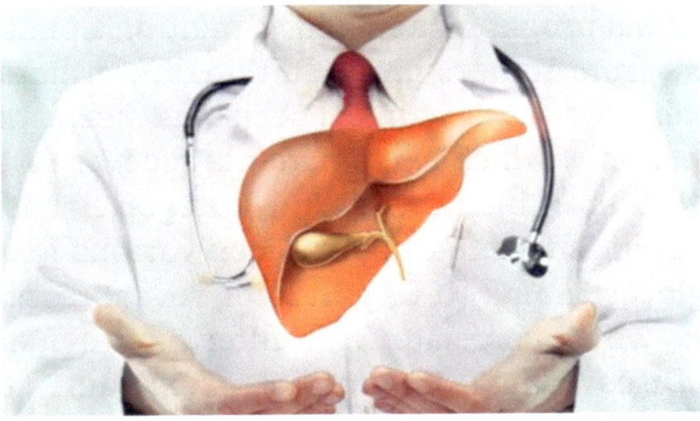

Figure 15.1. Overview of Hepatology

Source: https://www.gastropune.com/wp-content/uploads/2024/07/Untitled-design-2024-07-16T115210.358-1024x614.png.

Importance of Advances in Liver Health

Advances in liver health are of utmost importance toward neutralizing the rising prevalence of liver diseases, which are major factors of worldwide public health. With diverse diseases like viral hepatitis, NAFLD, and HCC on the rise, the need for new diagnostic as well as therapeutic modalities comes to the forefront. Evolution in knowledge of liver disease has put into prominence various etiologies, particularly the global burden of hepatitis B and C, and an alarming increase in NAFLD secondary to lifestyle, including obesity and sedentary lifestyle. As CLD runs in the background, causing significant complications like cirrhosis and liver cancer, innovations like non-invasive biomarkers and sophisticated imaging technology are pivotal to making early detection possible and facilitating timely intervention (Wazir *et al.*, 2025). This innovation is a significant shift in liver disease management and patient outcomes. The role of immunotherapy and antiviral advancements cannot be overemphasized in liver health. Breakthrough developments in antiviral therapies have transformed the trajectory of viral hepatitis treatment, particularly in hepatitis C, where sustained virologic response can lead to the total annihilation of the virus. These advances in clinical practice not only minimized morbidity and mortality from chronic hepatitis infections but also held the prospect for enhancing liver health nationwide. On the other hand, immunotherapy offers not only HCC management but also treatment of many liver-related cancers. Advances in the immunological pathways of liver disease pave the way for novel therapeutic modalities with potential to optimize rates of response and decrease treatment-related complications (Wazir *et al.*, 2023). As liver diseases change, these new forms of treatment are vital in optimizing patient care and long-term impact on health. Gene therapy and the future of liver transplantation are yet another frontier in optimizing liver health. The demand for donor organs continues to outstrip supply, and new sources such as bioengineering of artificial organs and refinement of existing transplant protocols are being pursued. Gene therapies also promise to treat genetic liver diseases, including alpha-1 antitrypsin deficiency and hereditary hemochromatosis. Treatment would remedy the genetic defect, with a potential for normal liver function and arresting disease progression. With mounting research, the use of new technologies and treatment modalities will be the key to creating a path for better liver health and quality of life in patients with liver diseases (Wazir *et al.*, 2023, 2025). Thus, the concerted effort in the domain of hepatology not only reaffirms the importance of advancements in liver health but also underscores the need for further study and collective action towards resolving these vital health problems.

15.1. Biomarkers in Hepatology

The exploration of biomarkers in hepatology has significantly advanced the understanding and management of liver diseases, particularly hepatocellular carcinoma (HCC). By using biomarkers, it is possible to spot disease, monitor its development, and check how the patient responds to treatment, which helps doctors personalize care. Psychosocial factors influence the need for early detection and effective management protocols, as HCC's lethal prognosis demands a multidisciplinary approach to care (N/A, 2022). Tissue and fluid markers from tumors give additional information that goes beyond the results of standard imaging. Their ability to guide clinical decisions means that these biomarkers make it possible to act quickly and correctly, which helps patients recover faster in a complex medical setting. Furthermore, the classification of biomarkers into categories based on their molecular profiles has emerged as a critical tool in differentiating between various forms of liver cancers, such as HCC and intrahepatic cholangiocarcinoma (iCCA). Studies reveal distinct molecular characteristics associated with these cancers, which correlate with differing prognoses and therapeutic interventions (Friedman *et al.*, 2018). Discovering such biomarkers explains how cancer develops and how tumors change. Because adult hepatocytes may be the source of HCC, new treatments can now be developed to target certain genetic changes. It helps explain the causes of liver cancer and also supports the creation of new treatments that can be adjusted for each person's biomarkers. Also, using non-invasive biomarkers is now replacing some traditional LBx methods, which helps to reduce the dangers of invasive procedures. Scientists are working hard to develop and confirm reliable biomarkers, which are gaining more attention. Emerging technologies in genome profiling and next-generation sequencing (NGS) provide an innovative framework for identifying biomarkers associated with liver pathology, allowing for improved monitoring of disease progression and therapeutic efficacy (Friedman *et al.*, 2018). With these biomarkers in clinical use, hepatology is changing so that treatment and monitoring can be much more precise than was possible before. With more progress in biomarker research, hepatology could see better diagnosis, new treatments, and more involved patient care.

15.1.1. Definition and Role of Biomarkers

In the field of hepatology, biomarkers are now seen as key in helping diagnose, predict the outcome, and treat liver diseases. Biomarkers, which measure the condition of the body, can be obtained from blood, tissues, and images. Biomarkers are especially important for understanding how a disease develops, how much damage the liver has suffered, and selecting the right treatment. For instance, the evolution of NAFLD to its later stage, metabolic dysfunction-associated steatohepatitis (MASH), can be monitored by specific biomarkers that indicate both inflammation and fibrosis. As Elangovan *et al.* (2025) posit, the rising prevalence of metabolic liver disease necessitates a better understanding of the biomarkers and, therefore, is critical in maximizing clinical management and intervention. Also, non-invasive biomarkers are better than LBx in some ways, since LBx is known to be unreliable because of its variable results. The development of scoring systems, such as the Fibrosis-4 (FIB-4) index and the NAFLD fibrosis score, demonstrates how such biomarkers simplify the assessment of liver function and health to be easy to implement, thereby increasing patient compliance with screening schedules. The new guidelines point out that identifying at-risk patients for severe liver disease can help change the way treatment is given, adjusting to the fast-changing lifestyle-related changes in liver disease. Through the integration of such advanced non-invasive instruments into routine clinical use, clinicians can facilitate better patient outcomes, thereby emphasizing the importance of biomarkers as foundation cornerstones within today's hepatology, part of the increasing emphasis on patient-centered care strategies. The clinical environment for hepatitis research also emphasizes the central role that biomarkers play in the management of chronic viral diseases such as Hepatitis B and C (HBV and HCV). Biomarkers make it possible to detect people who may develop serious complications such as LC or HCC. The emphasis on screening programs in Asia, as described in (Kaewdech *et al.*, 2024), underscores the necessity of applying these biomarkers to enhance public health programs for reducing HBV and HCV-related morbidity and mortality. Person-centered care based on biomarkers can help distribute resources well and ensure that the most needy people get the best and most helpful care. Thus, the evolving patterns of disease management in hepatology not only underscore the utility of biomarkers in clinical practice but also the potential they can unlock in facilitating effective public health policy towards the eradication of viral hepatitis and promotion of liver health globally (Figure 15.2).

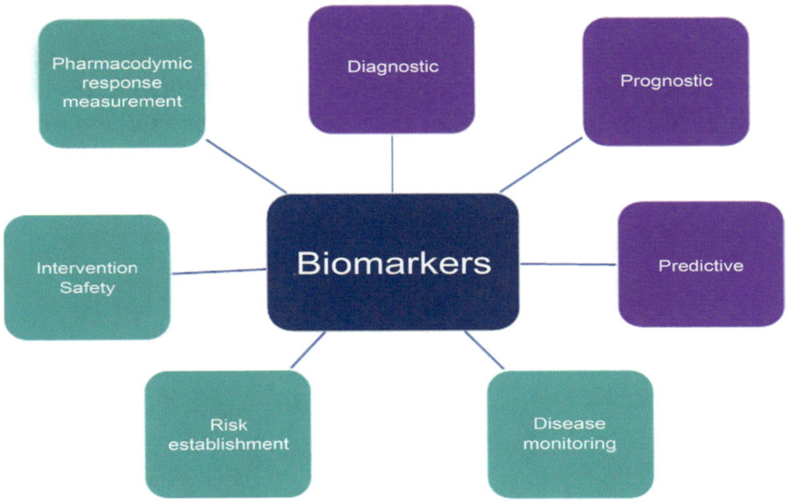

Figure 15.2. Biomarkers.

Source: https://www.wisecube.ai/wp-content/uploads/2023/06/image.png.

15.1.2. Current Biomarkers for Liver Disease

Looking into current biomarkers for liver disease is very important in hepatology, mainly for catching problems early and managing them accurately. Biomarkers such as alpha-fetoprotein (AFP), which is often elevated in HCC, play a crucial role in the diagnosis and monitoring of liver malignancies. Since AFP is good at predicting risks, it is now used in healthcare to help identify people who may need special care and support. New discoveries, such as new biomarkers, are now available to support the traditional biomarker AFP. Using imaging and circulating biomarkers together can help doctors make more accurate diagnoses, which affects treatment outcomes. With the progress of hepatology, these various biomarkers should be included in a unified, multidisciplinary strategy to deal with complex liver diseases, mainly in managing HCC, which is difficult to treat. Non-invasive biomarkers are now being used to monitor liver disease, which is becoming an important area in hepatology. Using platelet count, prothrombin time, and FibroTest has become popular for determining liver fibrosis without having to do invasive liver biopsies. Since these methods are gentle, patients feel more comfortable, and it allows doctors to monitor them more often. For example, the Model for End-Stage Liver Disease (MELD) score has been widely implemented to predict mortality risk, thereby guiding treatment decisions. In addition, recent studies suggest that including new biomarkers such as amino acid and glycoprotein changes can give more information about how the disease develops and responds to treatment. With the help of non-invasive biomarkers, clinicians are able to choose better therapies and improve the outcomes of their patients with liver disease. In the context of chronic hepatitis B (CHB), the identification and utilization of biomarkers are pivotal for achieving treatment goals, particularly the functional cure characterized by HBsAg loss. Current treatment regimens predominantly rely on nucleos(t)ide analogues that suppress viral replication but often fall short of eliciting a durable immune response necessary for HBsAg loss. Researchers have started to explore biomarker-driven strategies because of a better understanding of HBV and the immune system. New research shows that using antiviral therapies with immunotherapies can significantly lower antigen levels which is important for a functional cure. Regular biomarker monitoring helps predict how the treatment will work and reveals details about the immune system of chronic infections. As innovative therapeutic avenues continue to develop, a robust biomarker framework will be vital for personalizing treatment approaches in the diverse population affected by CHB (Baumert *et al.*, 2023) (Figure 15.3).

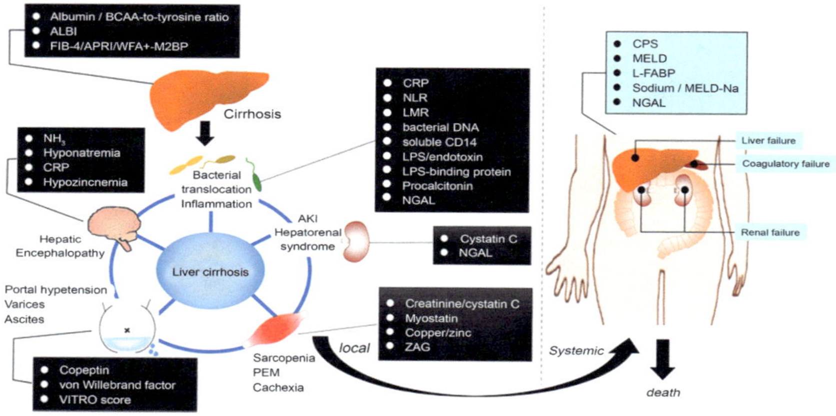

Figure 15.3. Blood-based prognostic biomarkers for advanced liver diseases.

Source: https://www.researchgate.net/publication/355783237/figure/fig2/AS:11431281181902246@1692207699258/Blood-based-prognostic-biomarkers-for-advanced-liver-diseases-BCAA-branched-chain-amino.png.

15.1.3. Future Directions in Biomarker Research

Directions in the future of biomarker research promise to reshape the field of hepatology through the refinement of the diagnosis and treatment of liver disease, particularly HCC. The application of multi-omics technologies, such as genomics, proteomics, and metabolomics, promises to permit more precise profiling of liver tumors. This profiling can make it possible to distinguish specific molecular signatures of different tumor types, like HCC and iCCA. Through the identification of these biomarkers, clinicians would not only be able to enhance early detection but also design treatment regimens that are specific to target particular molecular therapeutic pathways. In addition, advancements in technologies like liquid biopsies could enable non-invasive monitoring of disease progression and response to therapy, supporting the need for an integrated strategy in biomarker implementation into clinical practice, which is well in tandem with insights presented by experts in the management of HCC (N/A, 2022). The evolution of bioinformatics tools also plays an important part in the future of biomarker research, particularly in analyzing and interpreting sophisticated data being produced by multi-omics strategies. Machine learning (ML) algorithms can be utilized to enhance prognostic precision of biomarker profiles by integrating clinical parameters with genomic data to enable prognostication and therapeutic selection. For example, one can stratify between various subclasses of HCC, such as the proliferation-progenitor and TGF-β subclasses segregated based on genome profiling, to guide therapeutic interventions. This level of specificity in classifying patient populations on the basis of molecular traits could enhance treatment outcomes and extend survival rates for liver cancers, whose outcomes are famously dismal (Friedman *et al.*, 2018). Enhancing our understanding of the molecular mechanisms of liver tumorigenesis can then reveal novel therapeutic opportunities, confirming the necessity for further research into this field. In addition, interdisciplinary collaborations are essential in bridging knowledge from biomarker research to the clinic. As our knowledge of the cell-of-origin of liver cancer progresses, with the prime contributions being the role of adult hepatocytes and progenitor cells in carcinogenesis, a convergence of the research produced in oncology, hepatology, and molecular biology will increasingly become essential. The prospect of identifying specific genetic mutations for targeting, as has become available with the advent of sequencing technology, makes an integrated research strategy balancing laboratory findings with clinical practice imperative. Through facilitating collaboration among clinicians, researchers, and bioethicists, the hepatology community can maximize the effective utilization of biomarkers in clinical practice, which will ultimately benefit the development of the holistic management of liver disorders (N/A, 2022) (Figure 15.4).

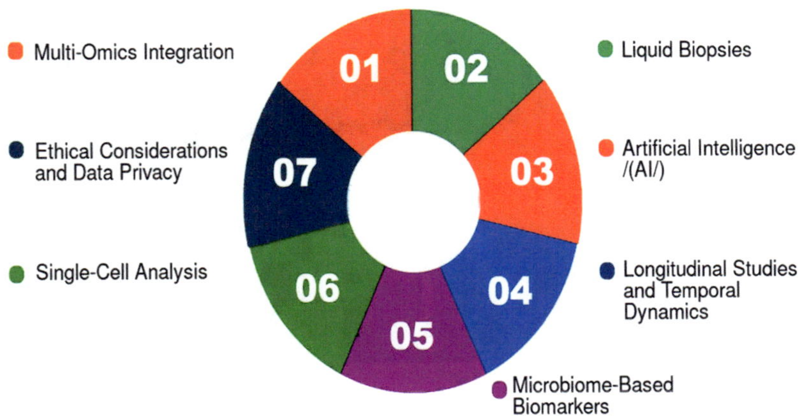

Figure 15.4. Future directions in biomarker discovery.

Source: https://fastercapital.co/i/Clinical-laboratory-biomarkers-Understanding-the-Role-of-Biomarkers-in-Disease-Diagnosis--Future-Directions-in-Biomarker-Discovery.webp.

15.2. Non-Invasive Fibrosis Assessment

It is now possible to check for fibrosis in the liver without using invasive methods, which is very helpful for patients and doctors. Even though traditional ways to test liver damage are accurate, they may cause bleeding or infection. Elastography, biomarkers in the blood, and imaging tests are considered good and safe replacements for biopsies. With these methods, doctors are able to measure fibrosis and notice changes in liver disease in patients with chronic issues, mostly those with hepatitis B and C. By employing these methods, clinicians can make informed treatment decisions, leading to improved patient management and outcomes, especially in cases where early detection of fibrosis is crucial for intervention and therapy (Gores *et al.*, 2018). Doctors can now use non-invasive methods to assess fibrosis, so they pay more attention to what is best for each patient. Transient elastography and magnetic resonance elastography are very effective at detecting fibrosis and cirrhosis. Furthermore, biochemistry-based scoring systems, like the Fibrosis-4 index (FIB-4) and the aspartate aminotransferase-to-platelet ratio index (APRI), rely on standardized laboratory metrics, eliminating the need for specialized equipment and making them accessible to a broader range of healthcare settings. Because of these changes, patients experience more comfort, can stick to their plans better, and medical expenses are reduced. As these methodologies continue to evolve, the non-invasive assessment of liver fibrosis will likely refine strategies to manage CLD effectively, paving the way for personalized medical approaches (N/A, 2022). Adding non-invasive fibrosis assessment to routine care allows doctors to select the most effective treatment for liver patients and results in better outcomes. Noticing fibrosis early makes it possible to treat it quickly, which could stop HCC and liver failure from developing in chronic diseases. Also, as biomarkers and imaging techniques keep improving, assessing fibrosis should become more precise and reliable. AI and ML advances might allow doctors to better understand non-invasive tests by providing personalized details from patient records. Ultimately, establishing robust non-invasive fibrosis assessment protocols within hepatology will not only facilitate better care for liver disease patients, but will also significantly contribute to the broader landscape of personalized medicine in this field (Gores *et al.*, 2018) (Figure 15.5).

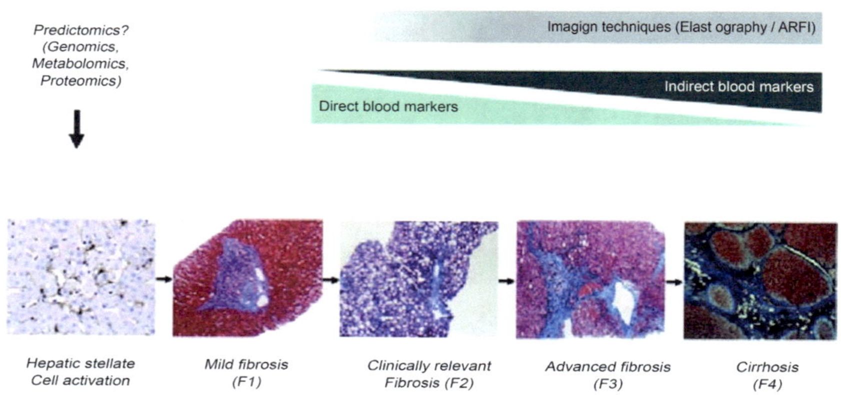

Figure 15.5. Noninvasive assessment of liver fibrosis. Most of the non-invasive methods currently used have a good accuracy to identify clinically relevant/advanced fibrosis (F ≥ 2/3). It is possible that in the near future the incorporation of genetic, metabolic and proteomic profiles could be a feasible strategy to allow the identification of liver fibrosis at its early stages. ARFI, acoustic radiation force impulse.

Source: https://www.researchgate.net/profile/Jose-Altamirano-2/publication/225375395/figure/fig1/AS:340595785650191@1458215771703/Noninvasive-assessment-of-liver-fibrosis-Most-of-the-non-invasive-methods-currently-used.png.

15.2.1. Importance of Non-Invasive Techniques

Use of non-invasive techniques in hepatology has the potential to be extremely hopeful as a method of improving patient care and diagnostic accuracy. Traditional assessment of liver disease is often rooted in invasive techniques such as liver biopsy, which may subject patients to complications and discomfort. Non-invasive techniques, including elastography and serum biomarker testing, have also emerged as an option that not only reduces patient risk but also renders the monitoring of liver diseases a standard procedure. These modalities allow clinicians to measure liver stiffness and fibrosis without tissue removal, thus promoting a patient-friendly strategy for hepatology. With further improvements in these techniques, it is hoped that they will introduce new biomarkers and better assessment methods, which will enhance the precision of diagnoses and the treatment of liver disease in the clinic, as has been stressed in recent publications emphasizing technological advancements in liver diagnosis (Kim *et al.*, 2024). The use of non-invasive approaches is at the forefront of future hepatology, particularly personalized medicine. Non-invasive biomarkers can inform personalized therapeutic strategies, ensuring that treatment regimens correspond to the individual profile of liver disease for each subject. Such a shift towards personalized medicine is facilitated by enhanced omics technologies that provide a greater understanding of the molecular underpinnings of liver diseases. In addition to non-invasive testing, these methods have the potential to accurately quantify disease progression and response to treatment without exposing patients to the hassles of invasive treatment. With the increasing prevalence of CLD, the inclusion of new non-invasive approaches is essential in designing strategies for treating such diseases effectively (Kim *et al.*, 2024). Furthermore, with increasing research efforts aimed at deciphering the complexities of liver pathophysiology, non-invasive approaches have promise for advancing disease mechanism understanding by way of more accessible real-time observation. This ability to visualize liver changes dynamically not only allows clinicians and researchers to make informed decisions, whether adjusting treatment regimens or conducting longitudinal studies assessing disease evolution, but also allows for the observation of changes in real-time. The development of liver organoids and advanced imaging modalities has the potential to further enhance non-invasive approaches by facilitating complex modeling of liver function and disease. This advancement is critical since it not only contributes to enhanced patient care but also facilitates significant research that will be crucial for future therapeutic advances in hepatology. The increasing acceptability of these approaches underlines their importance in the development of a novel generation of liver disease assessment and treatment (Alvarado-Tapias *et al.*, 2024).

15.2.2. Common Non-Invasive Assessment Methods

In this field, doctors use non-invasive techniques to check liver disease and its progression, instead of doing invasive biopsies. Elastography and serum biomarker panels are being used more often because they are good at predicting outcomes and are safe for patients. For example, transient elastography uses ultrasound to measure the stiffness of the liver, and this is related to the severity of fibrosis. It also means there are fewer risks from liver biopsies, and it is easier to track liver diseases over time. Consequently, the integration of these non-invasive methods into clinical practice aligns with the evolving landscape of hepatology, which emphasizes the need for safe and effective disease management strategies, particularly in light of the increasing prevalence of liver conditions, including HCC (Gores *et al.*, 2018). Serum biomarkers, in addition to elastography, are now important for non-invasive testing of liver problems. Various biomarker panels, such as the Fibrosis-4 (FIB-4) index and the aspartate aminotransferase to platelet ratio index (APRI), offer clinicians valuable insights into liver fibrosis progression. They gather standard clinical measures and turn them into tools for assessing risk, which helps choose the best treatment plan for each person. Using biomarkers helps find patients who are more likely to have serious liver disease and makes sure resources are used where they are most effective. Furthermore, as HCC continues to pose major clinical challenges, the development of reliable biomarkers becomes essential in refining surveillance strategies and improving patient outcomes (N/A, 2022). In the future, improving and confirming non-invasive assessment methods will probably have a big impact on hepatology. With more people needing early diagnosis of liver diseases, there is a strong reason to bring advanced technologies, such as AI, into the analysis of imaging and biomarker data. Being able to predict disease progression without invasive methods could change how patients are cared for and how doctors decide on treatment. Also, as research continues, linking these methods with new therapies may help intervene earlier and may also improve the success of current antiviral and immunotherapy strategies. By embracing developments in non-invasive assessments, the field of hepatology stands to improve overall patient care and outcomes in the face of persistent liver health issues (Gores *et al.*, 2018) (Figure 15.6).

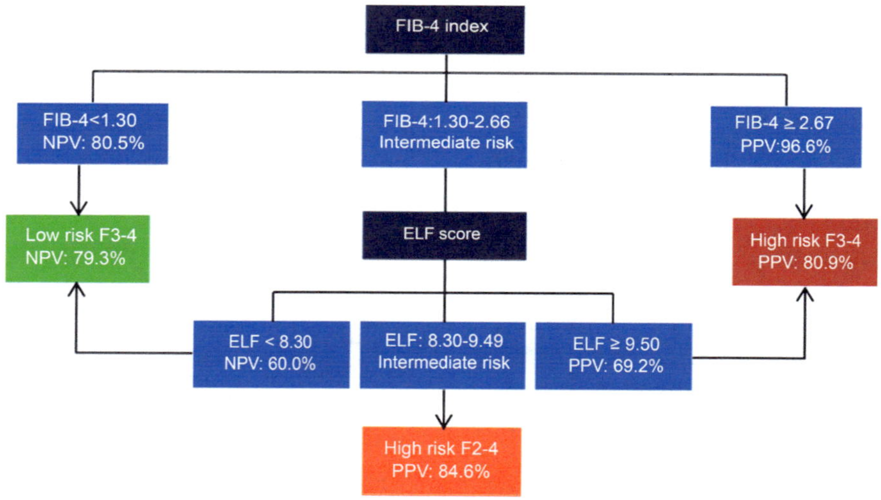

Figure 15.6. Fibrosis-4 (FIB-4) index.

Source: https://media.springernature.com/lw685/springer-static/image/art%3A10.1007%2Fs11739-023-03441-2/MediaObjects/11739_2023_3441_Fig1_HTML.png.

15.2.3. Limitations and Future Innovations

The advances in hepatology, particularly in the fields of biomarkers and measurement of non-invasive fibrosis, usher in a revolution in the management of liver diseases. However, even with these advances, there are wide limitations that inhibit their wide-scale acceptance. The first is the biomarker heterogeneity in performance across different groups of patients based on genetics, ethnicity, and comorbidity. This heterogeneity is likely to lead to misdiagnosis and unconventional treatment strategies, hence sustaining health disparities among communities. Additionally, the majority of non-invasive procedures, despite being promising, are never verified in longitudinal studies to establish their long-term validity and accuracy. Their validation requires rigorous, multicenter clinical trials for complete assessment of these biomarkers and measurement tools in various populations and phases of liver disease, thereby further establishing their clinical usefulness and patients' benefits. As science progresses, the search for innovative therapeutic strategies in antiviral as well as immunotherapy also encounters crushing odds. Their formation and use can be compromised by issues of drug resistance and heterogeneity of individual patients to the therapy. Furthermore, the cost of these new therapeutic modalities is also often an access limitation for patients, particularly in low-resource settings. The upcoming advancements must put more focus on developing cost-effective therapies and personalized medicine approaches that respond to treatment regimens based on individual patient profiles, including genetic predisposition and subtypes of liver disease. Interdisciplinary collaboration among researchers, physicians, and the pharmaceutical industry is critical in research advancement and offering equitable access to new treatments, which might, in turn, improve patient outcomes of CLD and open up doors to more intensive therapeutic interventions (Greten, 2018). Emerging liver support technologies have considerable potential for the treatment of liver failure and for the optimization of patient therapy; these systems are, however, not ideal. Current technologies, including bioartificial liver support systems, must be more optimized for the maximum exploitation of their potential in the clinical setting. Far too often, problems with biocompatibility, scalability, and complex regulatory pathways prevent their broader application. The future technologies must aim to integrate AI and ML to enhance the design and functionality of such support systems and achieve intelligent, efficient technologies with real-time monitoring and intervention. Further, keeping in view the advancements in gene therapy, the prospect of modulating the function of the liver at the genetic level brings about a paradigm shift. Overall, overcoming these limitations and driving innovations in liver support technologies can have a major impact on the treatment of liver diseases and enhance survival rates among involved patients (Greten, 2018) and lay a basis for personalized treatment regimens (Greten, 2018).

15.3. Advances in Antiviral Therapy

The recent developments in antiviral therapy have greatly changed the treatment of viral hepatitis, specifically hepatitis B and C, which are still major causes of liver disease globally. The invention of DAAs has changed the treatment of hepatitis C, with cure rates of more than 95% in the majority of populations. The drugs target the viral life cycle, interfering with replication processes without harming host cells, thus causing fewer side effects compared to the conventional therapies. Furthermore, research is still redirecting focus towards the identification of new antiviral compounds that target various stages of viral infection, expanding the therapeutic arsenal against hepatitis B and its subsequent progression to cirrhosis and HCC. These advances are indicative of a broader movement within hepatology, where individualized treatment and tailored medicine become increasingly feasible because of prevalent molecular studies in infectious disease environments (Kim *et al.*, 2024). The use of omics technologies such as genomics, proteomics, and metabolomics in hepatology is continuously revealing new avenues for the design and use of antiviral treatments. Utilization of these technologies can enable the researchers to characterize biomarkers for predicting treatment response and disease progression and thus optimize individualized therapeutic regimens. For instance, the ability to recognize specific genetic variations in patients can direct the selection of more potent antiviral regimens with reduced potential for resistance and treatment failure. Moreover, ongoing immunologic characterization of viral hepatitis-induced immune responses is coming up with new concepts for immunotherapies that can add to traditional antiviral measures. These therapeutic results suggest a multifaceted mechanism of the therapy for liver disease, complementing reports during the 5th Translational Hepatology Meeting emphasizing new biomarker discoveries and therapies to overcome current clinical limitations in liver pathologies (Alvarado-Tapias *et al.*, 2024). In addition to pharmaceutical development, the exploration of liver organoids and applications is ushering in a new era of antiviral therapy testing and design. These organoid three-dimensional tissues, which are stem cell-derived, are an *in vitro* model by which viral pathogenesis may be analyzed and antiviral efficacy can be assessed under human physiology-simulating conditions. The use of organoids in high-throughput screening allows for the rapid screening of numerous compounds, speeding the discovery of effective therapeutics. In addition, their potential application in personalized medicine is a platform upon which therapies may be customized based on differential patient responses observed *in vitro*. While challenges remain in the complete replication of liver tissue complexity, technology advances in organoids are proving to be pivotal in speeding up the quest for effective antiviral therapies as a modality within an integrated approach to the treatment of liver disease (Kim *et al.*, 2024).

15.3.1. Overview of Antiviral Treatments

The development of antiviral drugs has made it much easier to manage viral hepatitis, mainly hepatitis B and C, which are important causes of liver disease around the world. Because of direct-acting antivirals (DAAs), hepatitis C infections that were once long-term can now be treated and cured. Direct-acting antivirals (DAAs) work by interfering with certain stages of the virus's life cycle, which helps reduce the virus without the major side effects seen with older medicines such as interferon. Because DAAs are more tolerable and need less time to treat, they have made it possible for more people to receive the therapy. As the field of hepatology continues to evolve, there is a growing need for ongoing research into novel antiviral drugs that address drug-resistant viral strains and enhance therapeutic options for patients with complicated liver diseases (Kim *et al.*, 2024). Antiviral therapy is also heading in the direction of personalized medicine, which tries to match treatments to each patient's unique needs.

Biomarkers can help predict how well a person will respond to treatment and how the disease will develop, which will make antiviral treatments more effective and reduce the risk of side effects. New research has pointed out that genomic and proteomic technologies help find biomarkers that can lead to better decisions about therapy, which improves patient results. In addition, using non-invasive methods to assess liver fibrosis and inflammation is very important, as it enables monitoring of the disease without the need for invasive tests. These advancements not only democratize access to healthcare by eliminating the need for biopsies but also foster a more proactive approach to managing viral hepatitis (Alvarado-Tapias *et al.*, 2024). As well as discovering new drugs and using personalized medicine, combining different antiviral therapies is very important for improving the treatment of viruses. DAAs and Immunotherapeutics together may help get rid of viral infections and also repair the immune system in the liver, which is frequently damaged in chronic infections. The use of immune modulators might help maintain control over the virus and also manage any remaining inflammation. The results of current clinical trials are expected to explain whether these combination strategies are effective in liver care. As hepatology evolves, the implications of advanced antiviral treatments are far-reaching, with the potential to significantly reduce the burden of liver diseases and enhance the long-term quality of life for affected individuals (Kim *et al.*, 2024) (Figure 15.7).

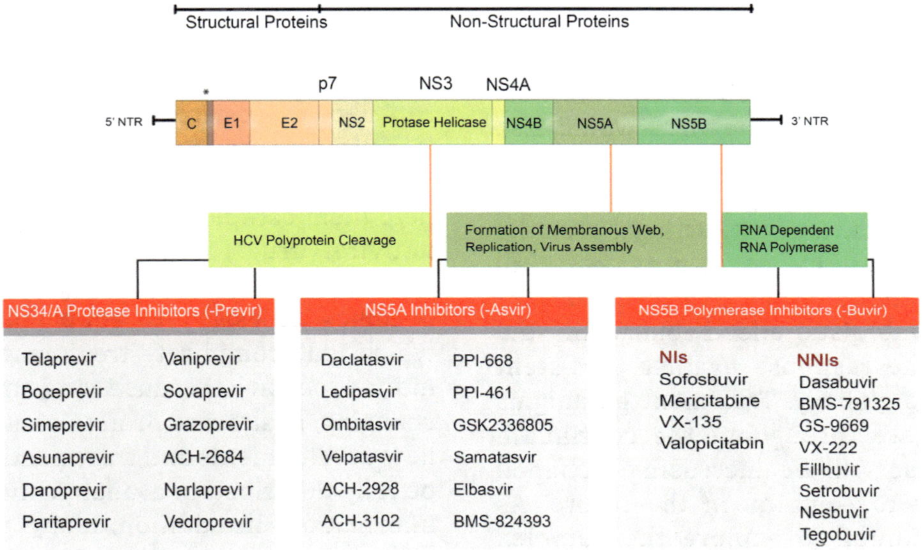

Figure 15.7. Direct-acting antiviral agents for treatment of hepatitis C virus infection.

Source: https://www.researchgate.net/profile/Seyed-Alavian-2/publication/305877907/figure/fig1/AS:391643644612615@1470386529847/Direct-Acting-Antiviral-Agents-for-Treatment-of-Hepatitis-C-Virus-Infection.png.

15.3.2. Recent Breakthroughs in Antiviral Drugs

New advances in antiviral treatment are the core of the practice of hepatology, with a very significant impact on the therapy of viral hepatitis, especially Hepatitis B and C. The introduction of DAAs revolutionized the treatment of these infections and offered highly potent therapy with the ability to induce long-lasting virological responses in most patients. These new therapies work by targeting individual stages of the viral life cycle, thus minimizing the chance for resistance—a major consideration for the treatment of chronic infection. Furthermore, the ability to modulate treatment regimens according to genetic profiling maximizes the effectiveness of these drugs, making targeted medicine a guiding principle of contemporary antiviral therapy. This modification not only improves the outcomes of patients but also reduces the economic burden of CLD, reinforcing the necessity for ongoing investigations into new antiviral drugs and mechanisms of action (Kim *et al.*, 2024). In addition to traditional antiviral drugs, the incorporation of new technologies, such as AI, is enabling unparalleled developments in the identification of antiviral medications. AI allows the discovery of new compounds by being able to make predictive modeling and data analysis stronger. For instance, ML algorithms can be applied to analyze complex genomic data to identify potential therapeutic targets, hence facilitating easier drug development. This is especially so in the situation involving new and rare hepatitis virus genotypes, where classic genotyping methods may not work. By providing glimpses into viral mutations and resistance patterns, AI facilitates the creation of more effective and scalable antiviral therapies targeted to individual patient profiles. Such developments point to the intersection of computer science and medicine in meeting global health challenges related to viral hepatitis (Kim *et al.*, 2024). Besides direct application in hepatitis treatment, the discoveries in antiviral drugs are also providing opportunities for the establishment of immunotherapy and liver transplantation. The development of antiviral drugs that can eliminate the virus would also enhance the success rate of liver transplantation by preventing the re-emergence of viral disease following transplantation. Furthermore, the synergy produced by combining antiviral therapy with immunotherapeutic modalities can lead to synergistic effects, enhancing the overall immune response against persistent viral infections globally. Treatment paradigms and patient care throughout the continuum of liver disease will be increasingly shaped by the ability to combine in the future. As research continues to explore the complex interactions between viruses, host responses, and therapeutic regimens, it is evident that advances in antiviral drugs are not only about meeting short-term viral challenges but also about laying the foundations for authoritative answers to the treatment of liver disease (Kumar *et al.*, 2024) (Figure 15.8).

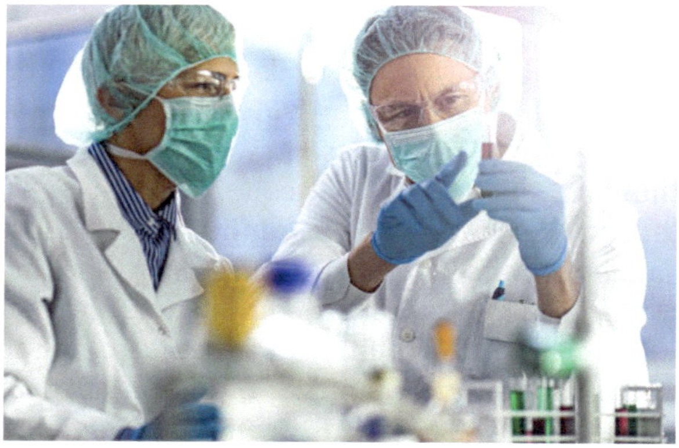

Figure 15.8. Antiviral Drugs

Source: https://media.istockphoto.com/id/1216332497/photo/chemists-cooperating-while-analyzing-chemical-substance-in-laboratory.jpg?s=612x612&w=0&k=20&c=5HkLIjl3tztxTceVDa5Uoc0EoEc7IzK-uG4JeRyhgLg=.

15.3.3. Challenges in Antiviral Therapy

There are many difficulties in antiviral therapy for hepatological diseases that hinder effective treatment. A major concern is that viruses can become resistant to drugs, which makes it harder to treat Hepatitis B and C. When viruses evolve, they can obtain mutations that help them escape the immune system or resist antiviral drugs, which can cause treatment to fail. Also, because viral genotypes vary, it becomes necessary to adapt antiviral drugs, which may complicate treatment and make it more expensive. Because viral infections keep changing, healthcare professionals must follow new developments and treatments that may not be fully described in available pharmacological information. In addition, many people find it hard to stick to antiviral treatment, which is a major problem for viral hepatitis. Because hepatitis infections are chronic, patients may have to take treatment for many months or even years. The long-term nature of treatment can cause patients to have trouble following the plan, which may be affected by side effects, the fear of becoming dependent, or the emotional stress of a long-term disease. Poor adherence to the treatment plan reduces the effectiveness of antiviral drugs and increases the chance of resistant viral strains appearing. The situation is further complicated by the socioeconomic status of patients with liver diseases; those from lower socioeconomic groups may not be able to get the healthcare resources they need, such as regular check-ups and needed medications. It is important to use many approaches, such as informing patients about the value of regular therapy and making mental health support available. In addition, there are problems in antiviral therapy besides drug resistance and patient compliance, such as the difficulty in correctly diagnosing and following viral infections. Biomarkers that do not require surgery and modern imaging techniques have helped a lot in spotting and following liver diseases early on. Still, using these technologies in daily medical care has been difficult because biomarkers do not always work the same in different laboratories. Proper management of antiviral therapy includes using reliable tests to check how the treatment is working and if the disease is getting better or worse, highlighting the importance of cooperation among different specialists in hepatology. By fostering cooperation among researchers, clinicians, and diagnostic professionals, healthcare systems can enhance their strategic approach to managing antiviral therapy challenges and improve patient outcomes significantly, as outlined in studies exploring HCC management strategies and associated risk factors (Friedman *et al.*, 2018).

15.4. Immunotherapy in Liver Disease

Managing liver diseases, especially HCC, is tough because of the disease's complex nature and the liver's complex environment. The unusual way the liver responds to immune cells usually prevents the immune system from working well, which has made it difficult for conventional therapies to be successful. Emerging evidence suggests that leveraging immune checkpoint inhibitors (ICI) and cellular therapies can re-establish immune surveillance against tumor cells, thereby enhancing the body's capacity to fight HCC.

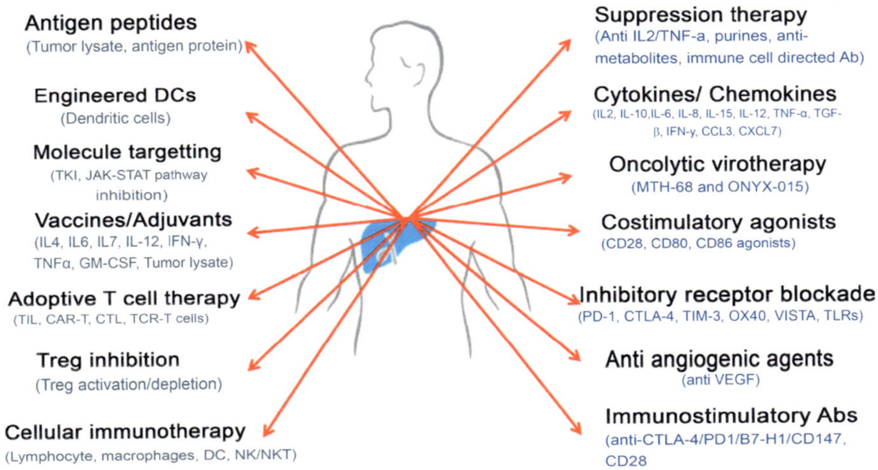

Figure 15.9. Various immunotherapeutic approaches for the treatment of liver diseases like HCC, NAFLD, ALD, DILI and autoimmune liver diseases.

Source: https://www.researchgate.net/profile/Pramod-Upadhyay-2/publication/310458850/figure/fig1/AS:440929237639168@1482137130220/Fig-2-Various-immunotherapeutic-approaches-for-the-treatment-of-liver-diseases-like.png.

By focusing on immunotherapy, the treatment of HCC is now more likely to combine surgical, medical, and palliative methods, leading to better patient outcomes. New progress in immunotherapy has made it clear that knowing biomarkers that predict treatment responses in liver diseases is very important. Finding and confirming biomarkers could lead to personalized ways of treating patients, which would improve immunotherapy. For example, the number and types of immune cells, as well as cytokines, in the tumor area, may indicate how well checkpoint inhibitors will work. Also, combining biomarker analysis with non-invasive fibrosis assessments gives a complete picture of the disease and aids in choosing the right treatment. As a result, clinicians are able to design immunotherapy plans that suit each patient, which is important for precision medicine in hepatology. Also, studies are being done to use immunotherapy with other therapies such as targeted drugs and antiviral treatments, which are improving the way HCC is managed. Trying these combinations in clinical trials has revealed better results against cancer, suggesting that they might help overcome the resistance found in HCC. As these studies continue, they may help change the usual treatment approaches for liver disease by making immunotherapy a key part of care. This synergistic approach could potentially lead to improved survival rates and quality of life for patients afflicted with liver malignancies, marking significant strides in the field of hepatology as it navigates the complexities of treatment (Figure 15.9).

15.4.1. Mechanisms of Immunotherapy

The immunotherapies' mechanisms have become increasingly prominent in the field of hepatology, particularly in liver cancer therapy and treatment of viral hepatitis. Immunotherapy employs the body's immune response to recognize and kill cancer cells, a strategy integral to combat against HCC, or the most prevalent form of liver cancer. With ICIs, such as anti-PD-1 and anti-CTLA-4 antibodies, researchers aim to prevent the cancer cells from exploiting the tumor-suppressing signals. The drugs restore T-cell function, making it easier for the body to recognize and destroy cancerous cells. The addition of these new therapies to the field of hepatology has spurred further research with a goal toward the explanation of some immunological aspects of liver cancers, thereby maximizing therapy and improving patient outcomes in the context of liver disease (Kim *et al.*, 2024). In addition, application of immunotherapy in the management of chronic viral hepatitis, namely hepatitis B and C, has made encouraging advances. The presence of viral antigens can provide an atmosphere of immune tolerance, which inhibits the functioning of the immune system. Immunotherapeutic approaches are focused on augmenting a better immune response against such pathogens by therapeutic vaccines and cytokine-based therapy. Immune-modulating agents in combination with antiviral therapies have been targeted in recent research on the dual front of viral multiplication and immunological reaction to achieve maximum treatment outcome. These dual strategies represent a step towards personalized medicine, where patient and disease profiles are used to design individualized immunotherapeutic protocols, ultimately aiming for virus eradication and liver function improvement (Kim *et al.*, 2024). Liver organoid development and advanced *in vitro* models also hold significance in figuring out the mechanisms of immunotherapy. Such models enable scientists to investigate liver-specific immune responses in a controlled setting, allowing for close inspection of the action of therapeutic compounds on liver cells and the immediate immune tissues. With continuing development in organoid technology, there is great promise in high-throughput screening of immunotherapeutic agents and exploration of their impact on liver pathology in a more representative model. Also, the systems encourage exploration of personalized treatment protocols because organoids can be derived from individual patients, thus facilitating individualized immunotherapeutic treatments. In this way, integration of organoid research into the area of liver immunotherapy not only consolidates knowledge of the underlying mechanisms but also accelerates translation of emerging therapies into the clinic (Alvarado-Tapias *et al.*, 2024) (Figure 15.10).

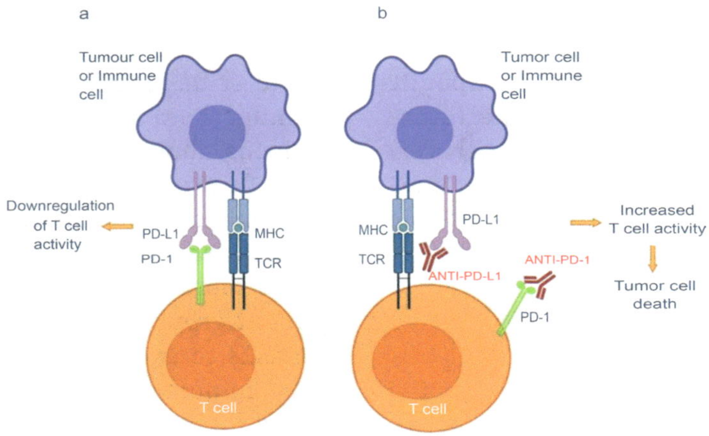

Figure 15.10. Schematic representation of PD-1 and anti-PD-1/PD-L1 mechanisms of action on T cell activity.

Source: https://www.researchgate.net/publication/342750704/figure/fig3/AS:11431281210515913@1702050475646/Schematic-representation-of-PD-1-and-anti-PD-1-PD-L1-mechanisms-of-action-on-T-cell.tif.

15.4.2. Current Applications in Hepatology

A major progress in hepatology is the use of new biomarkers to help diagnose liver diseases and monitor patient response to treatment. Biomarkers facilitate risk stratification and disease progression evaluation, making them essential in the management of conditions such as hepatitis B and C, alcoholic liver disease (ALD), and non-alcoholic fatty liver disease (NAFLD). Lately, researchers have looked into serum biomarkers, especially those related to fibrogenesis, which help assess liver fibrosis without requiring a liver biopsy. They make it possible to understand liver problems more completely and with less risk and discomfort for patients. Additionally, ongoing studies aim to identify further biomarkers that could predict treatment responses and long-term outcomes, paving the way for more personalized therapeutic approaches in hepatology and less reliance on invasive diagnostic techniques that carry potential complications (Kim *et al.*, 2024). Organoid technology is also being explored in hepatology, which could lead to major changes in the field. Researchers use organoids, which are made from liver stem cells, to study liver diseases because they closely resemble the human liver. Making liver organoids that self-organize helps scientists study diseases and test drugs on them, without the need for animal testing, and also increases knowledge about liver microenvironments and how cells interact with different drugs. The progress in organoid technology enables researchers to screen many samples and target drugs precisely, which is not possible with regular 2D cell culture systems. Furthermore, these organoids can be generated from patient-specific cells, providing invaluable insights into individual disease mechanisms and responses, thus advancing personalized medicine efforts in liver disease management (Kim *et al.*, 2024). Besides using diagnostics and research, there have been major improvements in treating liver diseases with antiviral drugs and immunotherapy, mainly for viral hepatitis. Because of new antiviral drugs, it is now possible for many people with hepatitis C to be cured by achieving SVR. In addition, immunotherapy, for example, with checkpoint inhibitors and therapeutic vaccines, is being noticed for its ability to boost the immune response to hepatitis B and HCC. They show how treatments are now designed to use the immune system to treat liver diseases. As ongoing research identifies new therapeutic agents and combination therapies, the future of liver disease treatment may increasingly rely on harnessing the immune system, ultimately improving patient outcomes and quality of life (Alvarado-Tapias *et al.*, 2024).

15.4.3. Future Perspectives on Immunotherapy

Because HCC is a difficult disease to treat, immunotherapy is expected to have a major impact on its management. Although ICI and similar treatments have improved patient results, some issues still exist, for example, the rise of drug resistance. Knowing the molecular changes in HCC has helped find important mutations that may be targeted with immunotherapy. Also, scientists are studying how to combine immunotherapy with other drugs, such as targeted therapies and antiviral agents, which could make them more effective. Addressing the unmet needs highlighted in recent studies, particularly regarding patient stratification through biomarkers, will be essential in tailoring immunotherapy treatments to individual patients, ultimately leading to better survival rates and quality of life improvements for those afflicted by this disease (Gores *et al.*, 2018). NGS is making it possible to study HCC at the genetic level, which is having a big impact on immunotherapy. NGS makes it possible to carefully study both viral and host genomes, which helps find the unique mutations that contribute to cancer and affect the response to treatment. If clinicians know the exact genetic changes, they can choose immunotherapeutic options that fit the patient's disease. With more resistance to therapies being seen, NGS makes it possible to create personalized treatments that address these resistant strains, so treatment is more effective. Furthermore, integrating AI to process NGS data holds the potential to enhance predictive modeling and treatment planning, ultimately pushing the boundaries of precision medicine in HCC management (Apte *et al.*, 2025). Advanced sequencing and immunotherapy working together are expected to bring about a new age in cancer treatment. The future of immunotherapy for HCC is influenced by technology, our knowledge of tumors, and by making clinical guidelines for these therapies better. Focusing on particular patient groups and using thorough biomarker systems to track how treatments work will be very important. These covers examine how liquid biopsies can give us instant information about the behavior of tumors and the immune system during treatment. Also, working together with pharmaceutical companies can help move new immunotherapeutic agents from research settings to use in the clinic. With a concerted effort directed towards overcoming existing barriers, the integration of immunotherapy into standard care pathways for HCC holds the promise of significantly improving outcomes and extending the therapeutic arsenal against this formidable cancer (Gores *et al.*, 2018).

15.5. Emerging Liver Support Technologies

In the past several years, hepatology has made tremendous strides in liver support technologies in response to the inadequacies of standard approaches to treating liver failure. Foremost among these advances are bioartificial liver (BAL) systems, intended to offer temporary liver function support until patients are candidates for liver transplantation or have resolved acute liver injury. These systems employ human liver cells or other biomaterials to perform the hepatic functions, such as detoxification and protein synthesis. Employment of sophisticated biomaterials has been indicated to be effective in enhancing the potency and biocompatibility of these systems to be translated into clinical applications that can possibly reduce ALF mortality. Therefore, bioartificial devices have emerged as an essential adjunct to the management of liver disease and demonstrated the central position of technology in providing new treatment possibilities and improving patient care in hepatology. Another intriguing potential with future liver support technologies is the development of ambulatory and wearable devices to monitor liver function in real-time. Such devices are made to offer real-time assessment through non-invasive biomarker analysis, hence allowing clinicians to customize treatment protocols according to individual patient requirements. An example includes incorporating molecular sensors to detect certain biomarkers associated with liver impairment as a groundbreaking leap ahead in tracking disease progression. Employing technology in this capacity not only raises patient engagement by providing them with real-time data about their health status but also allows health professionals to take action more proactively. With technology continuing to develop, such technologies could radically advance the control of liver ailments, ultimately leading to enhanced patient' outcomes as well as reduced healthcare costs in CLD management. Lastly, cell therapy advances are a revolutionary area for liver support technologies. Techniques such as stem cell therapy and hepatocyte transplant are gaining popularity as acceptable alternatives for patients with liver failure who are too ill to qualify for transplant or who are awaiting a donor organ. These procedures are aimed at the restoration of hepatic function through the exchange of failed liver cells with new cells derived from stem cells or other sources. Current reports have highlighted the regenerative potential of these treatments with promising results from initial clinical and preclinical trials. The future holds the promise of personalized medicine, and with such regenerative approaches on board, the landscape of treating liver disease can be revolutionized. The innovation of these technologies reflects a desire for creative solutions in hepatology in response to the need for ongoing research and development to offset the challenges that liver health issues present.

15.5.1. Overview of Liver Support Systems

The liver performs various physiological processes like metabolism, detoxification, and immune system regulation. Because of its complex functions, hepatic support systems become necessary to maintain hepatic function in patients with acute or chronic liver failure. Traditional therapy has predominantly involved organ transplantation; however, the unavailability of donor organs stimulated the quest for novel liver support technology. These technologies aspire to provide temporary or prolonged support for liver failure patients, thereby stabilizing their health until eventual transplantation or liver function restoration. Emerging new technologies in artificial liver support, such as BAL devices, are arising because they mimic the liver's metabolic and synthetic functions, thereby ultimately improving survival rates in individuals afflicted with severe hepatic privations. New liver support technologies extend beyond artificial systems by incorporating biomolecular approaches to enhance liver function and recovery. Recent observations indicate the promise of stem cell therapies and gene therapy as possible modalities in reconstructing liver tissue following injury or in correcting genetic abnormalities. The ongoing exploration of such new approaches is in accordance with the necessity of aggressive multidisciplinary treatment strategies in effectively treating liver diseases. A core aspect of enhancing liver support systems is the integration of biomarkers and non-invasive assessments. These may provide useful information regarding a patient's liver condition, in order that interventions can be instituted in a timely manner, and treatment regimens maximized. As emphasized in ongoing research, better biomarkers can enable therapy stratification, whereby patients are provided with individualized care according to their specific liver condition and status. Despite the significant advancements made in liver support systems, the best therapy protocols are still an issue as well as affording equal access to such developments. Clinical input from every specialty must come together in order to create a holistic management plan for liver disease patients, particularly HCC. It is worth noting that the global burden of HCC emphasizes establishing effective multidisciplinary treatment plans between clinicians to enhance patient outcomes. A foundation for this multimodal treatment is the Barcelona Clinic Liver Cancer staging system, through which clinicians can allocate appropriate treatments by disease stage and individual patient needs. The necessity for ongoing research and clinical creativity, creation of more advanced trial designs, and conjoining new therapeutic modalities are essential to address the unmet requirements in HCC care and for general liver health, as underscored in the liver support system literature (Gores *et al.*, 2018) (Figure 15.11).

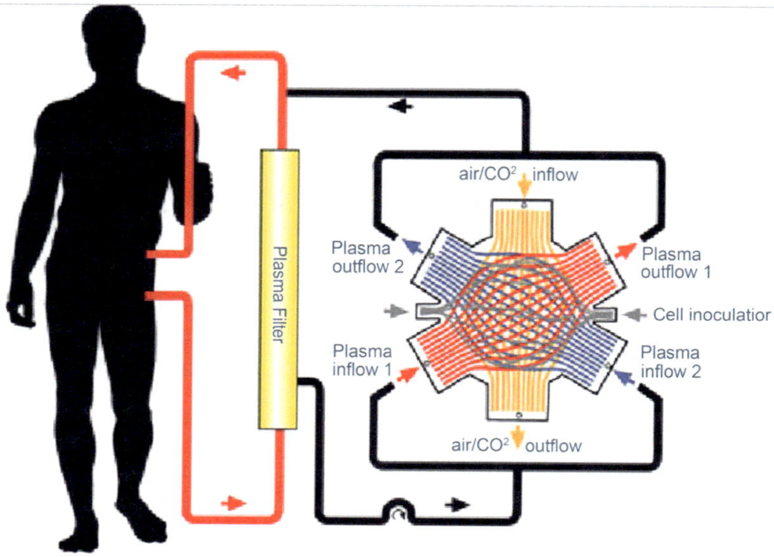

Figure 15.11. Extracorporeal liver support system based on a multicompartment bioreactor technology for high-density perfusion culture of liver cells.

Source: https://www.researchgate.net/profile/Thomas-Weiss-15/publication/50990780/figure/fig1/AS:394273674547206@1471013577375/Extracorporeal-liver-support-system-based-on-a-multicompartment-bioreactor-technology-for.png.

15.5.2. Innovations in Artificial Liver Devices

The area of artificial liver devices is experiencing fantastic progress, which is primarily centered on avoiding the organ shortage crisis faced during liver transplantation. The advancements involve a variety of technologies employed for temporary liver support to enable the patient to survive until a transplant is acquired. One such method involves bioengineered devices that replicate hepatic function by employing sophisticated bioreactor systems, which can provide essential metabolic and synthetic functions. The emerging use of organoids in this context has also been of much interest. These 3D cell cultures not only mimic liver function but also expand personalized medicine uses, with prospects for individualized therapies according to patients' individual needs. This application is particularly relevant considering limitations in the use of traditional donor organ availability and necessitating keeping up with treating ALF cases (Kim *et al.*, 2024). Further research on artificial liver devices has focused on greater integration of bioartificial technology using cellular components in conjunction with man-made materials. BALs attempt to create a more physiologically appropriate environment, hence better biocompatibility, and functional viability. The incorporation of stem cell-derived hepatocytes, for instance, in such devices guarantees greater metabolic functions and reduces immune rejection. With increasingly sophisticated multicellular systems being engineered, researchers are investigating how to amplify the dynamic interaction of liver cells with other vital anatomical components through organ-on-chip systems. Not only does this provide a prospect for drug screening but for the examination of sophisticated liver pathophysiology, thus playing central roles in new therapeutic interventions in hepatology (Alvarado-Tapias *et al.*, 2024). Recent advancements in artificial liver devices also involve the application of new biomaterials and nanotechnology, which have great potential for improving the performance of the device. Employing smart biomaterials that respond dynamically to the biochemical environment is the aim of researchers to enhance overall efficiency and lifespan of the devices. Nanotechnology, in particular, holds the potential to enhance the interaction of liver cells with the artificial substrates, marking a new era of optimized functionality. Moreover, the use of predictive analytics and ML in solution design can make it possible to customize therapeutic interventions, tailoring interventions that address particular pathologic conditions. As they mature, continual research is needed to address concerns such as scalability and regulation issues to allow them to be effectively utilized within clinical settings (Alvarado-Tapias *et al.*, 2024) (Figure 15.12).

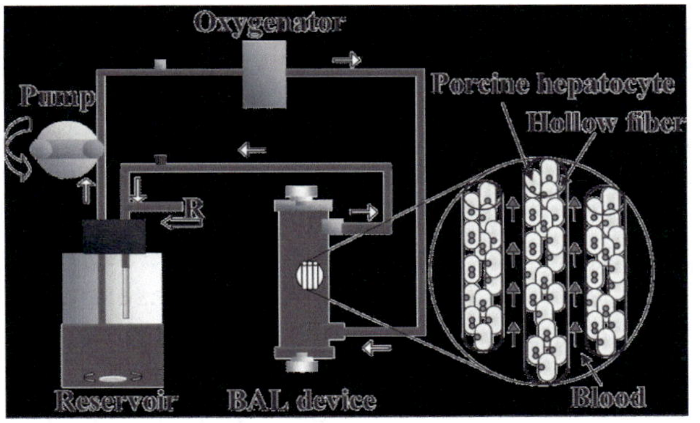

Figure 15.12. Schematic representation of the bioartificial liver (BAL) device and the *in vitro* circulating system used for evaluation of its function.

Source: https://www.researchgate.net/profile/Yuichiro-Ueda-2/publication/226755535/figure/fig1/AS:545650720731136@1507104677489/Schematic-representation-of-the-bioartificial-liver-BAL-device-and-the-in-vitro.png.

15.5.3. Future Trends in Liver Support Technologies

The creation of liver support technology is at the forefront of hepatology advancements, with state-of-the-art specializations such as synthetic biology playing a central role. As traditional liver support has a tendency to be restrictive, researchers have turned to the use of engineered organisms, the greatest being *Saccharomyces cerevisiae*. This yeast has developed from an accidental fermentation catalyst to a promising collaborator in the medical field, with potential applications such as live biotherapeutic products for the therapy of liver disease *in situ*. The prospect of using engineered yeasts as cell factories for therapeutics and vaccines foretells a new era for the treatment of liver diseases, perhaps both safely and effectively. These advancements, aided by synthetic biology, offer a route to personalized liver support therapies that have the potential to cure many types of liver diseases, altering clinical outcomes and patient courses in hepatology (Maneira *et al.*, 2025). Concurrent with synthetic biology advancements, current liver support technologies are being advanced to more complex, non-invasive modalities. The application of biomarkers with real-time sensing using biosensors is evolving as an important augmentation of traditional methodology. Such non-invasive sensors have the promise to advise clinicians with important information about liver function with fewer discomforts to patients than can be achieved with invasive methods. Using biomarkers, including proteins that are markers for inflammatory responses, diagnosis and therapy can be enhanced early on, potentially avoiding extensive damage to the liver. These advances not only reflect changes in medical practice but also highlight the need for patient-centered approaches to hepatology. As liver support continues to advance, technological innovation complementing clinical practice is essential in delivering timely and effective interventions, classically demonstrating dependence of patient care and research (Halldorsdottir, 2024). The potential of liver support technologies is also directly linked to advances in regenerative medicine and gene therapy. As it becomes better understood about liver regeneration processes and the cell biology behind them, scientists are ever more actively exploring methods of inducing liver repair and function through new gene-editing techniques. The potential to apply CRISPR-Cas9 and other gene editing tools offers a promising field in the treatment of genetic liver diseases through direct modification at the cellular level. Furthermore, the potential to combine gene therapy with liver support technologies may open a way for a synergistic effect where injured liver can be supported as well as functionally reconstituted. These advances foretell prospects for personalized therapies that would significantly alter patient outcomes. With the growing horizon of liver support, the integration of biotechnology, cellular therapy, and regenerative techniques will be crucial towards holistic treatment of patients with liver diseases, beginning a new era in hepatology (Figure 15.13) (Maneira *et al.*, 2025).

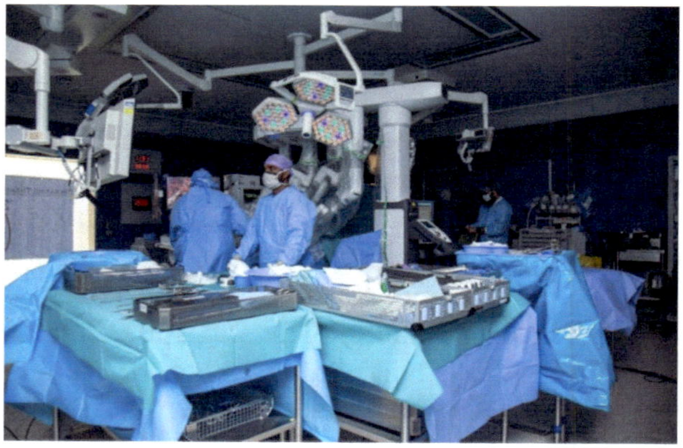

Figure 15.13. Future Trends in Liver Support Technologies

Source: https://www.saudigazette.com.sa/uploads/images/2023/09/27/2160520.jpg.

15.6. Future Directions in Liver Transplantation

The future of liver transplantation is being dictated more and more by regenerative medicine progress, specifically through the development of liver organoids. These three-dimensional structures formed through the self-organization of adult stem cells hold the promise to overcome the shortage crisis of allogeneic liver transplantation donor organs. Even though a fully functional liver organoid remains elusive, the impact of these technologies is already being felt in most fields of hepatology, including disease modeling and high-throughput drug screening. With researchers working on more complicated systems, such as multicellular assemblies and organoid-on-chip platforms, the ability for complex modeling of liver microenvironments expands. Though tumorigenicity and biocompatibility concerns remain, organoid technology advances are also revealing new approaches to transplantation with the promise to revolutionize patient outcomes and enable more personalized intervention in the treatment of liver disease, as observed in the advancements outlined in current research (Kim *et al.*, 2024). The integration of biomarkers and non-invasive tests in liver transplant plans is an important area for increasing post-transplant and pre-transplant surveillance. Emerging technologies such as transient elastography and ELF measurement provide valuable data regarding the fibrotic condition of transplant candidates. A new study revealed similar rates of fibrosis reversal and progression in HBsAg seroclearance patients and treatment-naive controls, noting that liver stiffness measurements are useful in determining the patients appropriately without subjecting them to invasive biopsy procedures. With biomarkers being increasingly used to establish the likelihood of successful transplant outcomes, advancing the development of these diagnostic tools will enable patients to receive treatment in a timely fashion, thus reducing the occurrence of post-transplant morbidity and enhancing graft survival. In addition to enhancing the usage of biomarkers, gene therapy is emerging as a revolutionary method in the future of liver transplantation. With scientists drawing nearer to being able to manipulate genetic material in order to correct underlying genetic defects, the optimism to be able to cure illnesses such as familial hypercholesterolemia (FH) and certain liver diseases becomes all the greater. The existence of adeno-associated viral vectors has already shown itself to be an effective means to get therapeutic genes directly into liver cells. This could potentially complement liver transplantation procedures to improve patient recovery and reduce dependency on long-term immunosuppression. Furthermore, combining gene therapy with sophisticated organoid technology would make pre-transplant evaluation and post-transplant recovery protocols optimal, making this procedure not only a life-saving procedure but also a pathway toward curative treatment for liver disease in the coming years (Kim *et al.*, 2024).

15.6.1. Advances in Transplant Techniques

The technique of liver transplantation has also improved tremendously over the recent years, resulting in improved patient outcomes among those suffering from liver disease. One key factor in such progress is the enhancement of surgical technique, particularly that of laparoscopic liver resection (LLR). The minimally invasive procedure has been seen to enhance periods of recovery and reduce postoperative complications, which was also found to be particularly beneficial to patients with HCC and other states of disease. The laparoscopic technique, in conjunction with innovations such as three-dimensional computed tomography (3D-CT) and indocyanine green near-infrared fluorescence imaging, facilitates surgical precision and planning during liver transection. With advancing surgical technique, the merit of individualized approaches that cater to the unique anatomical and pathological challenges faced by the patient is increasingly evident, uncovering innovations that are revolutionizing transplant procedures and patient management in hepatology at large (Alvarado-Tapias *et al.*, 2024). Another important area of development in transplant procedures is the use of novel biomarkers and non-invasive assessment tools, which would substantially enhance donor organ procurement and post-transplant management (Figure 15.14).

Traditional methods of monitoring the liver's function, as well as assessing organ donor viability, have been relying mostly on invasive methods that undermine the safety of patients. The introduction of new biomarkers in clinical practice allows capable, real-time evaluation of liver function, thus facilitating more rational transplantation decision-making.

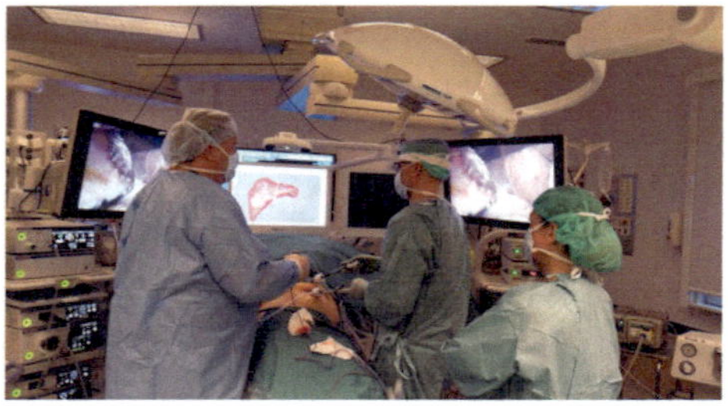

Figure 15.14. Advances in Transplant Techniques

Source: https://www.tandfonline.com/cms/asset/2a5d9e72-e7ff-4676-8008-32fbc672ce38/imit_a_1727524_f0001_c.jpg.

Emerging research presented at the 5th Translational Hepatology Meeting underscores the need for continued efforts to demystify such biomarkers in order to address the clinical challenges surrounding liver transplantation. As the field continues to progress, how technical advancement and surgical advancement work together will become central to optimizing outcomes and refining transplantation protocols (Alvarado-Tapias *et al.*, 2024). Lastly, gene therapy research provides a hopeful advantage in the arena of liver transplantation. Emerging evidence proposes that genetic manipulation may be utilized to promote liver regeneration and maximize transplant acceptance rates and offer solutions to the limitations imposed upon traditional pharmacologic immunosuppressive treatments. CRISPR-Cas9 methods provide assays for precise gene editing, holding promising opportunities to correct genetic disease and disposable transplantation complications. As these technologies continue to be refined, the potential of gene therapy in the future can revolutionize the field of liver transplantation. By enabling more effective incorporation of transplanted tissue and support of healthy liver function, gene therapy is a key player in the future of transplant techniques and hepatology (Figure 15.15).

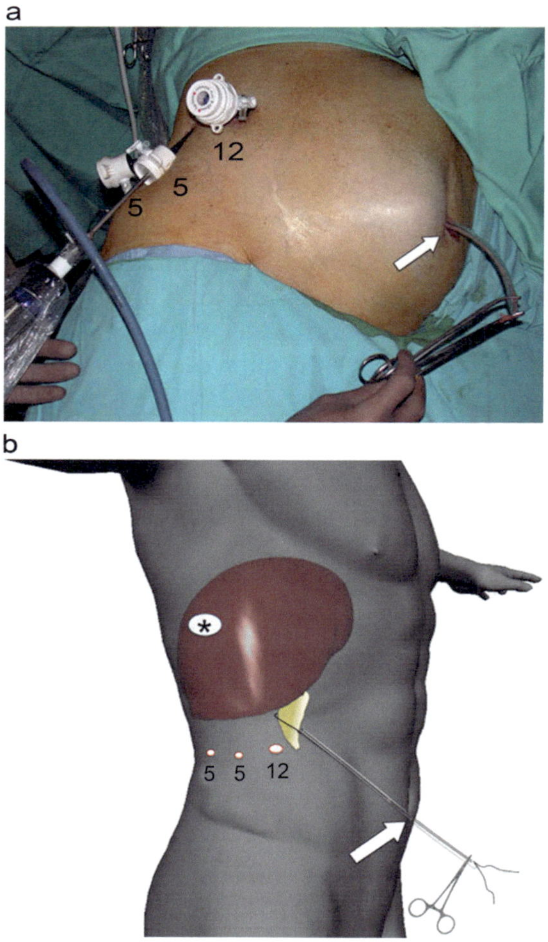

Figure 15.15. a Patient and trocar position for laparoscopic resection of lesions posteriorly located: segments 6 and 7 and posterior areas of segments 5 and 8; b schema of this position with the tourniquet in place. The asterisk indicates the lesion. The white arrow points the Tiemann catheter in the place where the tourniquet becomes extracorporeal.

Source: https://www.researchgate.net/profile/Fernando-Pardo-3/publication/51901415/figure/fig2/AS:601634031812608@1520452139031/a-Patient-and-trocar-position-for-laparoscopic-resection-of-lesions-posteriorly-located.png.

15.6.2. Innovations in Post-Transplant Care

In the past few years, developments in post-transplant management have dramatically improved the treatment and rehabilitation of liver transplant patients. An interesting development is the integration of telemedicine in the normal follow-up and monitoring regimen. This has the advantage of making the patients more accessible to healthcare professionals, allowing them to intervene in a timely manner in case of complications. By allowing patients undergoing transplants to have their vitals and transplant-related symptoms monitored remotely, telemedicine allows for increased patient compliance with follow-up visits and a reduction in the workload of the health facility. Furthermore, the integration of advanced data analytics with telemonitoring platforms can allow for patient health patterns to be understood, guiding individualized therapeutic management that may optimize recovery and improve long-term outcomes. These developments underscore a key shift to a more patient-centered model of care, aimed at optimizing post-transplant quality of life and ensuring graft longevity through preventive care strategies. Concurrent with telemedicine, the introduction of new biomarkers has changed the practice of post-transplant care. Biomarkers are at the hub of the early detection of allograft rejection and other complications. There has been work on the detection of specific protein profiles and genetic markers that predict impending rejection, allowing for early intervention before significant damage has occurred. Introduction of non-invasive blood tests to monitor liver function and status of transplant has been a giant leap away from the crude method of invasive biopsy, traditionally accompanied by associated complications. Through such advanced biomarker analysis, clinicians can more effectively tailor immunosuppressive therapy, minimizing toxicity and maximizing graft survival rates. In doing so, focus on biomarker-guided care not only underpins personalized medicine but also contributes to the overall prognosis among liver transplant patients, representing a significant advancement within hepatology and post-transplant care (Chu, 2018). Another significant area of innovation surrounds the development of advanced immunotherapy protocols for maximizing outcomes following transplant. Individualized immunosuppressive regimens are now the key to the prevention of graft rejection without the risk of infection and other complications of long-term immunosuppression. New drugs that modulate specific immune response pathways provide a vehicle for optimizing the protection of the grafts against side effects. Therapies that influence T-cell function, for instance, have been promising in generating adequate immunosuppression without additional complications. Moreover, ongoing clinical trials into the synergy from using these treatments in conjunction with antiviral drugs aim to treat co-infections that threaten transplant success. These developments in immunotherapy are a guarantee of hope for post-transplant therapy, and they provide an opening into improved patient outcomes and potentially new standards in liver transplant care (Chu, 2018) (Figure 15.16).

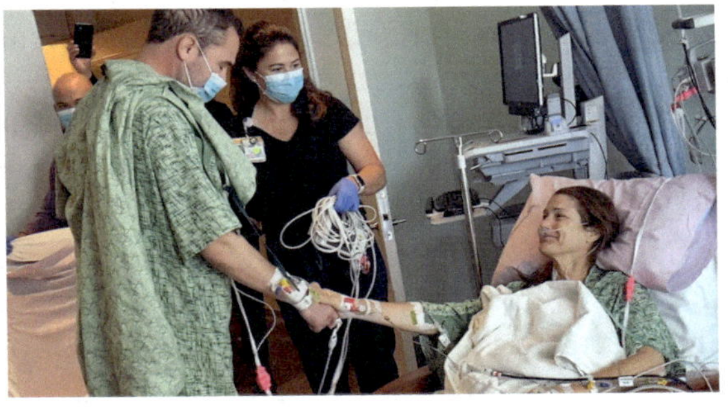

Figure 15.16. Post-Transplant Care

Source: https://health.ucsd.edu/globalassets/video-thumbnails/liver-transplant-living-donor-thumbnail.jpg?width=1920&quality=80.

15.6.3. Ethical Considerations in Transplantation

Because organ transplantation and especially liver transplantation involve many ethical issues, it is important to carefully examine the principles used for choosing donors, setting criteria, and making allocations. There is a major ethical concern about ensuring fairness in assigning donor organs because more people need them, and there are not enough. It brings up important issues about justice and fairness, such as who should get a transplant and why. Medical need, the chances of success, and psychosocial aspects play a major role in deciding who gets a transplant. Organizations such as the United Network for Organ Sharing (UNOS) attempt to normalize these criteria to bridge the gap between organs available and the needs of the patients. Even so, biases might affect the system, which can result in unfairness concerning social class, race, or place of residence. Because of this, the process of organ allocation should be open, fair, and accountable to represent these details. Besides organ allocation, ethical issues in transplantation are very similar to those involving informed consent, mainly for living donors. Making sure potential donors know exactly what their donation means is the main way to maintain ethical standards. It is not enough to inform; true informed consent means donors are not coerced to donate. The living donor-healthcare provider relationship demands a fine balance between promoting the donor's and recipient's medical needs and advocating for their welfare. Now that gene therapy and other new therapies are being developed in transplantation, the ethical questions about donor health, the long-term consequences and handling new technologies become more important. Recent issues have shown that each case is different and so needs careful and specific ethical attention in transplantation. In addition, ethics in transplantation are important in post-operative care and follow-up, not only in choosing who receives organs and getting consent. Even with better results in hepatology, there are still ethical issues in looking after patients after transplantation, mainly about following treatment and making changes in lifestyle. The need for patients to keep taking their medicine causes tension between their own freedom and what is good for everyone. In this case, healthcare professionals have to convince patients to follow the advice while still respecting their right to make their own decisions. Ethical guidelines should support patient-focused care and handle public worries about non-compliance, mainly because it can influence future access to organs for transplantation. Effectively handling these intricacies is important not just for the treatment of individual patients but for the overall integrity of transplantation as a medical field, eventually shaping ethical guidelines in the future (Wazir *et al.*, 2023, 2025).

15.7. Gene Therapy in Hepatology

With our understanding of the molecular pathophysiology of HCC becoming more complex, gene therapy emerges as a rich field for new therapies. As HCC accounts for approximately 90% of primary liver cancer cases and ranks among the top cancer-related causes of death globally, new therapeutic options are indispensable (Gores *et al.*, 2018). Gene therapy would possibly target individual genetic mutations and faulty signaling pathways involved in liver cancers. By using techniques such as CRISPR-Cas9 and RNA interference, scientists hope to repair genetic defects or suppress oncogene expression. This approach not only offers a specific therapeutic modality but also allows therapy to be tailored to the individual molecular signature of patients' tumors, which is an essential unmet need in the therapy of HCC. The integration of gene therapy into the broad vision of hepatology highlights the necessity of synergy among multidisciplinary specialties to deliver comprehensive care to patients with liver disease. As HCC is a multifaceted disease and liver function is a multifaceted process, the treatment of this disease requires consultation from several specialties, including hepatology, oncology, and surgery. Gene therapy can be combined with existing treatment regimens by providing an adjuvant strategy that complements current treatments like resection, liver transplantation, and local ablation. The combination of gene therapy with immunotherapy boosts the immune response to tumor cells, which also leads to improved outcomes. It is thus through the ongoing clinical trials that safety, efficacy, and side effects of the treatment regimens are evaluated, ultimately leading to more complex treatment strategies. In the future, future developments in gene therapy will transform the practice of hepatology and liver cancer therapy. The emphasis of current research is on utilizing biomarkers to enhance patient stratification as well as monitoring response to therapy for gene therapies. This scenario emphasizes the necessity for identifying established biomarkers with predictive significance for the success of therapy and guiding subsequent treatment (Gores *et al.*, 2018). Furthermore, as research uncovers new gene delivery vehicles like viral vectors and nanoparticles, the administration route for gene therapies can be enhanced with efficiency and reduced in toxicity. Effective application of gene therapy in clinical practice not only has the potential to cure HCC but also broadens its applicability to other liver diseases, thus opening new vistas for hepatology research and patient care (Figure 15.17).

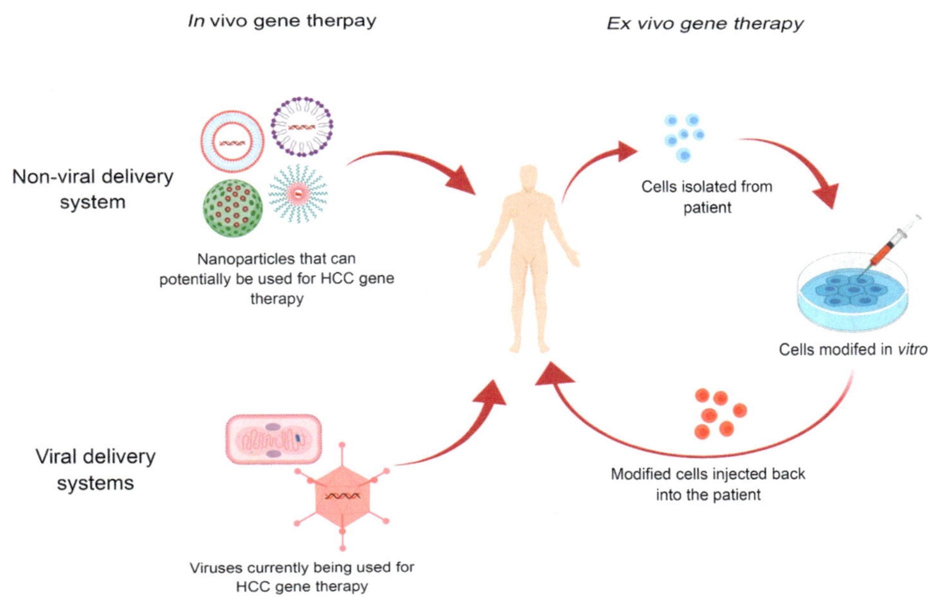

Figure 15.17. An overview of the types of gene therapy techniques used in HCC treatment.

Source: https://www.mdpi.com/cancers/cancers-11-01265/article_deploy/html/images/cancers-11-01265-g001.png.

15.7.1. Overview of Gene Therapy Approaches

Gene therapy has brought a new approach to treating liver diseases, especially as scientists work on finding new treatments for chronic diseases such as hepatitis and metabolic liver disorders. Gene therapy tries to fix genes that cause disease. It is possible by introducing corrected genes, using

CRISPR to fix errors in genes, and injecting RNA to stop disease-causing genes from working. They try to restore normal cellular functions and reverse harmful changes in the liver that lead to disruption. Surprisingly, gene therapy's potential goes beyond conventional therapies with possibilities for tailored medicine where therapies can be tailored to specific genetic profiles, thereby enhancing clinical outcomes in hepatology (Kim *et al.*, 2024). Researchers are working on useful gene therapy, and liver organoids have become popular because they can reproduce important liver functions and diseases in the lab. Liver cultures made from stem cells are like the liver's original cells and have its normal structures and functions. With organoids, scientists can better study diseases, see how drugs react, and handle gene editing cases, compared to using traditional cell culture or animal models. With these improvements, screening many samples at once and checking the cellular reaction to treatment in real time is now possible. With progress in the area, organoids are bound to make a significant advancement when it comes to comprehending liver pathophysiology and refining gene therapy for liver disease (Alvarado-Tapias *et al.*, 2024). Although gene therapy is promising, there are certain challenges. It is very difficult to safely direct therapeutic drugs to the liver cells, since their ability to reach their targets without harming the body is very important. Another issue is to handle the complex regulation of genes and ensure the gene modification remains stable over time. New ways, for example, using nanoparticles and viral vectors, are being looked into to address these issues. More studies are needed to perfect these methods, which makes gene therapy a good option for treating even more liver diseases. As the discipline advances, it can be expected that continuous breakthroughs will greatly impact the therapeutic scenario of hepatology in the next few years (Alvarado-Tapias *et al.*, 2024; Kim *et al.*, 2024).

15.7.2. Current Research in Gene Therapy for Liver Diseases

Scientists are moving forward rapidly with gene therapy for liver diseases, able to address genetic disorders, chronic hepatitis, and liver cancer. Researchers are considering using adeno-associated viruses (AAVs) to introduce therapeutic genes into liver cells directly, which has shown promise in preclinical models. Thanks to AAV gene therapy, people with hemophilia and α1-antitrypsin deficiency can now produce the necessary protein for a long period. CRISPR technology allows scientists to change genes more precisely, which might help address genetic changes that cause liver disease. Researchers are optimistic that such advances could mark the beginning of a new paradigm in the management of liver diseases, highlighting the importance of continued research in this promising area of hepatology, as seen in recent reviews taking into account the future of liver diseases (Wazir *et al.*, 2025) and the range of gene therapy strategies (Wazir *et al.*, 2023). At the same time, researchers are trying to improve how genes are delivered within the body. The liver's unique anatomical and physiological characteristics have a tendency to complicate the assays of efficient transfection rates without inducing unnecessary immune responses. The aim is to keep improving by making nanoparticles that can carry therapeutic genes and safely deliver them to hepatocytes. It is also being studied whether using certain ligands and antibodies that target receptors on liver cells can make gene therapy more accurate. Giving drugs to certain parts of the body will help the medicine work longer since global delivery can cause side effects elsewhere. The continued advancement of these technologies has the potential to enhance the translational value of gene therapy in the treatment of liver disease, underscoring the relevance of this area of study in hepatology (Wazir *et al.*, 2023). It is important in gene therapy studies to address ethical issues and obey the rules to keep patients safe and get accurate results. When gene therapy is used in practice, people will need to continue talking about informed consent, equal access, and what might happen in the long run from genetic changes. Regulatory authorities point out that gene therapy should be well evaluated to discover any possible effects of unexpected genetic changes on patients. Also, when clinical researchers, regulatory bodies, and ethics committees cooperate, it can help new treatments be approved more quickly. Discussing such ethical considerations, the field can not only foster public trust in gene therapy approaches for liver diseases but also pave the way towards novel treatments that are ethical according to society's expectations and healthcare objectives (Wazir *et al.*, 2023, 2025).

15.7.3. Future Prospects and Challenges

Because of progress in hepatology, both diagnosing and treating liver disease are expected to be bright, although the process may be complicated. The most important advance here is the creation of non-invasive biomarkers. They may greatly improve the way clinicians detect NAFLD and HCC. For a long time, doctors depended on invasive liver biopsies for diagnosis, which caused risks and discomfort for patients. It is also being studied how to create blood-based tests that can properly measure liver injury and the level of fibrosis. These innovations not only seek to improve patient safety and comfort but also seek to offer timely interventions that would dramatically enhance clinical outcomes in the treatment of liver disease, addressing associated complications that increase patient morbidity (Wazir *et al.*, 2025). Even with great progress in hepatology, there are many difficulties to overcome to ensure the best care for patients. The increasing global cases of viral hepatitis and NAFLD, which are mainly caused by unhealthy lifestyles, clearly call for focused public health actions. Since more patients are using the healthcare system, giving each one personalized therapy is now necessary. Treatments that consider a patient's genes, environment, and lifestyle may improve the treatment's effectiveness and adherence. But, for these strategies to be successful, the healthcare system needs strong infrastructure, more funding, and ongoing training of medical staff. Further, understanding the interfacing between liver pathology and extrinsic complications, such as socioeconomic status and access to health care, remains important in achieving overall solutions (Wazir *et al.*, 2023). As time goes on, using new liver support devices and therapies such as gene therapy and advanced immunotherapy will be very important for hepatology. Such advanced treatments increase hope for CLD patients and also help create ideas that can help prevent liver disease. Gene therapy research is helping to find new ways to cure genetic diseases, such as HCC. Also, as technology improves in liver transplantation, the chances of success are higher and complications are less likely, which benefits patients' well-being. While these exciting developments are met with regulation, ethical, and logistically complex challenges to navigate cautiously, so that such new treatments are provided to all patients in a fair way (Wazir *et al.*, 2025).

SUMMARY

These new discoveries in hepatology highlight the role of new technologies and methods in finding and treating liver disease. Finding new biomarkers and performing fibrosis tests without the need for invasive methods is a major change in how liver conditions are monitored and studied. With this change, patients feel better and specialists gain a clearer picture of how the liver works. As illustrated in recent proceedings like the 5th Translational Hepatology Meeting, there is a collective emphasis on integrating the latest molecular understanding and immunologic responses into daily care, further solidifying the foundation for upcoming models of managing liver disease (Alvarado-Tapias *et al.*, 2024). Advances in antiviral and immunotherapy give patients with chronic liver disease new hope. Targeted therapies have helped to improve how well hepatitis C and HCC are treated. Also, new liver support technologies give valuable help in treating ALF and allow for more options in liver transplantation. The ability to carry out more sophisticated surgical procedures, such as laparoscopic liver resection (LLR), signifies a greater inclination toward minimizing patient risk through optimizing the efficacy of surgical procedures, reflecting a better understanding of hepatic anatomy and physiology. Hepatology is set to make important progress in the future, especially in gene therapy and regenerative medicine. Gene-editing technology can help repair or replace liver tissues, which may change how we treat liver diseases. Further research on how well and safely these new therapies work over time will be very important for their use in medical practice. As hepatology advances, working together across different fields will be important for learning more, improving care for patients, and changing how liver diseases are managed and treated in the future.

Recent progress in hepatology has increased our knowledge and ways to manage liver diseases, mainly through biomarkers and non-invasive tests. Because of these developments, we can predict how much liver fibrosis there is and how likely it is for the liver to develop more serious diseases such as HCC. Using serum biomarkers and imaging techniques makes it possible for clinicians to find and treat liver disease early and track its progress without doing many liver biopsies. Using the latest literature, a wider, multidisciplinary approach to HCC treatment fits better with recent findings on how to treat patients, diagnose their condition correctly, and achieve the best outcomes. At the same time, new approaches to antiviral and immune therapy have been developed, mainly for people with CHB. The main goal of current treatments for CHB is to achieve a functional cure, which means losing HBsAg and stopping therapy. But current agents are not yet capable of reaching this goal. It points out that while reducing viral load is very important, this may not always be linked to a drop in HBsAg. Therefore, novel combinations of therapy with nucleos(t)ide analogues, immunomodulators, and new agents targeting antigen load are in development. Such approaches are intended to maximize patient outcomes by aligning therapy with biomarkers that forecast and monitor the efficacy of treatment (Baumert *et al.*, 2023). Also, new liver support technologies are making a big difference in treating advanced liver disease. They include new artificial liver devices that can help patients until they recover or need a transplant by giving their bodies temporary liver support. They become very important when standard medical care is not effective. Bioartificial approaches, which combine hepatocytes with biocompatible materials, have demonstrated potential in restoring liver function. Thanks to these developments, it is likely that patient care will improve, mainly for people dealing with ALF or end-stage liver disease. These technologies, being used in liver transplantation and gene therapy, will certainly shape the future of hepatology, showing that new approaches are still needed.

CLOSER LOOK

DIRECT-ACTING ANTIVIRAL AGENTS (DAAS)

DAAs are a class of medications that specifically target the hepatitis C virus (HCV) by inhibiting its replication cycle. These drugs are highly effective and well-tolerated, revolutionizing HCV treatment by achieving cure rates of over 95% in most patients (Figure 15.18).

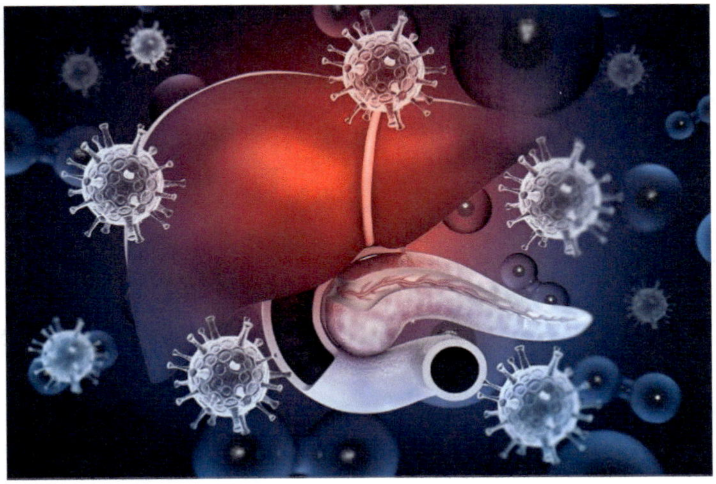

Figure 15.18. Direct-Acting Antiviral Agents (DAAs)

Source: https://scx2.b-cdn.net/gfx/news/2023/direct-acting-antivira.jpg.

Mechanism of Action

DAAs work by interfering with the HCV's ability to replicate, essentially disrupting its life cycle. They target different viral proteins, such as NS3/4A protease, NS5A, and NS5B polymerase, by inhibiting their functions.

DAA Classes:

- **NS3/4A Protease Inhibitors:** These DAAs target the HCV protease enzyme, which is essential for viral replication. Examples include simeprevir, grazoprevir, and voxilaprevir.
- **NS5A Inhibitors:** These DAAs target the NS5A protein, which plays a role in viral RNA replication and assembly. Examples include ledipasvir, elbasvir, and velpatasvir.
- **NS5B Polymerase Inhibitors:** These DAAs target the NS5B polymerase, which is responsible for replicating the HCV RNA genome. Examples include sofosbuvir.

Advantages of DAAs

- **High Efficacy:** DAAs achieve cure rates of over 95% in most HCV-infected patients.
- **Short Treatment Duration:** DAA therapy is typically shorter than previous HCV treatments, often 8 to 12 weeks.
- **Well-Tolerated:** DAAs are generally well-tolerated, with fewer side effects than older HCV treatments.
- **No Interferon Required:** Most DAA regimens are all-oral, meaning they do not require injections of interferon.
- **Available for Most Patients:** DAAs are suitable for a wide range of patients, including those who have previously failed other HCV treatments or who have advanced liver disease.

Examples of DAAs

- **Harvoni (ledipasvir/sofosbuvir):** A combination DAA targeting NS5A and NS5B polymerase.
- **Zepatier (elbasvir/grazoprevir):** A combination DAA targeting NS5A and NS3/4A protease.
- **Epclusa (sofosbuvir/velpatasvir):** A combination DAA targeting NS5B polymerase and NS5A.
- **Vosevi (sofosbuvir/velpatasvir/voxilaprevir):** A triple combination DAA targeting NS5B polymerase, NS5A, and NS3/4A protease.

References

1. Rahman Abdul, W. (2013). A study of novel biomarkers of hepatitis C related liver injury. https://core.ac.uk/download/41237537.pdf (accessed on 24 May 2025).
2. Alvarado-Tapias, E., Maya-Miles, D., Albillos, A., Aller, R., Ampuero, J., Andrade, R. J., Arechederra, M., *et al.* (2024). Proceedings of the 5th meeting of translational hepatology, organized by the Spanish Association for the Study of the Liver (AEEH). *Gastroenterología y Hepatología, 47*, 502207. https://doi.org/10.1016/j.gastrohep.2024.502207.
3. Apte, V., Bigogno, C. M., Boussios, S., *et al.* (2025). Precision oncology through next generation sequencing in hepatocellular carcinoma. https://core.ac.uk/download/647985564.pdf (accessed on 24 May 2025).
4. Baumert, T. F., Boni, C., Gane, E., *et al.* (2023). The scientific basis of combination therapy for chronic hepatitis B functional cure. https://core.ac.uk/download/558910901.pdf (accessed on 24 May 2025).
5. Chu, Q. D. (2018). *Hepato-Pancreato-Biliary and Transplant Surgery*. Beaux Books Publishing, LLC. https://play.google.com/store/books/details?id=lwLMDwAAQBAJ&source=gbs_api (accessed on 24 May 2025).
6. Elangovan, H., & George, J. (2025). Guidelines for the evolving landscape of liver disease: From viral hepatitis to MAFLD. *Chinese Medical Journal*. https://doi.org/10.1097/cm9.0000000000003616.
7. Friedman, S. L., Llovet I Bayer, J. M., Sia, D., Villanueva, A., *et al.* (2018). Liver cancer cell of origin, molecular class, and effects on patient prognosis. https://core.ac.uk/download/154917402.pdf (accessed on 24 May 2025).
8. Gores, G., Llovet I Bayer, J. M., Pikarsky, E., *et al.* (2018). Hepatocellular carcinoma. https://core.ac.uk/download/154917403.pdf (accessed on 24 May 2025).
9. Greten, T. F. (2018). *Immunotherapy of Hepatocellular Carcinoma*. Springer. http://books.google.com/books?id=rcvfwQEACAAJ (accessed on 24 May 2025).
10. Halldorsdottir, H. (2024). Heparin-binding protein and endothelin-1 in acute inflammation and trauma. https://doi.org/10.69622/27283959.v1.
11. Kaewdech, A., Charatcharoenwitthaya, P., & Piratvisuth, T. (2024). Asian perspective on hepatitis B virus and hepatitis C virus elimination. *Viruses, 17*, 34. https://doi.org/10.3390/v17010034.
12. Kim, Y., Kang, M., Mamo, M. G., Adisasmita, M., & Choi, D. (2024). Liver organoids: Current advances and future applications for hepatology. *Clinical and Molecular Hepatology*. https://doi.org/10.3350/cmh.2024.1040.
13. Kumar, A., Kumar, S., Kumar, S., Qureshi, H. A., & Naguib, J. S. (2024). AI-assisted genotype analysis of hepatitis viruses: A systematic review on precision therapy and sequencing innovations. *International Journal for Multidisciplinary Research, 6*. https://doi.org/10.36948/ijfmr.2024.v06i06.32058.
14. Maneira, C., Chamas, A., & Lackner, G. (2025). Engineering *Saccharomyces cerevisiae* for medical applications. *Microbial Cell Factories, 24*. https://doi.org/10.1186/s12934-024-02625-5.

15. N/A. (2025). Hepatocellular carcinoma. https://core.ac.uk/download/541039649.pdf (accessed on 24 May 2025).

16. Wazir, H., Abid, M., Essani, B., Saeed, H., Khan, M. A., Nasrullah, F., Qadeer, U., *et al.* (2025). Liver disease diagnosis and treatment: Current trends and future directions [Review]. https://assets.cureus.com/uploads/review_article/pdf/211919/20231201-1598-1gms5qe.pdf (accessed on 24 May 2025).

17. Wazir, H., Abid, M., Essani, B., Saeed, H., Khan, M. A., Nasrullah, F., Qadeer, U., *et al.* (2023). Diagnosis and treatment of liver disease: Current trends and future directions. *Cureus, 15*(12), e49920. https://www.cureus.com/articles/211919-diagnosis-and-treatment-of-liver-disease-current-trends-and-future-directions.pdf (accessed on 24 May 2025).

INDEX

D

E

F

G

H

I

N

R

S

T